Fundamentals of

Pharmacology for Midwives

Fundamentals of

Pharmacology for Midwives

EDITED BY

IAN PEATE, OBE, FRCN

Senior Lecturer, University of Roehampton; Visiting Professor of Nursing, St George's University of London and Kingston University London; Visiting Professor Northumbria University; Visiting Senior Clinical Fellow, University of Hertfordshir, Hatfield, UK

AND

CATHY HAMILTON, RGN, RM, PGDIP, PGCERT, MSC

Principal Lecturer, Lead Midwife for Education and Professional Lead (Midwifery), University of Hertfordshire, Hatfield, UK

WILEY Blackwell

This edition first published 2022

© 2022 John Wiley & Sons Ltd

Registered Offices

John Wiley & Sons, Inc., 111 River Street, Hoboken, NJ 07030, USA

John Wiley & Sons Ltd, The Atrium, Southern Gate, Chichester, West Sussex, PO19 8SQ, UK

Editorial Office

9600 Garsington Road, Oxford, OX4 2DQ, UK

For details of our global editorial offices, customer services, and more information about Wiley products visit us at www.wiley.com.

Wiley also publishes its books in a variety of electronic formats and by print-on-demand. Some content that appears in standard print versions of this book may not be available in other formats.

Library of Congress Cataloging-in-Publication Data applied for

Paperback ISBN: 9781119649236

Cover Design: Wiley

Cover Images: © sturti/Getty Images, Jose Luis Pelaez Inc/Getty Images

Set in 9/11pt MyriadPro by Straive, Chennai, India

Printed and bound by CPI Group (UK) Ltd, Croydon, CR0 4YY

C9781119649236_280622

Contents

Contributors

Dr Laura Abbott, FRCM, SFHEA, RGN, RM, BSc (hons), MSc, DHres

Dr Laura Abbott is a Senior Lecturer and Researcher in Midwifery at The University of Hertfordshire, a Senior Fellow of The Higher Education Academy and a Fellow of the Royal College of Midwives. Laura's doctorate examined the experiences of pregnant women in prison: *The Incarcerated Pregnancy: An Ethnographic Study of Perinatal Women in English Prisons.* She was awarded the Jean Davies award in 2014 and Midwives award in 2017 from The Iolanthe Midwifery Trust. She has presented at several international conferences and has published several research papers in high quality, international peer reviewed journals. Laura edited the book; Complex Social issues in Maternity Care published by Springer MacMillan in 2021. Laura volunteers with the charity Birth Companions and co-authored The Birth Charter for pregnant women in England and Wales published by Birth Companions in May 2016. She has been publicly recognised as one of the Nation's lifesavers from Made at Uni for her research, won the Vice Chancellors Award for Research success in 2020 and has been interviewed about her research by newspaper, radio and TV journalists. Laura has contributed to the review of Her Majesty's Prison and Probation Services operational policy for prison staff managing and caring for all women experiencing pregnancy, Mother and Baby Units (MBUs), and maternal separation in prison. In September 2020 Laura was awarded the Mildred Blaxter Post-Doctoral Fellowship from The Foundation for the Sociology of Health & Illness to continue with her research into the experiences of imprisoned perinatal women. More recently Laura has co-founded Pregnancy in Prison Partnership International (PIPPI) with academics in Australia, New Zealand and the USA and the UK wide Prison Midwives Action Group (PMAG).

Cathy Ashwin, PhD, MSc, PGCHE, RM, RN
Honorary Assistant Professor, University of Nottingham, Nottingham, UK

Cathy has worked predominantly in midwifery throughout her career, initially training and becoming a state registered nurse in Lincolnshire working in orthopaedics for a short period, and then undertaking midwifery training. Having worked in all areas specialising in community midwifery and smoking cessation for pregnant women and their families, she moved into midwifery education in 2005. Her key areas of interest are student education, public health and perinatal mental health. She has published and presented at national and international conferences. From 2014 to 2020, she was Editor of and Head of *MIDIRS Midwifery Digest*, an international midwifery journal and extensive reference database, and is currently a midwifery consultant supporting midwives in developing continuity of care midwifery.

Sam Bassett, DHC, MA, Bsc(Hons), DipHe Mid, RGN, PGSHSCE
Lead Midwife for Education/Head of Department Midwifery, Florence Nightingale Faculty of Nursing, Midwifery & Palliative Care, King's College, London, UK

Sam is an experienced midwife whose ongoing centre of clinical practice is high-risk pregnancies, having completed her doctorate, focusing on maternal high-dependency care in 2016. Currently working as lead midwife for education at King's College London, her areas of teaching expertise include medical complexities in childbirth, maternal high-dependency care and midwifery emergencies, across both pre- and post-qualification curricula. Clinical midwifery practice remains central to her work, and she is a recognised managing Medical and Obstetric Emergencies and Trauma and Resuscitation Council Newborn Life Support instructor, with a particular interest in the assessment of clinical skills using objective structured clinical examinations.

Jenny Brewster, RM, RN, BSc Health Studies, PGCert Higher Professional Education, MEd
Midwifery Lecturer, University of West London, London, UK

Jenny started her training as a nurse at King's College Hospital in 1978 and worked on a male medical ward before moving to St Peter's Hospital in Chertsey, where she completed her midwifery training. Having worked in the high-risk environment for several years, she then moved to work in a low-risk midwifery unit before being appointed as a practice development midwife at Wexham Park Hospital in Slough. This led to meeting the teaching team from the University of West London, where she has now been a midwifery lecturer for 11 years. She has also written for leading midwifery textbooks. One of her main interests is teaching obstetric emergencies, especially the support and resuscitation of the newborn baby.

Carl Clare, RN, Dip N, BSc (Hons), MSc (Lond), PGDE (Lond)
Senior Lecturer, Department of Adult Nursing and Primary Care, School of Health and Social Work, University of Hertfordshire, Hatfield, UK

Carl began his nursing a career in 1990 as a nursing auxiliary. He later undertook 3 years' student nurse training at Selly Oak Hospital in Birmingham, moving to the Royal Devon and Exeter Hospitals, then to Northwick Park Hospital, and finally to the Royal Brompton & Harefield NHS Trust as a resuscitation officer and honorary teaching fellow of Imperial College London. Since 2006, he has worked at the University of Hertfordshire as a senior lecturer in adult nursing. His key areas of interest are long-term illness, physiology, sociology, endocrinology and cardiac care.

Emma Dawson-Goodey, MA, DipHE, RM, RN
Senior Midwifery Lecturer, University of Hertfordshire, Hatfield, UK

Emma began her career in nursing in 1986 and worked on a coronary care unit. Having qualified as a midwife in 1990, she then worked in all areas of midwifery care at Chase Farm Maternity Unit. Since 2003, she has worked in midwifery education and her key interests are low-risk midwifery care, physical examination of the newborn, family planning, sexual health and global midwifery. Between 2009 and 2019 she worked as a part-time family planning nurse. Her volunteer work has taken her to Cambodia as part of the RCM Midwifery Global Twinning Campaign, and she continues to undertake volunteer work with the RCM and with midwives in Bangladesh. She was a registrant member of the NMC Fitness to Practise Committee for 8 years.

Kirsty Fishburn, BSc(Hons), MSc, INP, SFHEA
Programme Director for Mental Health, University of Hull, Hull, UK

Kirsty has been a mental health nurse since 2000, spending most of her career in forensic mental health and secure care. She has worked within private mental health service providers in many roles, such as nurse consultant, working up to director of nursing and then further to hospital director and a registered manager role. She completed her independent and supplementary prescribing qualification in 2007 and became an active prescriber, adding to her levels of competence by branching out into developing holistic prescribing practice. She completed her MSc in health professional education in 2011 and commenced her PhD in 2016. She left practice in 2015 to join the University of Hull, where she is the Programme Director for Mental Health and leads the Nurse Non-Medical Prescribing module.

Debbie Gurney, RN, RM, BSc, MA(Med Ed), FHEA
Senior Lecturer, University of Hertfordshire, Hatfield, UK

Debbie began her career in healthcare by training as an adult nurse at the University of Hertfordshire in 2000. Midwifery training followed and, once qualified, she worked in a rotational midwifery post at the QEII Hospital in Welwyn Garden City. She developed a passion for education and worked within NHS practice development teams while undertaking a Master's degree in medical education, before securing a post as a lecturer. Her key areas of interest include bridging the theory–practice gap, preceptorship, high-risk maternity care and perineal repair.

Cathy Hamilton, MSc, PGCert
Lead Midwife for Education, University of Hertfordshire, Hatfield, UK

Cathy Hamilton completed her nurse training at St Bartholomew's Hospital, London, in 1984, having undertaken an integrated degree programme at the City University. She later qualified as a midwife at the West Hertfordshire School of Nursing and Midwifery in 1987. She worked in all areas of the maternity unit and as a research assistant before becoming a lecturer at the University of Hertfordshire in 2001. She gained an MSc in midwifery at Southbank University, London, in 2001 and a postgraduate diploma in teaching and learning in higher education in 2003. She completed a doctorate in health research at the University of Hertfordshire in 2018. Since January 2018 she has been the lead midwife for education at the University of Hertfordshire.

Barry Hill, MSc, PGC Academic Practice, BSc(Hons) Intensive Care Nursing, DipHE Adult Nursing, OA Dip Counselling Skills, RN, NMC RNT/TCH, SFHEA
Programme Leader (Senior Lecturer) in Adult Nursing, Northumbria University, Newcastle, UK

Barry Hill is the Director of Employability for the Department of Nursing, Midwifery and Health at Northumbria University. He is on the editorial board for the *British Journal of Nursing* and the *Healthcare Inform* editorial advisory board. He leads and teaches on a range of higher education programmes and modules/courses. Prior to teaching at Northumbria University, he worked in both undergraduate and postgraduate programmes at the University of West London. He was also course leader for PGDIP nursing practice modules for all fields, and pre-registration adult nursing. Clinically, Barry worked at Imperial College NHS Trust for 10 years across all three adult intensive care units while undertaking a clinical Master's in advanced practice. Prior to joining higher education, Barry was a Band 8 (AfC) matron within the surgical division for plastics, orthopedics, ent and major trauma (POEM), managing and leading the ENT, airway, head and neck and plastics divisions, including breast surgery. He is a Fellow of the Higher Education Academy and a registered Teacher with the NMC.

Andrea Hilton, BPharm(Hons), MSc, PhD, PGCert, SFHEA
Senior Reader and Non-Medical Prescribing Programme Director, University of Hull, Hull, UK

Andrea is a pharmacist who has previously worked in primary care and in community pharmacy. She gained her undergraduate degree in pharmacy from the University of Bradford in 1999, before completing an MSc in clinical pharmacy while working in secondary care. She completed her PhD in 2006 while working on the MRC-funded RESPECT trial. She has been involved with non-medical prescribing at the University since 2006, and has extensive experience of Professional Statutory and Regulatory Bodies accreditation/validation requirements for non-medical prescribing.

Claire Leader, BSc(Hons), MA, PGCert
Senior Lecturer, Northumbria University, Newcastle, UK

Claire qualified as a registered nurse from York University in 1998, after which she moved to Leeds, working in the areas of cardiothoracic surgery and emergency nursing. In 2003, she commenced her midwifery education at Huddersfield University, where she was awarded a 1st Class BSc (Hons). Working initially at Sheffield Teaching Hospitals, she later moved to the north east, where she commenced her role as a staff midwife before moving into the area of research as a research nurse & midwife. She was awarded a distinction for an MA in sociology and social research at Newcastle University, with the focus of her dissertation being decision making in pregnancy following a caesarean section. She moved to Northumbria University in 2018 and is now a Senior Lecturer and Programme Lead for Pre-Registration Nursing programmes, while also studying for her PhD in the area of well-being for nurses and midwives.

Iñaki Mansilla, MSc, PGCE, RM, RGN
Senior Midwifery Lecturer/Practitioner, University of Hertfordshire, Hatfield, UK

Iñaki began his adult nursing studies in Spain, graduating and working for the same hospital where he did his placements. Although he worked across different wards while gaining knowledge and skills, he specialised in intensive care and resuscitation units. He also worked in orthopaedics in France as an adult nurse in a private hospital. He moved to the UK to become a midwife, his dream career. While working for almost 5 years as a community midwife facilitating home births, he researched why some women changed their place of birth, from the hospital to home, when they were offered an assessment at home in early labour. In early 2020, he achieved an internship award (Surrey University) from the HEE to commence his PhD studies (due to COVID, this was postponed). Later that year, he started his pathway in education.

Jayne E. Marshall, FRCM, PFHEA, PhD, MA, PGCEA, ADM, RM, RGN
Foundation Professor in Midwifery, Lead Midwife for Education and Deputy Head of School/ Director of Education, School of Healthcare, University of Leicester, Leicester, UK

With her internationally reputable career as a leader in midwifery education, Jayne has pioneered in partnership with University Hospitals of Leicester NHS Trust, an innovative 4-year undergraduate pre-registration Master in Science (MSci) Midwifery with Leadership programme for aspiring leaders of the midwifery profession. She was a member of the UK's Council of Deans of Health's Future Midwife Advisory Group that informed the 2019 Nursing and Midwifery Council Midwifery Standards, and is a coach on their student leadership programme. With a substantial international publishing history, Jayne is co-editor of the seminal textbook *Myles' Textbook for Midwives*, which is sold in over 75 countries and has been adapted for use in sub-Saharan Africa and translated into Korean and Greek. She is a member of the International Confederation of Midwives (ICM) Education Standing Committee and the ICM Research Advisory Network. Jayne is a Principal Fellow of the Higher Education Academy and an Aurora Role Model and mentor for the Leadership Foundation for Higher Education. In 2018, Jayne was awarded a Fellowship of the Royal College of Midwives for her service to midwifery education and the midwifery profession.

Helen McIntyre, BSc(Hons), RGN, RM, MSc, DHSci, SFHEA
Associate Professor of Midwifery, University of Leicester, Leicester, UK

Following graduation, Helen worked as a nurse on an acute mixed medical/surgical gastroenterology ward. Her midwifery career started in 1991, and she commenced in midwifery education in 2002, both of which have taken her across the UK and Asia. Her particular interests are enhancing physiology, infant feeding, postnatal care and change management. Her role as programme lead to an innovative MSci Midwifery with leadership programme embodies these passions. The development of the 'SNUBY', a skin-to-skin device for mother and baby, accentuates her desire for positive relationship building and physiology in the neonate.

Sinéad McKee, MPH, PGC, PGCert, FHEA, BSc(Hons), RN
Lecturer in Nursing (Advanced Practice), Glasgow Caledonian University, Glasgow, UK

Sinéad began her nursing career in Antrim, Northern Ireland. After qualifying as a staff nurse, she spent 2 years consolidating her nurse training, before moving to Edinburgh to pursue further academic qualifications. Following this, she focused on cardiology nursing, gaining clinical experience in medical, surgical and intensive care and then in a research capacity. She specialised in the management of patients with heart failure, initially clinically managing inpatients and outpatients before again returning to research in the National Heart Failure Service. She has worked in education since 2019 and has published widely. Her main areas of interest are advanced practice, research, managing patients with heart failure and the legal and ethical issues in healthcare.

Janet G. Migliozzi, RGN, BSc(Hons), MSc, PGD Ed, FHEA
Senior Lecturer, University of Hertfordshire, Hatfield, UK

Janet completed her initial training in London and commenced her career in 1988. She has worked at a variety of hospitals across London, predominantly in vascular, orthopaedic and high-dependency surgery, before specialising in infection prevention and control and communicable disease. She has worked in higher education since 1999 and is involved in teaching across a range of healthcare professional programmes at both undergraduate and postgraduate level. She is also involved in the research supervision of students undertaking advanced clinical practice pathways. Her key interests include clinical microbiology, particularly in relation to healthcare-associated infections, global communicable disease and public health. Patient safety at a local and global level is also an area of interest. She has published in journals and books on subjects including immunology, minimising risk in relation to healthcare-associated infection, and pathophysiology.

Karen Mills, BA, MA, PhD, CQSW, FHEA
Principal Lecturer in Social Work, University of Hertfordshire, Hatfield, UK

Karen Mills' practice experience is as a probation officer from 1988 to 2001. During this period, she held a range of roles: working with women, with high-risk offenders and ultimately specialising in practice education. In 2001, Karen moved to the University of Hertfordshire's Criminal Justice programme and has led that and later the MSc Social Work and Step up to Social Work programmes. Karen's research interest is in drugs, drug policy and safeguarding issues and she has researched and written extensively in this area. Karen's current research considers issues of compassion and empathy and the ways in which social workers and other practitioners engage with service users to build relationships of change.

Rebecca Murray, MRes, PGCertLTHE, RM, FHEA, BSc(Hons)
Senior Lecturer in Midwifery, University of Hertfordshire, Hatfield, UK

Rebecca graduated from Queen's University Belfast in 2012 with a BSc(Hons) in midwifery science. She moved to London to work as a research midwife, alongside clinical midwifery roles. She completed a MRes Clinical Research at King's College, London, in 2017 and began her midwifery education career. She is an NMC registered teacher and a fellow of the Higher Education Acadamy. She has interests in clinical simulation, medicines management and intrapartum care.

Emmanuel Ndisang, MSc, PGCert, BSc(Hons), RN(MH), ISP, FHEA
Senior Lecturer and MH MSc Field Programme Lead, University of Hertfordshire, Hatfield, UK

Emmanuel has extensive experience in healthcare as a clinical practice specialist and held positions as clinical manager and lead in mental health services. He has a background in medical biochemistry and his interests include psychopharmacology, perinatal mental health and treatment resistance with psychotropic medications. He has led graduate courses for pre-reg and advanced mental health practitioners. He is a fellow of the Higher Education Academy, and the mental health MSc field programme lead at the University of Hertfordshire.

Deborah Sharp, MSC, PGCHE, RM, FHEA
Programme Lead, University of Hertfordshire, Hatfield, UK

Deborah began her midwifery career in 1995 at Bedford Hospital NHS Trust. She has worked in all areas of midwifery and has extensive clinical and leadership experience. She moved into midwifery education in 2016 and is currently the programme lead for MSc in midwifery and women's health at the University of Hertfordshire. She has specialised in infant feeding, parent–infant attachment, clinical risk, governance and audit. Professional interests include the development of positive parent–child relationships, infant feeding, restorative clinical supervision and quality improvement. In 2015, Deborah was elected to be the maternity chair for the Hypoglycaemia Working Group, NHS Improvement Patient Safety Programme, to reduce admission of term babies to neonatal units. She is especially proud of leading an acute trust to achieve full UNICEF Baby Friendly accreditation in January 2015. Recently she has been extensively involved in the development and teaching of the professional midwifery advocate and leadership courses.

Chin Swain, RM, FHEA, MSc, BSc
Programme Leader, University of Hertfordshire, Hatfield, UK

Chin began her career in St Mary's Hospital in London as a junior midwife on the labour ward. She later took on the role of community midwife in Welwyn Garden City, rising to the role of antenatal, postnatal and labour ward sister. It was then that she took an interest in teaching and became a practice development midwife. She worked at the Rosie Hospital, Cambridge, through which she had the opportunity to contribute to maternity care in El Salvador, culminating in a presentation at St James's Palace. She started her career in education in 2017 at the University of Hertfordshire and became fellow of the Higher Education Academy in 2018.

Hema Turner, MSc, PGCHE, FHEA, LLB(Hons), BSc(Hons), RM, RGN
Senior Lecturer in Midwifery, University of Hertfordshire, Hatfield, UK

Hema began her nursing career as a registered general nurse at San Fernando General Hospital, Trinidad and Tobago, in 2000. She later migrated to the UK where she completed the 18 months shortened midwifery programme in 2003. Her midwifery career at Barking, Havering and Redbridge NHS Trust started as a staff midwife which then led to several different roles including an HDU specialist midwifery, labour ward co-ordinator, a Newly Qualified (NEWQUAL) clinical facilitator and education lead midwife. Prior to her present role as senior lecturer in midwifery, she worked as a programme lead and admissions tutor for the pre-registration shortened midwifery programme at the University of Hertfordshire, and as a senior lecturer in midwifery and practice learning at another UK higher education institute. Some of her significant achievements included being part of the NHS London NEWQUAL international project addressing the recruitment and retention crisis within the midwifery profession. This involved recruiting midwives from EU member states onto a 4-month clinical midwifery education and training programme to achieve full NMC registration. She also completed a full law degree (LLB Hons) at the University of London in 2011 and became a member of the Inner Temple, London. She has had experience and gained knowledge during her pupillage at a prestigious law chamber in London specialising in medico-legal cases and employment law cases with the Free Representation Unit, and successfully developed and co-lead the midwifery law and ethics module at another HEI.

Zoi Vardavaki, FHEA, PGCertLTHE, PhD candidate, MSc, BSc, RM
Senior Midwifery Lecturer, University of Hertfordshire, Hatfield, UK

Zoi has worked for the NHS as a midwife in both hospital and birth centre settings since 2014. She has also worked as a research midwife in fertility and maternity units. Since 2018, she has been a senior lecturer at the University of Hertfordshire, teaching undergraduate and postgraduate midwifery students. She is totally committed to supporting her colleagues and student midwives to maximise potential for all women to have a positive and satisfactory birth experience. As a midwife, she promotes normality in childbirth, and is interested in supporting alternative birth choices, advocacy and midwifery-led care. She is co-founder and one of the non-executive board members of the Hellenic British Midwifery Association (HBMA) in London, a role that enables her to serve the midwifery community and promote women's and birthing people's health at every level. She has been granted a fellowship in higher education and recently started her doctoral studies.

Amanda Waterman, MRes, BSc, RM, PGCert, FHEA
Senior Lecturer in Midwifery, University of Hertfordshire, Hatfield, UK

Amanda is a senior lecturer in midwifery at the University of Hertfordshire and previously worked as a registered midwife at West Hertfordshire Trust and University College London Hospital. She gained her BSc(Hons) in Medical Biochemistry at the University of Birmingham in 1997, before gaining a BSc(Hons) pre-registration midwifery degree at the University of Hertfordshire in 2015. In 2019, Amanda completed her MRes in Clinical Research at King's College, London. Amanda's interests include lecturing in research and she was a member of the James Lind Alliance Priority Setting Partnership Steering Committee and contributed to the publication in the *British Journal of Haematology* (2019) of 'The top 10 research priorities in bleeding disorders: a James Lind Alliance Priority Setting Partnership'. Other interests include high-dependency care and antenatal education.

Celia Wildeman, RGN, SCM, DipN, BEd(Hons), PGDip Counselling, MSc, PGDip Family Therapy
Senior Lecturer in Midwifery, University of Hertfordshire, Hatfield, UK

Celia began her nursing career at the Royal Free Hospital in London. She later undertook midwifery training at the Elsie Ingles Memorial Maternity Unit in Edinburgh. She has worked in midwifery education since 1986. Her key areas of interest include midwifery theory and practice, domestic violence and abuse, assessment and pastoral care of students and practice-based research.

Preface

The Fundamentals of Pharmacology for Midwives aims to provide the reader with an understanding of the essentials associated with pharmacology and the pregnant woman and in so doing enhance safety and care outcomes along with the woman's overall care experience. This book will help readers develop their competence and confidence within the field of pharmacology as related to the women in midwifery care settings, enabling them to recognise and respond compassionately to the needs of those women and their families. The contributors to the text are all experienced clinicians and academics who have expertise in their sphere of practice.

The Nursing and Midwifery Council (NMC) in the UK is required to establish standards of proficiency that each midwife must achieve prior to being admitted to the professional register, including demonstrating safe and effective practice. The Standards of Proficiency for Midwives (NMC, 2019) have been established to ensure that pre-registration midwifery students are deemed proficient in assessing, planning and providing care and support to women by using evidence-based techniques that include comfort measures, non-pharmacological and pharmacological methods when caring for the woman in pain.

The Okendon Report (2022), a review of maternity services at the Shrewsbury and Telford Hospital NHS Trust independently assessed the quality care to newborn, infant and maternal harm at the trust. In this report a number of references are made to the use of medicines and how they impact on care provison.

If undergraduate, pre-registration midwives are to offer care and support in relation to medicines management then they require a knowledge and understanding of pharmacology along with the ability to recognise the positive and opposing effects of medicines across the continuum of care; this includes allergies, drug sensitivities, side-effects, contraindications, incompatibilities, adverse reactions, prescribing errors and the impact of polypharmacy and over-the-counter medication usage (NMC, 2019).

The Fundamentals of Pharmacology for Midwives provides the reader midwife with the insight required to confidently and competently offer women and their families care that is woman centred, enabling them to practise as safe and accountable practitioners. This book will add to the student's repertoire of skills as they acquire appropriate pharmacological knowledge. Whilst much emphasis is placed on the principles of safe drug administration in midwifery curricula, there is also a need to ensure that students are equipped with the pharmacological foundations related to the larger issues associated with medicines management. This text provides the reader with an overview of the key issues that will enable them to begin to understand the complexities associated with pharmacology that they will face as well as the exciting challenges ahead of them.

Clause 18 of our Code of Professional Conduct (NMC, 2018) requires all of those whose name appears on the professional register to ensure that if they advise people, prescribe, supply, dispense or administer medicines, they must do this within the limits of their training and competence. They must do this with respect to the law and guidance produced by the NMC and other relevant policies and regulations. In order to comply with the NMC's requirements and other guidance, the midwife must have an understanding of the fundamentals of pharmacology. Professional guidance has been co-produced by the Royal Pharmaceutical Society and the Royal College of Nursing (2019) to ensure the safe administration of medicines and this has also been endorsed by the Royal College of General Practitioners.

There are 24 chapters in your book; the early chapters provide a broader discussion of pharmacology, including a general overview of medicines management, legal aspects, pharmacodynamics and pharmacokinetics. Information and discussion around the use of prescribing reference guides, the various medicinal formulations and the importance of preventing, noticing and responding effectively to adverse drug reactions are provided.

It could be that when you are looking at the table of contents, this could make you feel a little intimidated and you could be forgiven for thinking: 'How on earth am I going to remember, recall and apply all this information to the provision of high-quality, safe midwifery care?' We have provided a number of features in the text that will help you with your learning.

All the chapters are fully referenced and evidence based. Chapters begin with an aim and learning outcomes, providing you with an overall flavour of chapter content. At the beginning and the end of each chapter are a range of learning features that test your knowledge, including multiple choice questions. This approach has been adopted so as to enhance learning and recall.

In most chapters, there are boxed features that can assist the reader in applying this complex subject area to their practice. The clinical consideration boxes address clinical issues related to chapter content. The skills in practice feature offers a 'how to do. . .' component. The episodes of care feature uses a case study approach, linked to chapter content, that can occur in the care setting. There is a further reading list provided at the end of most chapters to encourage you to delve deeper.

As a healthcare student, your learning is not about rote learning and being able to simply recall. It is more than this – it is about applying that learning to the numerous situations that you will find yourself in, ensuring that the woman and her family, the people you have been given the privilege to offer care and support to, are at the heart of all that you do. The goal should be to take your learning further, to develop, to discover and to question. In this text, you will learn and develop your own strategies that will shape the way you study and learn, changing the way you think as you become a life-long learner with myriad transferable skills.

Life-long learning means just that – the continual pursuit of more knowledge as you develop personally and professionally. Learning does not stop once you have graduated and had your name entered on to the professional register. The acquisition of information does not stand still; new information is always being generated and applied in the midwifery, obstetric and medical fields. In the area of pharmacology, there are always new drugs being discovered and developed.

There are various terms that are used to describe receivers of health services. The Nursing and Midwifery Council refers to people, the General Medical Council refers to people treated by a doctor as patients, social workers refer to people using services, the British Psychological Society and the College of Occupational Therapists both refer to clients. In this text, the terms woman, patient, labourer, birthing or labouring person are used interchangeably in the chapters.

Ian Peate, London
Cathy Hamilton, Hertfordshire

References

Nursing and Midwifery Council (2018) The Code. Professional Standards of Practice and Behaviour for Nurses, Midwives and Nursing Associates. www.nmc.org.uk/globalassets/sitedocuments/nmc-publications/nmc-code.pdf (accessed February 2022).

Nursing and Midwifery Council (2019) Standards of Proficiency for Midwives. www.nmc.org.uk/globalassets/sitedocuments/standards/standards-of-proficiency-for-midwives.pdf (accessed February 2022).

Ockenden, D. (2020). Emerging findings and recommendations from the independent review of maternity services at the Shrewsbury and Telford Hospital NHS Trust. Retrieved from www.gov.uk/government/publications/final-report-of-the-ockenden-review (accessed March 2022).

Royal Pharmaceutical Society and Royal College of Nursing (2019) Professional Guidance on the Administration of Medicines in Healthcare Settings. www.rpharms.com/Portals/0/RPS%20document%20library/Open%20access/Professional%20standards/SSHM%20and%20Admin/Admin%20of%20Meds%20prof%20guidance.pdf?ver=2019-01-23-145026-567 (accessed February 2022).

Acknowledgements

Ian would like to thank Jussi, his partner, for his enduring encouragement and Mrs Frances Cohen for her ongoing support.

Cathy would like to thank her family and friends for their ongoing support and encouragement.

How to use your textbook and the companion website

Every chapter begins with **test your existing knowledge** questions.

Test your existing knowledge

- Describe the constituent parts and main functions of the gastrointestinal tract.
- What are the common routes for the administration of gastrointestinal medications?
- Write down the names of the hormones that influence gastrointestinal conditions in pregnancy.
- Write down the common gastrointestinal disorders you have seen in your practice.
- How is gastric acidity managed during labour where you are on placement?

Learning outcomes boxes give a summary of the topics covered in a chapter.

Learning outcomes

After reading this chapter, the reader will:
- Be able to relate the signs and symptoms of common gastrointestinal disorders of pregnancy to their underlying physiology and pathophysiology
- Demonstrate an understanding of gastrointestinal disorders of pregnancy, including their causes and clinical presentation
- Understand pharmacological treatment options for gastrointestinal disorders of pregnancy
- Understand the pharmacokinetics and pharmacodynamics of gastrointestinal medicines used in pregnancy.

Skills in practice boxes encourage the reader to apply the theory to everyday practice.

Skills in practice

Administration of medicines per rectum (PR)

Preparation and equipment
The midwife should understand the anatomy of the rectum before administering PR medications. All equipment should be available and within reach, including:

- prescription
- prescribed medication (warmed enema or suppositories – checking expiry date)
- water-based lubricant
- clean trolley or tray
- personal protective equipment – non-sterile gloves, disposable apron
- clinical waste bag
- disposable incontinence pad
- clean bed sheet.

Clinical considerations and **Episodes of care** features have been included to engage the reader and relate the discussion to care provision.

Clinical considerations

Half-life
The half-life of medication is how long it takes for the medication to be reduced by half of its blood concentration level. This is done through metabolisation. It can be affected by the individual's ability to metabolise, such as if the patient has renal failure and liver damage.

Episode of care

In pregnancy, women should be advised to continue using their medication as previously instructed but seek midwifery/medical support when symptomatic or suspecting a chest infection.
Extra information includes: frequency and nature of exacerbations, regular medication requirements and any additional medications presently available to Elizabeth.

Don't forget to visit the **companion website** for this book:

www.wiley.com/go/pharmacologyformidwives

There you will find interactive multiple choice questions and other self-test material designed to enhance your learning.

Part 1

Essentials of pharmacology

Chapter 1

Introduction to pharmacology

Jenny Brewster

University of West London, London, UK

Aim

The aim of this chapter is to introduce the reader to pharmacology and to consider specific applications related to pregnancy, labour and the postnatal period.

Learning outcomes

After reading this chapter the reader will:
- Have an understanding of the Code (NMC, 2018) and related documents that support the use of medicines in practice
- Consider the role of the pre-registration standards for midwifery programmes (NMC, 2019a) in relation to medicines management
- Be able to discuss the importance of medicines optimisation in relation to the pregnant woman
- Develop an awareness of the use of medicines during pregnancy, labour and the postnatal period, and the effect that some drugs may have on the developing fetus and/or newborn infant.

Test your existing knowledge

- Consider the role of the NMC in relation to the supply, keeping and administration of medicines.
- What does medicines optimisation mean?
- Define *teratogenic*.
- When is the period of greatest risk to the fetus from the administration of drugs?
- Where can information regarding the use of medication in pregnancy be accessed?

Introduction

Despite pregnancy and childbirth being a low-risk event for the majority of women, it is thought that 50% of women will be prescribed medication on at least one occasion during their pregnancy, with up to 90% of these being in the first trimester (Lassiter and Manns-James, 2017). This covers a

Fundamentals of Pharmacology for Midwives, First Edition. Edited by Ian Peate and Cathy Hamilton.
Companion website: www.wiley.com/go/pharmacologyformidwives

variety of medications, such as analgesics, antibiotics and antidepressants, but many women also enter pregnancy with an underlying health condition, such as epilepsy or a cardiac condition, requiring regular medication.

In planning for and during pregnancy, labour and breast feeding, when prescribing any drug, consideration also must be given to the fetus and newborn infant. It is known that certain drugs cross the placental barrier and cause harm to the fetus during its development, and some drugs will filter into breast milk, thus affecting the baby. The midwife should have a general understanding of the drugs that are used in this crucial period of a woman's – and fetus's – life and be able to work with both women and medical practitioners to ensure safety for women whilst achieving optimal clinical requirements.

Pharmacology

The word 'pharmacology' stems from *phaemakon*, the Greek word for medicine or poison (Brucker, 2017). Essentially, pharmacology is concerned with how drugs work and how they affect the chemistry of the body (British Pharmacological Society, 2021). It is important to have an understanding of the changes brought about by the use of different drugs in order to ensure that they are safe to use in a range of situations, and that side-effects which may be harmful can be reduced or eliminated. Recently, the importance of this has been seen in discussions regarding the new vaccines developed for COVID-19, in particular the Oxford/AstraZeneca vaccine where there were reports of blood clots in a minority of individuals receiving the vaccine (NHS, 2021). In line with this, the science of pharmacology helps to develop an understanding of why the action and reaction of and to various medications differ from one person to another (British Pharmacological Society, 2021).

Nursing and Midwifery Council (NMC)

As the regulatory body for the nursing and midwifery professions, the NMC sets standards for the training and conduct of nurses and midwives with the main aim of protecting the public. This includes its role in the management, supply and administration of medicines. In order to practise within the United Kingdom, nurses and midwives must be registered with the NMC following a period of training, and then provide evidence that they have maintained and updated their knowledge and skills through the revalidation process every 3 years (NMC, 2019b). They must also uphold the principles set out in the Code (NMC, 2018) related to both their practice and behaviour.

The Code (NMC, 2018) consists of four sections, clearly outlining the standards of professionalism that are required in order to support and protect the general public, putting the patient at the forefront of care and service provision (Figure 1.1).

This includes the role of the professional in the use of medicines, as set out in Clause 18, where nurses and midwives are guided to advise on, prescribe, dispense or administer medicines within the limits of their training and competence, the law, NMC guidance and any other policies, guidance or regulations (NMC, 2018). Only midwives who have completed further training post registration are able to prescribe medications.

Clear expectations of midwives at the point of qualification are also laid out by the NMC in the *Standards of proficiency for midwives* (2019c). The midwife is seen as the lead professional in the care of women throughout their pregnancy and the postnatal period, working in partnership with them to support their views and decisions with regard to their care as well as with the multidisciplinary team as and where appropriate. **Six domains are identified within these standards (NMC, 2019c).**

1. Being an accountable, autonomous, professional midwife.
2. Safe and effective midwifery care: promoting and providing continuity of care and carer.
3. Universal care for all women and newborn infants.
4. Additional care for women and newborn infants with complications.
5. Promoting excellence: the midwife as colleague, scholar and leader.
6. The midwife as a skilled practitioner.

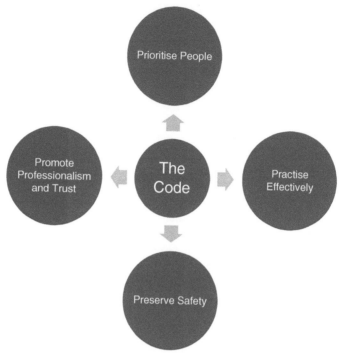

Figure 1.1 The Code.
Source: Based on NMC (2018)

The standards relating to the safe and effective use of medicines can be seen in Box 1.1.
Professional guidance on the safe handling of medicines in practice has been issued by the Royal Pharmaceutical Society (RPS, 2018) replacing the *Standards for Medicine Management* (2007) which were withdrawn by the NMC in 2019. Further guidance on the safe administration of medicines in practice has been produced jointly by the RPS and the Royal College of Nursing (RCN and RPS, 2019). Midwives and student midwives, as well as other health professionals, should be aware of these documents and the information provided within. Midwives also need to relate to the Human Medicines Regulation Act 2012, Section 17, which outlines the prescription-only medicines that can be given under Midwives' Exemptions.

Box 1.1   The *Standards of proficiency for midwives* related to the safe and effective use of medicines.

Domain 3.18 demonstrate knowledge and understanding of pharmacology and the ability to recognise the positive and adverse effects of medicines across the continuum of care; to include allergies, drug sensitivities, side effects, contraindications, incompatibilities, adverse reactions, prescribing errors and the impact of polypharmacy and over the counter medication usage

Domain 3.19 demonstrate knowledge and understanding of the principles of safe and effective administration and optimisation of prescription and non-prescription medicines and midwives exemptions, demonstrating the ability to progress to a prescribing qualification following registration

Domain 6 relates to the skills required for safe evidence-based practice

Domain 6.50 demonstrate the ability to work in partnership with the woman to assess and provide care and support across the continuum that ensures the safe administration of medicines

6.50.1 carry out initial and continued assessments of women and their ability to self-administer their own medications

6.50.2 recognise the various procedural routes under which medicines can be prescribed, supplied, dispensed and administered; and the laws, policies, regulations and guidance that underpin them

6.50.3 use the principles of safe remote prescribing and directions to administer medicines, including safe storage, transportation and disposal of medicinal products

6.50.4 demonstrate the ability to safely supply and administer medicines listed in Schedule 17 of the Human Medicines Regulations (Midwives' Exemptions) and any subsequent legislation and demonstrate the ability to check the list regularly

6.50.5 undertake accurate drug calculations for a range of medications

6.50.6 undertake accurate checks, including transcription and titration, of any direction to supply and administer a medicinal product

6.50.7 exercise professional accountability in ensuring the safe administration of medicines, via a range of routes, to women and newborn infants

6.50.8 administer injections using intramuscular, subcutaneous, intradermal and intravenous routes and manage injection equipment

6.50.9 recognise and respond to adverse or abnormal reactions to medications for the woman and the newborn infant, and the potential impact on the fetus and the breastfed infant

6.50.10 recognise the impact of medicines in breastmilk and support the woman to continue to responsively feed her newborn infant and/or to express breastmilk.

Source: Adapted from NMC (2019c).

Medicines optimisation

The most common intervention in healthcare is the prescription of medications (NICE, 2015), yet it is also recognised that up to half of the drugs prescribed are not taken as they should be (RPS, 2013). This is obviously concerning as not only are patients not benefiting from the treatment they should be having, but there is also a huge financial cost to the NHS. The aim of medicines optimisation is that, by involving patients in decision making regarding their medication, they will be more motivated to follow the treatment plan, thus achieving improved outcomes for them, as well as a reduction in the wasting of medicines and drugs across the board (RPS, 2013).

The principles of medicines optimisation are that there is an ongoing communication with the patient and multidisciplinary team, so that up-to-date evidence is given to the patient, and their views regarding both the drugs and their condition are taken into consideration (NICE, 2015). This could be particularly important for a woman planning a pregnancy where the medication she is taking for an established condition is known to be teratogenic.

Embryology

In order to understand the effects of medicines on the fetus, we first need to consider the development of the fetus from fertilisation to term. There are essentially three outcomes if the developing fetus is affected by medications taken by the mother, as indicated in Box 1.2. The fertilised ovum, the *zygote*, starts to undergo the process of mitosis, cell division. At the point where there are 12 cells, this is known as the *morula*, with the cells beginning to communicate with each other and moving to form the *blastocyst*. The cells of the blastocyst migrate to form an outer layer, the *trophoblast*, which will go on to develop into the placenta and chorion, and the inner cell mass which develops into the fetus. The blastocyst enters the uterus at around 4 days after fertilisation and embeds into the decidua. From implantation until 8 weeks gestation, the conceptus is known as the embryo. Initially, the cells are pluripotential, meaning that they have the potential to develop

Box 1.2   Effects of exposure to certain drugs on the developing fetus

Embryocidal – fetal death
Teratogenic – the development of the fetus is affected, leading to congenital abnormalities
Fetotoxic – the growth and/or development of the fetus is altered during the second and third trimesters

into any of the cells within the body (Mitchell and Sharma, 2005). During this preimplantation stage, if affected by any medication taken by the mother, the cells will either die or they will survive. The development of the cells is not affected if they survive at this stage.

Organogenesis, when the cells begin to differentiate into the various tissues and organs, begins at around 3 weeks post fertilisation and continues until 8 weeks, during which time the major organs will be formed. This period is known as the embryonic period (Webster and de Wreede, 2016) and is the time when the fetus is at maximum risk from teratogenic drugs with the potential for major developmental abnormalities (Lassiter and Manns-James, 2017). Table 1.1 shows fetal development and risks associated with exposure to teratogens.

From 8 weeks onwards, the fetus grows and develops until term, when the newborn is able to survive independently. This is the fetal period and although the chances of major developmental abnormalities are lower, the fetus is still at risk from drugs which can cross the placenta, altering its growth and development (Lassiter and Manns-James, 2017).

Although it is thought to act as a barrier, most drugs can cross the placenta to the fetal blood, although the majority of these are harmless to the fetus (Bailey, 2020). Initially there are several layers lining the chorionic villi through which substances must pass by diffusion: the syncytiotrophoblast membrane and cell, the cytotrophoblast and the endothelial lining of the fetal blood vessels (Lassiter and Manns-James, 2017). However, this barrier thins as pregnancy progresses. Some drugs, such as antibiotics and anaesthetics, diffuse easily across the placenta, whilst those with a high molecular weight, such as heparin, insulin and oxytocin, are not able to cross the barrier (Lassiter and Manns-James, 2017). A discussion on some of these drugs may be found further on in this text.

The use of medicines in pregnancy

Wherever possible, the use of medications in pregnancy should be avoided due to the risks to the developing fetus. However, as stated earlier, it is thought that at least 50% of pregnant women are prescribed drugs during their pregnancy (Lassiter and Manns-James, 2017), and many will take non-prescription medications, often before they even realise that they are pregnant.

There are actually very few drugs that are known to have teratogenic effects on the fetus (BNF, 2021a), with only about 1% of fetal abnormalities being related to the taking of drugs in pregnancy (Rang et al., 2016). The aim of this chapter is not to discuss each one individually. Although extensive trials are carried out on new drugs before they are used in practice, these trials do not generally involve pregnant women, so it is through trial and error that effects of drugs on the fetus may be discovered (Lassiter and Manns-James, 2017).

Two bodies are responsible for the safe and effective use of medicines in the UK; the Medicines and Healthcare products Regulatory Agency (MHRA) regulates the use of both medicines and medical devices to ensure that the benefits of the product outweigh any risks involved, whilst the Commission on Human Medicines (CHM) is the body that advises the government on all medicines and devices (MHRA, 2021).

The first drug to be recognised as causing teratogenic abnormalities was thalidomide in the 1960s. The drug was used for morning sickness in the UK from 1958 to 1961, when the link between the drug and the number of babies born with a variety of disabilities, including shortening of the limbs, was made (Thalidomide Trust, 2017). This led to the establishment of drug regulation agencies in many countries, including the Medicines Act 1968 in the UK (Rang et al., 2016).

Table 1.1 Fetal development and risks associated with exposure to teratogens. Source: Adapted from Webster and de Wreede (2016)

Weeks from fertilisation	1	2	3	4	5	6	7	8	9	10	16	32	40
Fertilisation / Embryonic period					Cleft lip								
							Heart							
							Limbs							
							Upper lip							
Fetal development									Eyes	Ears		Central Nervous system	
									Palate					
										External genitalia			

Not susceptible to teratogens

The embryo dies and spontaneous abortion occurs

Major congenital abnormalities

Minor abnormalities and Functional disorders

Pale violet – Systems highly sensitive to teratogens
Dark violet – Systems less sensitive to teratogens

The guiding principles for the use of medications in pregnancy are based around avoiding medications in the first trimester if at all possible. Where the use of medication is indicated, this should only be where the benefit to the woman is greater than the potential risk to the developing fetus, and the smallest possible dose of the drug should be prescribed (BNF, 2021a). The advice is also to avoid new drugs and use those that have previously been used during pregnancy, where no adverse effects have previously been noted (BNF, 2021a).

Pre-existing conditions

Those already taking medications for pre-existing conditions will, ideally, have a consultation with their GP and/or specialist consultant prior to conception. This may also involve a referral to an obstetrician. A plan would be made which would either involve staying on their existing treatment if this is not known to cause harm to the fetus or perhaps changing the medication if the one they are taking is known to be teratogenic. The principles of medicines optimisation certainly apply to the decisions made during these discussions. For the women who discover they are pregnant and have not made such plans, the medication should be continued and an urgent referral to a specialist is recommended to discuss the situation and the best options to take.

Where a drug is being taken that is known to have teratogenic potential, the advice is that these risks should be fully discussed with the woman, and that she should then be strongly encouraged to use an effective form of contraception that is suitable for her and her personal circumstances (MHRA, 2019). The medicines prescribed for epilepsy are known to have teratogenic properties, with the use of valproate in particular being highlighted in the British press over recent years (BBC, 2020). A review was published by the MHRA and CHM in January 2021 to establish the safety of antiepileptic drugs in pregnancy. The risks of taking valproate in pregnancy include spina bifida, facial and skull defects as well as deformities in the limbs, heart, kidneys and sexual organs (MHRA, 2021). These is also a risk of autism, and effects on speech, language and memory. Due to this, the recommendations are that if valproate is prescribed to any woman with child-bearing capacity, a pregnancy prevention programme must be in place (MHRA, 2021; BNF, 2021b). In the case of valproate, the effects on the fetus are teratogenic and fetotoxic (see Box 1.2).

Other epilepsy medications are also associated with birth defects, for example carbamazepine and phenobarbital, and data are still be collected on gabapentin, clobazam and zonisamide. In general, lamotrigine and levetiracetam are safer to use in pregnancy, as they do not appear to have teratogenic properties (MHRA, 2021). Chapter 17 of this text discusses medications and the nervous system.

The risk to the fetus of taking drugs in pregnancy varies as the pregnancy progresses and is also dependent on the drug itself. Many drugs are known to have teratogenic properties; that is, they are known to interrupt the fetal development process, leading to birth defects and abnormalities. As the pregnancy progresses, the risk of teratogenesis lessens but the fetus may still be susceptible to other forms of harm, such as growth retardation or underlying mental health issues, some of which are not identified for many years (Rang et al., 2016).

Another drug which a woman may be taking before planning a pregnancy is warfarin, as discussed in the following episode of care.

Episode of care

Susan is a 34-year-old para 1 who had a pulmonary embolism following the birth of her first baby 18 months ago. She has been taking warfarin since then and is now planning a second baby. She attends an appointment with the practice nurse at her local surgery to discuss the best way forward and is referred to the obstetric consultant. The risks of taking warfarin in pregnancy are explained to her as an increased risk of early miscarriage and, if taken in the first trimester, 'fetal warfarin syndrome', a condition resulting in a flat facial profile, defects in the spinal bones, arm and leg bones, and heart and brain defects. If taken throughout pregnancy, there is the potential for fetal bleeding (Best Use of Medicine in Pregnancy (BUMPS), 2021; BNF, 2021g). A plan is made for Susan to change from taking warfarin to using heparin.

As seen with valproate, there are also concerns that some drugs taken during the second and third trimesters can lead to restrictions in fetal growth. This may be due to interference with fetal hormones or a restriction in the supply of nutrients (Rang et al., 2016). Throughout the pregnancy, there is a risk of interference with the development of the brain and neurological system. Although the main development of the brain takes place between weeks 3 and 16, there is continual rapid growth and differentiation which can be affected by certain drugs (Moore et al., 2016), an example being valproate, as discussed earlier.

Occupational exposure

Occupational exposure to drugs and other forms of teratogens may also need to be taken into consideration when planning or discovering a pregnancy. A risk assessment should be carried out to identify any potential situations that may cause harm to the fetus, and reasonable adaptations to working practices put in place and adopted. An example is those working with x-rays and ionising radiation. A report published by the British Institute of Radiation (Temperton, 2009) found that the dose of radiation to those working in these areas was well below the recommended annual dose and that, when wearing a lead apron, the dose to the fetus would be even lower. Those working with MRI scanners are recommended to leave the room during the scan.

Pharmacists may also have to consider alterations to their practice when handling some drugs as some substances may be absorbed through the skin. An example is finasteride, a drug for treating enlarged prostate glands in men. Although no studies exist on humans, trials in animals suggested that there is an increased risk of miscarriage, and birth defects in the male sex organs. The recommendations are that gloves should be worn when handling this drug (MotherToBaby, 2020).

A further example of an occupational hazard is if the pregnant woman is working with chemical substances. Again, a full risk assessment would be needed as early in the pregnancy as possible, with suitable adjustments to working practices being established.

Drugs used in labour

Certain drugs are used on a regular basis in labour for a variety of reasons, with those related to labour itself being discussed in Chapter 10. With regard to induction of labour, there are no concerns that the use of vaginal progesterone or intravenous oxytocin will cause any long-term effect to the fetus (BNF, 2021c, 2021d).

Opioid analgesia may be administered in labour at the request of the woman, with the drug of choice varying in individual healthcare providors between morphine, diamorphine and pethidine. It is known that all opioids cross the placenta, pethidine within 2 minutes and diamorphine within an hour (Davey and Houghton, 2021). Due to the immaturity of the fetal liver, the drugs are metabolised more slowly in the fetus, and are not readily transferred back to the mother through the placenta due to the lower pH of the fetal blood. This can lead to respiratory depression in the fetus at birth and, as the excretion is slower, the newborn infant may also be slower to initiate and establish breast feeding (BNF, 2021e, 2021f).

Should a general anaesthetic be required for a caesarean section, the midwife and neonatologist present at the birth should be prepared for a newborn that is slow to establish respirations, depending on the time taken from initiation of the anaesthetic to the birth. As with opioids, the drugs used for a general anaesthetic will cross the placenta and depress the respirations of the newborn (Ritter et al., 2008).

Episode of care

Naga Mohan, a 40-year-old gravida 5, para 4, had had four previous caesarean sections, the last one 14 months previously. It was known that she already had scar tissue and that this would, in all probability, be a difficult caesarean section to perform, so, after discussion with Naga and her partner, it was decided that a general anaesthetic would be the best option.

Due to the potential difficulties in performing the surgery, plans were made for a senior experienced midwife and a neonatologist to be present at the birth. The resuscitaire was checked and in full working order, and naloxone was drawn up in preparation in case the baby did not respond at birth.

Following the general anaesthetic, it was almost 10 minutes until the baby was born. The male infant was wrapped and taken to the resuscitaire, dried and, as no respiratory effort was made, inflation breaths were given. These were effective and the heart rate remained above 100 beats per minute, but the baby was not breathing, so ventilation breaths were carried out. After 4 minutes, the baby was still not breathing spontaneously, so naloxone 200 μg was given intramuscularly. The baby started breathing very quickly following this and was then observed closely in the SCBU.

Group B streptococcus infection is an example of when antibiotics are given to the mother with the aim of preventing infection in the newborn. For those women identified as group B streptococcus positive in pregnancy, the risk is that the fetus will become infected as it passes through the birth canal, which can lead to sepsis within the first few hours of life. Intravenous antibiotics are given to the mother in labour with the aim that they will cross the placenta to protect the fetus from infection (Lowe et al., 2017).

Breast feeding

There have been few studies into the relative amounts of drugs that enter breast milk (Schaefer, 2015), meaning that there is minimal information available to support the theories that any medications taken by the mother whilst breast feeding will cause harm to the fetus (BNF, 2021h). Due to the fact that there is little information on many drugs, the guidance is that only essential medication should be given to the breast-feeding mother (BNF, 2021h). The majority of drugs taken by the breast-feeding mother transfer to the breast milk through diffusion, due to the balance of the drug in the mother's blood and the milk. As levels in the maternal system rise, the drug is then forced across into the milk (Baker and Hale, 2017).

On the whole, it is thought that there are seldom sufficient levels of a drug within the breast milk to cause harm to the infant, and this is especially relevant if the medication has been given parenterally or is not absorbed well when taken orally (BNF, 2021h). The risks are, however, increased in premature infants and those who are jaundiced. There is also a relatively small possibility that the infant may develop a sensitivity to the drug and have a reaction to this (BNF, 2021h).

The lack of in-depth evidence regarding the effects of many drugs related to breast feeding can lead to some confusion both for the professional and for the women using them. An example is tinzaparin, a low molecular weight heparin frequently administered postnatally as prophylaxis for women at risk of developing deep vein thrombosis or pulmonary embolism in the postnatal period. The BNF (2021i) advises that, as the molecular weight of this drug is relatively high, it is unlikely to pass into the breast milk, but also states that the manufacturers do not support its use during breast feeding. This information is readily available to the public and could lead to women not using the heparin they have been prescribed due to fears for the infant.

There are a number of drugs which will pass into breast milk and may affect the baby's ability to latch and feed effectively. As discussed above, opioids may affect the infant at birth, and the effects may last for a few hours as the drug is excreted from the infant's body. However, if morphine is given in the postnatal period, for example following a caesarean section, the dose given is thought not to be at a sufficient level to further depress the respirations of the infant or affect feeding (BNF, 2021j).

As with other medications, there is little evidence related to breast feeding regarding the use of drugs to treat anxiety and depression. Some of the symptoms reported in infants are thought to be related to the adjustment in the infant from the dosage in pregnancy to that at birth and is rarely seen as a reason not to take the medication (Schaefer, 2015). An exception to this is the benzodiazepine group, which includes diazepam. This is not recommended for use with breast-feeding mothers (BNF, 2021k) as neonatal respiratory depression has been noted, as well as associated tremors, hypertonicity of muscles, and diarrhoea and vomiting where the drug is used over a period of time (Schaefer, 2015). Associated with this is a reluctance to feed, and seizures have been reported.

For women taking antibiotics in the postnatal period, the amount of antibiotic that reaches the infant is negligible (Schaefer, 2015). However, the normal gut flora may be affected, leading to a more watery stool, but this is temporary and does not normally require any treatment. It has been recognised that metronidazole passes into the breast milk, but no adverse effects had been identified in infants (Schaefer, 2015). Chapter 9 of this text discusses antibiotics and Chapter 20 addresses medications and breast feeding in more depth.

Conclusion

Pharmacology is the study of drugs and the effect they have on the body. The use of any medication during pregnancy and the postnatal period should be treated with caution, with consideration of the suitability of the drug before it is prescribed. The principles of medicines optimisation apply during these times, ensuring that the woman is fully involved in the decision making regarding her treatment, that she is aware of the reasons for the medication, and the potential effects for both her and the fetus/newborn infant.

There is insufficient information on the majority of drugs related to pregnancy and breast feeding, with many manufacturers stating that a particular drug should not be used in these circumstances. However, some have been used with no ill effects, and are prescribed in practice. This may lead to confusion for the woman if she accesses conflicting information regarding the drug.

The guiding principles for both pregnancy and breast feeding should be that the need for medication should outweigh the risks to the fetus/newborn. At all times, the smallest possible dose of any drug should be prescribed. Although only a few drugs have been highlighted in this chapter, the principles of care apply to all medications.

Glossary

Blastocyst   The fertilised ovum enters the uterus at day 4

Embryo   From implantation of the blastocyst into the decidual lining of the uterus until 8 weeks from fertilisation

Embryonic period   The first 8 weeks following fertilisation

Fetal period   From 9 weeks until birth. A time of growth and development

Morula   Twelve-cell stage

Neurulation   The formation of the brain and spinal cord between days 19 and 25 following fertilisation

Organogenetic period   From 4 to 8 weeks following fertilisation when the formation of major organs occurs

Teratogen   Any substance which leads to a birth defect

Zygote   The oocyte and spermatozoa combined

Test yourself

Now review your learning by completing the learning activities for this chapter at www.wiley.com/go/pharmacologyformidwives.

References

Bailey, J. (2020) Chapters 5–7. In: Marshall, J. and Raynor, M. (eds) *Myles Textbook for Midwives*, 17th edn. Elsevier: Edinburgh.

Baker, T.E., Hale, T.W. (2017) Breastfeeding. In: Brucker, M.C., King, T.L. (eds) *Pharmacology for Women's Health*, 2nd edn. Jones and Bartlett Learning: Burlington.

BBC (2020) 'I didn't know epilepsy drug would harm my baby.' www.bbc.co.uk/news/uk-scotland-55149108 (accessed January 2022).

Best Use of Medicine in Pregnancy (BUMPS) (2021) Warfarin use in pregnancy. www.medicinesinpregnancy.org/Medicine--pregnancy/Warfarin-use-in-pregnancy/ (accessed January 2022).

British National Formulary (2021a) Prescribing in pregnancy. https://bnf.nice.org.uk/guidance/prescribing-in-pregnancy.html (accessed January 2022).

British National Formulary (2021b) Epilepsy. https://bnf.nice.org.uk/treatment-summary/epilepsy.html (accessed January 2022).

British National Formulary (2021c) Dinoprostone. https://bnf.nice.org.uk/drug/dinoprostone.html (accessed January 2022).

British National Formulary (2021d) Oxytocin. https://bnf.nice.org.uk/drug/oxytocin.html (accessed January 2022).

British National Formulary (2021e) Diamorphine hydrochloride. https://bnf.nice.org.uk/drug/diamorphine-hydrochloride.html (accessed January 2022).

British National Formulary (2021f) Pethidine hydrochloride. https://bnf.nice.org.uk/drug/pethidine-hydrochloride.html#pregnancy (accessed January 2022).

British National Formulary (2021g) Warfarin sodium. https://bnf.nice.org.uk/drug/warfarin-sodium.html (accessed January 2022).

British National Formulary (2021h) Prescribing in breastfeeding. https://bnf.nice.org.uk/guidance/prescribing-in-breast-feeding.html (accessed January 2022).

British National Formulary (2021i) Tinzaparin. https://bnf.nice.org.uk/drug/tinzaparin-sodium.html#breastfeeding (accessed January 2022).

British National Formulary (2021j) Morphine. https://bnf.nice.org.uk/drug/tinzaparin-sodium.html#breastfeeding (accessed January 2022).

British National Formulary (2021k) Diazepam. https://bnf.nice.org.uk/drug/tinzaparin-sodium.html#breastfeeding (accessed January 2022).

British Pharmacological Society (2021) What is pharmacology? www.bps.ac.uk/about/who-we-are-(2)/history-of-the-society (accessed January 2022).

Brucker, M.C. (2017) Modern pharmacology. In: Brucker, M.C., King, T.L. (eds) *Pharmacology for Women's Health*, 2nd edn. Jones and Bartlett Learning: Burlington.

Davey, L., Houghton, D. (2021) *The Midwife's Pocket Formulary*, 4th edn. Elsevier: Edinburgh.

Lassiter, N.T. and Manns-James, L.E. (2017) Pregnancy. In: Brucker, M.C., King, T.L. (eds) *Pharmacology for Women's Health*, 2nd edn. Jones and Bartlett Learning: Burlington.

Lowe, N.K., Openshaw, M., King, T.L. (2017) Labour. In: Brucker, M.C., King, T.L. (eds) *Pharmacology for Women's Health*, 2nd edn. Jones and Bartlett Learning: Burlington.

Medicines and Healthcare products Regulatory Agency (2019) Medicines with teratogenic potential: what is effective contraception and how often is pregnancy testing needed? www.gov.uk/drug-safety-update/medicines-with-teratogenic-potential-what-is-effective-contraception-and-how-often-is-pregnancy-testing-needed#download-print-and-use-new-table (accessed January 2022).

Medicines and Healthcare products Regulatory Agency (2021) Antiepileptic drugs: review of safety of use during pregnancy. www.gov.uk/government/publications/public-assesment-report-of-antiepileptic-drugs-review-of-safety-of-use-during-pregnancy/antiepileptic-drugs-review-of-safety-of-use-during-pregnancy (accessed January 2022).

Mitchell, B., Sharma, R. (2005) *Embryology: An Illustrated Colour Text*. Elsevier: Edinburgh.

Moore, K., Torchia, M., Persaud, T.V.N. (2016) *Before We Are Born*, 9th edn. Saunders: Philadelphia.

MotherToBaby (2020) Finasteride. https://mothertobaby.org/fact-sheets/finasteride/ (accessed January 2022).

National Health Service (2021) Coronavirus (COVID-19) vaccine. www.nhs.uk/conditions/coronavirus-covid-19/coronavirus-vaccination (accessed January 2022).

National Institute for Health and Care Excellence (2015) Medicines optimisation: the safe and effective use of medicines to enable the best possible outcomes. www.nice.org.uk/guidance/ng5/resources/medicines-optimisation-the-safe-and-effective-use-of-medicines-to-enable-the-best-possible-outcomes-pdf-51041805253 (accessed January 2022).

Nursing and Midwifery Council (2018) The Code: Professional standards of practice and behaviour for nurses, midwives and nursing associates. www.nmc.org.uk/globalassets/sitedocuments/nmc-publications/nmc-code.pdf (accessed January 2022).

Nursing and Midwifery Council (2019a) Realising professionalism: Part 3: Standards for pre-registration midwifery programmes. www.nmc.org.uk/globalassets/sitedocuments/standards-of-proficiency/standards-for-pre-registration-nursing-programmes/programme-standards-nursing.pdf (accessed January 2022).

Nursing and Midwifery Council (2019b) Revalidation. http://revalidation.nmc.org.uk/ (accessed January 2022).

Nursing and Midwifery Council (2019c) Standards of proficiency for midwives. www.nmc.org.uk/globalassets/sitedocuments/standards/standards-of-proficiency-for-midwives.pdf (accessed January 2022).

Rang, H.P., Ritter, J.M., Flower, R.J., Henderson, G. (2016) *Rang and Dale's Pharmacology*, 8th edn, Elsevier: Edinburgh.

Ritter, J.M., Lewis, L.D., Mand, T.G.K., Ferro, A (2008) *A Textbook of Clinical Pharmacololgy and Therapeutics*, 5th edn. Hodder Arnold: London.

Royal College of Nursing and Royal Pharmaceutical Society (2019) *Guidance on the Administration of Medicines in Healthcare Settings*. RCN and RPS, London.

Royal Pharmaceutical Society (2013) *Medicines Optimisation: Helping patients to make the most of medicines*. RPS: London.

Royal Pharmaceutical Society (2018) *Professional Guidance on the Safe and Secure Handling of Medicines*. RPS: London.

Schaefer, C. (2015) *Drugs During Pregnancy and Lactation: Treatment Options*. Elsevier: Edinburgh.

Temperton, D.H. (2009) *Pregnancy and Work in Diagnostic Imaging Departments*. British Institute of Radiographers: London.

Thalidomide Trust (2017) About Thalidomide. www.thalidomidetrust.org/about-us/about-thalidomide/ (accessed January 2022).

Webster, S., de Wreede, R. (2016) *Embryology at a Glance*. Wiley Blackwell: Chichester.

Further reading

Best Use of Medicine in Pregnancy (2021) www.medicinesinpregnancy.org (accessed January 2022).

Gov.UK (2021) Use of medicines in pregnancy and breastfeeding. www.gov.uk/guidance/use-of-medicines-in-pregnancy-and-breastfeeding (accessed January 2022).

Royal Pharmaceutical Society (2013) *Medicines Optimisation: Helping patients to make the most of medicines*. RPS: London.

Thalidomide Trust (2017) About Thalidomide. www.thalidomidetrust.org/about-us/about-thalidomide/ (accessed January 2022).

UK Drugs in Lactation Advisory Service www.sps.nhs.uk/articles/ukdilas/ (accessed January 2022).

United Kingdom Teratology Information Service www.uktis.org (accessed January 2022).

Chapter 2

How to use pharmaceutical and prescribing reference guides

Kirsty Fishburn and Andrea Hilton

University of Hull, Hull, UK

Aim

To give an overview of the resources available to those providing midwifery care and how to use to them in order to facilitate medicines optimisation and safe and effective administration of medicines.

Learning outcomes

Following completion of this chapter you will be able to:
- Use sources of information/reference guides such as the British National Formulary (BNF) to underpin and support your practice
- Recognise the limitations of sources of information/reference guides
- Acknowledge and understand the role that national guidelines provide in practice
- Apply academic knowledge to practical scenarios.

Test your existing knowledge

- What are the advantages of using the app to access the BNF?
- What does the acronym NICE stand for?
- Where in the BNF can information relevant to pregnancy be located?
- What is the role of the Medicines and Healthcare products Regulatory Agency?
- What are blacklisted medicines and where can these be located?

Fundamentals of Pharmacology for Midwives, First Edition. Edited by Ian Peate and Cathy Hamilton.
© 2022 John Wiley & Sons Ltd. Published 2022 by John Wiley & Sons Ltd.
Companion website: www.wiley.com/go/pharmacologyformidwives

Introduction

This chapter will explain why healthcare practitioners, including midwives, need to use prescribing guidelines and reference sources. It will identify how these resources can add to the knowledge needed to understand the role of the midwife in maintaining the safety of those women in their care who are in receipt of medication.

Issues surrounding midwifery and medication are complex, with much to be learnt and understood. It is not just about the tablet or the liquid in the syringe, it is also about how that drug works in the body and that this is the right medication to treat women. The resources discussed in this chapter will help with understanding and provide a source of reference and information to gather and apply knowledge.

Registered midwives (or potential registrants) are accountable to the people to whom they offer care and support (NMC, 2018). Standards of proficiency for midwives (NMC, 2019) in relation to regulatory body requirements have been published. These state that the midwife at the point of registration must possess an in-depth knowledge of medications that they encounter during their practice. They must also ensure that they have the necessary knowledge and skills to maintain competency under these standards.

British National Formulary and British National Formulary for Children

The British National Formulary (BNF) and the British National Formulary for Children (BNFc) are joint publications of the British Medical Association and Royal Pharmaceutical Society. The BNFc provides prescribing guidance to healthcare practitioners who work within the sphere of paediatrics, child health and neonates. Both resources offer advice on prescribing and pharmacology.

The BNF started in 1949 and was initially called the National Formulary but has since been revised and updated to its current form. The BNF initially was published three times yearly and is now published twice yearly. A major overhaul occurred in 1981 and by 2003 there were close to 3000 different drug interactions included. In the hard copy version, the front covers remain colourful and distinctive, helping to identify the latest version.

Paper versus electronic guides

The BNF and BNFc are available as paper books, a website and an app. As the world moves increasingly to the provision of online resources, the question is raised as to whether we still need a paper copy. Once the paper copy is published, it can be expensive and laborious to distribute paper updates and therefore as soon as it is published, it may potentially be out of date. This is the benefit of websites and apps which can readily be revised and updated.

The paper copies are currently published twice a year and are numbered with a coloured front to help identify the latest version. It is essential that healthcare practitioners use the most up-to-date version of the information. As an accountable practitioner, your practice must be defensible as your duty of care to your service user is paramount. This is something you need to be mindful of as old copies of this book do tend to accumulate in clinical areas. Since 1949, whole sections have been replaced, reformatted or removed, as the publication must reflect contemporary practice and the world of medicines tends to move quickly with frequent updates.

In order to ensure the safety of women, it is vital that the midwife's medicines knowledge is current and contemporary. The potential risk to women in passing on incorrect and outdated information could leave the midwife in a precarious position in regard to service user safety and their duty of care as stipulated by the NMC (2018). For these reasons, accessing medicines information via a website or app is recommended. It can help the health professional to highlight to patients how medication and treatment decisions are made and give an insight into how professional decisions are made, underpinned by clear guidance and standards. This in turn will help support women's care in relation to medication, including shared decision making, and supporting a person-centred approach.

Structure of the BNF

In its current version, the BNF is approximately 1748 pages, with the BNFc having 1180 pages. At first glance, these tomes may feel overwhelming as they contain so much detail and information. However, both the hard copy and electronic versions are separated into sections and chapters to help the reader navigate through the information. Signposting and appendices are included to help the reader locate the information needed in a timely and organised manner.

Front pages

This section presents how the BNF is constructed by incorporating all the advisory groups that feed into prescribing guidelines. It also examines the hierarchy of the evidence that is presented, which can give the reader an insight into how the BNF garners its information and how this is then weighted in its pages. The BNF does make reference to the BNFc. There is a further section that highlights what has changed in this version of the publication, a key signpost here being that the printed version shows the reader the way in which this printed copy is updated and where to find these updates, something the app and website do not need. References are also made here to the use of monographs within the BNF, explaining the structure and use when the BNF presents the drug in a systematic way that details all the information about that drug in one place. This was not previously the case in the BNF.

The front pages provide advice on prescribing, particularly in relation to security of prescriptions and Patient Group Directions (PGDs). A point to note is the inclusion of what makes a legal prescription. This demonstrates in pictorial format what the legal requirements for a prescription are. Included in this section is a detailed and clear sample prescription, which helps the reader to see quickly what is needed to make a prescription legally valid.

Nurses and midwives have been given the right to prescribe under the law. The NMC and Royal Pharmaceutical Society have developed standards and competencies for nurses and midwives to engage with and ultimately undertake university-level education to gain a non-medical prescribing qualification (within their area of competence) (NMC, 2018). If career progression into a non-medical prescribing (NMP) role is one of your goals, this helps to start developing your knowledge. These front pages include a wide range of topics from prescribing in pregnancy to prescribing in palliative care. In particular, the BNFc provides an overview on supply of medicines with emphasis placed on the child and/or the child's carer. This section also highlights the importance of safety and labelling of medications in the home if children are present in the environment.

There are sections in both the BNF and BNFc relating to Controlled Drugs (CD). As this class of medication is subject to legal restrictions, it is important to know the different Schedules these medications have under the Misuse of Drugs Act 1971. As registrants, you are accountable under the NMC rules for the safe storage, dispensing and administration of all medications, CDs included, so it is important to be aware of the role of the midwife in this respect. Throughout the BNF, CDs and their schedules are clearly noted on their monographs.

One of the last things to note in this front section is the overview of adverse drug reactions (ADR). This section explains the Yellow Card system and defines what is meant by an ADR. It explains how to recognise and report an ADR to ensure it is correctly documented and acknowledged in relation to the medication that has possibly caused it. Pharmacovigilance is a key area to ensure safe administration to all recipients who take these medications. Chapter 7 of this text also discusses the Yellow Card system. See the later section on the role of the Medicines and Healthcare products Regulatory Agency.

Chapters

There are 16 chapters which cover all areas of medicines. The content of the chapters follows a similar structure and the individual medications relating to that bodily system are included. This structure helps the reader to locate the information required and once familiarity with the structure is established, it is seen to follow a logical order.

Each chapter starts with the drug family, such as antibiotics, mood stabilisers, statins, etc. The next section will identify the drug name, for example ondansetron, sertraline, paracetamol. Each area will report drug interactions, dose and actions. This is to show what the drug does, how it does it and what it is prescribed and administered for. For each drug, specific reference is made to women who are pregnant and breast feeding, which must always be considered for women of child-bearing age. With respect to pharmacokinetics (what the body does to a drug) and pharmacodynamics (what the drug does to a body), the BNF includes details on hepatic and renal impairments and considerations for practitioners who not only administer and dispense medication, but who may also prescribe them.

An important area is that of drug interaction (covered in detail in Appendix 1 of the BNF). There are, however, further topics explored including side-effects and contraindications, cautions and costings, alternative drug brand names and formulations of that drug, such as oral tablets or capsules, intramuscular injections, intravenous injections and so on as these can alter how the drug works in the body and potentially what it is called and how much it costs.

Most people who are prescribed medication want to know why and what it is for. This is how the BNF/BNFc can help practitioners to offer advice and alleviate some concerns by providing information and answering potential questions. The importance of shared decision making when supporting people in their medication and treatment choices is highlighted. This can be achieved by promoting their right to choose (NHSE, 2021a). If you feel you are lacking the knowledge to provide information in regard to medications, it is important that you always refer to a more senior practitioner for appropriate advice and guidance.

Practitioners cannot be expected to know about all potential side-effects associated with drugs, but midwives should know the more common ones that they may be involved in administering. This is a clear part of the professional accountability required by the NMC (NMC, 2018). A key thought here is that as a midwife, you need to know how to access the right information at the right time. When dealing with side-effects, as this can be an emotive and troubling topic, it is important to support women in ensuring that they have all the facts. Discussing side-effects needs to be done in a measured and supportive manner but exercise caution here, as there is no need to scare people. Honesty and support are the key communication skills required for midwives to fulfil their roles in relation to medication. The BNF/BNFc can be used as a medical education tool.

It is worth noting the different names of medications, from their generic name (e.g. co-codamol) to their brand name (e.g. Kapake®). Co-codamol is a good example of a medication to explore in the BNF/BNFc as it comes in many formulations, dosages and costings. It may help the reader to navigate the structure of a BNF chapter, drug family and the details of the medication (Joint National Formulary, 2020, p.474; Joint National Formulary, 2020–21, p.290). Co-codamol is also a medication subject to the Misuse of Drugs Act (1971) as a licensed CD which is displayed clearly in the BNF/BNFc.

Appendices

Note that the BNFc only includes appendices 1, 2 and 3. There is no appendix 4 in the BNFc.

Appendix 1 Interactions

Any time a medication is taken with another one, whether as a prescription-only medication (POM), bought over the counter (OTC) or an herbal preparation such as St John's wort or oil of evening primrose, interactions should be checked. Many interactions will not cause serious harm but they can become serious, depending on the drug and the person's natural biological idiosyncrasies. As a registered practitioner, you have a professional responsibility to know how to find information on drug interactions. Drug interactions occur through pharmacokinetic and pharmacodynamics mechanisms. If we take more than one medicine at a time, they could perhaps affect not the body but each other. This means that they could counteract each other or just cancel each other out so that the therapeutic response is lost. For this reason, the interaction appendix in the BNF/BNFc is particularly detailed and robust.

Appendix 2 Borderline Substances

Borderline substances are nutritional or dermatological products that have been specially formulated to assist in managing medical conditions. The Advisory Committee on Borderline Substances (ACBS) recommends products that may be considered medications for the management of certain diagnosable symptoms. Some examples would be nutritional supplements for specific dietary requirements or topical treatment such as E45 and Aveeno as emollient bath oils. In the BNFc, there is a section covering specialised nutritional formulas for children.

Appendix 3 Cautionary and Advisory Labels

The medications in the BNF/BNFc have numerical codes written next to them, under the medicinal form section. For example, for ibuprofen, the tablet has the number 21, cross-reference this to Appendix 3 and it will state 'take with or just after food' (Joint National Formulary, 2020). For lansoprazole, the orodispersible tablet has the numbers 5 and 22 and upon checking Appendix 3, it states 'Do not take indigestion remedies 2 hours before or after you take this medication' (5) and 'Take 30–60 minutes before food' (22). This appendix has 32 different advisory and cautionary labels. You need to be able to access this information and advise the woman accordingly in order to maintain their safety. To be clear, not all medications have these labels but the ones that do must be understood by the registered accountable practitioner who administers, dispenses and may prescribe them.

Appendix 4 Wound Management

This appendix is only found in the BNF, not in the BNFc. These products require a prescription but relate mainly to wound care management products and garments such as tapes, dressings and bandages. To clarify, different types of wounds require different types of dressings to assist with healing. Some dressings work to dry the wound out or to improve the wound healing environment or assist in debridement of the wound itself. As with the main chapters of the BNF, there are brand names and costings included in this appendix, to facilitate decision making and support service user choice. Wound management is complex and is considered a specialist area.

Back section

The back section of the BNF/BNFc also contains valuable information; this section is something that midwives should be aware of and know how to use. It contains MHRA Yellow Cards, to be completed if there is a suspected ADR. There is also an algorithm on adult life support and in the BNFc there

Clinical considerations

Example: using dalteparin/Fragmin® (Joint National Formulary, 2020)

Pregnant women are 4–5 times more susceptible to developing blood clots than women of the same age who are not pregnant. They will be assessed for this risk and can be prescribed heparin.

How can a midwife find out more about dalteparin if a woman under her care is prescribed this medication?

Using the BNF, the first step is to locate the area of the BNF this medication is in. As a first step, check the index at the back in alphabetical order.

Under 'D' – Dalteparin, p.140 – Blood Clots; Thromboembolism. Chapter 2 Cardiovascular System, under Heparins.

Questions you would need to check out:

- Is the prescription correct? Check the indications and that the medication is prescribed in the right preparation, as in subcutaneous injection.
- What signs and symptoms have lead the woman to believe she may have a blood clot?

  Advise on side-effects, what to expect and how to report via Yellow Card and the MHRA.
  Check cautionary advisory labels and then Appendix 1 for interactions.
  Remember some key areas:

- Baby considerations: will this medication have an effect on the fetus?
- What are the risks and benefits?

Example: using the BNF to locate information about drug interactions

A woman is currently taking the contraceptive pill which contains desogsterel and is thinking of taking St John's wort. Appendix 1 of the BNF provides the following information.

'St John's wort is predicted to decrease the efficacy of desogestrel. MHRA advises avoid.'

The Faculty of Sexual and Reproductive Healthcare (of the Royal College of Obstetricians and Gynaecologists) guidance would also be useful here.

www.fsrh.org/standards-and-guidance/

is a newborn and paediatric life support algorithm. There is also further wording for the cautionary and advisory labels. The very back page contains symbols and abbreviations providing a reminder of what abbreviations used in medicines management stand for.

Index

The last section to note is the index, which is a list of every single medication in the BNF/BNFc in alphabetical order. It is very much a go-to section to locate what is being looked for.

Drug tariff

The following section is based on the information presented online regarding the Drug Tariff. This can be accessed at: www.nhsbsa.nhs.uk/pharmacies-gp-practices-and-appliance-contractors/drug-tariff

The Drug Tariff is mainly aimed at pharmacists and GPs but there are useful sections for midwives to review. Understanding and appreciating the roles of other healthcare professionals is an important aspect of multidisciplinary work for the benefit of patients, so it is useful to have an overview of information within the Drug Tariff.

The Drug Tariff is published monthly by the NHS Business Services Authority (Prescription Services) on behalf of the Department of Health and Social Care (NHS Business Services Authority, 2021a). The Drug Tariff can be viewed online and provides information for contractors on reimbursement and remuneration, as well as information on dispensing and prices. The NHS Business Services Authority has produced an online user guide as well as a PDF user guide and these can be accessed via the website (NHS Business Services Authority, 2021a). Another useful reference source for information about the Drug Tariff is the Pharmaceutical Services Negotiating Committee (PSNC) (Pharmaceutical Services Negotiating Committee, 2021a). The PSNC 'promotes and supports the interests of all NHS community pharmacies in England' (Pharmaceutical Services Negotiating Committee, 2021b). As of April 2021, in England the Drug Tariff will no longer be available in a paper format. Using the Drug Tariff online enables the search engine to be used.

Part XV lists the borderline substances which are prescribable at the NHS expense and FP10 prescriptions should be endorsed with 'ACBS' (see the BNF for further details). These substances are certain foods and toilet preparations. Of note, in midwifery practice and prescribing for children are products such as Aptamil Pepti 1 'For the dietary management of established cows' milk allergy with/without proven secondary lactose intolerance' and PKU Anamix infant 'For use in the dietary management of proven phenylketonuria in infants from birth to 12 months and as a supplementary feed up to 3 years of age'.

Part XVIIB(ii) is useful to note for non-medical prescribing and gives information about what can be prescribed by qualified non-medical prescribers within their sphere of competence. Part XVIIIA includes a list of 'drugs, medicines and other substances that may not be ordered under the National Health Service (General Medical Services Contracts) (Prescription of Drugs, etc.) Regulations 2004 and the National Health Service (General Medical Services Contracts) (Prescription of Drugs, etc.) (Wales) Regulations 2004' (NHS Business Services Authority, 2021b). Some examples within midwifery and prescribing for children include Benylin children's cough linctus, Farleys Rusks and Infaderm baby lotion; these products are listed in the Drug Tariff.

Electronic medicines compendium (eMC)

The eMC is a website which provides clear detailed guidance for healthcare professionals, including midwives, to gain knowledge about medications, licensing and prescribing guidelines for all medications in the UK – www.medicines.org.uk.

The eMC was launched in 1999 with the aim of establishing a trusted and reliable information source about medications. This resource was designed to be a 'go to' for everything about medicines and medication licensing. The webpage is set up as a search engine where you can search for the item you are looking for be, this a patient information leaflet, summary of product characteristics or safety alert.

The eMC works closely with pharmaceutical companies, the NHS and other healthcare organisations to ensure that the information presented is robust and informative, highlighting multiple perspectives of all things medicine related. There are approximately 14 000 different documents on this website that have all been checked and approved by the Medicines and Healthcare products Regulatory Agency (MHRA) and European Medicines Agency (EMA).

Types of information available on the eMC include:

- product information
- patient information leaflets (PIL)
- safety alerts
- Summary of Product Characteristics (SPC/SmPC)
- live chat and video.

Two of these will now be discussed in more depth.

SPC/SmPC

This provides healthcare practitioners with information around how to prescribe and use a medication effectively and safely. This information is contained within a detailed document that provides an overview of an officially approved use of a medicine including clinical trial data. They are specific to each medication and will usually include a range of dosages that the medicine is licensed for, with a detailed overview of the medicine's pharmacokinetic and pharmacodynamic properties.

It will provide the professional with a detailed account of the medicine's clinical trials with outcomes and licensing as authorised by the MHRA. It will detail contraindications, warnings and precautions for use, interactions with other products and how it affects fertility, pregnancy and women who breast feed. There will also be details on expected side-effects and undesirable effects. These are useful and informative resources for midwives to have to hand when wanting to know more about a medication.

Patient information leaflets

These are of vital importance when speaking to anyone about a medicinal product. These leaflets have an abundance of useful information to aid the midwife and person taking the medication to gain a wider understanding of the prescribed treatment. It is important to share this resource in order to ensure that women are making an informed decision about their treatment. Subjects included on the PIL include what the medication is for and why it is being taken, what to do before the medication is taken and what to do prior to it being stopped. It also includes side-effects and how the medication should be administered. This section will usually include advice from the BNF's cautionary advisory labels. The PIL will also signpost the woman to further services if needed and further resources to read about the medicine (MHRA, 2020a).

It is recommended to share this resource with women and their family members, using these leaflets to explore the medication/treatment prescribed and answer any questions. This will help people to feel assured that a safe course of action has been taken to promote recovery from the diagnosed medical condition. As an NMC registrant, you have an underlying duty of care and legal accountability to ensure that accurate information is given.

Medicines and Healthcare products Regulatory Agency

The following section is based on information presented on the Medicines and Healthcare products Regulatory Agency website which can be accessed at: www.gov.uk/government/organisations/medicines-and-healthcare-products-regulatory-agency. This section contains public sector information licensed under the Open Government Licence v3.0.

The Medicines and Healthcare products Regulatory Agency (MHRA) is an executive agency of the Department of Health and Social Care. The MHRA is the regulatory authority for the UK, regulating medicines, medical devices and blood components for transfusion. Safety, quality and effectiveness of medicines, medical devices and blood component are the responsibility of the MHRA. The agency was formed on 1st April 2003. Prior to 2003, there were other agencies which had responsibility for medicines and devices.

The MHRA is responsible for: 'helping to educate the public and healthcare professionals about the risks and benefits of medicines, medical devices and blood components, leading to safer and more effective use, supporting innovation and research and development that's beneficial to public health, and influencing UK, EU and international regulatory frameworks so that they're risk-proportionate and effective at protecting public health' (MHRA, 2021a).

There is a wealth of information on the MHRA website. In this chapter, the focus is on areas key to the professional role of the midwife, namely the Yellow Card reporting system and classifications of medicines.

Most medicines used in clinical practice will have a licence; licences for medicines in the UK are granted by the MHRA (National Health Service, 2020). Three categories of medicines are used in the UK: Prescription-Only Medicine (POM), Pharmacy (P) and General Sales list (GSL). The MHRA is involved in reclassification of medicines. The level of control (reflecting how much input is needed by a health professional) of a medicine determines its legal classification (MHRA, 2021b).

The MHRA also monitors the safety of marketed medicines, which is known as pharmacovigilance. At the time of a medicine receiving its licence, it may have only been tested in a small number of patients. Some adverse drug reactions may not be known at this stage. One aspect of this monitoring is using reports made on what is known as the Yellow Card scheme. Any possible relative or suspected side-effect should be reported to the MHRA by members of the public and health professionals. This is important as it means that midwives can report adverse drug reactions using the Yellow Card scheme and this is how further information is obtained about the safety of medicine. It also highlights when medicines and medical devices may need further investigation. Yellow Cards can be found in the BNF. 'Reports can be made for all medicines including vaccines, blood factors and immunoglobulins, herbal medicines and homeopathic remedies, all medical devices available on the UK market and reports of safety concerns associated with e-cigarette products. The MHRA is also able to investigate counterfeit or fake medicines or devices and if necessary, take action to protect public health' (MHRA, 2021c).

Some medicines in the BNF and BNFc have the symbol ▼next to their entry. This means that the medicine is under additional monitoring and reporting on the Yellow Card so any suspected adverse drug reactions are especially important. There are e-learning modules available for midwives and NMC registrants relating to the importance of reporting adverse drug reactions. The *Nursing Times* has developed this module (in close collaboration with the MHRA). It is free to access after you have registered.

Using the knowledge gained through pharmacovigilance, the MHRA will communicate with patients and health professionals, via safety alerts and fact sheets. An example within midwifery practice was the material sent to health professionals regarding valproate. This information highlights the pregnancy prevention programme. If this is not achieved then valproate is contraindicated in girls and women of child-bearing potential. Further information about this issue (correct at time of publication) can be sourced directly from the MHRA website (MHRA, 2020b).

National Institute for Health and Care Excellence

The National Institute for Clinical Excellence (NICE) was founded in February 1999. Its aim was to build, create and publish consistent evidence-based guidelines. All these guidelines and clinical pathways can be accessed at www.nice.org.uk. The name of the organisation is now the National Institute for Health and Care Excellence (NICE).

NICE collaborates with many professional, research and educational bodies in order to provide quality standards for healthcare professionals, carers, family members, service users and the general public. It provides a range of guidelines, clinical knowledge summaries (CKS) and pathways to help decision making and aid professionals to advocate recommendations for treatments. It also helps patients, carers, family members and members of the general public to become more informed and gain insights into treatment plans and prescribed medicines. NICE guidelines are another good resource to share with women and their families. Signposting to the CKS is particularly recommended as these are health-related topics listed in an A–Z format, thereby enabling the resource to be user friendly and relatively straightforward to navigate.

When using NICE as a resource to aid medications and prescribing guidance, a recommended link to follow is www.nice.org.uk/about/nice-communities/medicines-and-prescribing which provides an additional link to the BNF/BNFc. This section of NICE uses signposting to access other related areas within NICE, such as:

- medicines evidence advice – providing summaries of new research studies on medicines
- medicines and prescribing associates – supporting professionals with medicines optimisation
- NICE guidance – that relates particularly to prescribing standards
- alerts – a tool to assist in receiving the most up-to-date and evidence-based information relating to medications and prescribing.

Medicines optimisation is referenced in NICE (2015), BNF (2021) and BNFc (2020–21) as it is recognised that medicines are the most common intervention when treating and managing ill health. It is also recognised that multimorbidity is on the increase and the ageing population is living longer with more long-term conditions. This therefore increases pharmacological interventions and thus creates polypharmacy. With reference to the interaction section in the BNF/BNFc, it is important to think how polypharmacy can affect the medication regime of an individual. The more medications prescribed, the greater the potential for drug interactions or side-effects to manifest in a person's symptomology. A midwife needs to know about interactions, side-effects and the increased likelihood of these occurring due to polypharmacy. The essence of medicines optimisation is to promote a change in the way that patients are supported to get the best possible outcomes from their medicines, through the adoption of a patient-focused approach to medicines use (NHSE, 2021b).

NICE promotes a person-centred approach in its guidance and by using the medicines optimisation guideline (NICE, 2015), it gives all patients the opportunity to be involved in their treatment decisions, helping them to adopt a well-informed non-biased approach to their care by using the evidence base in order to inform their decision making

UK teratology information service

The UK Teratology Information Service (UKTIS) can be accessed via the following link: www.uktis.org/index.html.

The UKTIS was established in 1983 and became part of the Newcastle National Poisons Information Service in 1995. It is the 'sole dedicated UK provider of evidence-based information on fetal risk following pharmacological and other potentially toxic pregnancy exposures' (UKTIS, 2018). The service is commissioned by Public Health England. Only health professionals can access UKTIS whereas members of the public can access the Best Use of Medicines in Pregnancy (BUMPS) website on www.medicinesinpregnancy.org. This website contains a useful collection of leaflets, based on scientific material. The material on the website is evidence based, reliable and accurate. Some of the leaflets include information on exposure to substances that may not be thought of as causing a problem or potential problem when used during pregnancy, examples being eucalyptus oil, hair dye and vitamin A face cream. Also included in the leaflets is information about risks to the baby if the father has been exposed.

Further examples of how the BNF can be used in practice

1. As a student midwife, you are observing a consultation between a 35-year-old woman and her obstetric consultant. She is c30 weeks gestation and has been diagnosed with gestational hypertension; her blood pressure is 155/95 mm/Hg.

    Recognising you would not diagnose or treat this condition yourself but want to find out more information about gestational hypertension, use the BNF and NICE guidance to find out what medications could be used to treat this.

    Response: Labetalol can be used to treat gestational hypertension; nifedipine could be considered if labetalol is not suitable and also methyldopa if labetalol and nifedipine are not suitable www.nice.org.uk/guidance/ng133/chapter/recommendations#management-of-gestational-hypertension

2. The community midwife is consulting with a woman who is 28 weeks pregnant. She is asking for advice as she has hurt her foot running; when this has happened before, she usually takes ibuprofen.

    Using the BNF, what would you suggest in this scenario?

    Response: Ibuprofen should be avoided in the third trimester. Paracetamol is not known to be harmful in pregnancy (assuming there are no other contraindications to it).

3. The midwife is examining a woman who had a caesarean section 5 days ago; her wound shows clinical signs of an infection. She is currently breast feeding. The midwife decides to refer the case to a doctor who decides that antibiotic therapy is required.

    Review what antibiotics could be given using the latest local guidance and the BNF to check whether antibiotics are appropriate in breast feeding.

    Response: This will depend on local guidance. Check your local trust infection guidelines and cross-reference with the BNF.

4. A woman is 32 weeks plus 2 pregnant with a suspected preterm labour. She is to receive betamethasone 12 mg via intramuscular injection. Using the Electronic Medicines Compendium and the information from Chapter 5, discuss the pharmacokinetics and pharmacodynamics.

    Response:
    www.medicines.org.uk/emc/product/9097/smpc

Conclusion

This chapter has provided guidance for midwives and other healthcare professionals around how to locate reliable, accurate information which will support their practice associated with medication use. The importance of ensuring that any information used is based on the latest, most up-to-date guidance has been emphasised throughout. Accurate knowledge is essential in order to ensure that the best available treatment is given to women and their babies during pregnancy, labour and beyond.

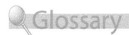 Glossary

Adverse drug reaction   An unwanted or harmful reaction which occurs after administration of a drug or drugs

Blood components   Those parts of a unit of blood which are separated by physical or mechanical means

Compendium   A collection of concise but detailed information about a particular subject, especially in a book or other publication

Contraindication   A specific situation in which a drug, procedure or surgery should not be used because it may be harmful to the person

Controlled Drug   A drug or other substance that is tightly controlled by the government because it may be abused or cause addiction

E Number   Artificial substances which are added to some foods and drinks to improve their flavour or colour or to make them last longer

Gestational hypertension   High blood pressure in pregnancy

Homeopathic remedy   A 'treatment' based on the use of highly diluted substances, which practitioners claim can cause the body to heal itself

Immunoglobulin   Any of a class of proteins present in the serum and cells of the immune system, which function as antibodies

Medicines optimisation   A person-centred approach to safe and effective medicines use, to ensure people obtain the best possible access to medication

Multimorbidity   The co-occurrence of two or more chronic conditions

Patient Group Directions   Allow healthcare professionals to supply and administer specified medicines to predefined groups of patients, without a prescription

Pharmacovigilance   Medicines and vaccines have transformed the prevention and treatment of diseases. In addition to their benefits, medicinal products may also have side-effects, some of which may be undesirable and/or unexpected. Pharmacovigilance is the science and activities relating to the detection, assessment, understanding and prevention of adverse effects or any other medicine/vaccine-related problem

Polypharmacy   The prescribing of multiple medications appropriately or inappropriately, or where the intended benefit of the medication is not realised (inappropriate)

Symptomology   The set of symptoms characteristic of a medical condition or exhibited by a patient

Teratology   The science that studies the causes, mechanisms and patterns of abnormal fetal development

Test yourself

Now review your learning by completing the learning activities for this chapter at www.wiley.com/go/pharmacologyformidwives.

References

Joint Formulary Committee (2020–21) *British National Formulary for Children*. Joint Formulary Committee: London.

Joint Formulary Committee (2021) *British National Formulary 80*. Joint Formulary Committee: London.

Medicines and Healthcare products Regulatory Agency (2020a) Best Practice Guidance on patient information leaflets. www.gov.uk/government/publications/best-practice-guidance-on-patient-information-leaflets (accessed January 2022).

Medicines and Healthcare products Regulatory Agency (2020b) Valproate (Epilim▼, Depakote▼) pregnancy prevention programme: updated educational materials. www.gov.uk/drug-safety-update/valproate-epilim-depakote-pregnancy-prevention-programme-updated-educational-materials (accessed January 2022).

Medicines and Healthcare products Regulatory Agency (2021a) About us. www.gov.uk/government/organisations/medicines-and-healthcare-products-regulatory-agency/about (accessed January 2022).

Medicines and Healthcare products Regulatory Agency (2021b) Medicines: Reclassify your product. www.gov.uk/guidance/medicines-reclassify-your-product (accessed January 2022).

Medicines and Healthcare products Regulatory Agency (2021c) About Yellow Card. https://yellowcard.mhra.gov.uk/the-yellow-card-scheme/ (accessed January 2022).

National Health Service (2020) Medicines Information. www.nhs.uk/conditions/medicines-information/ (accessed January 2022).

National Institute for Health and Care Excellence (2015) Medicines Optimisation: the safe and effective use of medicines to enable the best possible outcomes. www.nice.org.uk/guidance/ng5 (accessed January 2022).

National Institute for Health and Care Excellence (2021) Medicines and Prescribing. www.nice.org.uk/about/nice-communities/medicines-and-prescribing (accessed January 2022).

NHS Business Service Authority (2021a) Drug Tariff. www.nhsbsa.nhs.uk/pharmacies-gp-practices-and-appliance-contractors/drug-tariff (accessed January 2022).

NHS Business Service Authority (2021b) Part XVIIIA – Drugs, Medicines and Other Substances not to be ordered under a General Medical Services Contract. www.drugtariff.nhsbsa.nhs.uk/#/00799927-DD/DD00799841/Part%20XVIIIA%20-%20Drugs,%20Medicines%20and%20Other%20Substances%20not%20to%20be%20ordered%20under%20a%20General%20Medical%20Services%20Contract (accessed January 2022).

NHS England (2021a) Shared decision making. www.england.nhs.uk/shared-decision-making (accessed January 2022).

NHS England (2021b) Medicines optimisation. www.england.nhs.uk/rightcare/useful-links/medicines-optimisation/ (accessed January 2022).

Nursing Midwifery Council (2018) The Code: professional standards of practice and behaviour for nurses, midwives and nursing associates. www.nmc.org.uk/standards/code/ (accessed January 2022).

Nursing and Midwifery Council (2019) Standards of Proficiency for Midwives. www.nmc.org.uk/globalassets/sitedocuments/standards/standards-of-proficiency-for-midwives.pdf (accessed January 2022).

Pharmaceutical Services Negotiating Committee (2021a) *Virtual Drug Tariff*. https://psnc.org.uk/dispensing-supply/drug-tariff-resources/virtual-drug-tariff/ (accessed January 2022).

Pharmaceutical Services Negotiating Committee (2021b) About PSNC. https://psnc.org.uk/psncs-work/about-psnc/ (accessed January 2022).

UK Teratology Information Service (2018) About Us. www.uktis.org/html/about_us.html (accessed January 2022).

Chapter 3
Legal and ethical issues

Hema Turner
University of Hertfordshire, Hatfield, UK

Aim

The aim of this chapter is to examine the legal and ethical considerations related to pharmacology and medicines management in midwifery practice.

Learning outcomes

By the end of this chapter the student midwife will be able to:
* Demonstrate an understanding of the law that governs pharmacology in midwifery practice
* Identify and name the medicines on the midwives' exemption list
* Define commonly used medico-legal concepts and ethical principles applied to pharmacology in midwifery practice
* Explain the legal and ethical role of the student midwife during safe medicine management.

Test your existing knowledge

* What is the law that governs medicinal products for human use in the UK?
* What is the most common category of allegation referred for fitness to practise at the NMC?
* Can a partner consent to treatment on behalf of their wife during childbirth?
* Do women in active labour lack capacity to consent to treatment?
* Can service users accessing maternity care under the age of 16 give consent to treatments?

Introduction

This chapter will introduce you to the fundamental legal and ethical principles governing midwives' practice relating to the broader pharmacological aspects of medicines management. This will also include a brief introduction to the law and the basic principles of clinical negligence applied to medicines management in midwifery. Midwives are autonomous practitioners who are highly skilled and knowledgeable and are required to provide high-quality, respectful and compassionate care to women, newborn infants and their families across the pregnancy continuum, ranging from pre-pregnancy, pregnancy, labour and birth to the postpartum period (NMC, 2019b).

Fundamentals of Pharmacology for Midwives, First Edition. Edited by Ian Peate and Cathy Hamilton.
© 2022 John Wiley & Sons Ltd. Published 2022 by John Wiley & Sons Ltd.
Companion website: www.wiley.com/go/pharmacologyformidwives

Incorporated into this role, midwives and student midwives are expected to uphold the duties outlined in the Code and 'advise on, prescribe, supply, dispense or administer medicines within the limits of [their] training and competence, the law, our guidance and other relevant policies, guidance and regulations' (NMC, 2018, section 18, p. 16). Therefore, any clinical decisions made about the broader pharmacological aspects of medicines management require careful consideration of the professional and legal role and responsibilities of the midwife, including the guidance of local organisational policies, the ethical principles underpinning professional practice and the assessment and clinical status of the service user such as consent and mental capacity. These issues are now considered in turn.

The law

Britain is governed by an 'unwritten constitution' composed of laws and rules. The law is a system of rules laid down by a body or persons with the power and authority to make law. This process is achieved in Parliament. In the UK, a Bill is proposed as a new law or a change in the existing law and is first presented in either the House of Lords or the House of Commons. The Bill once debated must be approved by both Houses before receiving Royal Assent, becoming an Act of Parliament (Cabinet Office, 2013). Once enacted, the Act of Parliament becomes statute, i.e. law. In the UK, there is little statutory regulation of medical care. An example of this is the Nursing and Midwifery Order 2001 and the repealed 1902 Midwives Act that previously existed. However, the Supply of Goods and Services Act 1982 c 29; Part ii- Supply of Services, expects that in a contract for the supply of a service where the supplier is acting in the course of a business, such as the National Health Service (NHS), including any private and independent health sectors, the supplier (healthcare professional) performs their professional services with reasonable skill and care. The laws governing healthcare services are also found in case law. Case law are disputes resolved in a court of law and are referred to as judicial precedent. Case laws are therefore created by judges during their judgement of a case and are found in the *ratio dicidendi* or reason for the decision which is then later applied to similar disputes (cases) when presented to the courts.

Laws applied to healthcare exist to safeguard service users and the public from harm. In the UK, clinical negligence is a process where a service user can take action against a health professional in a civil court for compensation. Since 2007 clinical negligence cases have rapidly increased, forcing healthcare professionals to defend their practice (NHSI, 2019), with maternity care resulting in almost 50% of all NHS negligence claims, of which drug errors accounted for 1.63%, costing the NHS £8^759^430.00 in 2011 (NHS Litigation Authority, 2012). It will also be discussed later in this chapter that prescribing and medicines management has topped the list of all allegations of harm by midwives and nurses referred to the NMC for investigation (NMC, 2021a).

Clinical negligence and duty of care

However, in order to bring a claim of negligence against a healthcare professional. three criteria need to be fulfilled.

- It must first be proven that the healthcare professional owed a duty of care to the claimant (service user).
- Second, the healthcare professional had breached that duty of care.
- Third, in breaching that duty of care, the claimant suffered harm, a loss or injury as a result (Herring, 2018).

Duty of care is defined as a 'legal obligation imposed on individuals or organisations that they take reasonable care in the conduct of acts that could foreseeably result in actionable harm to another' (Samanta and Samanta, 2011, p. 89). The concept of 'duty of care', also referred to as the 'neighbour principle', was developed in Donoghue v Stevenson (1932) and then later affirmed in Caparo Industries plc v Dickman (1990). In these case laws, the judicial precedent identified that anyone directly affected by a careless or unreasonable act is owed a duty of care. In the law of tort, this concept has been applied to the 'special relationship' that exists between a health professional and their service user. The NMC identifies that midwives have a professional duty to put the interests of service users in their care first and to safeguard them from harm (NMC, 2019a). Duty of care owed is also judged by the same standard for student midwives in a learning capacity (Nettleship v Weston 1971). In Wilsher v Essex Area Health Authority (1988) the court of appeal rejected the claim that a junior unexperienced health professional owed a lower duty of care.

Healthcare organisations across the UK are also not exempted. The statutory duty of candour applies to all healthcare organisations across the NHS and independent healthcare providers (Health and Social Care Act 2008 (Regulated Activities) Regulation 20) to which they are held responsible or face possible prosecution for a breach of parts 20 (2) and 20 (3) of the Regulation. They are to ensure that they uphold their duty of being open and transparent to service users regarding the care or treatment they receive, including providing factual information regarding incidents when things go wrong, apologise and provide reasonable support as required.

The Bolam test and Bolitho principles

The second criterion used to establish clinical negligence is whether the healthcare professional had breached their duty of care. Normally, a person is considered to breach a duty of care owed if they behave in a way in which a reasonable person in the same situation would not act. In clinical negligence, to determine whether a duty of care owed is breached, the healthcare professional needs to satisfy the Bolam test. The Bolam test applied in a court of law will identify whether the healthcare practitioner or healthcare organisation in question acted in accordance with a practice accepted as proper by a body of health professionals specialising in the specific field under scrutiny.

The relevant case (Bolam vs Friern Hospital Management Committee, 1957) involved a patient who had suffered a fractured hip during electroconvulsive therapy. No relaxant or other restraint had been given to the patient in preparation for the treatment. The case explored this, along with the information the patient had been offered. The question was asked of a group of similar professionals and it was assessed that the practitioner had not been negligent as he had acted in accordance with accepted practice at that time. This set the standard and the Bolam test is now used in cases of negligence as a benchmark for whether the professional concerned acted in a reasonable manner. In the case of Whitehouse v Jordan (1981), despite a child suffering severe brain damage as a result of the use of forceps by a senior medical professional, it was found that the decision to use forceps would have been made by any reasonable professional in the same circumstances. The judge later identified that 'in a professional person, an error of judgement is not necessarily negligent'.

However, the Bolam test was criticised for being too protective of healthcare professionals and that it allowed them to set their own standards rather than these being set by a court of law. As a result, the Bolam test was clarified and reaffirmed in Bolitho v City and Hackney Health Authority (1997). The legal principle supporting Bolitho identified that a court can decide that a body of opinion is not reasonable or responsible if it can be demonstrated that the professional opinion is not capable of withstanding logical analysis.

Episode of care

Jenna is a second-year student midwife working on a midwifery-led unit. During her labour and birth, Jenna cared for Annabel who was a low-risk primigravida at 38 weeks and 4 days. Jenna gave birth to a healthy male infant weighing 3.4^kg with an Apgar score of 9 at 1 minute, 10 at 5 minutes and 10 at 10 minutes. After completing care during the third stage of labour, Jenna proceeded to perform the newborn's first examination. Jenna saw that her midwife supervisor had documented that Annabel consented for her baby to have Konakion® 1^mg intramuscularly (IM) at birth. Once Jenna had completed her newborn examination, she administered the Konakion 1^mg IM to the baby. Jenna then dressed the baby and handed him over to Annabel to initiate breast feeding; Annabel asked if the baby had had 'the injection' and why it was needed. The midwife supervisor then entered the room, advising Jenna that once she had completed the newborn examination, she would need to get the Konakion prescribed prior to it being administered under supervision.

This scenario highlights several issues. First, it is clear Jenna owed Annabel and her newborn baby a duty of care. Second, we need to examine whether Jenna breached that duty of care. Jenna was required to obtain informed consent prior to administering the Konakion to the baby. Jenna therefore needed to ensure Annabel was competent, had been sufficiently informed about the drug, including any side-effects and any alternative route or options available if declined, was not subjected to coercion or undue influence and had reached a clear decision. This was not evident when Annabel asked Jenna why the 'injection' was needed. Third, was there any harm as a result of Jenna's action of administering the Konakion to the baby? If the answer is no, in law, all three criteria must be met in order for Annabel to claim clinical negligence. If yes, Jenna could be facing possible suspension of her training with the case being referred for investigation.

This is an example where in a court of law, the Bolam and Bolitho principles would be applied. The question will be considered whether Jenna acted in accordance with accepted practice at that time (Bolam, 1957). However, the court can decide that the 'body of opinion' is not reasonable or responsible if it can be demonstrated that the professional opinion is not capable of withstanding logical analysis (Bolitho, 1997). The issue also remains that Jenna did not work within the guidance of the Code (NMC, 2018) in ensuring that informed consent was obtained prior to administration of the medication. Jenna is also in breach of the NMC (2021b) guidance where she was not permitted to administer the Konakion without a prescription and under direct supervision of her midwife supervisor.

It is important that as student midwives you understand that you owe the same duty of care as your midwife supervisor to women, babies and their families. You will need to ensure you keep up to date and are fully aware and informed of the law, guidance and policies surrounding pharmacology in midwifery practice and uphold the NMC Code in doing so.

The law relating to midwives and medicines

In 2016, the Human Medicines Regulation 2012 was amended to ensure the law provided a comprehensive document that governs the administration, sale and supply of medicinal products for human use in the UK. Included in this regulation are the guidance and scope of practice for midwives regarding medicines management. The scope of practice relates to Patient-Specific Directions (PSD), Patient Group Directives (PGD) and midwives' exemptions. Paragraph 18 of the Code requires all nurses and midwives who 'advise on, prescribe, supply, dispense or administer medicines to do so within the limits of their training and competence, the law, NMC guidance and other relevant policies, guidance and regulations'. On successful completion of an approved NMC midwifery education programme and entry onto the NMC register, all midwives are required to uphold the Code (NMC, 2018) regarding medicines management (Table 3.1) and are deemed competent to safely select, acquire and administer a range of permitted drugs consistent with the Human Medicines (Amendment) Regulations 2016.

The three categories identified for prescribing medicinal products are General Sales list (GSL), pharmacy (P) medicines and prescription-only medicines (POMs). Within their scope of practice, midwives can supply all GSL and P medicines. Medicines not included in midwives' exemptions (this includes GSL, P and specified POM medicines) require a prescription, a PSD or PGD. However, unless a medicine is included on the list of midwives' exemptions, the sale or supply of POM by a midwife may only be permitted in receipt of a prescription from a suitable prescribing practitioner. Only midwives who have successfully completed an NMC-approved independent and supplementary prescribing qualification (V300) and have had that qualification recorded on the NMC's register may prescribe medicines, within the limits of those qualifications (NMC, 2021b). Schedule 17 of the Human Medicine Regulations lists the limited list of POMs referred to as the midwives' exemptions, which midwives can also supply and administer only during their professional practice. The list identifies POMs for parenteral administration that contain (a) diamorphine, (b) morphine and (c) pethidine hydrochloride. It is important that midwives keep up to date on the list of medicines in the exemption. Schedule 17 of the Human Medicine (Amendment) Regulations 2016 also identifies circumstances when midwives can lawfully administer P and supply and administer POM.

It is important that midwives are also aware of their local organisational policies and guidance on medicines management relating to their scope of practice in supplying and dispensing of

Table 3.1   The Code related to medicines.

Section	Code
18.1	prescribe, advise on, or provide medicines or treatment, including repeat prescriptions (only if you are suitably qualified) if you have enough knowledge of that person's health and are satisfied that the medicines or treatment serve that person's health needs
18.2	keep to appropriate guidelines when giving advice on using controlled drugs and recording the prescribing, supply, dispensing or administration of controlled drugs
18.3	make sure that the care or treatment you advise on, prescribe, supply, dispense or administer for each person is compatible with any other care or treatment they are receiving, including (where possible) over-the-counter medicines
18.4	take all steps to keep medicines stored securely
18.5	wherever possible, avoid prescribing for yourself or for anyone with whom you have a close personal relationship Prescribing is not within the scope of practice of everyone on our register. Nursing associates don't prescribe, but they may supply, dispense and administer medicines. Nurses and midwives who have successfully completed a further qualification in prescribing and recorded it on our register are the only people on our register that can prescribe

Source: NMC (2018).

medicines, such as the giving of paracetamol and administration of nitrous oxide and oxygen using Entonox apparatus (NMC, 2021b).

The Code

Advise on, prescribe, supply, dispense or administer medicines within the limits of your training and competence, the law, our guidance and other relevant policies, guidance and regulations. To achieve this, see Table 3.1.

The law relating to student midwives and medicines

The NMC (2021b) provides a clear and comprehensive statement on the advice given to student midwives and their supervisors relating to medicines management in clinical practice.

> 'All midwives who support, supervise and assess student midwives should ensure that they are familiar with the law in relation to the supply of medicines, including the midwives' exemptions, in order to safely support and supervise student midwives who may administer medicines to women in their care. In accordance with Part 3 of Schedule 17 of the Regulations student mid-wives can administer the drugs included within the midwives' exemptions (with the exception of controlled drugs) under the direct supervision of a midwife. Student midwives are not permitted to administer controlled drugs using midwives' exemptions, including Diamorphine, Morphine and Pethidine Hydrochloride. They may participate in the checking and preparation of controlled drugs under the supervision of a midwife. Student midwives may administer prescribed drugs (including controlled drugs) parenterally if prescribed by a doctor or an appropriate practitioner according to their directions for administration. This must be under the direct supervision of a midwife. A registered nurse during their clinical placement on the shortened programme acts as a student midwife for the purposes of all drug administration.'

The regulatory body: the Nursing and Midwifery Council

In the UK, the NMC is the professional regulator for nurses and midwives and in England for nursing associates. The role of the NMC as a regulator serves to safeguard service users and the public, support the nursing and midwifery profession and influence health and social care (NMC, 2019a). All practising nurses and midwives are required to be registered with the NMC and are referred to as registrants. All practising registrants are required to follow the Code (NMC, 2018) which sets out the standards of practice and behaviour. Registrants are deemed 'fit to practise' if they possess the necessary skills, knowledge, good health and character to provide safe, high-quality care to their service users.

Table 3.2   NMC fitness to practise. The three most common categories of allegations.

Allegation level one (% of total allegations)	Allegation level two
Prescribing and medicines management (25%)	• Patient or clinical records • Drugs or medication records • Other record-keeping issues • Care plan
Patient care (18%)	• Not administering or refusing to administer medication • Other drugs administration or medicines management errors • Administered incorrect dosage • Inappropriate or incorrect delivery of medication
Record keeping (12%)	• Patient or clinical records • Drugs or medication records • Other record-keeping issues • Care plan

Source: NMC (2021).

In an event where clinical care falls below the expected standard or concerns are raised that cannot be resolved at a local level, the registrant's employer, a fellow colleague, the service user or the public can report this behaviour or concern to the NMC for further investigation. The NMC encourages registrants to raise and escalate concerns appropriately (NMC, 2019a) and midwives to practise the professional duty of candour in being open and honest with women and their families, their colleagues and employer when something goes wrong that may result in harm (NMC, 2019c). The NMC then investigates the registrant's 'fitness to practise (ftp)'. Concerns that are investigated further include cases of misconduct (including clinical misconduct), lack of competence, criminal convictions, serious ill health, not having the necessary knowledge of the English language and cases where someone has gained access to the register fraudulently or incorrectly (NMC, 2021a). In 2020–2021 a total of 176 midwives were referred to the NMC for further investigations. This figure has remained unchanged and is reflective of a steady 5% of the total number of registered midwives referred to the NMC in 2019–2020 and 2018–2019.

The annual ftp report 2020–2021 also highlighted the top three most common categories of allegations which remained unchanged from 2019–2020, of which prescribing and medicines management topped the list with a total of 25% of all allegations. Table 3.2 taken from the NMC annual ftp report 2020–2021 shows the most common allegations within each of the three categories. Level one is the headline allegation category and level two provides more detail about the allegation type. Information presented in allegation two clearly highlights the need for this chapter and the importance of adhering to the Code (NMC, 2018); ensuring the practice of safe medicines management is paramount.

Ethical principles

Ethics are rooted within midwifery care. Our professional values, beliefs, morals and theories of ethics applied to our decision making are at the heart of becoming a midwife. The guiding ethical principles in healthcare initially identified by Beauchamp and Childress (2009) are beneficence, non-maleficence, autonomy and justice and later included veracity and fidelity.

The ethical principle of *beneficence* expects that midwives, along with all other healthcare professionals, endeavour to do good. The international code of ethics for midwives promotes women as individuals, recognising that they are to be respected, to uphold their human rights, be treated fairly and with dignity, making healthcare equally accessible to all (International Confederation of Midwives (ICM), 2014). In clinical practice, midwives are expected to put women, babies and their family first, acting in their best interest at all times. At times, this can be very challenging as midwives will need to work through a number of complex ethical dilemmas whilst upholding their professional values. As a result, the principle of beneficence is tested through careful considerations in weighing up the risks of harm when making clinical decisions relating to midwifery/obstetric interventions.

The principle of *non-maleficence*, which means 'to do no harm', is interconnected with beneficence. Midwives are faced daily with the competing quandary of ensuring their decisions and actions do not cause harm to either the woman or their fetus. For example, midwives administer prescribed oxytocic drugs to women either to induce or augment their labour which can cause adverse reactions such as fetal distress, leading to possible fetal mortality. A balance between the beneficence of doing good to assist with the progression of labour for medical reasons against the risk of harm (non-maleficence) to the fetus requires careful consideration along with respecting the woman's decision.

The principle of *autonomy* encourages midwives to uphold and respect the rights of women, respect their choices and support them in their decisions. Justice Hale, in her judgment of Montgomery v Lanarkshire Health Board (2015), reinforced that 'Gone are the days when it was thought that, on becoming pregnant, a woman lost, not only her capacity, but also her right to act as a genuinely autonomous human being'. The principle of autonomy is therefore rooted in the doctrine of informed consent (see section on consent for further information linked to this principle). The NMC (2018) advises registrants to respect and encourage shared decision making with service users on the treatments and care they receive. This also includes respecting their choice to decline recommended treatment or care offered. An example of this is a case where a woman with epilepsy refuses to take her antiepileptic drug during pregnancy after being advised that it is safe to do so by midwives and the interprofessional healthcare team. It is important to remember that although some women may decide that they do not wish to be concordant with their recommended treatment, the midwife is required to support the woman and to provide non-judgemental and compassionate care.

Justice is concerned with the belief that as health professionals, we are expected to treat people in our care fairly, equally and reasonably. In healthcare, this is not always straightforward and can pose some difficulty when applying the concept of equality. An example of this is the fair and equal distribution of fertility resources referred to as 'distributive justice'. Infertility has the potential to have a long-lasting devastating impact on women, couples and families. Women and couples requesting treatment for fertility, referred to as in vitro fertilisation (IVF), must endure the unfairness of resource distribution. In England, fertility services are commissioned by the Clinical Commissioning Groups (CCGs) and it is estimated that less than 1 in 5 CCGs are meeting national standards for providing fertility treatments (HFEA, 2020; Smith and Marshall, 2020). NICE (2013) identified that IVF is cost-effective up to age 43, highlighting the importance of CCGs reviewing current policies in ending the postcode lottery and allowing a fairer distribution of fertility treatment.

The *veracity* principle encourages healthcare professionals to be open, honest and accurate when communicating with service users. It is the condition in which our service users demonstrate trust and confidence in the care they receive (NMC, 2018). The 'duty of candour' guidance for health professionals (NMC and GMC, 2015) is a working example of the application of the veracity principle. In midwifery at times mistakes can happen. An example of this includes medication errors which can have severe consequences. It is important when this happens that health professionals are truthful in fully disclosing the error to the service user, apologising and offering any remedy (Francis, 2013). The principle of veracity is also applied to the concept of informed consent to any form of treatment or intervention. For example, midwives are required to be truthful to women when discussing requests for analgesia at any stage of labour and to provide unbiased information about the different options for pain relief, the mechanism of action and any side-effects (Royal College of Midwives (RCM), 2012).

Midwives are autonomous practitioners who are predominantly the first contact for women in pregnancy, provide continuity of care throughout pregnancy and the postnatal period and facilitate access to secondary or specialist services when required. As a result, midwives develop professional relationships with women and their families which in turn creates trustworthiness and loyalty, referred to as the principle of *fidelity*. The issues surrounding this principle include the ongoing conflict of health professionals' professional and organisational obligation and upholding the trust of service users when faced with ethical dilemmas. An example of this is a woman disclosing to her midwife a situation of substance misuse. The midwife must use her clinical judgement in disclosing pertinent information to other health professionals, including discussing any social care arrangements which will provide the necessary treatment required in pregnancy to prevent harm to the woman and safeguard the unborn fetus.

Use of unlicensed medicines and further ethical considerations

The term 'unlicensed' covers the use of drugs that have not been evaluated or approved outside the terms of the manufacturer's licence (Aronson and Ferner, 2017). This includes the use of drugs administered in an alternative form other than the licensed use; for example, a drug that has been manipulated from a solid form to be administered as liquid solution. The use of unlicensed medicine in obstetrics is very common and it is important to note that unlicensed drugs are considered safe and effective to use. It is referred to as unlicensed when the drug is administered to a category of service users that were not approved for use by the regulatory authority. However, robust information on the safety of medicines used in pregnancy is limited and this can be attributed to the ethical implications of including pregnant women in clinical trials (Ayad and Constantine, 2015; Phillippi and Hartmann, 2018).

In 1962, the thalidomide tragedy highlighted significant birth defects following use of the antiemetic drug which was licensed to be used in pregnancy. Safety concerns about fetal development and the impact of the physiological changes in pregnancy on pharmacokinetics led to the exclusion of pregnant women from participating in clinical drug trials (Vargeeson, 2015). Further research and robust clinical drug trials are therefore needed and are often conducted in evaluating the effectiveness of the unlicensed drug specific to that service user.

This then raises ethical dilemmas surrounding the healthcare practitioner's duty of care to prevent unforeseen harm. We have seen earlier that in order to uphold the principles of beneficence, healthcare professionals endeavour to do good and not cause harm (non-maleficence). In clinical practice, healthcare professionals undergo a complex interplay of ethics, professional and legal duty in making clinical decisions to provide safe care to service users.

The *utilitarian or consequentialism theory* examines whether an act causes more harm than good for the greatest number of people. In applying this to pharmacology and the use of unlicensed medicines, healthcare professionals will weigh the potential benefits of using unlicensed drugs against the risks posed and use these drugs as required to reduce the risk of unnecessary harm. Application of the utilitarian principle disregards the principle of autonomy of the individual because the use of unlicensed drugs seeks to do good and provide treatment for the greater good of that category of service user. As a result, this affects the process of obtaining informed consent. Healthcare professionals must therefore ensure the correct provision is implemented in obtaining informed consent when using unlicensed drugs, providing open, honest and truthful information on the efficacy and safety of drugs used along with any other alternative options available (Sinclair et al., 2016).

Another guiding principle is *deontology* which is concerned with rules and duties. For example, in applying the deontological concept, healthcare professionals will consider whether the administration of unlicensed medication to their service user is the right thing to do regardless of 'the consequences' or safety and efficacy of the unlicensed drug. As a result, duty of care here is of paramount importance in ensuring that healthcare professionals 'do no harm'. Nevertheless, there will be instances where conflict will arise, and these principles, along with the healthcare professional's professional and legal obligations, will be examined more closely during clinical decision making to ensure the best possible care is provided to service users.

Midwives and student midwives are therefore advised to keep up to date with the law, the Code and local trust guidelines and polices governing the supply, administration and use of medicines, including the midwives' exemptions.

Consent for treatment: adults

The concept and process of informed consent has been well established in law (Schloendorf v Society of New York Hospitals, 1914) and its guiding principles have been embodied within guidelines and polices to which all healthcare professionals are required to adhere. More recently and pertinent to maternity care, Montgomery v Lanarkshire Health Board (2015, para 87) reinforced that:

> 'An adult person of sound mind is entitled to decide which, if any, of the available forms of treatment to undergo, and her consent must be obtained before treatment interfering with her bodily integrity is undertaken. The [healthcare professional] is therefore under a duty to take reasonable care to ensure that the [service user] is aware of any material risks involved in any recommended treatment, and of any reasonable alternative or variant treatments. The test of materiality is whether, in the circumstances of the particular case, a reasonable person in the [service user's] position would be likely to attach significance to the risk, or the [healthcare professional] is or should reasonably be aware that the particular [service user] would be likely to attach significance to it.'

Informed consent is an integral part of medicines management. The Code (NMC, 2018) encourages healthcare professionals to obtain and document informed consent prior to providing any treatment. Obtaining informed consent provides legal justification for care and forms the basis of trust with service users. Without consent, a healthcare professional may be committing the crime of battery or assault (Re W, 1992). An example of battery was identified in Potts v NWRHA (1983) when a woman consented to what was described as a routine postnatal vaccination but in fact was a long-acting contraceptive.

Therefore, for a service user to give informed consent, it is not enough that they say 'yes'. In gaining informed consent, ensure that the service user:

- is competent
- has been sufficiently informed
- has not been subjected to coercion or undue influence
- has reached a clear decision.

Midwives supervising students are required to be accountable for any delegated duties in obtaining informed consent. Student midwives are expected to fully understand the instructions in gaining informed consent and supervisors are required to ensure that students midwives are adequately supervised and supported to provide safe and compassionate care when obtaining informed consent prior to any treatment or drug administration (NMC, 2018).

Capacity and consent

An adult service user with capacity has an absolute right to decline medical treatment even if their life depends on it (St George's Healthcare NHS Trust v S, 1998) or choose one treatment rather than another being offered. The right for that choice or decision is not limited to decisions which others or even health professionals may regard as sensible (Re T, 1992). However, when capacity is uncertain, the duty is on the healthcare professional to satisfy the requirements in law outlined in the Mental Capacity Act (MCA) 2005. The NMC requires that all registrants keep up to date with the laws governing mental capacity and rights and best interests are at the centre of the decision-making process for those service users who lack capacity (NMC, 2018).

Section 3(1) of the MCA sets out the criteria for health professionals to assess the ability of an adult to make decisions. A person is able to make a decision for themselves if they are able to:

- understand the information relevant to the decision
- retain that information
- use or weigh that information as part of the process of making the decision
- communicate their decision (whether by talking, using sign language or any other means).

Clinical Considerations

Mental capacity in labour

According to the Mental Capacity Act 2005, an adult lacks capacity if there is an impairment or disturbance in the function of their mind or brain and they fail to:

- understand relevant information
- retain that information
- use or weigh information as part of the process of making the decision
- communicate their decision.

It has been questioned on several occasions whether labour affects a woman's mental capacity during labour. In the case of MB (1997), the court questioned the impact of fatigue, pain and drugs as factors that could possibly affect mental capacity in labour. The court was of the opinion that most women have capacity in labour and retain the ability to make decisions and to consent to or decline care. Further prospective studies also identified that women in active labour experiencing mild, moderate or severe pain whilst giving informed consent for an epidural were able to recall the risks of an epidural (Affleck et al., 1998) with a high degree of reliability (Gerancher et al., 2000).

Types of consent

The various types of consent will now be considered.

Expressed

- Verbal
- Written

Verbal consent is when a service user agrees to the care or treatment being proposed. This type of consent is not set out in any specific form or in writing (Re T, 1992). An example of this in practice is when midwives obtain verbal consent from parents to administer vitamin K prophylaxis for neonates. Written consent is a written record of the consent process with the service user. Apart from special circumstances which are examined later, there is no obligation in law for consent to be formally written. Consent to treatment is therefore equally valid in the verbal, implied or written form. It is, however, recommended practice implemented in all healthcare organisations that prior to any procedure, consent forms are signed. Conversely, a signature on a consent form does not indicate valid consent unless the benefits, risks and alternative options are discussed with the service user.

Implied

In law, implied consent has been well established as an appropriate form of gaining consent as it indicates from a person's conduct what their state of mind is, if not explicitly expressed. The courts rejected a claim of battery when a woman joined a queue of 200 passengers waiting for the smallpox vaccination. The court ruled that the woman had implied consent for the vaccination after she rolled up her sleeve and voluntarily held up her hand to be vaccinated without objection (O'Brian v Cunard SS co, 1891).

Statutory requirements

There are some limitations to the doctrine of gaining informed consent. These are listed below.

- For life-saving procedures where the service user is unconscious and cannot indicate their wishes (R v. Brown, 1993).
- Where there is a statutory power requiring the examination of a service user under the Public Health (Control of Diseases) Act 1984.
- In certain cases where a minor is under the supervision of court protection. The court decides whether a specific treatment is in the best interest of the child.
- Treatment for service users who are detained under the Mental Capacity Act 2005.

- Treatment for a physical disorder where the service user is incapable of giving consent due to impaired to mental health and the treatment is in the best interest of the person.
- In the UK, service users cannot consent to all interventions and some are not in the public interest and have statutory provisions prohibiting them, such as female circumcision and tattooing of minors, for example.

Special circumstances: consent for treatment: children – Gillick competence

In law, service users age between 16 and 17 years with capacity can consent to both medical and dental treatment and those who lack capacity will require someone with parental responsibility to consent on their behalf (Family Law Reform Act, 1969 s 8 (1)). Service users under the age of 16 years are assessed for capacity to consent or not by determining whether they possess sufficient understanding of what the treatment involves (Gillick v West Norfolk and Wisbech Area Health Authority, 1985). This assessment is referred to as Gillick competence and the onus of proof is on the service user to prove that they are competent to make that decision, including the repercussions of they are agreeing to, or refusal of the treatment. In cases where a Gillick-competent child refuses consent, this may be overruled by the authority of the court. In Re E (1993) the court ruled that a 15-year-old Jehovah's Witness should be treated after refusing a life-saving blood transfusion. Children under 16 years who are not deemed Gillick competent cannot give consent. Decisions regarding consent through parental responsibility may also be overruled and settled in court if the proposed treatment is in the best interest of the child.

Episode of care

Lilly-Ann is a 15-year-old primigravida with a RHD negative blood type who attended the day assessment unit at 28 weeks gestation as advised by her community midwife for administration of her anti-D immunoglobulin. Lilly-Ann attended the unit with her mother. Midwife Janice gained informed consent and performed routine antenatal care to Lilly-Ann which included a full set of observations, assessment of fetal well-being and the recommended blood test screening as per local trust guidelines. According to the NMC (2021b) guidance and in line with the midwives' exemptions, Janice ensured that the anti-D immunoglobulin was prescribed by an appropriate professional prior to administration. As Janice proceeded to gain informed consent, Lilly-Ann's mother intervened, advising Janice that she was not happy for Lilly-Ann to receive the drug because of a personal experience of miscarriage which she believed was linked to the drug. Janice was aware that Lilly-Ann was 15 years of age and so in order to gain informed consent without parental consent, Janice needed to assess whether Lilly-Ann was Gillick competent to make the decision about accepting the anti-D immunoglobulin injection, including the repercussions she was agreeing to, or refusal of the treatment. Janice asked Lilly-Ann's mother if she could get Lilly-Ann a drink from the water dispenser outside in the waiting room. This provided an opportunity for Janice to assess Lilly-Ann's capacity whilst discussing the proposed treatment with her, providing her with the benefits, side-effects andrepercussions of declining the treatment along with any alternative options available.

Research

The importance and contribution of research in healthcare cannot be overstated. In relation to pharmacology, research through clinical drug trials has enabled new discoveries of medicinal products to treat a range of illness. One recent example is the ability to create a vaccine to help fight against the global coronavirus disease.

However, there are legal and ethical standards that govern research into pharmacological treatments. The Nuremberg Code (1947), comprising 10 international ethical principles, was developed in response to atrocities conducted on Jewish prisoners in the Nazi concentration camps during the

Second World War. Jewish prisoners were used involuntarily as human subjects in medical experiments which lead to permanent physical and psychological morbidity and mortality. The Code includes guiding principles on the importance of informed consent, non-coercion and the right to withdraw along with robust protocols underpinned by beneficence. Later, in 1964, the Nuremberg Code (1947) was used to develop the Declaration of Helsinki which provides guidance on ethical principles involving human subjects (World Medical Association, 2008).

Despite the development of the Declaration of Helsinki in 1964, the Tuskegee study of untreated syphilis in the African American male instigated the Belmont Report in 1978 (United States National Commission, 1978). The study has been condemned as highly unethical, violating the principles of beneficence, informed consent, non-coercion, the right to withdraw and robust protocols. Over 600 male human subjects were coerced into obtaining free medical care and were enrolled in the study. They were informed that the study would only last 6 months, but it continued for 40 years until 1972. Of the 600 men, 399 were diagnosed with latent syphilis while the other 201 men in the control group were not infected. The 399 men were never informed of their syphilis diagnosis, were treated with disguised placebos, ineffective methods and diagnostic procedures and were not treated with the standard treatment of penicillin when this became widely available in 1947. During the study, 28 men died directly from syphilis, 100 from complications related to the disease, 40 of the men's wives became infected and 19 children were born with congenital syphilis. Whistleblowing led to the study being terminated in November 1972 (Bishop, 2017).

The Belmont Report lists the primary ethical principles for the protection of human subjects of research and includes beneficence, freedom from harm and exploitation, respect for human dignity, right to self-determination and full disclosure and justice, right to fair treatment and privacy. Today, further protection enshrined in legislation such as the Data Protection Act 2018, Human Tissue Act 2004, Medicines for Human Use (Clinical Trials) Regulations 2004 and the Human Rights Act 1998 complements these guiding principles in ensuring the safety of human participants in clinical trials.

Further safeguarding is also entrusted to research ethics committees (RECs). RECs independently and objectively review any proposed research in health and social care and have a significant role in preserving the rights, safety, dignity and well-being of research participants/subjects. Presently, there are over 80 RECs across the NHS and each REC consists of approximately 15 members, of which a third are 'lay', meaning that they are not registered health are professionals, nor do they have any professional link to research. It is an essential requirement that any research and in the case of pharmacology any research regarding drug trials, will need REC approval. Importantly, as the study progresses, the researcher will need to gain ethical approval for any amendments to the original proposed research in line with Good Clinical Practice (GCP) principles (MHRA, 2021). This will include any form of change regardless of how minor this may appear. Examples can include changes to wording contained in a patient information sheet to changes in dosage of medication.

Unfortunately, despite the governance surrounding research in health and social care, there have been examples where participants suffered harm. In 2006, information from the Northwick Park drug trials publicly reported that six of the research participants became seriously ill from the medication, suffering a severe immune response leading to organ failure, with one participant needing amputation of his fingers. As a result, findings following a full investigation allowed further improvements in governance to be made, and safe practices implemented to prevent future incidents (Expert Scientific Group on Phase One Clinical Trials, 2006).

Conclusion

This chapter has provided an overview of the fundamental legal and ethical considerations related to pharmacology and medicines management in midwifery practice. The relationship of how the law, professional regulation and ethics contribute to the safety and efficacy of pharmacology within midwifery practice was examined. The three criteria required to establish clinical negligence applied to pharmacology were explored, highlighting the application of relevant case laws and legislation. The role of the regulatory body, including pertinent documents such as the Code, provided an understanding of the role and remit of the midwife and student midwife when administering medications. An overview of the use of unlicensed medicine in obstetrics provided useful information for midwives to consider when administering unlicensed medicine.

The concept and principles of informed consent were discussed, introducing the type of consent used in healthcare and circumstances when special considerations are needed in cases of assessing capacity using the MCA 2005 and Gillick competence. A historical perspective of the introduction of the principles governing ethics in research was provided, highlighting the relevance of the Nuremburg Code (1947) in paving the way to develop further ethical guidance. This includes the Declaration of Helsinki (1964) and the Belmont Report (1978) that encompass the importance of informed consent, robust protocols, the safeguarding of human subjects, beneficence, freedom from harm and exploitation, respect for human dignity, right to self-determination and full disclosure and justice and the right to fair treatment and privacy.

It is important that midwives and student midwives keep up to date with current legislation and guidance surrounding pharmacology and medicines management to ensure they operate within their sphere of practice and ultimately provide safe, effective care to women, babies and their families.

Test yourself

Now review your learning by completing the learning activities for this chapter at www.wiley.com/go/pharmacologyformidwives.

References

Affleck, P., Waisel, D., Cusick, J., Van Decar, T. (1998) Recall of risks following labor epidural analgesia. *Journal of Clinical Anaesthesia*, **10**: 141–144.

Aronson, J.K., Ferner, R.E. (2017) Unlicensed and off-label uses of medicines: definitions and clarification of the terminology. British Journal of Pharmacology, **83**: 2615–2625.

Ayad, M., Costantine, M.M. (2015) Epidemiology of medications use in pregnancy. *Seminars in Perinatology*, **39**: 508–501.

Beauchamp, T., Childress, J. (2009) *Principles of Biomedical Ethics*, 6th edn. Oxford University Press: Oxford.

Bishop, J.D. (2017) Principles, rules, and the deflation of the good in bioethics. *Ethics, Medicine and Public Health*, **3**: 445–451.

Bolam vs Friern Hospital Management Committee (1957) 1 WLR 583.

Bolitho v City and Hackney Health Authority (1997) 3 WLR 1151.

Cabinet Office (2013) Legislative process: taking a bill through Parliament. www.gov.uk/guidance/legislative-process-taking-a-bill-through-parliament (accessed January 2022).

Data Protection Act (2018) www.legislation.gov.uk/ukpga/2018/12/contents/enacted (accessed January 2022).

Donoghue v Stevenson (1932) UKHL 100.

Expert Scientific Groups on Phase One Clinical Trials (2006). Final Report. https://webarchive.nationalarchives.gov.uk/20130105143109/www.dh.gov.uk/prod_consum_dh/groups/dh_digitalassets/@dh/@en/documents/digitalasset/dh_073165.pdf (accessed January 2022).

Family Law Reform Act (1969) www.legislation.gov.uk/ukpga/1969/46 (accessed January 2022).

Francis, R. (2013) *Report of the Mid Staffordshire NHS Foundation Trust Public Enquiry*. Stationery Office: London.

Gerancher, J., Grice, S., Dewan, D., Eisenach, J. (2000) An evaluation of informed consent prior to epidural analgesia for labour and delivery. *International Journal of Obstetric Anaesthesia*, **9**: 168–173.

Gillick vs West Norfolk and Wisbech Area Health Authority and Department of Health and Social Security (1985) Landmark decision for children's rights. *Childright*, **22**: 11–18.

Health and Social Care Act (2008) (Regulated Activities) Regulations (2014). Duty of Candour. Regulation **20**. www.legislation.gov.uk/ukdsi/2014/9780111117613 (accessed January 2022).

Herring, J. (2018) *Medical Law and Ethics*. Oxford University Press: Oxford.

Human Fertilisation and Embryology Authority (2020) Fertility treatment 2018: trends and figures. www.hfea.gov.uk/about-us/publications/research-and-data/fertility-treatment-2018-trends-and-figures/ (accessed January 2022).

Human Medicines (Amendment) Regulations (2016) www.legislation.gov.uk/uksi/2016/186/made (accessed January 2022).

Human Rights Act (1998) www.legislation.gov.uk/ukpga/1998/42/contents (accessed January 2022).

Human Tissue Act (2004) www.legislation.gov.uk/ukpga/2004/30/contents (accessed January 2022).

International Confederation of Midwives (2014) International Code of Ethics for Midwives. www.internationalmidwives.org/assets/files/general-files/2019/10/eng-international-code-of-ethics-for-midwives.pdf (accessed January 2022).

Medicines and Healthcare products Regulatory Agency (2021) Good clinical practice for clinical trials. www.gov.uk/guidance/good-clinical-practice-for-clinical-trials (accessed January 2022).

Medicines for Human Use (Clinical Trials) Regulations (2004) www.legislation.gov.uk/uksi/2004/1031/contents/made (accessed January 2022).

Mental Capacity Act (2005) www.legislation.gov.uk/ukpga/2005/9/content (accessed January 2022).

Midwives Act (1902) 2 Edw. VII c. **17**.

Montgomery v Lanarkshire Health Board (2015) 1 AC 1430.

National Health Service Improvement (2019) Clinical negligence and litigation. https://improvement.nhs.uk/resources/clinical-negligence-and-litigation (accessed January 2022).

National Institute for Health and Care Excellence (2013) Fertility problems: assessment and treatment. www.nice.org.uk/guidance/cg156/resources/fertility-problems-assessment-and-treatment-pdf-35109634660549 (accessed January 2022).

Nettleship v Weston (1971) 2 QB 691.

NHS Litigation Authority (2012) Ten Years of Maternity Claims. An Analysis of NHS Litigation Authority Data. https://resolution.nhs.uk/wp-content/uploads/2018/11/Ten-years-of-Maternity-Claims-Final-Report-final-2.pdf (accessed January 2022).

Nursing and Midwifery Council (2018) The Code: Professional standards of practice and behaviour for nurses, midwives and nursing associates. www.nmc.org.uk/globalassets/sitedocuments/nmc-publications/nmc-code.pdf (accessed January 2022).

Nursing and Midwifery Council (2019a) Raising concerns. Guidance for nurses, midwives and nursing associates. www.nmc.org.uk/globalassets/blocks/media-block/raising-concerns-v2.pdf (accessed January 2022).

Nursing and Midwifery Council (2019b) Standards for proficiency for midwives. www.nmc.org.uk/globalassets/sitedocuments/standards/standards-of-proficiency-for-midwives.pdf (accessed January 2022).

Nursing and Midwifery Council (2019c).The professional duty of candour. www.nmc.org.uk/standards/guidance/the-professional-duty-of-candour/read-the-professional-duty-of-candour/#appendix_two (accessed January 2022).

Nursing and Midwifery Council (2021a) Annual Fitness to Practise Report 2020–2021. www.nmc.org.uk/globalassets/sitedocuments/annual_reports_and_accounts/2021-annual-reports/annual-ftp-report-2020-21 (accessed January 2022).

Nursing and Midwifery Council (2021b) Practising as a midwife in the UK. www.nmc.org.uk/globalassets/sitedocuments/nmc-publications/practising-as-a-midwife-in-the-uk.pdf (accessed January 2022).

Nursing and Midwifery Council and General Medical Council (2015) Guidance on the professional duty of candour. www.nmc.org.uk/standards/guidance/the-professional-duty-of-candour/ (accessed January 2022).

Nursing and Midwifery Order (2001) www.legislation.gov.uk/uksi/2002/253/article/25/made (accessed January 2022).

O'Brian v Cunard Steamship Co. (1891) 154 Mass. 272.

Phillippi, J.C., Hartmann, K.E. (2018) Differentiating research, quality improvement, and case studies to ethically incorporate pregnant women. *Journal of Midwifery and Women's Health*, **63**: 104–114.

Potts v NWRHA (1983) QB 384.

Public Health (Control of Diseases) Act (1984) www.legislation.gov.uk/ukpga/1984/22 (accessed January 2022).

R v. Brown (1993) 2 All ER 75.

Re E (1993) 1 FLR 386.

Re MB (Caesarean Section) (1997) 2 FLR.

Re T (adult: refusal of medical treatment) (1992a) 4 All ER 649.

Re W (A Minor) (Medical Treatment: Court's Jurisdiction) (1992b) 2 FCR 785.

Royal College of Midwives (2012) Evidence Based Guidelines for Midwifery-Led Care in Labour. Understanding Pharmacological Pain Relief. www.rcm.org.uk (accessed January 2022).

Samanta, J., Samanta, A. (2011) *Medical Law*. Palgrave Macmillan: Basingstoke.

Schloendorf v Society of New York Hospitals (1914) 105 N.E. 92, 93.

Sinclaire, S.M., Miller, R.K., Chambers, C., Cooper, E.M. (2016) Medication safety during pregnancy: improving evidence-based practice. *Journal of Midwifery and Women's Health*, **61**: 52–67.

Smith, S., Marshall, O. (2020) BPAS investigation into the IVF postcode lottery: an examination of CCG policy for the provision of fertility services. British Pregnancy Advisory Service. www.bpas.org/media/3369/bpas-fertility-ivf-postcode-lottery-report.pdf (accessed January 2022).

St George's Healthcare NHS Trust v. S. (1998) 3 All ER 673.

Supply of Goods and Services Act (1982) c 29; Part ii Supply of Services. www.legislation.gov.uk/ukpga/1982/29/part/II (accessed January 2022).

United States National Commission for the Protection of Human Subjects of Biomedical and Behavioral Research (1978) The Belmont Report: Ethical Principles and Guidelines for the Protection of Human Subjects of Research (Vol. 2). www.hhs.gov/ohrp/regulations-and-policy/belmont-report/read-the-belmont-report/index.html (accessed January 2022).

Vargesson, N. (2015) Thalidomide-induced teratogenesis: history and mechanisms. *Birth Defects Research Part C – Embryo Today*, **105**: 140–156.

Whitehouse v Jordan (1981) 1 All ER 267.

Wilsher v Essex Area Health Authority [1988] 1 AC 1074.

World Medical Association (2008) World Medical Association Declaration of Helsinki. Ethical Principles for Medical Research Involving Human Subjects. www.wma.net/wp-content/uploads/2016/11/DoH-Oct2008.pdf (accessed January 2022).

Chapter 4

Medicines management

Rebecca Murray

University of Hertfordshire, Chigwell, UK

Aim

The aim of this chapter is to give the reader a better understanding of medicines management and the responsibilities of the midwife in relation to this.

Learning outcomes

After reading this chapter, the reader will be able to:
- Gain an understanding of medicines management in midwifery
- Understand the regulations and relevant regulatory bodies that are related to medicines management in healthcare
- Consider the appropriate use of midwives' exemptions in midwifery practice
- Apply the knowledge of medicines management to clinical practice.

Test your existing knowledge

- Which legislation is related to medicines management?
- Name the 9 Rs of medicines administration.
- What are midwives' exemptions?
- What are Patient Group Directions (PGD)?
- Can student midwives administer medication under midwives' exemptions and PGDs?

Introduction

In the UK, nurses and midwives must work in accordance with and uphold the standards set out by the Nursing and Midwifery Council in the Code (NMC, 2018). The Code states that midwives must prioritise people, practise effectively, preserve safety and promote professionalism and trust, all within the scope of their professional practice. According to the Code, midwives must 'Advise on, prescribe, supply, dispense or administer medicines within the limits of your training and competence, the law, our guidance and other relevant policies, guidance and regulations'. This is further expanded upon in the NMC *Standards of proficiency for midwives* (2019) which state that midwives

---

Fundamentals of Pharmacology for Midwives, First Edition. Edited by Ian Peate and Cathy Hamilton.
Companion website: www.wiley.com/go/pharmacologyformidwives

must 'demonstrate knowledge and understanding of the principles of safe and effective administration and optimisation of prescription and non-prescription medicines and midwives' exemptions, demonstrating the ability to progress to a prescribing qualification following registration'.

This chapter provides the reader with an understanding of these principles, the appropriate regulations and guidelines that midwives can use as they practise as autonomous midwives.

Medicines management and optimisation

The UK Medicines and Healthcare products Regulatory Agency (MHRA, 2014) describes medicines management as 'the clinical, cost-effective and safe use of medicines to ensure patients get the maximum benefit from the medicines they need, while at the same time minimising potential harm'. Medicines management is also known as medicines optimisation. However, the Royal Pharmaceutical Society (RPS, 2013) states that there is a difference between medicines management and medicines optimisation. Medicines optimisation focuses not only on safe processes and systems but on outcomes and how patients use medicines. Four principles of medicine optimisation are described by the RPS (2013) (Table 4.1).

The principles set out in the Medicines Optimisation Guidance (RPS, 2013) can be linked to the findings of the National Maternity Review (Cumberlege, 2016) which considered ways of improving care for women, babies and their families during pregnancy and the postpartum period. Women stated they wanted personalised, safer care with continuity of carer and better MDT working to improve their experience and outcomes. Having a patient-centred approach to prescribing medicines may help the client understand the importance of taking medication in pregnancy.

Pregnant women are often worried about continuing medication or starting new medication during pregnancy because they are concerned about the effects on the fetus. This is largely due to the thalidomide scandal in the 1960s (Dathe & Schaefer, 2019). However, according to *Mothers and Babies: Reducing Risk through Audit and Confidential Enquiries* (MBRRACE) (Knight, 2020), discontinuing or not taking essential medication can lead to morbidity and mortality. Midwives are in a unique position to help women understand the importance of continuing their medication. Other chapters in this book will cover specific conditions and the implications of medicines during pregnancy.

Clinical consideration

You are a student midwife working in the antenatal booking clinic alongside your practice supervisor. A client informs you that she has epilepsy, but she has stopped taking her medication as she is worried about the risks to her baby. What are your actions following this disclosure?

Table 4.1   The four guiding principles of medicines optimisation.

Principle	Description
Aim to understand the patient's experience	Midwives and other members of the multidisciplinary team (MDT) need to have open conversations with women about the choices, experiences of using medicines to manage their conditions and how they can work together to change these if needed
Evidence-based choice of medicines	The MDT needs to select the most appropriate and cost-effective medicine to treat the condition and meets the needs of the client
Ensure medicines use is as safe as possible	Open discussion with the client to make sure the medicine is effective, there are no unwanted side-effects or interactions, and that the client is taking it as appropriate
Make medicines optimisation part of routine practice	Midwives and the MDT should discuss with the client the medicines they are taking at each clinical appointment. This allows for open dialogue between the client and the team

Source: Based on RPS (2013).

Medicines regulations

There are two laws that govern medicines management in the UK: the Medicines Act 1968 and the Misuse of Drugs Act 1971.

The Medicines Act 1968 provides the legal framework for manufacturing, licensing, prescribing, supplying and administering medicines. This act further splits medicines into three groups: prescription only medicines (PoM), pharmacy only (P) medicines and General Sales List (GLS) (Table 4.2). However, it is important to know that some medicines can be included in two or more categories, as the category they are classified under is dependent on the dose (MHRA, 2014). For example, ibuprofen 200 mg tablets are GSL but ibuprofen 400 mg tablets are a P medication (Table 4.3).

The Misuse of Drugs Act 1971 provides the regulations related to Controlled Drugs. According to the National Institute for Health and Care Excellence (NICE, 2016), a Controlled Drug is any medicine that can cause addiction or harm or can be used illegally rather than for medical purposes. Controlled Drugs include strong pain medicines such as pethidine or diamorphine and benzodiazepines such as diazepam.

The MHRA is charged by the Medicines Act 1968 with determining quality and purpose of drugs used in the UK. The Human Medicines Regulations 2012 consolidate the acts of law in relation to the rules on prescribing, supplying and administering medicines. The MHRA is responsible for providing guidance to midwives and other healthcare professionals on exemptions to PoMs which can be used in their clinical practice.

Midwives can find further guidance for the safe handling, management and administration of medicines in the RPS *Professional guidance on the safe and secure handling of medicines* (RPS, 2018) and *Professional guidance on the administration of medicines in healthcare settings* (RPS, 2019).

Table 4.2   Description of medicines classifications.

Classification	Description
Prescription only medicines (PoM)	Prescription only medication can only be supplied by a pharmacist or administered by a midwife in the presence of a prescription from a doctor or appropriate non-medical prescriber. The list of PoMs is found in article 3 of the Prescription Only Order 1997. Examples of PoMs in midwifery practice are antibotics, labetalol and magnesium sulfate
General Sales List (GSL)	GSL medicines are those which can be purchased from any shop, without a prescription or authorisation from a pharmacist. Midwives can supply and administer all GSL medicines if it is within their scope of midwifery practice (NMC, 2019). Examples of a GSL medicine used in midwifery practice are paracetamol 500 mg tables or clotrimazole 2% cream. Patients only ever have enough medication for 2–3 days of use
Pharmacy only (P)	These are medicines that are not PoMs but do need to be supplied under the supervision of a pharmacist or a member of their team. Pharmacy medicines need more guidance upon supply and the pharmacist will assess the client's need for the medication. Pharmacy medicines may be stronger than GSL medicines or a larger amount supplied

Table 4.3   Examples of medicines classification based on dosage.

Drug	Dose	Classification
Ibuprofen	200 mg tablets	GSL
Ibuprofen	400 mg tablets	P
Co-codamol	8/500 mg tablets	P
Co-codamol	15/500 mg tablets	PoM

The 'rights' of medicines administration

According to a study by Elliot et al. (2018), there are approximately 237 million medication errors in England per year. Seventy-two percent of these errors cause little or no harm, but the cost to the NHS for these errors can be anything from as little as £67.93 to £6.9 million. Medicines errors can happen at any point in the process hence the need for good practice principles for administration of medicines. The NMC Code (2018) states that the midwife must be aware of, and reduce as far as possible, any potential for harm associated with their practice, so it is important for midwives to understand ways of reducing medication administration errors. It is reported that there is anything between five and nine principles (Bhavee et al., 2018) but this chapter will cover the 9 'Rights' of medicines administration as described by Elliot and Liu (2010) (Box 4.1).

Box 4.1   The 9 'rights' of medicines administration

1. Right patient

2. Right drug

3. Right route

4. Right time

5. Right dose

6. Right documentation

7. Right action/indication

8. Right response

9. Right to decline

Right patient

It is important that the right patient receives the medication they are prescribed and need. When approaching a client to administer medication, ask them to tell you their full name and date of birth. This should be checked against the patient drug chart and the wristband they are wearing. You should never ask a client 'Are you Mrs Khan?' because there may be a number of clients on the ward with the same surname.

Right drug

Medicines should be prescribed using the generic name of the drug and not the brand name. The aim of this is to minimise any errors due to similarities between brand names. It is the responsibility of the midwife administering the medicine to know what it is prescribed for, the writing on the drug chart must be clear and any uncertainty should be checked with the prescriber. Caution should be exercised when medicines are from the same group of medication but have different names, for example temazepam and diazepam. The midwife should also ask the client if they have any allergies, as this may not be recorded in the healthcare records (MHRA, 2018).

Right route

The medicines that midwives administer often have more than one route of administration. It is the midwife's responsibility to check that the route of administration is appropriate, as this can affect the action and absorption of the drug. Intravenous (IV) and oral liquid medication should never be drawn up in similar syringes. Following an incident where an oral medication was administered IV, there were changes in clinical practice to ensure there were different syringes for oral and IV administration of medicine and that oral syringes could not attach to IV giving sets.

Right time

It is important to check the medication chart to determine when medicines should be administered, at what intervals and if there are any time-critical medications. Time-critical medications include antibiotics and antiepileptic drugs.

Right dose

Check that the dose is clearly written using the correct unit. Midwives should be aware of the dosage of medications they administer and should check this in the British National Formulary (BNF) or organisational guidelines. Anything that is not clearly written should be checked with the prescriber. The prescriber should also avoid using, for example, µg but should use mcg for micrograms. When prescribing drugs that have unit dosage, they should write 10 units, not 10U, as the U could be mistaken for a 0.

Right documentation

For medicines to be administered, the appropriate documentation should be in place. This includes a prescription, an appropriate exemption or a PGD.

Prescribing

According to the Medicines Act 1968, at the point of registration midwives are unable to prescribe medicines; only doctors and dentists can prescribe at the point of registration. However, the Medicines for Human Use *Order* 2006 extended the list of appropriate practitioners to midwives, following completion of an independent prescribing course. A prescription is a written order by an appropriate prescriber, which authorises the treatment of a patient with a medicinal product (Griffith, 2010). To ensure patient safety, prescriptions should be clear, full name and date of birth must be present and it should be clearly signed and dated by the prescriber. The RPS (2016) has published a competency framework to promote best practice in prescribing.

Exemptions

A list of specific PoMs, GSL and P medicines that certain healthcare professionals can sell, supply and/or administer during their professional practice is specified by the Human Medicines Regulations 2012. Midwives have their own exemptions listed in Schedule 17 of the Human Medicines Regulations 2012. This states that midwives can supply all GSL and P medicines in accordance with their scope of practice. It also lists specific PoM medicines related to midwifery practice that midwives can supply and administer. The Secretary of State has the authority to change this list of exemptions as and when required (NMC, 2019). The list can be found in Tables 4.4 and 4.5.

PGDs

Patient Group Directions allow healthcare professionals to administer medications without a prescription to a predefined group of patients rather than to a specific patient. The development of a PGD involves a pharmacist, doctor and a representative of the professional group administering the

Table 4.4   Midwives' exemptions – prescription only medicines (POM).

Persons exempted	Prescription only medicines to which the exemption applies	Conditions
Registered midwives	Prescription only medicines containing any of the following substances: (a) Diclofenac (b) Hydrocortisone acetate (c) Miconazole (d) Nystatin (e) Phytomenadione	The sale or supply shall be only in the course of their professional practice

Table 4.5 Exemptions from restriction on administration of prescription only medicines.

Persons exempted	Prescription only medicines to which the exemption applies	Conditions
Registered midwives and student midwives	Prescription only medicines for parenteral administration containing any of the following substances but no other substance that is classified as a product available on prescription only: (a) Adrenaline (b) Anti-D immunoglobulin, (c) Carboprost (d) Cyclizine lactate (e) Diamorphine (f) Ergometrine maleate (g) Gelofusine (h) Hartmann's solution (i) Hepatitis B vaccine (j) Hepatitis immunoglobulin (k) Lidocaine hydrochloride (l) Morphine (m) Naloxone hydrochloride (n) Oxytocins, natural and synthetic (o) Pethidine hydrochloride (p) Phytomenadione (q) Prochloperazine (r) Sodium chloride 0.9%	The medicine shall, in the case of lidocaine and lidocaine hydrochloride, be administered only while attending on a woman in childbirth, and where administration is: • by a registered midwife, administered in the course of their professional practice • by a student midwife: (a) administered under the direct supervision of a registered midwife; and (b) not including diamorphine, morphine or pethidine hydrochloride (which are Controlled Drugs)

Clinical consideration

You are working in the postnatal ward alongside your practice supervisor. The woman in your care needs an anti D injection before discharge. You ask your mentor if you can administer the injection. The practice supervisor informs you that anti D is given under a PGD in this hospital, not a midwives' exemption. Are you still able to administer the anti D?

medication under a PGD. This working group will discuss the appropriate circumstances which need to be in place for administration of the drug, the roles and responsibilities of the MDT and the training needed. PGDs are often in place for 2 years and will be reviewed. Before a midwife can administer a medicine under a PGD, they need to be trained, read the relevant guidelines and sign the appropriate paperwork (NICE, 2013). An example of a PDG used in midwifery practice is the administration of the flu vaccine to pregnant women.

It is also the responsibility of the midwife to document the time the medication was given or if the client declined medication in the appropriate section of the drug chart. It should be clearly signed by the midwife who administered the medication and the second checker if appropriate. It may be necessary to record the administration of medication, or cardiotocograph (CTG) if applicable, in the patient notes (NMC, 2018).

Right action/indication

The midwife administering the medication must check that the correct medication has been prescribed for its intended use; for example, an antacid would not be prescribed for sickness; that would be an antiemetic.

Right response

It is important that medicines are having their intended effect and the client is not having an adverse reaction to the medication. The midwife should check the woman's allergy status prior to administration, although adverse reactions can still happen if the client has not had the medication before or they have had a sensitising event; these will be discussed further in Chapter 7. It is important that the medicine is having the intended effect as certain conditions could cause serious harm if not treated. For example, labetalol is prescribed for high blood pressure in a client with pre-eclampsia; if the blood pressure does not decrease, it could lead to an eclamptic seizure. Therefore, the blood pressure should be checked at an appropriate interval following administration of the medication.

Right to decline

All care and treatment provided to clients must have informed consent. Clients also have the right to refuse care or treatment unless they lack capacity. If a client declines medication prescribed to them, it is important not to make a judgement but have a discussion to determine why they are declining. Are they aware of the risks of not taking the medication? The conversation should be documented in the client's clinical records and the matter should be escalated to the obstetric team or midwife in charge so they are aware of the situation (NMC, 2018).

Medication errors

Despite following the 9 'Rights' of medicines administration, medication errors can still happen, and it is important that they are managed appropriately. According to Aronson (2009), 'A medication error is an unintended failure in the drug treatment process that leads to, or has the potential to lead to, harm to the patient'. These can happen if the appropriate policies and guidelines are not adhered to or when the midwife is interrupted or distracted during the drug administration process (Ofosu and Jarrett, 2015). If a medicines error or near miss occurs, it is important that you assess the client's clinical condition, escalate to the obstetric team and midwife in charge. If there is an appropriate antidote for the drug, this should be administered as per the prescription. The client should be monitored closely and a clinical plan put in place. When appropriate, the medication error, escalation, care and plan should be clearly documented in the client's records and a incident report should be completed. Completing a incident report allows the incident to be investigated and helps prevent future incidents (Cathala and Moreley, 2020).

It is also important to explain what has happened to the client. Duty of candour legislation (UK Government, 2020) safeguards clients by ensuring that hospitals and healthcare providers are open and honest when there are errors or failings in their care. This guidance sets out the specific requirements that hospitals and healthcare providers must follow if an unintended or unexpected incident occurs and the support they need to put in place for the client.

Self-administration of medicines

Midwives can work in partnership with the women in their care to empower them to take ownership of the administration of their medication (NMC,2019). Self-administration while in hospital can make women feel in control and allows them to take time-critical medication without delays. It can also encourage compliance with new medications started in hospital, particularly subcutaneous injections, as women will have time to build confidence with administration while gaining knowledge and having the support of the midwife (Cooper, 2020). One example of this is low molecular weight heparin injections for venous thromboembolism prophylaxis, which are administered based on risk assessment.

Storage and disposal of medicines

As well as safely and appropriately administering medication, midwives are responsible for the safe storage and disposal of medicines. Storage must be in line with the manufacturer's instructions to ensure that the medication is effective in use. They should also be stored in a locked cupboard or trolley (Pegram and Bloomfield, 2015).

Any medication that is unused, stored inappropriately or expired needs to be disposed of to avoid it being given to a client. Medicines should be disposed of in the appropriate hazard bin and liquids should not be poured down the sink. If a Controlled Drug is not used or only part used, it should be disposed of with the use of a denaturing kit. This ensures that it cannot be retrieved and misused. There should also be a record of the disposal signed by the two registrants witnessing the process. Midwives should also encourage clients to return any unused medicines to their local pharmacist for disposal (Care Quality Commission (CQC), 2020).

49

Student midwives

At the point of entry onto the register, all midwives will have been deemed competent by the approved educational institution (university) to select, acquire and safely administer a range of permitted drugs consistent with the Human Medicines Regulations 2012, amended in 2016, applying knowledge and skills to the situation (NMC, 2019). Therefore, during their education, student midwives need to be exposed to medicines management processes to achieve these competencies.

Student midwives can administer any medicine under the direct supervision of a registered midwife when there is an appropriate prescription in place signed by a doctor or independent prescriber. Under direct supervision of a registered midwife, student midwives can also administer GSL, P and PoMs on the midwives' exemption list, with the exception of Controlled Drugs. Student midwives can also check Controlled Drugs where a second registrant is not present. However, it is important to check local guidelines, as healthcare organisations may require two registrants for checking. Student midwives cannot administer medicine under a PGD. Midwives supervising students in practice also need to check any local restrictions to administering medication. For example, some healthcare organisations require newly qualified midwives to complete IV competency assessments during their preceptorship, before they can administer IV drugs or fluids. Therefore, students would not be able to add additives or administer IV drugs as they would not have completed the competency assessments. A registered nurse undertaking a shortened midwifery programme acts as a student midwife for the purposes of all drug administration (NMC, 2019).

At all times, the registered midwife supervising the student is responsible for the administration of the medication (RPS, 2019).

Clinical consideration

You are on placement in a stand-alone birth centre caring for a client in labour with your practice supervisor. The client requests pethidine for pain relief and an antiemetic. The midwife will use the midwives' exemptions to provide the client with the requested medication.

As a student, are you able to administer the pethidine injection? Are you able to administer the prochlorperazine (antiemetic) injection?

Conclusion

This chapter has reviewed the legislation and guidelines in relation to medicines management. It has covered the importance of medicines management for the delivery of high-quality, safe and individualised care to women throughout pregnancy and the postpartum period, whilst also looking at the potential errors that can occur and how they should be managed. This chapter helps student midwives understand the different classifications of medicines and how they can administer these within the scope of their practice and the law.

50

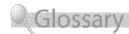
Glossary

Administration of medicines   The process of delivery mediciation into the body

Controlled Drug   The name given to any drug that has the potential for misuse

Duty of candour   Professional duty to be open and honest with patients

Low molecular weight heparin   Class of anticoagulated medication

Medicines and Healthcare products Regulatory Agency (MHRA)   UK government agency which regulates medicines, medical devices and blood components for transfusion

Medicines optimisation   Helps patients make the most of their medicines

Medicines Act 1968   UK legal framework for manufacturing, licensing, prescribing, supplying and administering medicines

Medication error   An unintended failure in the drug treatment process that leads to, or has the potential to lead to, harm to the patient

Midwives' exemptions   A list of exemptions for registered midwives which allows them to supply specific prescription only medicines on their own initiative in the course of their professional practice

Misuse of Drugs Act 1971   UK regulations related to Controlled Drugs

Patient Group Direction   PGDs allow healthcare professionals to supply and administer specified medicines to predefined groups of patients, without a prescription

Pharmacy only medication   Medicines that can only be supplied from a registered pharmacy, by a pharmacist or a person acting under their supervision

Prescription only medication   A treatment that must be prescribed by a doctor or independent prescriber and is not licensed for sale to the general public

Test yourself

Now review your learning by completing the learning activities for this chapter at www.wiley.com/go/pharmacologyformidwives.

References

Aronson, J.K. (2009) Medication errors: definitions and classification. *British Journal of Clinical Pharmacology*, **67**(6): 599–604.

Bhavee, P., Rachel, I., Pramodh, V. (2018) P28 Reducing medication errors – a tripartite approach. Small steps – better outcomes. www.researchgate.net/publication/322612916_P28_Reducing_medication_errors_-_a_tripartite_approach_small_steps_-_better_outcomes (accessed January 2022).

Care Quality Commission (2020) Disposing of medicines. www.cqc.org.uk/guidance-providers/adult-social-care/disposing-medicines (accessed January 2022).

Cathala, X., Moorley, C. (2020) Skills for newly qualified nurses 3: managing errors and mistakes. www.nursingtimes.net/clinical-archive/medicine-management/managing-errors-and-mistakes-guidance-for-newly-qualified-nurses-24-06-2020/ (accessed January 2022).

Cooper, A. (2020) *Self-administration of medicines*. Brief guidance and examples from practice. www.sps.nhs.uk/articles/self-administration-of-medicines/ (accessed January 2022).

Cumberlege, J. (2016) *Better Births. Improving Outcomes of Maternity Services in England*. www.england.nhs.uk/wp-content/uploads/2016/02/national-maternity-review-report.pdf (accessed January 2022).

Dathe, K., Schaefer, C. (2019) The use of medication in pregnancy. *Deutsches Arzteblatt International*, **116**: 783–790.

Elliott, M., Liu, Y. (2010) The nine rights of medication administration: an overview. *British Journal of Nursing*, **19**(5): 300–305.

Elliott, R., Camacho, E., Campbell, F. et al. (2018) *Prevalence and economic burden of medication errors in the NHS in England. Rapid evidence synthesis and economic analysis of the prevalence and burden of medication error in the UK.* Policy Research Unit in Economic Evaluation of Health and Care Interventions. Universities of Sheffield and York.

Griffith, R. (2010) Law, medicines and the midwife. In: Jordan, S. (ed.) *Pharmacology for Midwives: the evidence base for safe practice.* Macmillan International Higher Education: Basingstoke.

Human Medicines Regulations (2012) www.legislation.gov.uk/uksi/2012/1916/contents/made (accessed January 2022).

Knight, M. (2020) MBRRACE-UK update: key messages from the UK and Ireland Confidential Enquiries into Maternal Death and Morbidity 2019. *Obstetrician & Gynaecologist,* **22**(1): 93–95.

Medicines Act (1968) www.legislation.gov.uk/ukpga/1968/67/contents (accessed January 2022).

Medicines and Healthcare products Regulatory Agency (2014) Medicines: reclassify your products. www.gov.uk/guidance/medicines-reclassify-your-product (accessed January 2022).

Medicines and Healthcare products Regulatory Agency (2018) Drug-name confusion: reminder to be vigilant for potential errors. www.gov.uk/drug-safety-update/drug-name-confusion-reminder-to-be-vigilant-for-potential-errors (accessed January 2022).

Medicines for Human Use (Prescribing) (Miscellaneous Amendments) *Order* (2006) www.legislation.gov.uk/uksi/2006/915/contents/made (accessed January 2022).

Misuse of Drugs Act (1971) www.legislation.gov.uk/ukpga/1971/38 (accessed January 2022).

National Institute for Health and Care Excellence (2013) Patient Group Directions. *Medicines Practice Guideline* **2.** www.nice.org.uk/guidance/mpg2 (accessed January 2022).

National Institute for Health and Care Excellence (2016) Controlled drugs: safe use and management. www.nice.org.uk/guidance/ng46 (accessed January 2022).

Nursing and Midwifery Council (2018) The Code: Professional standards of practice and behaviour for nurses and midwives. www.nmc.org.uk/globalassets/sitedocuments/nmc-publications/nmc-code.pdf (accessed January 2022).

Nursing and Midwifery Council (2019) Standards of proficiency for midwives. www.nmc.org.uk/globalassets/sitedocuments/standards/standards-of-proficiency-for-midwives.pdf (accessed January 2022).

Ofosu, R., Jarrett, P. (2015) Reducing nurse medicine administration errors. *Nursing Times,* **111**(20): 12–14.

Pegram, A., Bloomfield, J. (2015) Medicines management. *Nursing Standard,* **29**(33): 36.

Royal Pharmaceutical Society (2013) Medicines optimisation: helping patients to make the most of medicines. www.rpharms.com/Portals/0/RPS%20document%20library/Open%20access/Policy/helping-patients-make-the-most-of-their-medicines.pdf (accessed January 2022).

Royal Pharmaceutical Society (2016) A competency framework for all prescribers. www.rpharms.com/Portals/0/RPS%20document%20library/Open%20access/Professional%20standards/Prescribing%20competency%20framework/prescribing-competency-framework.pdf (accessed January 2022).

Royal Pharmaceutical Society (2018) Professional guidance on the safe and secure handling of medicines. www.rpharms.com/recognition/setting-professional-standards/safe-and-secure-handling-of-medicines/professional-guidance-on-the-safe-and-secure-handling-of-medicines (accessed January 2022).

Royal Pharmaceutical Society (2019) Professional guidance on the administration of medicines in healthcare settings. www.rpharms.com (accessed January 2022).

UK Government (2020) Guidance: Duty of candour.www.gov.uk/government/publications/nhs-screening-programmes-duty-of-candour/duty-of-candour (accessed January 2022).

Further reading

Elliott, R.A., Camacho, E., Jankovic, D., Sculpher, M.J., Faria, R. (2021) Economic analysis of the prevalence and clinical and economic burden of medication error in England. *BMJ Quality & Safety,* **30**(2): 96–105.

NHS England (2020) *When Patient Group Directions (PGDs) are Not Required: Guidance on when PGDs should not be used and advice on alternative mechanisms.* NHS: London

NHS England and NHS Improvement (2019) *The NHS Patient Safety Strategy. Safer culture, safer systems, safer patients.* NHS: London.

Part 2

Introduction to pharmacology

Chapter 5

Medications and the gastrointestinal system

Barry Hill and Claire Leader

Northumbria University, Newcastle-upon-Tyne, UK

Aim

The aim of this chapter is to provide the reader with an introduction to pharmacokinetics and pharmacodynamics and the important issues surrounding medicines management within midwifery practice.

Learning outcomes

After reading this chapter, the reader will be able to:
* Acknowledge the professional responsibilities of midwives who administer drugs to women during pregnancy, labour and the postnatal period
* Define and understand the differences between pharmacodynamics and pharmacokinetics
* Appreciate the complexities associated with physiological changes during pregnancy and the post-natal period and how drugs may work differently as a result.
* Understand the additional considerations associated with medicines administration in relation to the developing fetus.

Test your existing knowledge

* Define pharmacodynamics.
* How many phases of pharmacokinetics are there?
* What are the phases of pharmacokinetics?
* Describe the professional responsibilities of the midwife who administers medication to pregnant women.
* Discuss drug interactions and some of the key considerations for the developing fetus and neonate.

Introduction

This chapter explores the pharmacokinetics and pharmacodynamics of drugs used within midwifery practice.

Fundamentals of Pharmacology for Midwives, First Edition. Edited by Ian Peate and Cathy Hamilton.
© 2022 John Wiley & Sons Ltd. Published 2022 by John Wiley & Sons Ltd.
Companion website: www.wiley.com/go/pharmacologyformidwives

Regulatory bodies
Royal pharmaceutical society

As new diseases emerge and older medicines, such as antibiotics, no longer work as well as they once did, the contribution of pharmacology to finding better and safer medicines becomes even more significant to improve the quality of life for patients. The Royal Pharmaceutical Society (RPS) is the body responsible for the leadership and support of the pharmacy profession within England, Scotland and Wales. The RPS is the leading society within the UK and believes that 'Pharmacological knowledge improves the lives of millions of people across the world'. It also recommends that all healthcare professionals have pharmacological knowledge, as it 'maximises their benefit and minimises risk and harm' (RPS and RCN, 2019). In 2019, the RPS and RCN published *Professional Guidance on the Administration of Medicines in Healthcare Settings* (RPS and RCN, 2019). This guidance has replaced all previously published NMC medicines management guidance and should be the key document for all healthcare professionals.

Nursing and Midwifery Council

The Nursing and Midwifery Council (NMC), which is the regulating body for nurses, nursing associates and midwives, requires utilisation of 'critical thinking' and 'clinical judgement' when working with medicines to provide patient safety. Midwives should be able to practise as autonomous professionals, exercising their own professional judgement, and should also be able to modify and adapt practice to meet the clinical needs of pregnant women, while maintaining the safety of the developing fetus (NMC, 2018).

Management of medicines is an increasingly important role for midwives. As the key professionals in pregnancy care, midwives are responsible for providing information on medicines throughout pregnancy, labour and the postnatal period. Consequently, for midwives to think critically, work within their scope of practice and, most importantly, improve safety when working with medicines, it is imperative that a comprehensive assessment has been made of the woman's past medical and obstetric history. This includes a full drug history, including over-the-counter medications, prescribed drugs and any illicit drug use (Jordan, 2010).

Teratogenesis and Fetotoxicity

When midwives directly prepare, administer or have any input into pharmacology and medicines management, it is vital that they understand how medicines work and how they will affect the woman receiving medicinal treatment as well as the fetus.

In the mid to late 1950s, a drug called thalidomide was widely prescribed in early pregnancy for nausea and vomiting. Evidence emerged of increasing cases of severe limb malformations which were subsequently attributed to the thalidomide drug. This led to changes in drug development regulation and increased awareness of the potential impact of drugs taken in pregnancy on the developing fetus.

A teratogen is a substance that leads to birth malformations, structural, metabolic or functional, through exposure during pregnancy. The greatest risk of a teratogenic effect is in weeks 3–11 of gestation (NICE, 2021). This critical period of structural development is also a stage where the woman may not be aware that she is pregnant or has not yet seen a midwife. Preconception advice regarding drugs and other substances to avoid while trying to conceive is paramount in facilitating the healthy development of the fetus in early pregnancy.

It is important to recognise that drugs can cause harmful effects on the developing fetus at any stage of gestation (Table 5.1). While teratogenesis is the greatest risk in early pregnancy, in the second and third trimesters some medicines can also cause fetotoxicity, leading to more subtle functional changes which may be more difficult to associate with specific drugs (NICE, 2021). For this reason, drugs should ideally be avoided altogether in the first trimester and prescribed with

Table 5.1   Examples of drugs known to cause teratogenic effects (BNF and NICE, 2021).

Drug	Use	Teratogenic effect
Antiepileptic (especially valproate)	Prevent occurrence of epileptic seizures	Lip and palate deformities, developmental delays and intellectual disability
Warfarin	Anticoagulant	Limb defects, central nervous system defects, growth restriction
Lithium	Treatment of depression, bipolar disorder, self-harm	Cardiac abnormalities
Tetracycline	Broad-spectrum antibiotics (commonly used for infections caused by chlamydia)	Impaired bone growth, teeth and bone staining, thin tooth enamel
Cytotoxic drugs	Treatment of cancer	Neural tube defects, cleft palate

caution throughout pregnancy, carefully balancing the benefits to the woman's health with the potential risks to the fetus (Henderson and Mackillop, 2011).

Pharmacokinetics

In its most basic form, pharmacokinetics is 'what the body does to drugs'. Pharmacokinetics can be considered as four processes: the absorption, distribution, metabolism and excretion (ADME) of drugs (Young and Pitcher, 2016), and their corresponding pharmacological, therapeutic or toxic responses.

Pharmacokinetic principles (the ADME process)

Pharmacokinetics describes the influence that the human body has on drugs or foreign chemicals over time (Young and Pitcher, 2016). The key concerns of pharmacokinetics are what the body does to the drug, how drugs are absorbed by the body, how they are distributed to the tissues, how drugs are metabolised by the body (with the liver being the primary organ for drug metabolisation) and elimination (primarily by the kidneys and lungs) (Box 5.1).

Pharmacokinetics is important to our understanding of why drugs are administered via different routes. For example, why is a drug administered orally (PO) via tablet or liquid suspension form, or into the tissues by subcutaneous injection (SC), intramuscularly (IM) or directly into the bloodstream by intravenous (IV) injection? Chapter 6 discusses drug formulations.

Pharmacokinetics also helps us appreciate the frequency of drug administration. For example, why are some drugs administered once a day and others administered twice a day, three times a day or four times a day, or even continuously by SC, IM or IV infusion via a mechanical pump? When thinking about the organs that work with drugs during the process of ADME, it becomes clear why organs that are absent, diseased or changed by pregnancy would affect the metabolisation of drugs.

Figure 5.1 integrates the four main features of pharmacokinetics (ADME) and the main routes or administration of medication. Note that the IV route bypasses absorption and the topical route is used to achieve a local effect and minimise absorption.

Box 5.1   Four stages of pharmacokinetics: ADME

- Absorption of drugs into the body. How does the drug get into the body?
- Distribution of drugs to the tissues of the body. Where will it go?
- Metabolism of drugs in the body. How is it broken down?
- Elimination of drugs from the body. How does it leave?

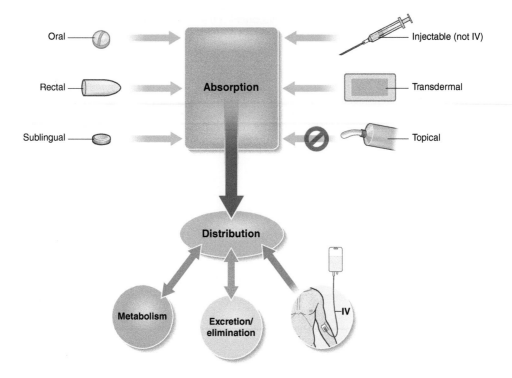

Figure 5.1   An integration of ADME and the routes of administration.
Source: Adapted from Young and Pitcher (2016).

Phase 1: Absorption

Absorption is defined as the process by which a drug proceeds from the site of administration to the site of measurement (usually blood, plasma or serum) (Table 5.2). Absorption is the process of a drug entering the blood circulation. Le (2019) suggests that drug absorption is determined by the drug's physicochemical properties, formulation and route of administration, i.e. enteral or parenteral. Dosage forms (e.g. tablets, capsules, solutions), consisting of the drug plus other ingredients, are formulated to be given by various routes (e.g. oral, buccal, sublingual, vaginal, rectal, parenteral, topical, inhalational). Regardless of the route of administration, drugs must be in solution to be absorbed. Thus, solid forms (e.g. tablets) must be able to disintegrate and disaggregate.

Unless given IV, a drug must cross several semi-permeable cell membranes before it reaches the systemic circulation. Cell membranes are biological barriers that selectively inhibit the passage of drug molecules. The membranes are composed primarily of a bimolecular lipid matrix, which determines membrane permeability characteristics.

How drugs cross the cell membrane

Many drugs need to pass through one or more cell membranes to reach their site of action. A common feature of all cell membranes is a phospholipid bilayer, about 10 nanometers (nm) thick. Spanning this bilayer or attached to the outer or inner leaflets are glycoproteins, which may act as ion channels, receptors, intermediate messengers (G-proteins) or enzymes. Cells obtain molecules and ions from the extracellular fluid, creating a constant in-and-out flow. The interesting thing about cell membranes is that relative concentrations and phospholipid bilayers prevent essential ions from entering the cell. Therefore, for drugs to move across the membrane, these problems must be addressed. In general, this is completed by facilitated diffusion or active transport. In facilitated diffusion, relative concentrations are used to transport in and out. Active transport uses energy (ATP) to transfer molecules and ions in and out of the cells.

Table 5.2 Factors that affect absorption of drugs.

Route	Factors Affecting Absorption
Intravenous (IV)	None: direct entry into the venous system
Intramuscular (IM)	Perfusion of blood flow to the muscle Fat content of the muscle Temperature of the muscle: cold causes vasoconstriction and decreases absorption; heat causes vasodilation and increases absorption
Subcutaneous (SC)	Perfusion of blood flow to the tissues Fat content of the tissue Temperature of the tissue: cold causes vasoconstriction and decreases absorption; heat causes vasodilation and increase absorption
Oral (PO)	Acidity of the stomach Length of time in the stomach Blow flow to the gastrointestinal tract Presence of interacting foods or drugs
Rectal(PR)	Perfusion of blood flow to the rectum Lesions in the rectum Length of time retained for absorption
Mucous membranes (sublingual, buccal)	Perfusion or blood flow to the area Integrity of mucus membranes Presence of food or smoking Length of time retained in area
Topical (skin)	Perfusion or blood flow to the area Integrity of skin
Inhalation	Perfusion or blood flow to the area Integrity of lung lining Ability to administer drug properly

Source: Karch (2017)/with permission of Wolters Kluwer.

Concept of drugs crossing the cell membrane

Cellular signals cross the membrane through a process called signal transduction. This three-step process proceeds when a specific message encounters the outside surface of the cell and makes direct contact with a receptor.

1. A receptor is a specialised molecule that takes information from the environment and passes it throughout various parts of the cell.
2. Next, a connecting switch molecule, a transducer, passes the message inward, closer to the cell.
3. Finally, the signal gets amplified, therefore causing the cell to perform a specific function, such as moving, producing more proteins or sending out more signals.

Methods of drugs crossing the cell membrane

Passive transport The most common way that drugs cross the cell membrane is by passive diffusion. Drug molecules will diffuse down their concentration gradient without expenditure of energy by the cell. However, membranes are selectively permeable, so the membrane has different effects on the rate of diffusion of different drug molecules. The rate of diffusion can also be enhanced by transport proteins in the membrane by facilitated diffusion. There are two types of transport proteins that carry out the facilitated diffusion: channel proteins and carrier proteins.

Active transport Active transport is an energy-requiring process. There are also two types of active transport: primary active transport and secondary active transport.

- *Primary active transport* directly uses energy to transport molecules across a membrane. Occasionally the carrier protein can be an electrogenic pump.
- *Secondary active transport* (or co-transport) also uses energy to transport molecules across a membrane.

Absorption depends on the administration route and can be either (i) *enteral*, entering the gastrointestinal (GI) tract by oral administration, feeding tubes or rectal suppositories, or (ii) *parenteral*, not into the GI tract, such as via injection or topical medicine (such as creams or patches).

To be absorbed, a drug given orally must survive encounters with low pH and numerous GI secretions, including potentially degrading enzymes. Peptide drugs (e.g. insulin) are particularly susceptible to degradation and are not given orally. Absorption of oral drugs involves transport across membranes of the epithelial cells in the GI tract. Absorption is affected by:

- differences in luminal pH along the GI tract
- surface area per luminal volume;
- blood perfusion;
- presence of bile and mucus
- the nature of epithelial membranes.

The oral mucosa has a thin epithelium and rich vascularity, which favour absorption; however, contact is usually too brief for substantial absorption. A drug placed between the gums and cheek (buccal administration) or under the tongue (sublingual administration) is retained longer, enhancing absorption.

The stomach has a relatively large epithelial surface, but its thick mucus layer and short transit time limit absorption. Because most absorption occurs in the small intestine, gastric emptying is often rate limiting. Food, especially fatty food, slows gastric emptying (and rate of drug absorption), explaining why taking some drugs on an empty stomach speeds absorption.

Drugs that affect gastric emptying (e.g. parasympatholytic drugs) affect the absorption rate of other drugs. Food may enhance the extent of absorption for poorly soluble drugs (e.g. griseofulvin), reduce it for drugs degraded in the stomach (e.g. penicillin G), or have little or no effect.

The small intestine has the largest surface area for drug absorption in the GI tract and its membranes are more permeable than those in the stomach. For these reasons, most drugs are absorbed primarily in the small intestine. The intraluminal pH is 4–5 in the duodenum but becomes progressively more alkaline, approaching 8 in the lower ileum. GI microflora may reduce absorption. Decreased blood flow (e.g. in shock) may lower the concentration gradient across the intestinal mucosa and reduce absorption by passive diffusion. Intestinal transit time can influence drug absorption, particularly for drugs that are absorbed by active transport (e.g. B vitamins), that dissolve slowly (e.g. griseofulvin) or that are polar (i.e. with low lipid solubility. e.g. many antibiotics).

In adolescents and adults, most drugs are given orally as tablets or capsules primarily for convenience, economy, stability and acceptability. Because solid drug forms must dissolve before absorption can occur, the dissolution rate determines the availability of the drug for absorption. Dissolution, if slower than absorption, becomes the rate-limiting step. Manipulating the formulation (i.e. the drug's form as salt, crystal or hydrate) can change the dissolution rate and thus control overall absorption.

Enteral medicines Enteral medicines are medicines that enter the GI tract. Oral medicines, such as a tablet or liquid suspension, would normally be administered directly into the mouth and would pass into the GI tract. If the oral route is not an option, enteral medications may also be administered via nasogastric tube (NGT) or orogastric tube (OGT). From here, medicine would be absorbed via the GI tract wall and would enter plasma. Any substances that are absorbed via the GI wall will be transported by plasma to the liver via the hepatic portal vein (HPV); this is completed prior to being delivered to the body's tissues and organs. In pharmacology, this process is known as first-pass metabolism.

Parenteral medicines Drugs given IV enter the systemic circulation directly (Le, 2019). However, drugs injected IM or SC must cross one or more biological membranes to reach the systemic circulation. If protein drugs with a molecular mass >20 000 g/mol are injected IM or SC, movement across capillary membranes is so slow that most absorption occurs via the lymphatic system. In such cases, drug delivery to the systemic circulation is slow and often incomplete because of first-pass metabolism (metabolism of a drug before it reaches the systemic circulation) by proteolytic enzymes in the lymphatic system.

Perfusion (blood flow/gram of tissue) greatly affects capillary absorption of small molecules injected IM or SC. Thus, the injection site can affect the absorption rate. Absorption after IM or SC injection may be delayed or erratic for salts of poorly soluble bases and acids (e.g. parenteral form of phenytoin) and in patients with poor peripheral perfusion (e.g. due to pre-eclampsia, during hypotension or shock).

Topical medicines Applying medication to the skin or mucus membranes allows it to enter the body from there. Medication applied in this way is known as topical medication. It can also be used to treat pain or other problems in specific parts of the body.

Topical medication can also be used to nourish the skin and protect it from harm. Some topical medications are used for local treatment and some are meant to affect the whole body after being absorbed through the skin.

Additional factors that can affect how the drug is absorbed include the drug's formulation, extended release versus immediate release, blood flow to the area of absorption and GI motility for enteral medications. A common example of enteral medication would be paracetamol. Common parenteral medications include insulin and heparin. Some medications, such as penicillin, have both enteral and parenteral formulations.

Key concerns in pregnancy relating to absorption are primarily around the GI changes occurring because of hormonal increases in progesterone and oestrogen. This, in addition to the increased gastric pH due to reduced gastric secretions, theoretically impacts absorption of drugs. However, there is a paucity of evidence to demonstrate that either of these factors significantly alters drug absorption (Ansari et al., 2016) and there are other compensatory mechanisms occurring in pregnancy, such as increased cardiac output and intestinal blood flow, which allow for improved absorption. Nausea and vomiting in pregnancy (NVP) decreases the bioavailability of drugs taken orally, and oral medications should be given when the nausea is minimal (Feghali et al., 2015). Koren and Pariente (2018) identify that gastrointestinal changes during pregnancy have an overall minimal effect on the bioavailability and therapeutic effect of most oral drugs, especially with repeated dosing. Additionally, there may be reduced efficacy of some drugs such as antiepileptics and analgesia where a fast response is required from a single dose, which should be a consideration when prescribing or administering to pregnant women. Intramuscular or subcutaneous administration may lead to a delay in reaching peak concentration, although increased blood flow and vasodilation may support absorption. However, there is relatively little evidence relating to the impact on changes to absorption for these routes (Feghali et al., 2015).

Phase 2: Distribution

Distribution is dispersal of the drug through the body's fluids and tissues as it travels to its site of action (usually blood or plasma). This is dependent on blood flow, both to the area where the drug is to be administered and how perfusion occurs to other areas of the body, as well as protein binding. If a drug binds to protein, they become attached and therefore the drug cannot exert its effect on the body. The more a drug binds to protein, the less of the drug there is available for distribution.

During pregnancy, there is up to a 50% increase in circulating blood volume by the third trimester. Theoretically, this increased volume could decrease peak concentrations of medications, even after multiple doses. However, any effect has not been established as clinically important in research studies (Anderson, 2005).

Protein binding

Most drugs are bound to proteins in the blood and transported around the body by venous circulation. When drugs bind to protein, they become enlarged and cannot enter capillaries and then into tissues to react. Some drugs are tightly bound and are released slowly, meaning that they have a longer duration of action as they are not broken down or excreted by the kidneys. Some drugs are in competition with other drugs at the same protein-binding site, which will change the effectiveness of the drug, or cause toxicity when two or more drugs of the same group are administered together (Karch, 2017).

Benet and Hoener (2002) found that there were clinically significant effects for only two types of highly protein-bound drugs during pregnancy: low-extraction ratio drugs such as sodium valproate (administered for epilepsy) and high-extraction ratio drugs such as fentanyl and midazolam. However, the effect of pregnancy on these has not been evaluated.

Blood–brain barrier

The blood–brain barrier (BBB) prevents entry of most drugs into the brain from the blood. The BBB is a protective system of cellular activity that keeps many things out, such as foreign invaders and poisons. Drugs that are highly lipid soluble are more likely to pass through the BBB and reach the central nervous system (CNS). Drugs that are not lipid soluble are not able to pass the BBB. This is clinically significant in treating brain infections. For example, antibodies are too large to cross the BBB and only certain antibiotics can pass. The BBB becomes more permeable during inflammation, allowing antibiotics and phagocytes to move across it. However, this also allows bacteria and viruses to infiltrate the BBB. Most antibiotics are not lipid soluble and therefore cannot treat brain infections as they are unable to cross the BBB. IV medications such as rifampicin would be used in such cases.

The presence of the BBB makes the development of new treatments for brain diseases, or new radiopharmaceuticals for neuroimaging of the brain, extremely complex. All the products of biotechnology are large-molecule drugs that do not cross the BBB.

Placenta and breast milk

The placenta is the lifeline of the developing fetus (Figure 5.2). It is a semi-permeable barrier through which all nutrients and waste products must pass. Several factors affect a medication's ability to cross the placenta; although many drugs are transported by passive diffusion based on the concentration gradient, if a medication is hydrophilic, ionised in maternal serum and highly protein bound, little to no medication will cross. If there is little to no published safety data for a medication, the pharmacist can evaluate these details of a medication to predict the possibility of fetal exposure.

The transfer of medication into human milk shares some of the same principles as crossing the placenta, by passive diffusion. A medication may cross through the placenta into fetal circulation and back on the concentration gradient, just as a drug may pass into milk and diffuse back into the bloodstream as serum concentrations decrease. Certain properties of some medications may cause them to be sequestered into or actively excreted into breast milk (Hale, 2012). Drugs should only be given to pregnant or breast-feeding women when the benefit clearly outweighs any risk. Drugs are likely to be secreted into breast milk and therefore have the potential to affect the neonate. All drugs must be checked prior to administration; this includes utilising the British National Formulary (BNF), organisation-approved guidelines and published contemporary medication guides.

Throughout gestation, dynamic changes in the maternal–placental–fetal unit influence the pharmacokinetic processes of drug absorption, distribution, metabolism and elimination. Maternal and fetal drug exposure and response are influenced by three factors: (i) maternal pharmacokinetics influenced by pregnancy-induced physiological changes; (ii) the amount of drug that crosses the placenta; and (iii) distribution, metabolism and elimination by the fetus. Drug transfer across the

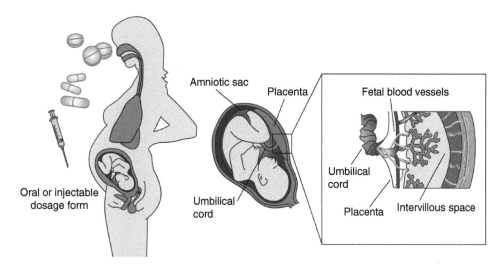

Figure 5.2   Medication delivery to the baby during gestation.
Source: Peate and Hill (2021)/with permission of John Wiley & Sons.

placenta depends on the physiochemical properties of the drug as well as the mechanism of transfer across the placental barrier, blood flow to the placenta, metabolism and binding by the placenta, differential plasma protein binding between the mother and fetus, and the pH of the maternal and fetal circulations. Fetal drug response will depend on how much drug crosses the placenta as well as how the fetus distributes, metabolises and eliminates the drug.

By better understanding the pharmacokinetics and pharmacodynamics of medications during lactation, midwives can assist mothers to make well-informed decisions about medication use during lactation. The most important factor in infant exposure through breast milk is the amount of medication in the mother's serum.

Phase 3: Metabolism (biotransformation)

Metabolism, sometimes referred to as biotransformation, is recognition by the body that the drug is present and the transformation of the drug into useable parts. Most drugs are metabolised in the liver via the cytochrome P450 family of enzymes. Other organs involved may include the kidneys and intestines.

Drugs can be metabolised by oxidation, reduction, hydrolysis, hydration, conjugation, condensation or isomerisation; whatever the process, the goal is to make the drug easier to excrete. The enzymes involved in metabolism are present in many tissues but generally are more concentrated in the liver. Drug metabolism rates vary among different people. Some people metabolise a drug so rapidly that therapeutically effective blood and tissue concentrations are not reached; in others, metabolism may be so slow that usual doses have toxic effects. In pregnancy, the key issue is the increase in the hormones oestrogen and progesterone. These can variously create a stimulatory or inhibitory impact on the metabolism of drugs which will increase or decrease liver metabolism, depending on the nature of the drug.

Individual drug metabolism rates are influenced by genetic factors, co-existing disorders (particularly chronic liver disorders and advanced heart failure) and drug interactions (especially those involving induction or inhibition of metabolism).

For many drugs, metabolism occurs in two phases.

- *Phase I* reactions involve formation of a new or modified functional group or cleavage (oxidation, reduction, hydrolysis); these reactions are non-synthetic.
- *Phase II* reactions involve conjugation with an endogenous substance (e.g. glucuronic acid, sulfate, glycine); these reactions are synthetic. Metabolites formed in synthetic reactions are more polar and thus more readily excreted by the kidneys (in urine) and the liver (in bile) than those formed in non-synthetic reactions.

Some drugs undergo only phase I or phase II reactions; thus, phase numbers reflect functional rather than sequential classification.

According to Young and Pitcher (2016), certain drugs only undergo phase I metabolism, others only phase II metabolism and some drugs have no metabolism at all. Some drugs underdo phase II metabolism and then phase I. Certain drugs are inactive in the body until biotransformation takes place (for example, codeine which converts to morphine). These drugs are known as pro-drugs. Certain drugs, such as the antidepressant fluoxetine, are transformed into metabolites that are also active and these metabolites are partially responsible for the therapeutic activity of the drug agent.

Rate
For almost all drugs, the metabolism rate in any given pathway has an upper limit (capacity limitation). However, at therapeutic concentrations of most drugs, usually only a small fraction of the metabolising enzyme's sites are occupied and the metabolism rate increases with drug concentration (Le, 2019). In such cases, called first-order elimination (or kinetics), the metabolism rate of the drug is a constant fraction of the drug remaining in the body (i.e. the drug has a specific half-life).

First-pass metabolism
The first-pass effect (also known as first-pass metabolism or presystemic metabolism) (Figure 5.3) was the term coined by Rowland (1972) for the phenomenon of drug metabolism whereby the concentration of a drug is greatly reduced before it reaches the systemic circulation.

1. The drug is absorbed by the GI tract.
2. Drug absorbed from the GI tract travels immediately to the liver through the HPV.
3. The first-pass effect occurs at this stage. Hepatic first pass occurs when drug absorbed from the GI tract is metabolised by enzymes within the liver to such an extent that most of the active agent does not exit the liver and, therefore, does not reach the systemic circulation.
4. The remaining drug is distributed around the body within blood cells and plasma.

The process of drug metabolism is part of the body's normal response to removal of drugs and chemicals from the circulating system. Hepatic metabolism, or biotransformation, is the main site and method of the process of elimination. This is followed by excretion of the drug and its metabolites

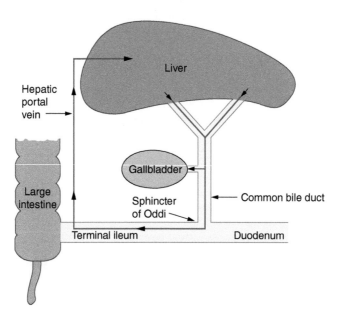

Figure 5.3   Hepatic first-pass metabolism (first-pass effect).
Source: Peate and Hill (2021)/with permission of John Wiley & Sons.

64

from the body. The liver plays an extremely important role in drug removal. When drug molecules are distributed in the bloodstream, the plasma flow through the functional units of the liver presents these molecules for biotransformation. This occurs after administration by any route.

The oral route of drug administration is by far the most used route. It is normally accessible and the least invasive route available in most cases. This route is well tolerated and convenient. Many common drugs are available in oral formulations as well as in preparations suitable for administration by other routes. There are very few drugs in the BNF that have no oral formulation.

Drugs given by the oral route are absorbed from the stomach and small intestine into the HPV, the blood vessel that goes directly to the liver. The process of biotransformation begins, and the drug will start to be metabolised in preparation for excretion from the body. The drug molecules in the plasma move through circulating volume. The molecules are now metabolised by liver enzymes. The 'first-pass effect' reduces the fraction of the dose which then goes on to reach the systemic circulation and become available for therapeutic effect. This process occurs in the hepatic microsomal enzymes and includes the cytochrome P450 enzymes.

For drugs given orally, the amount of first-pass metabolism known to occur has been factored into oral dosing by pharmaceutical companies. This means that the bioavailability, which is a known factor, has been considered when dose and dose ranges are advised in the BNF. However, these are largely based on standard adult doses for healthy and mostly male individuals (Thomas and Yates, 2012). Koren and Pariente (2018) note that unlike for renal failure or children, there are currently no dose alteration schedules specifically for pregnancy, meaning that the complex physiological changes that impact pharmacokinetics are not easily navigated by prescribers, and may inadvertently lead to reduced efficacy or toxicity, depending on the drug.

Altered hepatic clearance in pregnancy is caused by circulating hormones which may induce or inhibit metabolic enzymes. The implications of this differ depending on the drug in question (Koren and Pariente, 2018). It is important, therefore, that prescribers and people who administer medication must consider this altered physiology in pregnancy as well as establishing any other hepatic dysfunction for those receiving oral medications.

If there is compromised liver function or a disease such as cirrhosis, obstetric cholestasis or haemolysis elevated liver enzymes and low platelet count (HELLP syndrome), then first-pass metabolism will be compromised. This could lead to more active drug entering the systemic circulation due to reduced liver enzyme functionality and may cause side-effects, adverse effects or toxicity. Drug dosing may need to be reduced in patients in this situation.

Some drugs are destroyed by liver enzymes at this first-pass stage and will not enter the general systemic circulation. An example of such a drug is glyceryl trinitrate (GTN), which is metabolised completely by the liver and inactivated. Consequently, you will find GTN being given via non-oral routes, sublingual being a very good alternative.

Not all oral drugs are destroyed by the liver at first pass, but many clinically significant drugs do undergo an extensive first-pass effect. Therefore, the doses of some drugs are considerably higher when given by the oral route compared to their dosing if given intravenously.

Two drugs given together may change the absorption of either one or both drugs. For example, a drug that may change the acidity of stomach acid is likely to affect a drug that is dissolved in the stomach. Other drugs can interact and form an insoluble compound that cannot be absorbed. Sometimes an absorption interaction can be avoided by separating the administration of each drug by at least 2 hours (Gersh et al., 2016).

Phase 4: Elimination

Elimination is the irreversible loss of drug from the site of measurement (blood, serum, plasma). Elimination of drugs occurs by excretion, metabolism or both.5

Excretion

Excretion is the irreversible loss of a drug in a chemically unchanged or unaltered form. The two principal organs responsible for drug elimination are the kidney and liver. The kidney is the primary site for removal of a drug in a chemically unaltered or unchanged form (i.e. excretion) as well as for metabolites. The liver is the primary organ where drug metabolism occurs. The relationship between increased excretion of drugs in pregnancy via the liver and kidneys is well established (Davison and Dunlop, 1980) and leads to a lower concentration of some drugs such as aspirin. The lungs, occasionally, may be an important route of elimination for substances of high vapour pressure

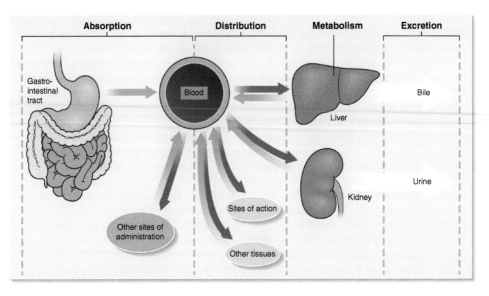

Figure 5.4   Pharmacokinetics (ADME) and the main anatomical structures/physiological systems that are responsble for executing those processes.
Source: Adapted from Young and Pitcher (2016).

(i.e. gaseous anaesthetics, alcohol). Another potential route of drug removal is via breast milk. Although not a significant route for elimination of a drug for the mother, the drug may be consumed in enough quantity to affect her baby or infant (Figure 5.4).

Physiological changes take place during pregnancy which may affect the absorption, distribution, metabolism and elimination of medications. These pharmacokinetic changes may result in lower psychotropic drug levels and, in some cases, loss of clinical effectiveness.

An example of the pharmacokinetics of aspirin (acetylsalicylic acid)

Aspirin is a medication generally used for pain, fever and inflammation but its use for these indications in pregnancy is advised against, with teratogenesis more of a concern in the first trimester before organogenesis. Aspirin is also an antiplatelet agent (blood thinner) and is prescribed at lower doses for prevention of cardiovascular and cerebrovascular disease. Its use in pregnancy is more commonly associated with its antiplatelet properties for women at high risk of cardiovascular disease. Guidance now indicates that daily low-dose aspirin (75–150 mg) should be considered from 12 weeks gestation until birth for women at risk of pre-eclampsia (NICE, 2019). Meta-analyses of data have shown that aspirin is associated with a significant reduction in preterm pre-eclampsia (Rolnik et al., 2017), fetal growth restriction and perinatal death (Bujold et al., 2010; Roberge et al., 2013). However, as with many other medications used in pregnancy, there is doubt surrounding the optimum dose for achieving these therapeutic benefits and studies have variously examined aspirin resistance in pregnancy and adherence to regimens as reasons for possible ineffectiveness (Vinogradov et al., 2020).

The pharmacokinetics of aspirin can be seen in Box 5.2.

Box 5.2   Pharmacokinetics of aspirin during pregnancy

A Aspirin is available in oral forms. When taken, it is absorbed in the gastrointestinal tract. Gastrointestinal motility is delayed because of the effects of progesterone and this can increase gastric emptying and decrease gastric acidity which may affect its absorption. Although the evidence around this is contradictory, studies have shown greater efficacy where the upper limit of 100–150 mg daily is administered (Shanmugalingham et al., 2019).

D It is distributed to all tissues of the body. In pregnant women, it does cross the placenta to the fetus. It is also passed through breast milk to a nursing infant. Pregnant women have up to a 50% increased circulating blood volume which can result in a decreased peak serum concentration of aspirin.

M In the body, it quickly breaks down into salicylic acid and the liver changes it into metabolites. The half-life of aspirin is only 15–20 minutes. Half-life is the amount of time it takes to decrease the concentration of the drug in the body by half. Once aspirin is broken down into salicylic acid, it has a half-life of 6 hours. In higher doses, half-life increases and in toxic doses (overdose) it may exceed 20 hours.

E It is then excreted by the kidneys. In pregnancy, glomerular filtration rate increases by up to 50% with a decrease in the final 3 weeks of gestation. This appears to lead to a lower peak concentration of aspirin. Based on the available data, aspirin requires up to a 45% dosage adjustment to account for this. Further trials comparing 100 mg to 150 mg daily doses are required to ascertain optimal dosages throughout pregnancy.

Source: Based on Shanmugalingham et al. (2019).

Clinical considerations

Half-life
The half-life of medication is how long it takes for the medication to be reduced by half of its blood concentration level. This is done through metabolisation. It can be affected by the individual's ability to metabolise, such as if the patient has renal failure and liver damage.

Steady state
A steady state (SS) is when the amount of drug administered is equal to the amount of drug eliminated within a one-dose interval, resulting in a plateau or constant serum drug level. Drugs with a short half-life reach steady state rapidly, while drugs with a long half-life can take days to weeks to reach steady state. Alterations in drug clearance during pregnancy can significantly affect steady-state concentrations of drugs. Hepatic clearance is dependent on protein binding, activity of the metabolic enzymes and liver blood flow. The enzyme activity is affected by an interplay of genetic, physiological and environmental factors (Anderson, 2005).

Routes of drug administration
The sites of drug administration include:

- oral
- sublingual
- rectal
- vaginal
- parenteral: intravenous, intramuscular, subcutaneous
- topical – an illustration can be seen in Figure 5.5 (see Chapter 6 for further information).

Pharmacodynamics
Pharmacodynamics explores what the drug does to the body; specifically, how the drug molecules interact within the body, what they interact with and how they cause their effects (Young and Pitcher, 2016, p. 21). To expand on this, a drug exerts its biological effects by interacting with the

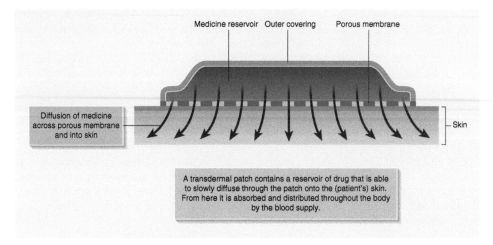

Figure 5.5　How a transdermal patch works.
Source: Adapted from Young and Pitcher (2016).

Clinical consideration

Termination of action

A termination of action is when the medication has stopped its action at the site where it is required. This may be seen in analgesic control; when pain returns, the medication has stopped acting.

receptors located on tissues and organs throughout the body. The effects of the drug are dependent upon the drug's ability to bind to a variety of the body's receptors (Gersh et al., 2016). For example, if a drug's concentration is increased where many receptors are located, the intensity of the drug's effect will be improved. Therefore, the pharmacological response depends on the drug's ability to bind to its target. The concentration of the drug at the receptor site influences the drug's effect.

One of the key challenges for midwives when studying pharmacodynamics is that drugs are affected by a woman's physiological changes during pregnancy, disease, genetic mutations, ageing and/ or other drugs. These changes are likely to alter the level of binding proteins or decrease receptor sensitivity (Campbell and Cohall, 2017). It is important that midwives recognise that some drugs acting on the same receptor (or tissue) differ in the magnitude of the biological responses that they can achieve (i.e. their 'efficacy') and the amount of drug required to achieve a response (i.e. their 'potency'). Drug receptors can be classified based on their selective response to different drugs. Constant exposure of receptors or body systems to drugs sometimes leads to a reduced response, for example desensitisation.

All medications act in one of four ways (Karch, 2017).

- To replace or act as a substitute for missing chemicals.
- To increase or stimulate certain cellular activities.
- To depress or slow cellular activities.
- To interfere with the functioning of foreign cells, such as invading micro-organisms or neoplasms leading to cell death (drugs that act in this way are called chemotherapeutic agents).

Agonists and antagonists

The terms *agonist* (a molecule that binds to a receptor causing activation and resultant cellular changes) and *antagonist* (a molecule that attenuates the action of an agonist) apply only to receptors. See Figure 5.6.

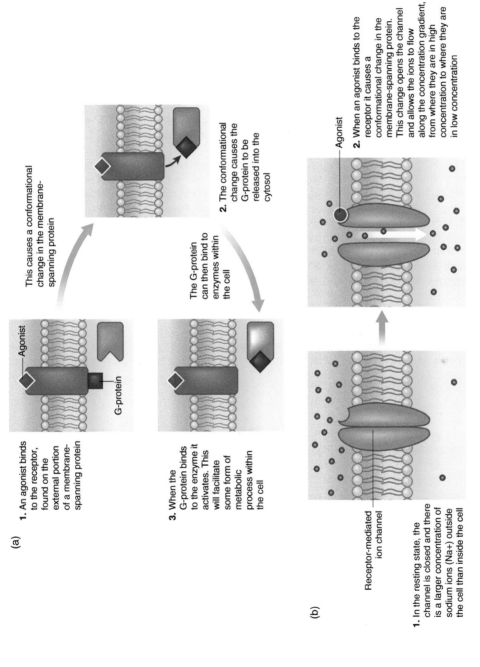

Figure 5.6 (a) The step-by-step process of a second messenger system. (b) Step-by-step receptor-mediated ion channel. Source: Adapted from Young and Pitcher (2016).

Agonist

An agonist is an example of a drug that interacts with receptors. Agonist drugs are attracted to receptors and stimulate them. Once stimulation has occurred, the agonist binds to the receptor and the drug effect occurs; the outcome of this activity is known as intrinsic activity.

Agonists can be full, partial or inverse. Some drugs act on a variety of receptors; these are known as non-selective and can cause multiple and widespread effects (Gersh et al., 2016). Pleuvry (2004) notes that a full agonist can produce the largest response that the tissue can give.

The term 'efficacy' has been used to describe the way in which agonists can vary in the response they produce even when occupying the same number of receptors. A high-efficacy agonist produces a maximum response even when occupying a small proportion of the available receptors. The magnitude of response to an agonist is usually proportional to the fraction of receptors occupied. As the concentration of an agonist at its site of action increases, so the fraction of occupied receptors rises and, in turn, the magnitude of response rises. A partial agonist cannot fully activate the receptors, irrespective of the concentration available. In contrast to a full agonist, a partial agonist cannot exert a maximal response. Finally, an inverse agonist: the simplest definition is that the compound binds to a receptor but produces the opposite effect from an accepted agonist.

An example of a widely used agonist is salbutamol which is a $\beta2$ agonist. One way to remember the location of $\beta1$ and $\beta2$ cells simply and quickly is that humans have one heart and two lungs. $\beta1$ cells are mainly based around the heart (one heart) and $\beta2$ cells are mainly based around the lungs (two lungs). Therefore, salbutamol, being a $\beta2$ agonist, would have its main effects on the receptors based within the lungs. $\beta1$ receptors, along with $\beta2$, $\alpha1$ and $\alpha2$ receptors, are adrenergic receptors primarily responsible for signalling in the sympathetic nervous system. β agonists bind to the β receptors on various tissues throughout the body. $\beta2$ agonists are used for both asthma and COPD, although some types are only available for COPD. $\beta2$ agonists work by stimulating $\beta2$ receptors in the muscles that line the airways, which causes them to relax and allows the airways to widen (dilate). Hence why salbutamol is known as a bronchodilator.

Table 5.3 gives examples of opioids by receptor binding.

Antagonist

The opposite of an agonist is an antagonist. An antagonist is a type of receptor ligand or drug that blocks or dampens a biological response by binding to and blocking a receptor rather than

Table 5.3   Examples of opioids by receptor binding.

Full Agonist	Partial Agonist	Mixed Agonist	Antagonist (also known as blockers or reversals)
Codeine	Buprenorphine	Buprenorphine	Naloxone
Fentanyl	Butorphanol	Butorphanol	Naltrexone
Heroin	Pentazocine	Nalbuphine	
Hydrocodone	Tramadol	Pentazocine	
Levorphanol			
Meperidine			
Methadone			
Morphine			
Oxycodone			
Oxymorphone			

Source: Peate and Hill (2021)/with permission of John Wiley & Sons.

70

activating it, like an agonist. They are sometimes called blockers; examples include alpha blockers, beta blockers and calcium channel blockers.

Antagonists can be competitive or non-competitive.

- A *competitive* antagonist binds to the same site as the agonist but does not activate it, thus blocking the agonist's action.
- A *non-competitive* antagonist binds to an allosteric (non-agonist) site on the receptor to prevent activation of the receptor.

71

Clinical considerations

Confidence in the drug

In clinical practice, all drugs have been tested through rigorous research trials prior to being made available for safe prescription and administration (unless patients have provided informed consent and are actively enrolled on early human clinical trials) (see Chapter 3). These drugs are licensed for use within a recommended dose range. This ensures that patients achieve a good response to their medication, without the need for constant review and titration of their prescription. This is known as the therapeutic index. It is important to recognise, however, that many drugs are not licensed for use in pregnancy. This is largely due to the practical, regulatory and ethical challenges of researching and developing drugs for use in pregnancy and the decisions made by pharmaceutical companies are generally led by commercial interests (RCOG, 2015). Prescribers are reliant on custom and practice which means women may receive doses that are either ineffective or potentially toxic. This paucity of information also has the potential to deprive women and babies of treatments which may be of benefit.

Drug potency and efficacy

The concepts of potency and efficacy are often confused and used interchangeably within the scientific and pharmaceutical industry. It is important that the distinction between the two is understood and that the terms are defined within their correct context. Potency is an expression of the activity of a drug in terms of the concentration or amount of the drug required to produce a defined effect, whereas clinical efficacy judges the therapeutic effectiveness of the drug in humans. Drug potency is also used to compare two drugs. For example, if Drug A and Drug B both produce the same response, but Drug A does this at a lower dose, that means Drug A is more potent than Drug B.

Therapeutic index

The therapeutic index is the range at which a medication is therapeutic to the individual. A drug with a low or narrow therapeutic index (NTI) has a narrow range of safety between an effective dose and a lethal one. Alternatively, a drug with a high therapeutic index will have a wide range of safety and fewer risks of toxic effects. It should be noted that doubling a dose of a drug does not mean that the therapeutic effect will be doubled but will most likely double the toxic effect. Furthermore, administration above the dose at which the maximum effect is observed will produce no added benefit.

Therapeutic drug monitoring (TDM) is commonly recommended to optimise drug dosing regimens of various medications. It has been proposed to guide therapy in pregnant women, in whom physiological changes may lead to altered pharmacokinetics resulting in difficulty in predicting the appropriate drug dosage. Ideally, TDM may play a role in enhancing the effectiveness of treatment while minimising toxicity of both the mother and fetus. Monitoring of drug levels may also be helpful in assessing adherence to prescribed therapy in selected cases. Limitations exist as therapeutic ranges have only been defined for a limited number of drugs and are based on data obtained in non-pregnant patients. TDM has been suggested for anticonvulsants, antidepressants and antiretroviral drugs, based on pharmacokinetic studies that have shown reduced drug concentrations. However, there is only relatively limited (and sometimes inconsistent) information regarding the clinical impact of these pharmacokinetic changes during pregnancy and the effect of subsequent dose adjustments. This process can be affected by the patient's health and organ condition/s, particularly the patient's liver and kidney function. For example, the liver is the principal site of drug metabolism. Although metabolism typically inactivates drugs, some drug metabolites are pharmacologically active.

An inactive or weakly active substance that has an active metabolite is called a pro-drug, especially if designed to deliver the active moiety (the molecule or ion responsible for the physiological or pharmacological action of the drug) more effectively. It is important to recognise that even slight changes in medication dose or blood concentration level need to be carefully monitored and recorded (see Boxes 5.3 and 5.4 for examples).

Box 5.3   Narrow therapeutic index examples

Drug name	Indication	Drug group
Phenytoin	Tonic-clonic seizures, Focal seizures	Anticonvulsants
Carbanazepine	Focal and secondary generalized tonic-clonic seizures, Primary generalized tonic-clonic seizures	Anticonvulsants
Gentamicin	Infection	Aminoglycoside antibiotics
Vancomycin	Infection	Glycopeptide antibiotics
Teicoplanin	Serious infection caused by gram-positive bacteria	Glycopeptide antibiotics
Lithium	Treatment and prophylaxis of mania, Treatment and prophylaxis of bipolar disorder, Treatment and prophylaxis of recurrent depression, Treatment and prophylaxis of aggressive or self-harming behaviour	Antimanic agents
Digoxin	Rapid digitalization, for atrial fibrillation or flutter	Cardiac glycosides
Aminophylline and Theophylline	Severe acute asthma or sever acute exacerbation of COPD in patients not previously treated with Theophylline.	Xanthines

Source: Joint Formulary Committee (2019). From Peate and Hill (2021)/with permission of John Wiley & Sons.

Box 5.4   Example of monitoring requirements of oxytocin for augmentation of labour in term pregnancy

Oxytocin (Syntocinon®) is administered as a slow continuous infusion via an infusion pump for the induction of labour or for augmentation of labour where delay in the first stage has been identified in accordance with NICE intrapartum guidelines (2017). There is no consensus on oxytocin dosing and infusion rates and local policy and guidelines should be followed. The commencement of oxytocin will increase the strength and frequency of contractions and options for analgesia should be discussed with the woman in anticipation of this.

Once a decision has been made between the woman, the midwife and obstetrician to commence active management of labour, amniotomy is recommended prior to the commencement of oxytocin if membranes are intact. Key concerns in relation to monitoring throughout the administration of oxytocin are the potential risks associated with hyperstimulation of the uterus. This is defined as the presence of more than five uterine contractions in 10 minutes, lasting up to 60 seconds with accompanying abnormal fetal heart rate.

Monitoring should include the following.

- Continuous fetal monitoring to observe for signs of fetal distress.
- Uterine contractions should be palpated and recorded, and infusion titrated accordingly.
- Infusion to be increased in 30-minute intervals until contractions are stabilised at 4–5 in 10 minutes.
- If contractions exceed five in 10 minutes, infusion should be reduced to the incremental dose.
- If contractions do not establish despite optimum dose, request obstetric review.
- Four-hourly abdominal and vaginal examinations should be performed to ensure labour is progressing.
- Regular monitoring of vital signs to ensure the woman remains haemodynamically stable, including fluid balance because of risk of fluid retention associated with oxytocin.

Oxytocin infusion should be stopped immediately and a medical review requested if any of the following occur.

- Pathological CTG trace
- Intrapartum haemorrhage
- Suspected uterine rutpture
- Signs of obstructed labour
- Cord prolapse
- Abnormal fetal presentation (e.g. breech, arm)
- Contractions of more than 5 in 10 with fetal compromise.

Episode of care

Emma is a 32-year-old woman who is pregnant with her second child. Her first son is now 18 months old. At 16 weeks gestation, she was complaining of fatigue, dyspnoea and headaches. Her serum ferritin was 13 µg/L and her haemoglobin was 90 g/L. She was diagnosed with iron deficiency anaemia and prescribed ferrous sulfate 200 mg twice a day. Emma returned for her 28-week antenatal appointment and her breathlessness and headaches had returned. She was also feeling irritable and finding it difficult to focus but had attributed this to pregnancy. She was advised to increase the ferrous sulfate to 200 mg three times a day.

When Emma returns for her 34-week appointment her haemoglobin is still 90 g/L and her ferritin is 14 µg/L. She reports that she has been skipping some doses of her ferrous sulfate because she has been suffering with nausea and epigastric pain as well as constipation. Her headaches and dyspnoea have alleviated but remain.

Clinical considerations

Key points
- The UK prevalence of iron deficiency anaemia in pregnancy is 23%.
- Serum ferritin level is considered to be a reliable indicator of iron deficiency anaemia in the first trimester in the absence of infection or inflammation. However, it is of limited use in the third trimester.

- Serum ferritin of less than 15 µg/L indicates iron depletion at any stage of pregnancy. Treatment should be considered when levels fall below 30 µg/L as this indicates early iron depletion which will continue to fall unless treated.
- In pregnant women anaemia is defined as a haemoglobin below 110 g/L.
- Physiological iron requirements are three times higher in pregnancy, with increasing demand as pregnancy advances.
- The aim of iron supplements is to restore haemoglobin levels and replenish iron stores.
- Dietary advice should accompany prescribing of iron supplements to ensure an iron-rich diet.
- Haemoglobin should be checked 2–4 weeks following commencement of iron supplements and should rise by approximately 2 g/100 mL over 3–4 weeks.

Side-effects

The side-effects of medication can be wide ranging, especially when people start a new medication; as a registrant you must understand medicines management, including side-effects and monitoring the effects of medication. You should report/take action where there is a possible or actual side-effect.

In this case Emma was reluctant to take the medication because of nausea, epigastric pain and constipation which are all common side-effects of iron supplements. The midwife should consider the following points.

- Side-effects should be addressed to increase adherence with iron supplementation.
- Nausea may be alleviated by taking the medication with or after food.
- Antacids may be used but absorption of iron may be reduced with medication containing zinc or magnesium salts found in some antacids.
- Usual advice for avoiding constipation should be offered, i.e. balanced diet, high in dietary fibre, keep well hydrated and exercise.
- Laxatives such as bulk-forming agents, stool softeners, may be considered as they have minimal systemic absorption so do not affect the fetus (Trottier et al., 2012).

Adverse effects

The International Union of Basic and Clinical Pharmacology (IUPHAR, 2019) suggests that the adverse effects of drugs are often dose related in a similar way to the beneficial effects. Drugs have multiple potential adverse effects but the concept of the therapeutic index is usually reserved for those requiring dose reduction or discontinuation. Drugs with low therapeutic indices are more difficult to prescribe and may be hazardous to pregnant women and/or the fetus (such as antiepileptic drugs; see Box 5.5), but they are still preferred if there are no alternative drugs with similar efficacy. The doses of such drugs must be titrated carefully for individual patients to maximise benefits but avoid adverse effects. This is done by monitoring drug effects, either clinically or using regular blood tests (often known as therapeutic drug monitoring – TDM).

Box 5.5 Therapeutic drug monitoring of antiepileptic drugs (AED) in pregnancy

The pharmacokinetics of AED may be altered in pregnancy due to physiological changes which impact absorption, distribution, metabolism and excretion. These changes may have consequences for the frequency of seizures during pregnancy. The risks to the mother and fetus of less stable epilepsy must be balanced with the teratogenic risk to the fetus of AED exposure. Appropriate dose modification must be considered, and close therapeutic drug monitoring must be carried out to ensure optimum efficacy and minimisation of risk (Arfman et al., 2020).

While there is variability in the pharmacokinetics of AEDs, there are standard recommendations around their monitoring. Arfman et al. (2020) undertook a review of AEDs and highlight the following key points.

- An increase in clearance and a decrease in the concentrations of lamotrigine, levetiracetam, oxcarbazepine's active metabolite licarbazepine, topiramate and zonisamide.
- Carbamazepine clearance is unchanged during pregnancy.
- No evidence for changes in clearance or concentrations for clobazam, gabapentin, lacosamide, perampanel, valproate (although valproate should be avoided altogether due to increased teratogenic effects).
- Elimination rates post partum resumed to pre-pregnancy values within the first few weeks following pregnancy for lamotrigine, levetiracetam and licarbazepine.

When women who are known to have epilepsy are planning to conceive, it is advised that two pre-pregnancy AED reference concentration (RC) levels are recorded as a baseline. Dose adjustments throughout pregnancy should be guided by these reference ranges and where there are symptoms such as increased convulsions, a change of 15–25% from RC dose should be considered. Where concentrations change more than 25% the dose should be adjusted accordingly.

General guidance around the use of AEDs during pregnancy includes the following points.

- Prescribe the lowest possible effective dose.
- Changes in doses should factor in RC in addition to clinical signs, seizure risk and pre-pregnancy doses.
- AED concentrations should be gradually adjusted over 0–21 days post partum to prevent overdose.
- Postpartum AEDs may not return to pre-pregnancy doses for optimum efficacy because of the effect of sleep deprivation and stress associated with caring for a newborn which may exacerbate epilepsy.

As with many drugs used in pregnancy, more research on the pharmacokinetics of AEDs is needed (also see Chapter 17).

Conclusion

This chapter has introduced the reader to the pharmacodynamics and pharmacokinetics of medicines. The reader should now be able to acknowledge the professional responsibilities of registered healthcare professionals who administer drugs to patients; define and understand the differences between pharmacodynamics and pharmacokinetics; and appreciate the complexities of how drugs work differently in every individual. The reader should now be able to recognise that pregnancy involves various changes in maternal physiology and disease. It logically follows that drug disposition and effects are altered in pregnancy.

Test yourself

Now review your learning by completing the learning activities for this chapter at https://www.wiley.com/go/pharmacologyformidwives.

References

Anderson, G. (2005) Pregnancy induced changes in pharmacokinetics: a mechanistic-based approach. *Clinical Pharmacokinetics*, **44**(10): 989–1008.

Ansari, J., Carvalho, B., Shafer, S., Flood, P. (2016) Pharmacokinetics and pharmacodynamics of drugs commonly used in pregnancy and parturition. *Anesthesia & Analgesia*, **122**(3): 786–804.

Arfman, I.J., Wammes-van der Heijden, E.A., ter Horst, P.G.J. et al. (2020) Therapeutic drug monitoring of antiepileptic drugs in women with epilepsy before, during, and after pregnancy. *Clinical Pharmacokinetics*, **59**: 427–445.

Benet, L.Z., Hoener, B.A. (2002) Changes in plasma protein binding have 2A6 (CYP2A6) gene: implications for interindividual differ – little clinical relevance. *Clinical Pharmacology and Therapeutics*, **71**: 115–121.

BNF and NICE (2021) https://bnf.nice.org.uk/ (accessed January 2022).

Bujold, E., Roberge, S., Lacasse, Y. et al. (2010) Prevention of preeclampsia and intrauterine growth restriction with aspirin started in early pregnancy: a meta-analysis. *Obstetrics and Gynecology*, **116**: 402–414.

Campbell, J.E., Cohall, D. (2017) Pharmacodynamics – a pharmacognosy perspective. In: Badal, S., Delgoda, R. (eds) *Pharmacognosy: Fundamentals, Applications, and Strategies* pp. 513–525. Elsevier: New York.

Davison, J.M., Dunlop, W. (1980) Renal hemodynamics and tubular function normal human pregnancy. *Kidney International*, **18**: 152–161.

Feghali, M., Venkataramanan, R., Caritis, S. (2015) Pharmacokinetics of drugs in pregnancy. *Seminars in Perinatology*, **39**(7): 512–519.

Gersh, C., Heimgartner, N., Rebar, C., Willis, L. (2016) *Pharmacology Made Incredibly Easy!* 4th edn. Wolters Kluwer: Philadelphia.

Hale, T.W. (2012) *Medication and Mother's Milk*, 15th edn. Hale Publishing: Amarillo.

Henderson, E., Mackillop, L. (2011) Prescribing in pregnancy and during breast feeding: using principles in clinical practice. *Postgraduate Medical Journal*, **87**(1027): 349.

International Union of Basic and Clinical Pharmacology (2019) Introduction to pharmacodynamics. www.pharmacologyeducation.org/introduction-pharmacodynamics (accessed January 2022).

Jordan, S. (2010) *Pharmacology for Midwives: The evidence base for safe practice*. Macmillan Education: London.

Karch, A. (2017) *Focus on Nursing Pharmacology*, 7th edn, pp. 18–19. Wolters Kluwer: Philadelphia.

Koren, G., Pariente, G. (2018) Pregnancy-associated changes in pharmacokinetics and their clinical implications. *Pharmaceutical Research*, **35**(3): 1–7.

Le, J. (2019) Drug metabolism. www.msdmanuals.com/en-gb/professional/clinical-pharmacology/pharmacokinetics /drug-metabolism (accessed January 2022).

National Institute for Health and Care Excellence (2017) Intrapartum care for healthy pregnant women. www.nice.org.uk/guidance/cg190/chapter/Recommendations#first-stage-of-labour (accessed January 2022).

National Institute for Health and Care Excellence (2019) Hypertension in pregnancy: diagnosis and management. www.nice.org.uk/guidance/ng133/chapter/recommendations (accessed January 2022).

National Institute for Health and Care Excellence (2021) Prescribing in pregnancy. https://bnf.nice.org.uk/guidance/prescribing-in-pregnancy.html (accessed January 2022).

Nursing and Midwifery Council (2018) The Code. www.nmc.org.uk/globalassets/sitedocuments/nmc-publications/nmc-code.pdf (accessed January 2022).

Peate, I., Hill, B. (2021) *Fundamentals of Pharmacology for Nursing and Healthcare Students*. Wiley, Chichester.

Pleuvry, B. (2004) Pharmacology: receptors, agonists and antagonists. *Anaesthesia and Intensive Care Medicine*, **5**(10): 350–352.

Roberge, S., Nicolaides, K.H., Demers, S., Villa, P., Bujold, E. (2013) Prevention of perinatal death and adverse perinatal outcome using low-dose aspirin: a meta-analysis. *Ultrasound in Obstetrics and Gynaecology*, **41**: 491–499.

Rolnik, D., Wright, D., Poon, C. et al. (2017) Aspirin versus placebo in pregnancies at high risk for preterm preeclampsia. www.nejm.org/doi/full/10.1056/nejmoa1704559 (accessed January 2022).

Rowland, M. (1972) Influence of route of administration on drug availability. *Journal of Pharmaceutical Sciences*, **61**(1): 70–74.

Royal College of Obstetricians and Gynaecologists (2015) Developing new pharmaceutical treatments for obstetric conditions. *Scientific Impact Paper No.* **50**. www.rcog.org.uk/globalassets/documents/guidelines/scientific-impact-papers/sip-50.pdf (accessed January 2022).

Royal Pharmaceutical Society and Royal College of Nursing (2019) Professional guidance on the administration of medicines in healthcare settings. www.rpharms.com/Portals/0/RPS%20document%20library/Open%20access/Professional%20standards/SSHM%20and%20Admin/Admin%20of%20Meds%20prof%20guidance.pdf?ver=2019-01-23-145026-567 (accessed January 2022).

Shanmugalingam, R., Wang, X., Münch, G. et al. (2019) A pharmacokinetic assessment of optimal dosing, preparation, and chronotherapy of aspirin in pregnancy. *American Journal of Obstetrics and Gynecology*, **221**(3): 255.e1–255.e9.

Thomas, S.H., Yates, L.M. (2012) Prescribing without evidence – pregnancy. *British Journal of Clinical Pharmacology*, **74**(4): 691–697.

Trottier, M., Erebara, A., Bozzo, P. (2012) Treating constipation during pregnancy. *Canadian Family Physician*, **58**(8): 836–838.

Vinogradov, R., Boag, C., Murphy, P. et al. (2020) Aspirin non-response in pregnant women at increased risk of pre-eclampsia. *European Journal of Obstetrics & Gynecology and Reproductive Biology*, **254**: 292–297.

Young, S. and Pitcher, B. (2016) *Medicine Management for Nurses at a Glance*. Wiley Blackwell: Chichester.

Chapter 6

Formulations

Sinéad McKee[1] and Cathy Hamilton[2]

[1]Glasgow Caledonian University, Glasgow, Scotland, UK

[2]University of Hertfordshire, Hatfield, UK

Aim

The aim of this chapter is to review the various medication formulations available and the issues to consider when offering care to women.

Learning objectives

After reading this chapter, you will be able to:
- Identify the various formulations in which medicines are available
- Explain the rationale for prescribing certain formulations
- Recognise and contemplate the challenges of administering medications using different routes
- Recognise and contemplate the risks and considerations involved when altering medication dose form by crushing/dissolving
- Recognise and apply your professional responsibilities as a registered healthcare professional when administering medications.

Test your existing knowledge

- What are the different formulations used in midwifery practice?
- Why is it important to consider the specific formulation of medications?
- What are the key considerations when deciding which route of administration to use?
- What is meant by parenteral administration of medication? Name some drugs relevant to midwifery practice that may be administered via this route.
- Explain the advantages and disadvantages of administering medications intravenously in midwifery practice.

Introduction

Medications should be administered only when the benefit of doing so outweighs any risks involved; this is especially relevant in pregnancy where the safety of the mother and baby is paramount. Whilst

Fundamentals of Pharmacology for Midwives, First Edition. Edited by Ian Peate and Cathy Hamilton.
© 2022 John Wiley & Sons Ltd. Published 2022 by John Wiley & Sons Ltd.
Companion website: www.wiley.com/go/pharmacologyformidwives

prescribing in pregnancy generally should be avoided, consideration of any concomitant conditions is important; managing the complexity of such health conditions requires access to a range of medications in different formulations or 'forms'. In order to develop medicinal products, a multistep pharmaceutical formulations process is carried out where the active drug is mixed with other components (Ukeje and Schmidt, 2013). The resulting formulations are available as liquids, solids or semi-solids which can be administered using a variety of routes either locally or systemically.

Systemic medications are those that enter the blood circulation and therefore can have an effect on the whole body, depending on the mode of action of the medication. The blood circulation carries the drug to the appropriate part of the body. For example, a beta-blocker used for the management of hypertension, taken orally, is absorbed and travels via the bloodstream through the cardiovascular system to target beta receptors that then relax blood vessels, so leading to a reduction in blood pressure. In contrast, medications that are administered locally or topically to the site where the action is indicated have a direct effect on that specific area only, with no effect elsewhere in the body. An example of a topical medication is an emollient for atopic eczema which is applied directly to the area of dry skin to cover it with a protective film and reduce water loss. There is no benefit of application of an emollient to any other organ in the body.

The choice of formulation to be prescribed depends on the physiological state of the woman, her age, the speed of action required and the route of administration to be used. Intravenous (IV) administration avoids first-pass metabolism, resulting in a very high level of bioavailability. IV administration is therefore the most efficient route, giving medication direct entry to the systemic circulation. Many drugs can be administered intravenously in different clinical situations, all of which have advantages and disadvantages; these will be discussed in this chapter.

Oral administration of medicines, in the form of tablets or liquids, is via the mouth and they are generally absorbed in the gastrointestinal tract (GI) before entering the bloodstream and travelling to their target site of action. Bioavailability varies from formulation to formulation as well as from drug to drug; consequently, the oral route is less potent and has a slower effect than the IV route. However, oral administration is the most convenient route for most people and is widely used in healthcare today.

Regardless of which formulation or route of administration is used, the woman's safety should be central to the process; all medications should be prescribed in accordance with the Royal Pharmaceutical Society (RPS, 2021) competencies and administered in accordance with the Nursing and Midwifery Council (NMC) Code (NMC, 2018). This chapter explores the different formulations available, the routes by which they can be administered, the rationale for prescribing formulations in specific conditions and the wider issues involved in decision making in midwifery practice.

Oral route of administration

Tablets

Tablets are available in several formulations.

Dispersible (soluble/effervescent) tablets

These are solid dosage forms that dissolve in a liquid (usually water) to form a suspension or solution (Lui et al., 2014). An example of medication in this form that may be taken by women during pregnancy or the postpartum period is dispersible paracetamol which can be used safely to relieve mild-to-moderate pain such as headache, pain from perineal trauma, engorged breasts or uterine 'afterpains'. These tablets are dissolved in water prior to ingestion. Taking paracetamol in this form is beneficial for women who may have difficulty swallowing whole tablets. However, women should be informed that after swallowing the solution, they should add extra water to the container and drink this too, to ensure that any residual drug particles have been administered. If they do not do this, they may receive an incomplete dose of medication which may be ineffective in relieving their discomfort (Underdown and Clipperton, 2021).

Soluble formulations make taking larger doses less challenging to administer as a solution and for many people, are easier to consume than a large tablet or multiple tablets. However, sometimes a particularly large volume of fluid is needed to ensure that the tablet dissolves fully, possibly up to 200 mL. The woman may find this difficult to ingest particularly if she feels nauseous or she finds the taste of the solution unpleasant. Adding flavoured squash or cordial to the solution may make it more palatable.

Enteric-coated/gastro-resistant tablets

These tablets have a special coating on the outside which does not dissolve directly in stomach acid; instead they dissolve in the more alkaline environment found within the intestines. This may protect the stomach lining from irritating effects of the drug and conversely may protect the drug from being destroyed by stomach acid. An advantage is that tablets with this type of coating take much longer to dissolve, sometimes up to 2 hours after ingestion. This makes them good for use with medicines that require delayed action (Singh et al., 2012). Drugs with enteric coating should never be crushed as doing so may cause the drug to be released into the body too soon or may cause irritation of the stomach lining; furthermore, the drug can be damaged by gastric acid, thereby reducing its effect. This makes them unsuitable for women who are unable to swallow whole tablets. Medicines with enteric coatings usually have the initials EC or 'gastro-resistant' at the end of their name. An example frequently prescribed to relieve moderate pain during the postnatal period is diclofenac gastro-resistant.

Modified-release (MR) and sustained/slow-release (SR) formulations

These are tablets or capsules that deliver the dose over a prolonged period as they have a long half-life. Capsules, along with tablets, are the most frequent formulations used to produce MR medications. MR and SR formulations are particularly advantageous for people with long-standing chronic disease as just one dose lasts for a longer time without the need for additional doses. A disadvantage of these formulations is that adverse side-effects cannot be readily resolved as the medicine is released over a prolonged period (Ummadi et al., 2013). Again, these tablets must never be crushed or broken in half as to do so would lead to an immediate release of the full dosage, which could be harmful. An example of medication that is available in MR form and may be used during pregnancy for the treatment of diabetes is metformin hydrochloride SR. The use of this medicine will be discussed further in Chapter 13.

Immediate-release (IR) tablets

As the name implies, these tablets act rapidly after ingestion for a specific time period depending on the half-life of the individual drug. A disadvantage of this type of preparation is that repeated doses may be required in order to maintain the therapeutic effect. However, there are also advantages in that due to the short-acting nature of the drug, any adverse side-effects are quickly resolved by not giving repeat doses. An example of an IR medicine is propranolol which may be prescribed for the management of migraine during pregnancy. This drug reaches peak plasma concentration in just 1–2 hours after administration and is very quickly distributed by the body (Electronic Medicines Compendium (EMC), 2021a).

Capsules

Capsules contain a solid dosage form of a medicine surrounded by a soluble shell which may be hard or soft in consistency. The medicine contained within capsules is absorbed by the body after the capsule coating has dissolved. The capsules may be gelatine, starch or liquid filled. Some women have a preference for capsules rather than tablets as they are usually quicker to dissolve once ingested and if they have a smooth shape, this may make them easier to swallow. However, they do tend to be more expensive to produce and if they contain animal products such as gelatine, this makes them an unsuitable choice for women who adhere to a vegan or vegetarian diet.

Episode of care

Sharon is 34 years old, has mild learning difficulties and is 28 weeks pregnant with her first baby. She has reported symptoms of a urinary tract infection and her GP has prescribed amoxicillin capsules 250 mg three times a day. When Sharon sees her community midwife, she tells her that her symptoms are not getting any better. On further discussion, Sharon tells her midwife that she is unable to swallow large capsules as they make her gag. She has spat out the prescribed capsules and doesn't know what to do. Her boyfriend suggested that she crush the capsules and dissolve them in water, but she has been unable to do that as the outer coating of the capsule will not dissolve. The midwife explains to Sharon that this is not a good thing to do as it will affect the way the medication works. The midwife contacts Sharon's GP and asks for the prescription to be amended to liquid form. She also telephones the local pharmacist where Sharon will collect her prescription and asks them to show Sharon how to measure the prescribed dose using the plastic spoon supplied. Once Sharon has the liquid form of her prescribed medication, she is able to take it three times a day and her symptoms subside. The midwife asks the GP to make a note in Sharon's medical records to avoid the issue in future.

Chewable tablets

Chewable tablets are compacted wet granulations of active ingredients (Dahab, 2020) as well as pharmaceutical excipients that disintegrate when chewed or dissolve in the person's mouth. They usually contain flavourings to enhance the taste and make them palatable so that an unpleasant aftertaste is avoided (Nyamweya and Kimani, 2020). They are not designed to be swallowed whole as, generally, they are bigger in size and therefore too large to swallow whole. They can be administered without water and, as such, are convenient; additionally, they may be a good alternative for women who have difficulty swallowing tablets whole, although they need to be able to safely swallow small particles.

Absorption occurs in the GI tract and begins as soon as the woman chews the tablet, breaking it down into smaller particles which dissolve. The increased surface area enables quick absorption which in turn causes increased bioavailability of the medication. This is a major advantage of this formulation and is therefore recommended for conditions where a fast response is required.

As with all medications, it is important to offer clear instructions to women and ensure that they understand them. It is essential that women know to chew the medication before swallowing it. Whilst it is unlikely to be harmful to swallow tablets whole instead of chewing them, many chewable tablets require the action of chewing to release the active ingredients (Food and Drug Administration Center for Drug Evaluation and Research, 2018). If, however, they are swallowed in their entirety, absorption and therefore effect will be much slower.

Many chewable tablets are available without prescription in pharmacies and supermarkets. Examples include multivitamins, antacids and antiflatulence tablets. An example of a chewable tablet which is safe to use in pregnancy and when breast feeding is Gaviscon Advance Mint Chewable Tablets, for the relief of indigestion or reflux (EMC, 2021a).

Buccal/sublingual formulations

Buccal and sublingual formulations are available as tablets or sprays. Sublingual medications are placed in the floor of the mouth, under the tongue, while buccal medications are placed in the buccal mucosa, the inner lining of the cheek, where they dissolve. Advantages of these routes are rapid effectiveness as first-pass metabolism is avoided and the highly vascular area enables quick absorption (Hood and Khan, 2020), providing local or systemic effects. As with all medications, it is important to give clear instructions to women; with the sublingual and buccal route it is important that they know not to swallow the medication as this would render it ineffective. If the woman's mouth is dry, she should be advised to take a drink prior to administration; additionally, she should be advised to avoid eating and drinking until the medication has completely dissolved. Repeated use of this route for medication administration may cause local irritation and the oral cavity should therefore be regularly reviewed.

An example of a buccal formulation is prochlorperazine, an antiemetic, which can be used in pregnancy up to the start of the third trimester (EMC, 2020a) after which it should be avoided due to the withdrawal symptoms that may occur in the newborn baby if the medication is taken by the pregnant woman 2 weeks prior to birth. An example of a sublingual formulation which may be used during pregnancy for the treatment of hypertension is nifedipine.

See Figure 6.1 for an illustration of sublingual and buccal routes.

(a)   (b)

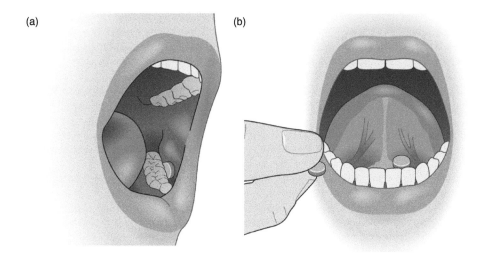

Figure 6.1   (a) Buccal routes and (b) sublingual.
Source: Peate & Wild (2017)/with permission of John Wiley & Sons.

Liquid formulations

Liquid formulations include medicines in suspensions, syrups, solutions and mixtures and are administered via the mouth and absorbed in the GI tract. They contain at least one active ingredient and are available either as powder which must be reconstituted before use or suspended throughout an excipient which supports stability until the medication is ready for administration. In addition, many liquid formulations contain sweeteners or flavourings to improve palatability. In order to ensure the active ingredients are adequately dispersed, the bottle should be mixed well before administration. It should be stored and disposed of in accordance with the manufacturer's instructions.

Liquid medications are prescribed for a variety of reasons, including for people with dysphagia or who dislike the taste of tablets, or because that is the most appropriate formulation for the condition. An example that is commonly prescribed in pregnancy is lactulose, a laxative for the treatment of constipation (EMC, 2017a).

Topical route of administration

Eye drops and ointments

Eye drops and ointments are administered to the anterior segment of the eye, either directly into the eye or onto the eye surface from where the active agent is absorbed through the epithelium of the conjunctival sac to produce a therapeutic effect (Henderson et al., 2018). If a higher drug concentration is required, topical administration is not appropriate as the active ingredients do not remain in the eye for a sufficient length of time, nor do they reach the posterior segment of the eye (British National Formulary (BNF), 2020).

Most of the active ingredient has a local effect; however, some may cause a systemic effect if excess medication has drained into the nasal cavity via the tear ducts (Vaalanen and Vapaatalo, 2017). This is an important consideration when women have contraindications to medications because of concomitant health conditions; an example is timolol which contains a beta-blocker, for the management of ocular hypertension; beta-blockers are generally contraindicated in those who have asthma or bradycardia (EMC, 2020b) and the use of timolol may cause bronchospasm or worsening bradycardia. To reduce systemic effects and therefore unwanted side-effects, following administration of eye drops, the woman should be encouraged to press on the lacrimal punctum for 1 minute to reduce drainage into the nasal cavity (BNF, 2020).

The eye has a mechanism to clear foreign substances, acting like a barrier in order to maintain visual acuity (Soni et al., 2019). This is an important function of the eye but can prove challenging when it comes to administering medications using this route. Encouraging the woman to close her eyes after administration of eye drops or blink after administration of eye ointment will help overcome this barrier.

Adherence with eye therapies can be poor due to difficulty in self-administration; however, eye drop dispenser devices are available to help administer drops from plastic bottles (BNF, 2020). If more than one drop is prescribed, deliver one drop and allow approximately 3 minutes before applying the second (Stanford, 2020). Advising women on how to use eye drops themselves or how to apply them to their baby is of the utmost importance, including emphasising the need for stringent hand hygiene before and after the administration of eye drops. When using eye ointments, temporary blurring of vision can occur and the woman should therefore be advised not to drive or operate machinery until her vision improves.

An example of an eye drop is chloramphenicol which is a broad-spectrum antibiotic prescribed for the treatment of conjunctivitis in either the woman or newborn baby. It should be stored upright in a cool, dry place, usually in a refrigerator; any remaining medication should be discarded after 5 days of treatment (EMC, 2017b).

Ear drops and ointments

Aural medications, either drops or ointments, are prescribed for the treatment of infection or to dislodge cerumen (ear wax) that is impairing hearing (BNF, 2020). They have a predominantly localised effect and as such, side-effects are minimal. Prior to prescribing ear drops or ointment, a thorough examination of the ear by a competent healthcare practitioner is essential, and the tympanic membrane must be visualised. If the tympanic membrane is ruptured, ear drops should not be prescribed as they will flow into the middle ear, resulting in an increased risk of ototoxicity (NICE, 2018).

Administration of ear drops or ointment can be challenging. As the woman needs to lie on her unaffected side, if possible, someone else should administer them and, following the application, the woman should be encouraged to remain in this position for approximately 3 minutes (Rosenfield et al., 2014). Gentle manipulation of the ear lobe will allow the drops to trickle into the ear canal. An example of ear drops is gentamicin for the treatment of otitis externia; although no safety data is currently available, it can be prescribed in pregnancy or when breast feeding if, on balance, the benefit of treatment to relieve infection outweighs the risk of, for example, a detrimental impact on the woman's hearing as a result of the actual infection (EMC, 2020c).

Ear drops should be stored in a cool dark area; they should be discarded after 28 days of first opening them (EMC, 2020c).

Nasal drops and sprays

Intranasal drops or sprays can be administered for the treatment of many conditions including nasal congestion, nasal polyps, rhinitis and sinusitis (BNF, 2020). They are absorbed by the nasal mucosa and cause a local effect with some systemic effect (EMC, 2020c); a systemic effect is thought to be higher with nasal drops, if treatment is prolonged or high doses are used (BNF, 2020). As with all medications, intranasal treatments should be administered at the dose and for the duration prescribed.

Before and after administration, good hand hygiene is required. The head should be tilted forward and downward prior to administering the treatment and following administration, the woman should breathe in gently through her nose (Scadding et al., 2017). She should be encouraged to clean the delivery device after each use. An example of a nasal spray is fluticasone for the treatment of allergic rhinitis.

Ointments, cream, lotions and gels

Cutaneous administration of medications is used when a local effect is desirable. Generally, topical treatment reduces unwanted systemic side-effects that may arise when other routes are used; however, adherence with treatment may be negatively affected because of inconvenience or difficulty with administration. Furthermore, the efficacy of topical drugs is dictated by their ability to infiltrate the epidermis of the skin; the 'vehicle' or base in which the drug is carried influences this infiltration (Waller and Sampson, 2018). In addition, skin hydration is important for drug absorption; the more hydrated the skin is, the easier it will be for drugs to penetrate it.

Four different 'vehicles' are used for the administration of topical agents: ointments, creams, lotions and gels. Many of these come with an applicator which should be used as instructed to help administer the medication dose to the appropriate area and reduce exposure of the hands/fingers to unnecessary substances. Furthermore, healthcare professionals should wear gloves when administering these products in order to reduce their exposure. Appropriate hand hygiene should be carried out before and after administration of products regardless of whether an applicator is used.

Ointments

Ointments are greasy preparations which are normally anhydrous, meaning they do not contain water, and are insoluble in water. They are more occlusive than creams and as such, they work by forming a protective layer on the skin surface, creating a barrier which prevents moisture loss. This makes them especially valuable in the treatment of chronic, dry lesions. Ointment bases consist predominantly of soft paraffin or a combination of soft, liquid and hard paraffin. As well as the active ingredient, they often have a mild anti-inflammatory effect. Women should be advised about the risk of fire associated with using any product containing paraffin, regardless of the percentage; they should therefore be advised to avoid smoking and naked flames due to the risk of clothing being contaminated and subsequently igniting (MHRA, 2020).

An example of an ointment is hydrocortisone for the management of contact dermatitis or mild-to-moderate eczema. Providing it is used sparingly and as prescribed, there are no known issues in pregnancy or when breast feeding (EMC, 2020d).

Creams

Creams are emulsions with a combination of oil and water, along with the active ingredient, which have a cooling and emollient effect on the skin. Generally, they are more acceptable to use as they are less greasy than ointments and are well absorbed into the skin, thereby reducing the chance of contamination of clothing. Many creams have an antimicrobial preservative unless the active ingredient or basis is intrinsically bactericidal and fungicidal; care is therefore required to avoid overuse which may result in allergic contact dermatitis (Waller and Sampson, 2018).

An example of a cream commonly used in the management of dry and pruritic skin is Dermol; there are no issues using it in pregnancy or while breast feeding (EMC, 2019a).

Lotions

Lotions are water-like suspensions containing aqueous medicinal preparations which cause cooling of the skin. For areas that have a lot of hair, lotions are often preferred as they can penetrate through the hair and tend to cause less mess. If skin is broken, care must be taken to avoid lotions containing alcohol as this can cause discomfort. An example of a lotion is Dalacin® T Topical which is used for the treatment of acne vulgaris. It is safe to use in pregnancy; no information is currently available for use when breast feeding (BNF 2020).

Gels

Gels have a high water content and contain suspensions of insoluble drugs as well as gelling agents, for example pectin, starch or carbomer, which encourage drug absorption (Kar et al., 2019). They are especially valuable for application to the face or scalp. An example is Dovobet® gel which is used for the treatment of scalp psoriasis. In pregnancy, the potential risk of using this medication is uncertain and therefore Dovobet gel should only be used when the benefit outweighs the risks (EMC, 2019b). Betamethasone, which is contained in Dovobet gel, passes into breast milk; however, providing it is used at the correct dose and not applied onto breast tissue, it is safe to use when breast feeding (EMC, 2019b).

Transdermal route of administration

The transdermal delivery of medication enables diffusion through layers of skin to either the blood or systemic circulation (Mishra et al., 2019). A limited number of medications can be delivered in the form of non-invasive patches which produce a steady rate of delivery by slowly releasing medication to cause a therapeutic effect (Mishra et al., 2019). The active ingredient is incorporated in a stick-on patch which can be easily applied and removed. Additionally, in the event of adverse effects, the patch can be quickly removed.

Appropriate hand hygiene should be performed before and after applying patches. Patches should be applied to clean, dry and non-hairy areas of skin. Areas that have any evidence of skin abnormalities, for example psoriasis or dermatitis, should be avoided as the patch may cause further harm. It is important to rotate the sites used to reduce skin irritation and damage to the epidermis.

An example of a patch that may be used during pregnancy is nicotine replacement therapy. Smoking cessation in pregnancy or whilst breast feeding is important and if possible, should be achieved without treatment as nicotine passes to the fetus, possibly affecting breathing and movement, and via breast milk (NICE, 2020). However, this is a balance of risks; the risk is thought to be less when using nicotine patches as an aid to smoking cessation than from second-hand smoke should the mother continue to smoke (EMC, 2020e).

Rectal application

The rectal route is used to administer medications that require a local effect, for example steroids for the treatment of ulcerative colitis, or a systemic effect, for example antiemetics in women who are vomiting or paracetamol in those who are fasting or unable to swallow. It is the preferred route of administering treatment for constipation and haemorrhoids. The rectal mucosa can absorb many soluble drugs into the blood circulation and therefore can be useful in many situations. However, absorption can be unpredictable, especially if faeces are present or the medication administered is an irritant causing defaecation, therefore interrupting the absorption process. Bioavailability is higher than with orally administered medications as approximately half of it is absorbed by the external haemorrhoidal veins and therefore avoids first-pass metabolism (Arivazhahan, 2019).

Some women may find administration of medications via the rectal route unacceptable due to embarrassment, discomfort, leakage and for cultural reasons (Hua, 2019). This is important to consider as it may impact on concordance. As with all medications, a clear explanation must be given to the woman as to why rectal administration is preferred and her understanding should be evaluated in order to obtain consent prior to administration. Furthermore, it is essential to maintain the woman's comfort and dignity throughout the administration procedure. The formulations available for use via the rectal route are suppositories and enemas.

Suppositories

Suppositories are solid pellet-shaped forms of medication often containing hydrogenated fats as well as the active ingredient. The fat dissolves at body temperature once inserted into the rectum via the anus, releasing the active medication which is absorbed by the rectal mucosa. It is therefore important when administering suppositories for systemic effect to ensure, if possible, that no faecal matter is present which may hinder absorption. Therefore, the woman should be asked, if possible, to defaecate prior to insertion of the suppository. The removal of faeces by the practitioner from the rectum may be necessary if the woman is unable to do so. For a woman who is constipated, this will be essential as there will be no beneficial effect of inserting a suppository into faeces in the rectum.

Suppositories have a pointed end (apex) and a blunt end; much debate around the correct way to insert suppositories is evident in the literature and as yet there is no conclusion (Peate, 2015). It is therefore recommended to follow local guidelines in conjunction with manufacturers' instructions and discuss with local experts prior to administering suppositories.

Suppositories are generally contraindicated in people who have had recent colon or rectal surgery and in those with undiagnosed abdominal pain. If appendicitis is the cause of the abdominal pain, peristalsis following insertion of a suppository may cause the appendix to rupture (Archer et al., 2003). They should also be avoided in women with cardiac arrhythmias or recent myocardial infarction as the vagus nerve, which innervates the heart (Davenport and Manji, 2018), is stimulated following insertion of suppositories, which may result in reduced heart rate and blood pressure, often referred to as a vasovagal syncope.

Enemas

Enemas are a liquid form of medication administered into the rectum to stimulate bowel action to treat constipation or in preparation for bowel investigations; the latter is used less commonly now due to the availability of oral preparations (Ness, 2017). Enemas can also be administered to treat inflammatory bowel conditions such as ulcerative colitis or Crohn's disease. In these conditions, the upper gastrointestinal tract is often affected so absorption of medications taken orally may be impeded, and the use of enemas is recommended (Lamb et al., 2019).

Enemas are presented in a plastic container with a small applicator which is inserted into the rectum. The volume varies from medication to medication and the enema is administered by inserting the applicator into the rectum and gently squeezing the container to expel all its contents while the woman is lying on her left side, ensuring local policy and procedures are adhered to. The woman should be encouraged to remain in this position for as long as possible to promote drug absorption.

85

Vaginal application

Pessaries and gels are available for vaginal administration.

Pessaries

Pessaries are generally solid forms containing the active medication and other excipients which can be administered using an applicator or fingers. In pregnancy, the use of an applicator is not recommended (EMC, 2017c). Using the body temperature and moisture within the vagina, the pessary dissolves and is gradually absorbed into the vagina, providing a local effect. As the peak plasma concentrations are low, medications administered intravaginally have no detectable systemic effects or side-effects. They can be used for candida vaginitis or dryness or to induce labour. Some prostaglandin drugs can be administered via the vaginal route, in conjunction with an oral dose, in order to induce labour. They should be placed as high as possible in the vagina and the woman should be advised to remain lying recumbent for at least 30 minutes.

Gels

Some antibiotics, if not tolerated using the oral route, can be administered intravaginally. An example is metronidazole for bacterial vaginosis although this should be used with caution in pregnancy (NICE, 2018). In women who are breast feeding, consideration should be given to stopping feeding or stopping treatment even though blood levels are lower than when used systemically.

Inhalation route of administration

Administration via inhalation delivers medication directly to the lungs with very few systemic side-effects. The large surface area of the respiratory membrane and extensive blood supply in the lungs allow rapid absorption and onset of action, justifying this route for the management of conditions such as asthma and chronic obstructive airways disease. Medications can be delivered by nebuliser or inhaler.

Nebulisers

Nebulisers deliver a fine aerosol of medication over a short period of time (approximately 10–15 minutes) deep into the lungs. The liquid medication is inserted into the nebuliser chamber and then, using pressurised air, it is converted into a fine aerosol of very small particles which the woman inhales through a mask or sometimes a mouthpiece. Instead of air, oxygen may be prescribed and used to 'drive' the nebuliser in women with asthma, providing their SaO_2 is >94% (BTS/SIGN, 2019).

An example of a medication administered by nebuliser is ipratropium. This is a type of anticholinergic which, absorbed locally in the lungs, causes bronchodilation of the smooth muscles, alleviating reversible bronchospasm (EMC, 2020f) and increasing air flow. Caution is advised in pregnancy and breast feeding due to the limited availability of data on ipratropium, and it should only be used after careful risk/benefit analysis (BNF, 2020). Salbutamol, some corticosteroids and antibiotics can also be administered by nebuliser; a mouthpiece rather than a mask is recommended for nebulised corticosteroids to reduce the risk of harm to the eyes or skin.

Nitrous oxide mixed with oxygen, as an inhaled gas, is self-administered via a mask or mouthpiece as an analgesic and is commonly used during childbirth. It also has anaesthetising properties; however, as it has a demand valve, the woman needs to be alert enough to use it which significantly reduces the chance of overuse. If used during delivery, however, it may decrease neonatal respiration (BNF, 2020); close monitoring is therefore essential.

Inhalers

Inhalers enable delivery of a single dose of medication from a pressurised container deep into the woman's lungs, and as such, the dose of inhaled medication administered is lower than that administered by nebuliser. Inhalation of medication such as bronchodilators and corticosteroids has local effects on the bronchial mucosa or smooth muscle in the respiratory tract (EMC, 2018). With some inhalers, an additional 'holding' device can be attached – a spacer – which is particularly useful for women who find it difficult to synchronise holding their breath on inspiration after actuating their inhaler. The addition of a spacer has been shown to be as effective as a nebuliser in the management of mild-to-moderate asthma exacerbation (BTS/SIGN, 2019). The inhaler is attached to the spacer, allowing the medication to be delivered into the chamber, and the woman can then inhale and exhale a few times as required, ensuring she receives the full dose of medication (Figure 6.2).

Inhalers are generally split into two groups – 'relievers' and 'preventers'; as the name suggests, 'relievers' are designed to treat acute exacerbations and should be administered as required. The most widely used in the UK is salbutamol, a β2 agonist, which acts by relaxing the muscles in the lungs, thereby allowing airway dilation and relief of symptoms. It is short-acting and therefore repeat dosing is required (EMC, 2018). 'Preventers' are administered daily or twice daily as prescribed, to reduce/prevent the exacerbation of symptoms and usually contain corticosteroids which reduce the inflammation and swelling commonly associated with chronic lung disease. An example of a preventer inhaler is beclometasone which is absorbed by the lungs. Mouth care is required after administration to reduce the risk of developing oral candidiasis.

The management of asthma to control symptoms is vital throughout pregnancy. The use of inhalers, both preventers and relievers, is safe during pregnancy and breast feeding (BNF, 2020) and should therefore be encouraged.

Injection route of administration

Intravenous (IV)

This is the administration of medication into the bloodstream usually via a peripheral vein. It is the fastest route of administration and is the most appropriate method to use during an emergency (such as a postpartum haemorrhage or eclamptic seizure). One hundred percent bioavailability is achieved following administration of medications, ensuring a rapid increase in therapeutic levels and therefore effect.

Intramuscular (IM)

This is the administration of medication directly into a muscle (Figures 6.3 and 6.4). Intramuscular injections lead to a slow, even absorption when compared with the intravenous route. Oxytocic

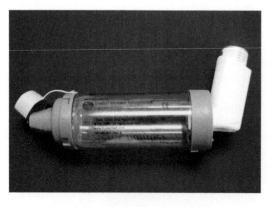
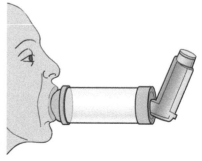

Figure 6.2   Aerosol holding chamber (spacer).
Source: Thomas (2015)/with permission of John Wiley & Sons.

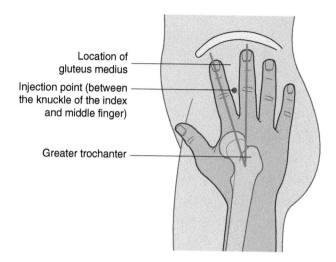

Figure 6.3   Location of the gluteus medius muscle.
Source: Peate & Wild (2017)/with permission of John Wiley & Sons.

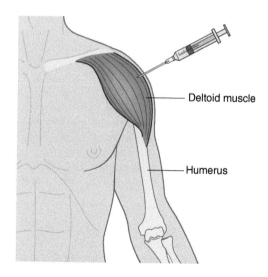

Figure 6.4   Location of the deltoid muscle.
Source: Peate & Wild (2017)/with permission of John Wiley & Sons.

drugs such as Syntocinon may be administered via the intramuscular route during active management of the third stage of labour.

Subcutaneous (SC)

This route of administration involves injecting medication just below the surface of the skin into the adipose (fat) layer of tissue. Sites for SC injections include the outer aspect of the upper arm, the abdomen within 1 inch of the umbilicus, the anterior aspect of the thighs, upper back and upper ventral gluteal area (just below the iliac crest on the side of the thigh) (Figure 6.5). This is a slower method of absorption and may be used to administer insulin and anticoagulants such as heparin (Lynn, 2011). Women can be taught to self-administer SC injections, for example insulin SC injections for the management of diabetes.

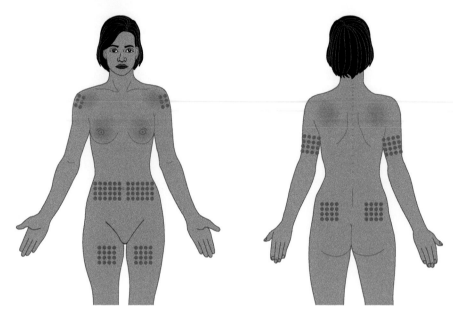

Figure 6.5   Subcutaneous injection sites.

Intradermal (ID)

This route of administration involves injection of a drug into the dermis of the skin just below the epidermis. It is much less commonly used than the IV, IM or SC routes and has the longest absorption time of all the parenteral routes. Intradermal injections may be used for sensitivity tests such as for tuberculosis, allergy and local anaesthesia tests. The advantages of using an ID injection for these types of tests is that it is relatively easy to visualise the body's reaction and the degree of reaction can then be assessed accordingly. Common sites used for ID injection are the inner surface of the forearm and the upper back beneath the scapula (Lynn, 2011).

Intraosseous (IO)

This is the injection of medication, fluids or blood products directly into the bone, so providing a non-collapsible entry point into the blood circulatory system. Administration of medication via this route is outwith the scope of midwives' practice. However, its use by obstetricians and anaesthetists has been described in the treatment of life-threatening conditions where access to the circulatory system is of major importance, such as massive postpartum haemorrhage, cardiopulmonary arrest, shock, sepsis, major trauma and burns. In these emergency situations, the use of drugs, blood products and large amounts of fluids is often required (de Vogel et al., 2011).

Conclusion

This chapter has provided information about different formulations of medication that are available and their various uses in midwifery practice. The reader should now understand why different formulations are available and have a wider awareness of the issues involved that will enhance their ability to provide safe, effective, high-quality care to women and their babies in the clinical setting.

Find out more

The following is a list of some common conditions that you may encounter during midwifery practice requiring a variety of medications to be administered via a variety of routes using different drug formulations. Take some time to write notes about each of the conditions. Think about the medications, treatments or therapies that the woman may need, how these might be administered, what formulations they are available in and which route of administration is most appropriate. Think about what may be used in order to treat these conditions and be specific about the pharmacokinetics and pharmacodynamics. Remember to include aspects of the woman's care. If you are making notes about women to whom you have offered care and support, you must ensure that you have adhered to the rules of confidentiality.

The condition	Your notes
Nausea and vomiting	
Eczema	
Asthma	
Vaginal *Candida*	
Constipation	

Glossary

Bioavailability   The degree and rate at which a drug is absorbed into the blood and circulatory system

Digest   The breakdown of material in the gastrointestinal tract that can then be absorbed by the body

Dispensing   Includes activities that occur between the time a drug prescription is presented to the pharmacy and the time the prescribed drugs are given to whoever collects them from the pharmacy

Excipient   An inactive substance that is included in a pharmaceutical dosage form not for a therapeutic effect but to aid the manufacturing process, protect, support or enhance stability of the product or for bioavailability or acceptability to the consumer

First-pass metabolism   A phenomenon of drug metabolism where the concentration of a drug, usually when given orally, is much decreased before it reaches the systemic circulation

Formulation   A combination of ingredients prepared in a specific way and used for a particular purpose

Half-life   The time it takes for the total amount of a drug in the body to be reduced by half

Ingest   To take something into the body by swallowing or absorbing it

Plasma concentration   The minimum concentration of a drug at the receptor site to achieve the required therapeutic effect

Systemic circulation   The system providing the blood supply to all tissues and organs in the body

Test yourself

Now review your learning by completing the learning activities for this chapter at www.wiley.com/go/pharmacologyformidwives.

References

Archer, E.A., Brady, C.L., Byrne, M. et al. (2003) *Medication Administration Made Incredibly Easy.* Lippincott, Williams and Wilkins: Philadelphia.

Arivazhahan, A. (2019) Principles and modes of drug administration. In: Raj, G.M., Raveendran, R. (eds) *Introduction to Basics of Pharmacology and Toxicology,* pp. 69–79. Springer: Singapore.

BNF (2020) *British National Formulary.* https://bnf.nice.org.uk/ (accessed January 2022).

British Thoracic Society/Scottish Intercollegiate Guidelines Network (2019) British Guideline on the Management of Asthma. SIGN Clinical Guideline. www.brit-thoracic.org.uk/quality-improvement/guidelines/asthma/ (accessed January 2022).

Dahab, A.A. (2020) Drug formulations. In: Hood, P., Khan, E. (eds) *Understanding Pharmacology in Nursing Practice*, pp. 57–88. Springer: Cham.

Davenport, R., Manji, H. (2018) The nervous system. In: Innes, J.A., Dover, A.R., Fairhurst, K. (eds) *Macleod's Clinical Examination*, pp. 119–150. Elsevier: Edinburgh.

de Vogel, J., Heydanus, R., Mulders, A.G., Smalbraak, D.J., Papatsonis, D.N., Gerritse, B.M. (2011) Lifesaving intraosseous access in a patient with a massive obstetric haemorrhage. *American Journal of Perinatology Reports*, **1**(2): 119–122.

Electronic Medicines Compendium (2017a) Lactulose. www.medicines.org.uk/emc/product/2796/smpc (accessed January 2022).

Electronic Medicines Compendium (2017b) Chloramphenicol eye drops. www.medicines.org.uk/emc/product/9662/smpc#SHELF_LIFE (accessed January 2022).

Electronics Medicine Compendium (2017c) Canesten pessary. www.medicines.org.uk/emc/product/2205/smpc#gref (accessed January 2022).

Electronic Medicines Compendium (2018) Salbutamol Easyhaler. www.medicines.org.uk/emc/product/6339/smpc#PHARMACOLOGICAL_PROPS (accessed January 2022).

Electronic Medicines Compendium (2019a) Dermol. www.medicines.org.uk/emc/product/5558 (accessed January 2022).

Electronic Medicines Compendium (2019b) Dovobet. www.medicines.org.uk/emc/product/5690/smpc (accessed January 2022).

Electronic Medicines Compendium (2020a) Prochlorperazine. www.medicines.org.uk/emc/product/11729/smpc (accessed January 2022).

Electronic Medicines Compendium (2020b) Timolol. www.medicines.org.uk/emc/product/10889 (accessed January 2022).

Electronic Medicines Compendium (2020c) Gentamicin. www.medicines.org.uk/emc/product/4218 (accessed January 2022).

Electronic Medicines Compendium (2020d) Hydrocortisone. www.medicines.org.uk/emc/product/1557/smpc (accessed January 2022).

Electronic Medicines Compendium (2020e) Nicorette. www.medicines.org.uk/emc/product/6437/smpc (accessed January 2022).

Electronic Medicines Compendium (2020f) Ipratropium bromide. www.medicines.org.uk/emc/product/3213 (accessed January 2022).

Electronic Medicines Compendium (2021a) Propranolol. www.medicines.org.uk/emc/product/5853/smpc (accessed January 2022).

Electronic Medicines Compendium (2021b) Gaviscon. www.medicines.org.uk/emc/product/73 (accessed January 2022).

Food and Drug Administration Center for Drug Evaluation and Research (2018) *Quality Attribute Considerations for Chewable Tablets; Guidance for Industry; Availability*. Federal Information & News Dispatch, LLC: Washington, DC.

Henderson, G., Flower, R.J., Loke, Y.K., Ritter, J.M., MacEwan, D., Rang, H.P. (2018) *Rang and Dale's Pharmacology*, 9th edn. Elsevier: St Louis.

Hood, P., Khan, E. (2020) *Understanding Pharmacology in Nursing Practice*. Springer: Cham.

Hua, S. (2019) Physiological and pharmaceutical considerations for rectal drug formulations. *Frontiers in Pharmacology*, **10**: 1196.

Kar, M., Chourasiya, Y., Maheshwari, R., Tekade, R.K. (2019) Current developments in excipient science: implication of quantitative selection of each excipient in product development. In: Tekade, R.K. (ed.) *Basic Fundamentals of Drug Delivery*, pp. 29–83. Academic Press: Malaysia.

Lamb, C.A., Kennedy, N.A., Raine, T. et al. (2019) British Society of Gastroenterology consensus guidelines on the management of inflammatory bowel disease in adults. *Gut*, **68**(Suppl 3): s1–s106.

Liu, F., Ranmal, S., Batchelor, H.K. et al. (2014) Patient-centred pharmaceutical design to improve acceptability of medicines: similarities and differences in paediatric and geriatric populations. *Drugs*, **74**(16): 1871–1889.

Lynn, P. (2011) *Photo Atlas of Medication Administration*, 4th edn. Lippincott, Williams & Wilkins: Philadelphia.

Medicines and Healthcare Products Regulatory Authority (2020) Emollients and risk of severe and fatal burns: new resources available. www.gov.uk/drug-safety-update/emollients-and-risk-of-severe-and-fatal-burns-new-resources-available (accessed January 2022).

Mishra, D.K., Pandey, V., Maheshwari, R., Ghode, P., Tekade, R.K. (2019) Cutaneous and transdermal drug delivery: techniques and delivery systems. In: Tekade, R.K. (ed.) *Basic Fundamentals of Drug Delivery*, pp. 29–83. Academic Press: Malaysia.

National Institute for Health and Care Excellence (2018) Bacterial vaginosis. https://cks.nice.org.uk/topics/bacterial-vaginosis/ (accessed January 2022).

National Institute for Heath and Care Excellence (2020) Smoking: stopping in pregnancy and after childbirth. www.nice.org.uk/guidance/ph26 (accessed January 2022).

Ness, W. (2017) Administration of an enema. www.clinicalskills.net/node/116

Nursing and Midwifery Council (2018) *The Code*. NMC: London.

Nyamweya, N., Kimani, S. (2020) Chewable tablets: a review of formulation considerations. *Pharmaceutical Technology*, **44**(11): 38–44.

Peate, I. (2015) How to administer suppositories. *Nursing Standard*, **30**(1):34–36.

Peate, I. (2021) *The Nursing Associate's Handbook of Clinical Skills*. Wiley: Chichester.

Peate, I., Wild, K. (2017) *Nursing practice: Knowledge and care 2nd edn*. John Wiley & Sons: Oxford.

Rosenfeld, R.M., Schwartz, S.R., Cannon, C.R. et al. (2014) Clinical practice guideline: acute otitis externa. *Otolaryngology – Head and Neck Surgery*, **150**(1 Suppl): S1–S24.

Royal Pharmaceutical Society (2021) *Prescribing Competency Framework*. Royal Pharmaceutical Society: London.

Scadding, G.K., Kariyawasam, H.H., Scadding, G. et al. (2017) BSACI guideline for the diagnosis and management of allergic and non-allergic. *Clinical and Experimental Allergy*, **47**(7): 856–889.

Singh, D.H., Roychowdhury, S., Verma, P., Bhandari, P. (2012) *A review on recent advances of enteric coating*. www.iosrphr.org/papers/v2i6/Part_1/B0260511.pdf (accessed January 2022).

Soni, V., Pandey, V., Tiwari, R., Asati, S., Tekade, R.K. (2019) Design and evaluation of ophthalmic delivery formulations. In: Tekade, R.K. (ed.) *Basic Fundamentals of Drug Delivery*, pp. 475–538. Academic Press: Malaysia.

Stanford, P. (2020) Instillation of eye medication. www.clinicalskills.net/node/120 (accessed January 2022).

Thomas, R. (2015) *Practical medical procedures at a glance*. John Wiley & Sons: Oxford.

Ummadi, S., Shravani, B., Rao, N.G., Reddy, M.S., Sanjeev, B. (2013) Overview on controlled release dosage form. www.semanticscholar.org/paper/Overview-on-Controlled-Release-Dosage-Form-Ummadi-Shravani/4f8cc6d6a4be78324b5c2e9179071a90aca53c2b (accessed January 2022).

Ukeje, A.M., Schmidt, K. (2013) *Predevelopment tasks for drug making*. www.pharmamanufacturing.com/articles/2013/017/#:~:text=Formulation%20is%20the%20process%20in,final%20medicinal%20product%20%5B6.5%5D (accessed January 2022).

Underdown, H., Clipperton, N. (2021) Drug formulations. In: Peate, I., Hill, B. (eds) *Fundamentals of Pharmacology for Nursing and Healthcare Students*, pp.91–107. John Wiley: Chichester.

Vaajanen, A., Vapaatalo, H. (2017) A single drop in the eye – effects on the whole body? *Open Ophthalmology Journal*, **11**(1):305–314.

Waller, D.G., Sampson, T. (2018) *Medical Pharmacology and Therapeutics*, 5th edn. Elsevier: St Louis.

Further reading

British Pharmaceutical Society. www.bps.ac.uk

National Institute for Health and Care Excellence (2018) Medications management. www.nice.org.uk/guidance/health-and-social-care-delivery/medicines-management

Nursing and Midwifery Council. www.nmc.org.uk

Royal College of Nursing/Royal Pharmaceutical Society (2019) Professional guidance on the administration of medicines in healthcare settings. www.rpharms.com/Portals/0/RPS%20document%20library/Open%20access/Professional%20standards/SSHM%20and%20Admin/Admin%20of%20Meds%20prof%20guidance.pdf?ver=2019-01-23-145026-567

Royal Pharmaceutical Society. www.rpharms.com www.pharmapproach.com/routes-of-drug-administration/

Chapter 7

Adverse drug reaction

Cathy Hamilton

University of Hertfordshire, Hatfield, UK

Aim

The aim of this chapter is to provide the reader with an understanding of the implications of an adverse drug reaction (ADR) for women receiving care during pregnancy, birth and the postnatal period.

Learning outcomes

After reading this chapter the reader will:
- Understand what the term ADR means and why it is important in healthcare
- Understand the different classifications of ADR
- Be able to recognise the signs and symptoms of ADR.
- Recognise the role of the midwife in caring for a woman who develops an ADR, including how to report an ADR.

Test your existing knowledge

- What is the definition of an ADR?
- What are the main symptoms associated with an ADR?
- What factors may contribute to an ADR?
- How do you report an ADR?
- How would you recognise an anaphylactic reaction?

Introduction

An ADR is defined as an unwanted or harmful response occurring after the administration of a drug (or drugs) that is suspected or known to be due to the drug (Medicines and Health Care products Regulatory Agency (MHRA), 2006). It is further defined as an unwanted response to a drug that occurs at the dosage normally prescribed for the treatment or diagnosis of a medical condition or for the modification of a physiological function (Tan, 2014). Since 2012, the definition has expanded to include reactions occurring as a result of error, misuse or abuse and suspected reactions to

Fundamentals of Pharmacology for Midwives, First Edition. Edited by Ian Peate and Cathy Hamilton.
© 2022 John Wiley & Sons Ltd. Published 2022 by John Wiley & Sons Ltd.
Companion website: www.wiley.com/go/pharmacologyformidwives

unlicensed medicines or those being used 'off-label' as well as the authorised use of medicine in normal doses (European Directive, 2010; Coleman and Pontefract, 2016).

The terms 'adverse reaction' and 'adverse effect' are often used interchangeably in the context of pharmacology but in reality, they reflect different viewpoints (National Institute for Health and Care Excellence (NICE), 2017). A drug may have an adverse effect but it is the individual who experiences the adverse reaction (Aronson and Ferner, 2005).

Global studies have found that 3–7% of all hospitalisations are caused by ADRs and 10–20% of inpatients suffer from ADRs (van der Linden et al., 2010; Edwards and Aronson, 2000). During pregnancy, women are at increased risk of an ADR (Kaufman, 2016). This is due to the physiological changes of pregnancy that may lead to an alteration in the way the body responds to a drug (da Silva et al., 2019). It is estimated that 80% of pregnant women will take additional medication to get relief from the discomforts and medical conditions associated with pregnancy (McElhatton, 2006). Drugs commonly used during pregnancy include antihypertensives, hypoglycaemic agents, analgesics, antibiotics, antiemetics and antispasmodics (da Silva et al., 2019).

For ethical reasons, extensive research into ADRs during pregnancy is limited but the studies that have been undertaken estimate a 10% incidence of ADRs amongst pregnant women (da Silva et al., 2019). It was found that ADRs in high-risk pregnancy are usually of mild severity. The risk was increased the less advanced in pregnancy the woman was and the use of parenteral drugs such as scopolamine, ceftriaxone and insulin demonstrated a higher risk for the development of ADR (da Silva et al., 2019). These findings highlight the importance of midwives being aware of the potential for women to experience an ADR when they are taking medicines to treat conditions occurring during pregnancy that they may never have taken before.

Classification of ADR

In order to differentiate between the different types of ADR, they are categorised into five subtypes using the mnemonic ABCDE (MHRA, 2015).

Type A reactions

Augmented and related to the pharmacological action of the drug. They are dose dependent and can be reversed by reducing the dose or withdrawing the treatment. Examples of type A reactions include the depression of respiration that may occur with opioids and excessive bleeding that may occur with warfarin. They also include reactions that are unrelated to the required pharmacological action of the drug; for example, a dry mouth may occur with tricyclic antidepressants. They are the most common ADR and account for over 80% of all reactions (Pirmohamed et al., 1998).

Type B reactions

Bizarre and idiosyncratic, meaning that they are related to the individual response rather than the action of the drug. They are uncommon in relation to type A and account for about 20% of all ADR (Pirmohamed et al., 1998). However, they are likely to be more serious with the potential to be fatal if they are not recognised and managed quickly. An example of this is the anaphylaxis that may occur with penicillin and the skin rashes that some women develop following antibiotic treatment.

Type C reactions

Chronic or continuing as they may persist for a long time. They arise from biological characteristics and can be predicted from the drug's chemical structure (Park and Mitchell, 2021). An example is osteocronosis of the jaw with bisphosphonates. These drugs, used to treat conditions affecting the bones, slow the rate of growth and dissolution, so reducing the rate of bone turnover.

Type D reactions

Delayed effects which usually only become apparent when some time has elapsed after drug administration. As a result, they can be difficult to detect. An example is leucopenia which may be noted up to 6 weeks after the administration of lomustine (a drug used to treat certain types of cancer).

93

Type E reactions

End of use reactions occurring when a medicine is stopped. An example is insomnia and anxiety following the withdrawal of benzodiazepines, the most commonly used sedatives (MHRA, 2015).

Recognising an ADR

Crouch and Chapelhow (2008) state that causes of ADR are often multifactorial, with common factors including:

- poor prescribing practices, including prescribing drugs that interact adversely with each other
- poor understanding of medicines management on the part of healthcare practitioners
- individual susceptibility to a certain medicine
- individual perceptions of the risks of using medicines.

The challenge of recognising an ADR in the first place is acknowledged (Beard and Lee, 2006). In maternity care, the midwife has the most regular and frequent contact with women throughout their pregnancies and therefore is well placed to notice that if something is wrong, it may be due to an ADR. It is important that any ADR is identified quickly in order to avoid the prescribing of further drugs to correct what is already a drug-induced disorder. The main challenge lies in distinguishing the ADR from the worsening of an existing condition or the development of a new condition which may or may not be pregnancy related. As Park and Mitchell (2021) highlight, in order to identify an ADR, the practitioner must first realise that it may be a possibility, otherwise potentially harmful signs may be missed. Drugs that pregnant women may be prescribed that most commonly cause ADRs include:

- diuretics
- tranquillisers
- antibiotics
- steroids
- antihypertensives.

Predisposing factors for ADRs

Certain individuals are likely to be more vulnerable to ADRs than others and pregnancy is already a risk factor. Other possible risk factors relevant to women during pregnancy and the postnatal period include the following.

- *Polypharmacy*: women who take several different medicines are more likely to experience an ADR as effects linked to one drug may influence another, causing a drug reaction.
- *Age*: individuals at either end of the life span are at increased risk of an ADR (Beard and Lee, 2006). Of relevance to midwifery is the fact that neonates are particularly susceptible because the way their bodies respond to drugs is different (Kaufman, 2016).
- *Gender*: pregnancy aside, women are already at greater risk of an ADR than men. The reason for this remains unclear but immunological and hormonal factors are believed to play a part as are differences in pharmacokinetics (Alder et al., 2016). The biological differences between the male and female body, including differences in body composition, weight, liver metabolism, gastrointestinal tract and renal function, may all influence drug action.
- *Genetic factors*, including those governing ethnicities, can determine an individual's unique susceptibility to an ADR and may lead to the drug acting in a distinctive and abnormal way. One example is that deficiency of the enzyme glucose-6-phosphate dehydrogenase is common in parts of Africa, Asia and southern Europe. This enzyme deficiency protects an individual's red blood cells from the harm caused by the antibiotics nitrofurantoin and quinoline, both of which are known to cause haemolytic anaemia (Alder et al., 2016).
- *Environmental factors*: it is thought that certain factors such as smoking, diet and alcohol consumption may have an influence on the way the body responds to a drug (Park and

Mitchell, 2021). For example, smoking is a known risk factor for many diseases, including cancer, cardiovascular disease and peptic ulcer. It is known to affect metabolic processes and by affecting liver enzymes, it may induce hepatic cytochrome. Alomar (2014) highlights that as many drugs are substrates, their metabolism can be induced in people who smoke, leading to a potentially significant decrease in pharmacological effect. It is not nicotine per se that instigates the drug interaction but rather tobacco which stimulates the body's sympathetic nervous system (Alomar, 2014).

- *Current state of health*: if a woman already has a pre-existing heath condition or develops one during pregnancy then this may predispose her to experiencing an ADR. For example, reduced renal function and impaired liver function may increase an individual's risk of an ADR (Alder et al., 2016). These reactions tend to occur more in the type B category. Other examples of health conditions making an individual more susceptible to ADR include glandular fever and human immunodeficiency virus (Kaufman, 2016).

Clinical consideration

Metabolism of codeine to morphine

The analgesic effect of codeine occurs following metabolism of codeine to morphine. The enzyme CYP2D6 is the main catalyst for the metabolism of opiates (Tharpe, 2011). Where individuals are genetically predisposed to having variations in the amount of this enzyme circulating in their blood, the rate of transformation from codeine to morphine will be altered. This genetic variation is believed to be present in up to 29% of the population (Tharpe, 2011). In people who are so-called 'ultra-metabolisers', codeine is rapidly converted to morphine, which may lead to an overdose. Where only a small amount of the drug is converted to morphine, the individual may be exposed to codeine toxicity without the desired analgesic effect (Smith, 2009). In the presence of this genetic variation in the woman who has just given birth, where there are high levels of circulating morphine in the body, this is readily transferred via breast milk to the baby, leading to a possible opiate overdose or toxicity in the baby (Koren et al., 2006). It is suggested that preventing neonatal opiate overdose can be achieved by prescribing non-steroidal anti-inflammatory drugs such as ibuprofen to breast-feeding women in preference to codeine, limiting codeine use following delivery to no more than 48–72 hours, ensuring close observation of women and breastfed babies when codeine is prescribed and obtaining genotyping when potential symptoms of overdose are noted (Koren et al., 2006).

Episode of care

Sita gave birth to her first baby in a midwife-led maternity setting after a 15-hour labour. She sustained a second-degree perineal tear during the delivery and was prescribed co-dydramol (containing 10 mg of dihydrocodeine and 500 mg of paracetamol per tablet), 1–2 tablets every 4 hours as required for perineal pain. Sita felt very drowsy following the first dose of this medication but attributed this to the hard work of giving birth. She was discharged home the next day but continued to take co-dydramol as prescribed as her perineum remained bruised and sore and it helped relieve her discomfort. Her baby breast fed very well and both mother and baby slept deeply between feeds.

On day 2, the community midwife visited the home to find Sita sleeping and her baby lethargic and drowsy and now uninterested in feeding. The midwife was concerned about the condition of the baby and referred both mother and baby back into the maternity unit for further observation. The paediatrician, having examined the baby, suspected morphine overdose secondary to ultra-rapid maternal metabolism of the codeine. This diagnosis was confirmed when the baby quickly became alert and active following administration of naloxone (an antidote to opiates). Sita underwent further blood tests, including one to detect a genetic polymorphism leading to ultra-rapid metabolism of codeine. The midwife documented the adverse event in Sita's records and notified it via the Yellow Card scheme.

Source: Based on Tharpe (2011).

Physical signs and symptoms of ADR

Symptoms may be relatively mild, for example red, itchy, dry or flaky skin, or severe and life threatening in nature, requiring the implementation of resuscitation measures.

Symptoms that may occur as an adverse reaction can include (but are not limited to):

- gastrointestinal bleeding
- heartburn
- fatigue/sleepiness
- nausea
- light-headedness or dizziness
- diarrhoea or constipation
- skin rashes.

In relation to skin reactions, a flat, red area covered with small bumps may develop on the skin. More severe symptoms include blistering and peeling skin, problems with vision and severe swelling or itching. Severe reactions include a condition called toxic epidermal necrolysis (TEN). This may be the result of an ADR to anticonvulsant medication or antibiotics. The main symptom is severe skin peeling and blistering leading to a large raw area that may ooze and later become infected.

Anaphylaxis is a sudden, life-threatening hypersensitivity reaction that requires immediate emergency treatment (NICE, 2020). Acute anaphylaxis may be caused by certain foods (for example eggs, nuts and fish), insect stings or contact with latex rubber. Penicillin is a drug notable for causing an anaphylactic reaction in susceptible individuals (Park and Mitchell, 2021).

Signs of an anaphylactic reaction include:

- feeling faint and light-headed
- feeling confused and anxious
- tachycardia
- wheezing
- clammy skin
- raised itchy skin (hives)
- collapse and loss of consciousness
- nausea and vomiting
- swelling (known as angio-oedema)
- stomach pain (Park and Mitchell, 2021).

Management of a suspected ADR

If a midwife suspects that a woman is demonstrating signs of an ADR, initial steps should include an investigation as to whether the drug concerned is known to cause a reaction, exclusion of other potential causes for the symptoms and establishing a link between the administration of the drug and the onset of symptoms.

Some ADRs, for example anaphylaxis following parenteral administration of medication, occur within minutes of the drug being given. Other symptoms such as TEN are due to delayed-type hypersensitivity and may occur days or even weeks after initial administration (Ferner and McGettigan, 2018). This means that ADRs, particularly those causing minor, non-threatening symptoms, can be challenging to diagnose as women do not always link the symptoms they are experiencing to a drug that they have taken. This highlights the importance of the midwife's role in informing women of possible adverse effects to medication that they are prescribed, making sure that they know what an ADR is and taking a careful drug history if women complain of symptoms indicating a potential ADR (Ferner and McGettigan, 2018).

These steps should lead to a quick identification and subsequent management of the ADR. However, communication needs to be undertaken in a careful and sensitive way to avoid women feeling overly anxious about experiencing an ADR. The relative risk of adverse effects versus the benefits of treatment needs to be emphasised by the midwife in these conversations.

Clinical consideration

Questions for the midwife to ask women if an ADR is suspected.

- Have you taken this drug before without experiencing an adverse reaction?
- Did the symptoms occur after the drug was taken?
- Did anything else change around the time of the suspected ADR, e.g. did you start any other treatment, develop any other medical condition?

Source: Based on Coleman and Pontefract (2016).

If the ADR is minor and non-life threatening, it is usually safe for the woman to be managed in the community setting under the care of the GP and midwife. The midwife should refer the woman to the GP, who will need to review and discuss potential treatment options with the woman. Options may include stopping the drug if the reaction is causing serious discomfort to the woman or at her request. If treatment for the original condition is still required, then the doctor will need to consider alternative medicines. If the drug is still needed for treatment, the dose may be reduced or the drug may be stopped temporarily to allow adverse symptoms to subside. Managing the symptoms of the ADR by prescribing another drug may be appropriate (for example, antihistamine may be prescribed to relieve itching of the skin). However, if other drugs are prescribed, the woman needs to be made aware of any potential risks and benefits of introducing further medication.

The ADR should be included in the woman's personal health records and reported through the Yellow Card scheme (NICE, 2017). The process for doing this will be described later in this chapter.

If a midwife observes an ADR in a woman that is considered serious or life threatening (for example, an anaphylaxis reaction following the administration of an intravenous drug or vaccine), they must remain with the woman and call for urgent help. In the hospital setting, this will be done by pressing the emergency buzzer and summoning the resuscitation team. In the community or stand-alone birth centre, this will be done by ringing the emergency services. If applicable, drug administration should be stopped by turning off the intravenous infusion. Emergency resuscitation and life support procedures may be required if the reaction is life threatening. See Chapter 23.

Anaphylaxis should be considered if all three of the following criteria are met (Resuscitation Council United Kingdom (RCUK), 2020).

- Sudden onset of symptoms and rapid deterioration of condition.
- Airway and/or breathing and/or circulation difficulties.

Box 7.1   Symptoms of anaphylaxis.

Airway problems	Breathing problems	Circulation problems
• Airway may swell, causing difficulty in swallowing and breathing • Throat may feel as though it is closing up • Voice may become hoarse • Stridor may be heard	• Increased respiratory rate and shortness of breath • Wheeze and persistent cough • Woman becomes tired due to effort of breathing • Woman may become confused due to hypoxia • Cyanosis (late sign) • Recognised as a blue/grey tongue or lips in dark skin • Respiratory arrest	• Signs of shock • Pale, clammy skin • Lighter skin on palmar creases and pale conjunctiva in dark skin • Tachycardia • Arrhythmia • Hypotension causing faintness, dizziness and eventual collapse • Loss of consciousness • Cardiac arrest

Source: RCUK (2020).

Episode of care

Management of anaphylaxis in a community setting

Tania is 25 weeks pregnant. She attends her GP surgery to receive her flu vaccination from the midwife. This is the first time she has received a flu vaccine. The midwife ensures that Tania knows why she is having the vaccine, highlights potential side-effects associated with the vaccine and gains consent for administration. After administering the injection in her upper arm, the midwife asks Tania to rest for 15 minutes before leaving the surgery.

Five minutes after receiving the vaccine, Tania starts to feel unwell. She feels faint and her breathing becomes laboured and wheezy. Tania has dark skin and when the midwife examines her hands, lightened skin is noted in the palmar creases. The conjunctiva of her eyes also appears pale. Tania feels clammy to the touch and swelling is noted around her lips. The midwife recognises the onset of an anaphylactic reaction and calls for urgent help from her colleagues. She stays with Tania and speaks calmly, telling her what is going on and what is being done to care for her and her unborn baby. The GP attends immediately, bringing with her the emergency vaccination pack while the receptionist rings for the emergency services and clearly states 'ANAPHYLAXIS' to the call handler. The midwife informs Tania that she is going to move her into another position that is better for the baby and then helps Tania to lie down and turns her on her left side to relieve aortocaval compression. Meanwhile the doctor draws up and administers an intramuscular dose of 1 mg of adrenaline in 1 mL. The midwife applies an oxygen mask in order to deliver high-flow oxygen, takes Tania's blood pressure (BP) and pulse and applies a pulse oximetry probe. The midwife stays by her side throughout, monitoring her condition by observing her demeanour and taking BP and pulse recordings every 5 minutes initially. The midwife ensures that contemporaneous records are maintained. The paramedic team arrives within 20 minutes and by this time Tania's condition has improved. She is transferred to the maternity unit with the midwife for continued monitoring and assessment.

The midwife reports the reaction via the Yellow Card scheme and ensures that details of the incident are recorded in the medical records. Tania is informed that she should tell healthcare professionals of this reaction when she is offered vaccination in the future.

Source: Based on NICE (2020).

- Skin and/or mucosal changes, for example itching, flushing, swelling and urticaria. For women with dark skin, flushing may be indicated by the skin adopting a red/purple hue with a burgundy overtone and swelling which pulls the skin tight and may lead to a smooth and shiny appearance (Mukwende et al., 2020).

Reporting ADRs

Despite modern medicines being tested systematically and extensively before becoming commercially available, prelicensing trials are usually not large enough to reveal important but uncommon reactions that medication may have on susceptible individuals (Ferner and McGettigan, 2018). In this context, reporting schemes are significant in developing our knowledge and understanding of drugs and the effect they may have on the body. This information is required in order to maximise therapeutic effects and minimise harm (Kaufman, 2016). However, despite the easy accessibility of ADR reporting schemes in the UK and elsewhere and their potential to reduce the number of patients being harmed by ADRs, the system is known to be underutilised, with less than 5% of ADRs being reported in practice (Coleman and Pontefract, 2016; Potlog Shchory et al., 2020). Inadequate ADR reporting may lead to the loss of important clinical information that has the potential to prevent harm to patients. Pharmacovigilance is defined as the scientific process of detecting, assessing, understanding and preventing ADRs or other drug-related problems (World Health Organization, 2002). Reporting on the basis of a suspected ADR is a vital aspect of pharmacovigilance. Coleman and Pontefract (2016) argue that if in doubt about an ADR, it is always best to submit a report.

The Yellow Card Scheme was introduced in the UK in 1964 following the thalidomide incident in the early 1960s when a significant number of babies born to women who had taken thalidomide to treat morning sickness were found to have significant congenital abnormalities. Through the Yellow Card scheme, data on all suspected ADRs is collected (including reactions to prescribed drugs and over-the-counter medications) and reported to the MHRA.

Yellow cards can be completed by healthcare professionals, service users, patients and their carers for any of the following treatments:

- all medicines
- vaccines
- blood factors
- immunoglobulins
- complementary medicines (herbal/homeopathic remedies) (NICE, 2017).

Reporting should be undertaken as soon as possible after a suspected ADR. The Yellow Card system can be accessed in many ways (Box 7.2).

Figure 7.1 shows an example of a standard Yellow Card form that a midwife may use to report an ADR. There is another version available for members of the public to use.

Box 7.2   The yellow card scheme (UK).

- Report online through the MHRA website: www.mhra.gov.uk/yellowcard
- Using a free mobile phone Yellow Card app
- In writing, to FREEPOST YELLOW CARD
- By email to yellowcard@mhra.gsi.gov.uk
- By telephone to the National Yellow Card Information Service: 0800 731 6789

Source: Based on MHRA (2021).

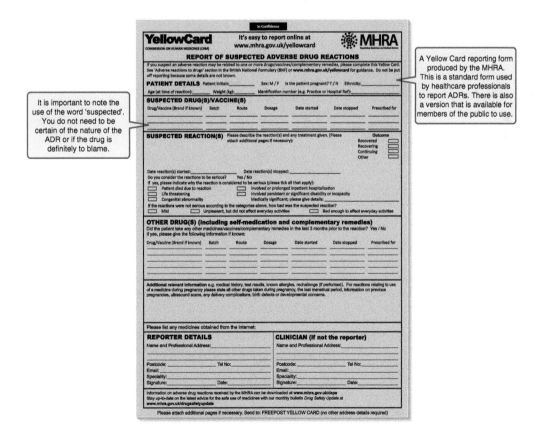

Figure 7.1   Yellow Card notification for suspected adverse drug reactions. Source: Yellow Card reporting form. © Crown copyright. Reproduced under OGL 3.0.

Skills in practice

How to complete a Yellow Card form

- The person completing the form should include their name and work contact details so that follow-up information can be obtained if needed. The MHRA will also acknowledge receipt of the form.
- As much information as is known about the drug suspected to have caused the ADR including dose and frequency. Dates of administration and, if known, the brand and batch number of the drug.
- Detailed information about the ADR, for example when it was first noticed, how serious it is, if any treatment was given and the outcome of the reaction.
- At least one of the following pieces of patient information: age, weight, initials, hospital number. This information is required so that the woman can be identified by the midwife and it does not breach client confidentiality.
- Any test results (printouts can be included).
- Medical history including allergies.
- Information about other drugs taken in the 3 months prior to the ADR (including any over-the-counter medicines and herbal remedies).
- State if the woman was not taking any other medicines at the time of the ADR.
- If no other relevant information is available, this should also be indicated on the form.

Source: NICE (2017).

Any suspected ADR should be documented in the woman's notes with a copy of the completed Yellow Card form included. Other forms of documentation may be required, depending on the medicines management policy in the organisation, for example, a requirement to report the incident to other members of the multidisciplinary team including the ward or unit manager or the pharmacy team.

Following reporting of the incident via the Yellow Card scheme, the MHRA will analyse and collate the relevant data. Reports are then produced and distributed widely to ensure that advice, recommendations and warnings are available nationally. Possible recommendations made by the MHRA depending on ADR include the following.

- Restrict subsequent use of the drug.
- Amend the status of the drug, for example from over the counter to prescription only.
- Update the warning information provided in patient and prescriber information leaflets.
- If risks are found to outweigh benefits of the drug, the MHRA may decide to remove the drug from the market.

Conclusion

Adverse drug reactions, how to recognise them, their impact on women's mortality and morbidity and the importance of reporting them have been discussed in this chapter. It is acknowledged that ADRs are an anticipated aspect of drug therapy. In view of this, it is important that the midwife is aware of the potential for a woman to experience an ADR which may have serious consequences for her health and the health and well-being of her baby. It is also known that pregnant women are at increased risk of experiencing ADRs. Midwives need to ensure that they are fully versed in any potential adverse effects and contraindications for medicines that pregnant women may be prescribed. They need to work in partnership with women and other healthcare practitioners (such as doctors and pharmacists) to ensure the earliest detection of an ADR in order to minimise harmful effects.

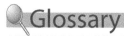

Glossary

Adverse drug reaction   An unwanted response to a drug that occurs at the dosage normally prescribed for the treatment or diagnosis of a medical condition or for the modification of a physiological function

Anaphylaxis   An acute allergic response to an antigen (e.g. an insect sting or medication) to which the body has become hypersensitive

Angio-oedema   Swelling of the deeper layers of the skin, caused by an accumulation of fluid. The symptoms can affect any part of the body, but swelling commonly affects the eyes and lips

Arrhythmia   When the heart beats with an irregular or abnormal rhythm

Glandular fever   A reaction caused by the Epstein–Barr organism. It is found in the saliva of infected individuals and can be spread through kissing and/or exposure to coughs and sneezes

Human immunodeficiency virus (HIV)   A virus that attacks the body's immune system. If untreated, it may lead to AIDS (acquired immunodeficiency syndrome).

Osteonecrosis   A disease affecting the bones, also called avascular necrosis, aseptic necrosis or ischaemic bone necrosis. The condition leads to the disintegration of bone cells. If the process involves bones situated close to a joint, it may lead to collapse of the joint surface, resulting in arthritis caused by the irregular joint surface

Stridor   An abnormal, high-pitched breathing sound. Caused by a blockage in the throat or voice box (larynx)

Toxic epidermal necrolysis   An acute-onset condition affecting the skin. It has the potential to be life-threatening. It may occur after commencement of a new medication

Urticaria   A rash of round, red welts on the skin that itch intensely, sometimes associated with swelling, caused by an allergic reaction, often to food or medication. Commonly known as 'hives'

Yellow Card scheme   The system in the UK for collecting information on suspected adverse drug reactions to medicines

Test yourself

Now review your learning by completing the learning activities for this chapter at www.wiley.com/go/pharmacologyformidwives.

References

Alder, J., Astles, A., Bentley, A. et al. (2016) Essential pharmacology: therapeutics and medicines management for non-medical prescribers. In: Nuttall, D., Rutt-Howard, J. (eds) *The Textbook of Non-Medical Prescribing*, 2nd edn, pp. 148–182. Wiley-Blackwell: Chichester.

Alomar, A.J. (2014) Factors affecting the development of adverse drug reactions. *Saudi Pharmaceutical Journal*, **22**(2): 83–94.

Aronson, J.K., Ferner, R.E. (2005) Clarification of terminology in drug safety. *Drug Safety*, **28**(10), 851–870.

Beard, K., Lee, A. (2006) Introduction. In: Lee, A. (ed.) *Adverse Drug Reactions*, 2nd edn, pp. 1–22. Pharmaceutical Press: London.

Coleman, J J., Pontefract, S.K. (2016) Adverse drug reactions. *Clinical Medicine*, **16**(5), 481–485.

Crouch, S., Chapelhow, C. (2008) *Medicines Management: A Nursing Perspective*. Routledge Taylor and Francis: London.

da Silva, K.D.L., Fernandes, F.E.M., de Lima Pessoa, T. et al. (2019) Prevalence and profile of adverse drug reactions in high-risk pregnancy: a cohort study. *BMC Pregnancy and Childbirth*, **19**: 199.

Edwards, I.R., Aronson, J.K. (2000) Adverse drug reactions: definitions, diagnosis, and management. *Lancet*, **356**(9237): 1255–1259.

European Directive 2010/84/EU of 15 December 2010, amending, as regards pharmacovigilance, Directive 2001/83/EC on the Community code relating to medicinal products for human use. https://eur-lex.europa.eu/LexUriServ/LexUriServ.do?uri=OJ:L:2010:348:0074:0099:EN:PDF (accessed January 2022).

Ferner, R.E., McGettigan P. (2018) Adverse drug reactions. *British Medical Journal*, **363** :k4051.

Kaufman, G. (2016) Adverse drug reactions: classification, susceptibility and reporting. *Nursing Standard*, **30**(50): 53–56.

Koren, G., Cairns, J., Chitayat, D., Gaedigk, A., Leeder, S.J. (2006) Pharmacogenetics of morphine poisoning in a breastfed neonate of a codeine-prescribed mother. *Lancet*, **368**(9536): 704.

McElhatton, P. (2006) Adverse drug reactions in pregnancy. In: Lee, A. (ed.) *Adverse Drug Reactions*, 2nd edn, pp.75–124. Pharmaceutical Press: London.

Medicines and Healthcare products Regulatory Agency (2006) Healthcare professional reporting of suspected adverse drug reactions. www.mhra.gov.uk (accessed January 2022).

Medicines and Healthcare products Regulatory Agency (2015) Guidance on adverse drug reactions: classification of adverse drug reactions. www.gov.uk/government/uploads/system/uploads/attachment_data/file/403098/Guidance_on_adverse_drug_reactions.pdf (accessed January 2022).

Medicines and Healthcare products Regulatory Agency (2021) Yellow Card scheme. https://yellowcard.mhra.gov.uk/the-yellow-card-scheme/ (accessed January 2022).

Mukwende, M., Tamony, P., Turner, M. (2020) *Mind the Gap. A handbook of clinical signs in black and brown skin.* St George's University: London.

National Institute for Health and Care Excellence (2017) Adverse drug reactions. https://cks.nice.org.uk/topics/adverse-drug-reactions/management/adverse-drug-reactions/ (accessed January 2022).

National Institute for Health and Care Excellence (2020) Anaphylaxis: assessment and referral after emergency treatment. www.nice.org.uk/guidance/CG134 (accessed January 2022).

Park, L., Mitchell, M. (2021) Adverse drug reaction. In: Peate, I., Hill, B. (eds) *Fundamentals of Pharmacology for Nursing and Health Care Students*, pp. 111–126. John Wiley and Sons: Chichester.

Pirmohamed, M., Breckenridge, A.M., Kitteringham, N.R., Park, B.K. (1998) Adverse drug reactions. *British Medical Journal*, **316**(7140): 1295–1298.

Potlog Shchory, M., Goldstein, L.H., Arcavi, L. et al. (2020) Increasing adverse drug reaction reporting – how can we do better? *PLoS One*, **15**(8): e0235591.

Resuscitation Council United Kingdom (2020) Management of anaphylaxis in the vaccination setting. file:///C:/Users/Owner/Downloads/MANAGEMENT%20OF%20ANAPHYLAXIS%20IN%20THE%20VACCINATION%20SETTING%20Guidance%20Aug%202021%20(2).pdf (accessed January 2022).

Smith, H.S. (2009) Opioid metabolism. *Mayo Clinic Proceedings*, **84**(7): 613–624.

Tan, K., Petrie, K.J., Faasse, K., Bolland, M.J., Grey, A. (2014) Unhelpful information about adverse drug reactions. *BMJ (Clinical Research Ed.)*, **349**: g5019.

Tharpe, N. (2011) Adverse drug reactions in women's health care. *Journal of Midwifery & Women's Health*, **56**(3): 205–213.

van der Linden, C.M., Jansen, P.A., van Marum, R.J., Grouls, R.J., Korsten, E.H., Egberts, A.C. (2010) Recurrence of adverse drug reactions following inappropriate re-prescription: better documentation, availability of information and monitoring are needed. *Drug Safety*, **33**(7): 535–538.

World Health Organization (2002) *The Importance of Pharmacovigilance.* World Health Organization: Geneva.

Chapter 8
Analgesics

Iñaki Mansilla
University of Hertfordshire, Hatfield, UK

Aim

This chapter aims to introduce the reader to pharmacological and non-pharmacological approaches that may be used by women during pregnancy, labour and the postnatal period.

Learning outcomes

Following completion of this chapter, you will be able to:
- Describe how pain impulses in pregnancy, labour and the puerperium are transmitted to the brain and the differences in the type of pain
- Demonstrate how analgesia is metabolised up until the point at which the analgesic is excreted
- Understand the role of the midwife in administering analgesia safely
- Demonstrate an awareness of the use of common analgesics in midwifery, their side effects and contraindications.

Test your existing knowledge

- What types of analgesia might you administer in pregnancy? List as many as you can.
- What are the main differences between pain during pregnancy and pain in labour?
- List as many non-pharmacological forms of analgesia as you can.
- What advice would you give to a woman in early labour with regard to pain control?
- What metabolic processes are involved in an intramuscular injection of pethidine?

Introduction

With the exclusion of pain experienced during labour and birth, it is not uncommon for pregnant women to experience a degree of pain during pregnancy and the puerperium. What makes labour pain different is that the pain experienced is not associated with a specific pathology but rather is perceived as a physiological process. This chapter discusses how analgesia can help with pain not only in labour but also during pregnancy and the puerperium, and how the physiological changes that occur during these periods play an important role for analgesia to be effective.

Fundamentals of Pharmacology for Midwives, First Edition. Edited by Ian Peate and Cathy Hamilton.
© 2022 John Wiley & Sons Ltd. Published 2022 by John Wiley & Sons Ltd.
Companion website: www.wiley.com/go/pharmacologyformidwives

Providing women with pain control can be complex and challenging. A thorough assessment and a clinical evaluation must be undertaken to provide the best pharmacological and non-pharmacological methods possible, thus improving the experience of pregnancy, labour and puerperium.

Inappropriate management of pain relief during the antenatal, intrapartum and postnatal periods may have a detrimental impact on the ability of women to care for their babies and themselves; anxiety, depression and psychological problems are associated with pain mismanagement (Virgara et al., 2018). Midwives must have a sound understanding of pharmacology and be able to explain how analgesia works and the possible side effects, as well as recognising the potential for adverse reactions to the women they are looking after.

It is well documented (Illamola et al., 2020; John and Shantakumari, 2015; Lupattelli et al., 2014; Servey and Chang, 2014) that many women will increase their consumption of over-the-counter medication or herbal remedies when pregnant; this chapter will therefore also explore non-pharmacological methods of analgesia (also referred to as complementary and alternative thera-pies). Such therapies include hydrotherapy, hypnosis, acupuncture/acupressure, aromatherapy and massage.

Midwives must be familiar with UK legislation regarding the administration of medicines, includ-ing the Human Medicines Regulation 2012, Schedule 17, and the standards issued by the Nursing and Midwifery Council (NMC, 2021).

Physiological changes in pregnancy and the puerperium that may require pain management

In pregnancy and the puerperium, pain may be experienced due to postural changes to accom-modate pregnancy or positions adopted while breastfeeding. In addition, increased body weight and mechanical load on axial joints and ligaments, pelvic floor changes, hormonal fluctuation, psychosocial issues or a combination of these (Zaghw et al., 2018) may lead to the perception of pain. These changes in pregnancy and the puerperium can affect all organ systems, including the respiratory system, gastrointestinal system and cardiovascular system; they also have an impact on hormone levels in the body and circulating fluid volume.

Hormonal levels

During pregnancy, concentrations of hormones in the body are dramatically changed, in particular progesterone and oestrogen. In a non-pregnant woman, the progesterone concentration level after ovulation is 10–35 ng/mL, whereas during pregnancy this typically rises to 100–300 ng/mL. Oestro-gen levels also increase significantly, as does oestradiol. These changes will affect the metabolism of analgesics in the body (Costantine, 2014).

Fluid volume

Throughout pregnancy, plasma volume and red blood cell mass increase by 40% of baseline. This increase in fluid leads to a reduction in maternal plasma protein and tissue concentration when compared to a non-pregnant woman, which will also affect the distribution of analgesia around the body. This reduction leads to a higher concentration of a free drug, which can be clinically significant in efficacy and toxicity (Feghali et al., 2015).

Cardiovascular system

Cardiac output increases due to the rise in heartbeats per minute and stroke volume to compen-sate for the diversion of 12–20% of cardiac output to the placenta (Meah et al., 2016). This is closely related to the fluid volume increment in which a greater volume may necessitate a higher initial and maintenance dose of drugs to obtain the therapeutic plasma concentration needed (Costantine, 2014).

Respiratory system

Due to an increase in hormonal changes, the respiratory system is also affected; there is nasal congestion and a significant increment of tidal volume by 30–50%, partially compensated by respiratory alkalosis, which affects protein binding of some drugs. There is therefore, the need for adjustment of the drug dose (Costantine, 2014). Moreover, certain medications (for example, steroids) may be more easily absorbed by pregnant patients (Pacheco et al., 2013).

Pain management approaches

Midwives will adopt both pharmacological and non-pharmacological pain management approaches that have numerous modes of action; a sound understanding of pain pathways is therefore necessary to understand and adapt the analgesia required for each woman and each situation, thus optimising the analgesic effect and reducing the potential for complications.

Transduction, transmission, modulation and perception are the processes involved in the pain pathway to the sensory cortex within the brain (Osterweis et al., 1987). First, pain starts in the tissue surrounding the traumatic stimuli, activating the nerve endings – this is known as *transduction*. The stimuli generate inflammation which involves a reaction from specific cell types (macrophages, monocytes) as well as the chemicals released from the mast cells (cytokines, chemokines, histamine, proteases, prostaglandins, leukotrienes, serglycin proteoglycans) (Chen et al., 2018).

Next, *transmission* occurs which is the communication between Aδ fibres (myelinated), C-fibres (unmyelinated) nociceptors, and the central nervous system via the spinal cord dorsal horn (DH) (Hudspith, 2016). Generally, a sharp pain is caused by activation of Aδ fibres, while dull, aching pain is caused by activation of C-fibres (Prescott and Ratté, 2017). Neurotransmitters such as glutamate and substance P act on the spinal cord DH, causing synaptic signalling in confluence with the relay neurons arriving at the somatosensory cerebral cortex (Yam et al., 2018).

Following this, *pain modulation*, occurs which is the process by which the body modulates the traumatic stimuli received when transmitted via the pain pathway process. Hence why individuals will react differently when subjected to the same painful stimulus. Most importantly, pain modulation explains the mechanisms of the actions underlying analgesia (Kirkpatrick et al., 2015). During modulation, the gate control theory of Melzack and Wall (1965) strengthens since the brain can inhibit (modulate) the pain transmission information carried by the pain fibres, should a larger diameter of afferent pain receptors be activated (Braz et al., 2014).

Finally, *perception* is the signal received by the brain which may be affected by different factors including cultural beliefs, emotions, past experiences, and age, thus altering the intensity of pain perception (Shankland, 2014) and influencing the descending inhibitory system via the spinal cord. This descending inhibition implicates the release of neurotransmitters that block or attempt to block the transmission of pain impulses, producing natural analgesia. The neurotransmitters involved in modulation are endogenous opioids (natural painkillers), which are endorphins and enkephalins, serotonin, noradrenaline, acetylcholine and oxytocin (Tocher, 2011). Since neurotransmitters release endogenous opioids, the perception of pain will differ depending on the number of endogenous opioids produced.

Pain transmission during pregnancy, labour and puerperium

It is of paramount importance to ascertain whether the pain experienced during this transition to parenthood is chronic or acute, related to pregnancy, labour, the puerperium or lactation period. This will help the midwife to understand how to pharmacologically treat the pain. Generally, this occurs by ruling out obstetric causes; non-obstetric causes are more common amongst pregnant women (musculoskeletal, rheumatological or neuropathic) and can be debilitating if not treated appropriately (Shah et al., 2015). In pregnancy, it is common for the woman to experience lower back pain, headaches or pelvic pain. In the puerperium, however, there is the added complication of reduced mobility, leading to an increased risk of venous thromboembolism (VTE), breathing difficulties or even pneumonia (Bisson et al., 2019).

According to Yam et al. (2018), there are three types of pain: nociceptive, neuropathic and inflammatory. Nociceptive pain can be further classified as visceral and somatic, and inflammatory pain as acute and chronic (Figure 8.1).

The use of pharmacological analgesia during pregnancy, labour (including early labour) and the puerperium will depend upon an individual's perception of pain and their capacity to cope with it. The pain in pregnancy and the puerperium is visceral, whereas pain associated with labour has two main components: visceral, which is when pain occurs during the first stage of labour, and somatic (Figure 8.2), which occurs during the second stage of labour (Labor and Maguire, 2008).

Pain management

Pain management in pregnancy and the puerperium can be a challenge for midwives and other clinicians since almost all medicines cross the placenta and are present in breast milk, therefore exposing the fetus to drugs (Castro-Garcés, 2019). Treating the symptoms will help women to manage their pain but failure to treat the pain will affect women, their environment and their babies. Pharmacological groups of analgesia most commonly used during pregnancy and the puerperium are analgesics, antipyretics, antibiotics, laxatives, and vitamin and mineral supplements (Orueta Sánchez and López Gil, 2011).

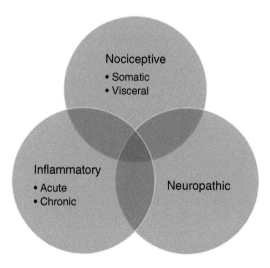

Figure 8.1   Types of pain in general.

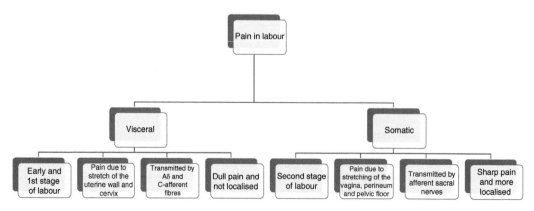

Figure 8.2   Types of pain in labour.

In pregnancy, the difficulty in evaluating pain could be due to various factors: some pregnant women and clinicians opt for a weaker analgesia to reduce risk to the fetus (Harris et al., 2017) and other clinicians are reluctant to prescribe pain relief, especially during the organogenesis stage of pregnancy (4–14 weeks of gestation). This inevitably leads to an increase in the use of over-the-counter analgesic and herbal remedies (Bisson et al., 2019); correct pain assessment during pregnancy and puerperium is therefore essential to reduce the risks of adverse outcomes for women and their babies. Castro-Garcés (2019) suggests that because of these challenges, whenever possible, a non-pharmacological treatment should be considered as an option to complement the prescribed pharmacological medicine, always using the smallest effective dose and less pharmacological interaction between drugs.

Additionally, during the first weeks of pregnancy, when organogenesis occurs, analgesia or any other medicine could expose the fetus to possible negative consequences and have an undesirable or adverse outcome. The European Medicines Agency (EMA) states that:

- from conception to 4 weeks, if a woman takes uncontrolled medication, this may result in early miscarriage
- from 4 to 16 weeks, organogenesis is at its maximum and medication can interfere with development, resulting in major birth defects. Furthermore, each congenital abnormality has its own critical period, such as a neural tube defect that affects gestation from 29 to 42 days
- from 16 weeks until delivery, medicines may affect minimal structural anomalies and also impact the growth of the fetus or cause neurodevelopmental disorders
- in late pregnancy or during delivery, medicines could physically affect the fetus by causing premature closure of the ductus arteriosus, acute renal insufficiency and drug withdrawal reaction
- during pregnancy, exposure to medicines or environmental agents (tobacco, air pollution or chemicals exposure (Nieuwenhuijsen et al., 2013)) may result in pregnancy loss or stillbirth (EMA, 2019).

BUMPS (Best Use of Medicines in Pregnancy) is a website that can support decision making regarding the use of pharmacological analgesia during pregnancy and the puerperium. This is a non-profit organisation funded by Public Health England on behalf of the UK Health Departments, providing scientific information to healthcare providers on the effects that drugs or chemicals used during pregnancy may have on the fetus.

Labour pain (including early labour) is experienced as a result of stretching of the cervix during the dilation period, ischaemia of the muscle wall of the uterus and broadening of the vagina and perineum in the second stage (Ebirim et al., 2012). During the latent phase (early labour) and first stages of labour, the pain stimuli are transmitted via the Aδ and C-afferent fibres through the sympathetic nerves to the sympathetic chain (Chu et al., 2017). Pain is conducted by the visceral uterocervical C-afferent fibres through the 10th, 11th and 12th thoracic vertebrae (T10, T11 and T12) and the first vertebra in the lumbar region (L1) and terminates at the dorsal and ventral horn, crossing the midline to the contralateral side (Hein, 2018). This type of pain is dull and not well localised (Labor and Maguire, 2008).

During the second stage of labour, the pain impulse is due to stretching of the pelvic floor, cervix, vagina and perineum. These stimuli are conducted via the sensory and motor pudendal nerve through the second and fourth anterior rami of the sacral plexus (S2–S4) (Njogu et al., 2021). This pain is sharper than the first stage of labour and better localised (Shnol et al., 2014).

Pain relief in labour is a key responsibility for every midwife and student midwife. Women whose pain is managed well typically require minimal support, and report positive experiences, whilst others may feel less able to cope and therefore request pain relief (Whitburn et al., 2014). Thus, inappropriate management of pain relief may not only influence women's satisfaction but also affect their birthing experience.

The World Health Organization (WHO, 2018) recommends that women should have access to the analgesia of their choice in labour, either pharmacological, such as epidural, systemic opioids (pethidine, fentanyl and more recently remifentanil (Nanji & Carvalho, 2020)), or non-pharmacological approaches, such as relaxation and massage techniques. A comprehensive list of opioid and non-opioid medication is shown in Tables 8.1 and 8.2.

Table 8.1 Systemic non-opioid analgesia (note: the route of administration and dosage will be the most common used in midwifery).

Medication name	Paracetamol	Aspirin	Ibuprofen	Diclofenac	Entonox
Medication type	Acetaminophen	Salicylate	Propionic acid derivate	Monocarboxylic acid	Oxygen and nitrous oxide gas (50%/50%)
Antidote	Acetylcysteine IV	Activated charcoal and sodium bicarbonate	Activated charcoal and sodium bicarbonate	Activated charcoal and gastric lavage within 1 hour of ingestion	Not available
Classification	P/GSL	GSL/P/POM	GSL	POM	P
Route of administration	Oral, rectal or intravenous (IV)	Oral	Oral or topical	Oral, intramuscular injection, rectal, topical, IV	Inhalation
Dose (oral) and frequency	0.5–1 g every 4–6 hours up to 4 g per day	75–150 mg once daily from 12 weeks onwards	300–400 mg 3–4 times a day, increase to 600 mg 4 times if needed	75–150 mg daily in 2–3 divided doses	Self-administration – as required
General side effects	Thrombocytopenia, skin reaction, tachycardia	Asthmatic attack, bronchospasm	Gastrointestinal discomfort, headache, hypersensitivity, nausea, rash, skin reaction	Oedema, skin reactions, hypersensitivity, nausea, vertigo, vomiting, diarrhoea	Disorientation, dizziness, euphoric mood, nausea, vomiting, paraesthesia
Breastfeeding	Amount too small to be harmful	Avoid – possible risk of Reye syndrome	Amount too small to be harmful but some manufacturers advise avoid	Amount too small to be harmful	No contraindication

Table 8.1 (Continued)

Medication name	Paracetamol	Aspirin	Ibuprofen	Diclofenac	Entonox
Absorption (A)	Has 88% oral bioavailability and reaches its highest plasma concentration 90 minutes after ingestion. Absorbed in the gastrointestinal tract	Rapidly by passive diffusion in the gastrointestinal tract and proximal small intestine	Rapidly absorbed in 1–2 hours from the upper gastrointestinal tract	Absorbed in the gastrointestinal tract but due to first-pass metabolism, only 60% of the drug reaches systemic circulation unchanged	Not available
Distribution (D)	The volume of distribution is 0.9 L/kg. 10–20% of the drug is bound to red blood cells. Binding to plasma protein is low when given at therapeutic doses	Binds to plasma protein and distributes rapidly into body tissues shortly after administration	Bound to plasma protein – the volume of distribution is 0.1 L/kg	99.7% bound to albumin in the plasma – the volume of distribution is 0.1–0.2 L/kg	Not available
Metabolism (M)	Mainly in the liver by conjugation with glucuronide, with sulfate and oxidation through the cytochrome P450 enzyme pathway	Hydrolysed in plasma to salicylic acid in the liver	Rapidly metabolised and biotransformed in the liver for major metabolites	Predominantly in the liver by conjugation with glucuronic and sulfuric acid and taurine	Not available
Excretion (E)	Excretion mainly in the urine. Less than 5% excreted as free and 90% excreted in 24 hours	Excretion through the kidneys by glomerular filtration (urine)	Excreted in the urine, accounting for more than 90% of the administered dose	Via metabolism. 60–70% is eliminated in the urine and 30% in the faeces	Not available

GSL, General Sales List; P, pharmacy; POM, prescription only medicine.

Table 8.2 Opioid analgesia.

Medication name	Codeine phosphate	Dihydrocodeine	Diamorphine hydrochloride	Morphine	Pethidine hydrochloride	Lidocaine 1%	Tramadol
Antidote	Naloxone hydrochloride	Naloxone hydrochloride	Naloxone hydrochloride	Naloxone hydrochloride	Naloxone hydrochloride	Naloxone hydrochloride	Naloxone hydrochloride
Classification	Controlled Drug (CD)	CD	CD	CD	CD	POM	CD
Route of administration	Oral/IM	Oral/IM	IM/IV	IM/Oral/IV	SC/IM	IM/SC	Oral
Dose and frequency	30–60 mg every 4 hours, max 240 mg per day	30 mg every 4–6 hours as required	(IM) 5 mg every 4 hours if required (IV)1.25–2.5mg every 4 hours	10 mg every 4 hours	50–100 mg, followed by again 50–100 mg, max 400 mg per day	5–15 mL of 1% lidocaine to a max of 20 mL for perineal suturing	50–100 mg every 4–6 hours, max 400 mg a day
General side effects	Nausea and vomiting, constipation, arrhythmias, confusion, dizziness, drowsiness, dry mouth, hallucinations, flushing	Nausea and vomiting, constipation, arrhythmias, confusion, dizziness, drowsiness, dry mouth, hallucinations, flushing	Nausea and vomiting, constipation, arrhythmias, confusion, dizziness, drowsiness, dry mouth, hallucinations, flushing	Nausea and vomiting, constipation, arrhythmias, confusion, dizziness, drowsiness, dry mouth, hallucinations, flushing	Nausea and vomiting, constipation, arrhythmias, confusion, dizziness, drowsiness, dry mouth, hallucinations, flushing,	Nausea and vomiting, constipation, arrhythmias, confusion, dizziness, drowsiness, nystagmus, psychosis, seizure	Respiratory depression and constipation but can also cause psychiatric disturbances. Important to note that more than 10% of the general population do not tolerate tramadol because of the adverse effects experienced

Table 8.2 (Continued)

Medication name	Codeine phosphate	Dihydrocodeine	Diamorphine hydrochloride	Morphine	Pethidine hydrochloride	Lidocaine 1%	Tramadol
Breastfeeding	Manufacturer advises avoid. Risk for toxicity in infant	Caution. Lowest effective dose for the shortest period. Monitor baby for sedation, feeding and poor weigh gain	Therapeutic dose unlikely to affect infant	Therapeutic dose unlikely to affect infant	Present in milk but not known to be harmful	Present in milk but not known to be harmful	Amount too small to be harmful but some manufacturers advise avoid
Absorption (A)	Absorbed by the GI tract, with a maximum plasma concentration 1 hour after	Bioavailability is low if administered orally due to poor GI absorption	Absorption is less than 35% with oral intake	In the upper intestine and rectal mucosa. Bioavailability is 80–100%	Bioavailability is 50–60% due to extensive first-pass metabolism. Less effective if administered orally	Absorbed across mucous membranes and damaged skin but poorly through intact skin	Administered with both negative and positive forms of both tramadol and the M1 metabolite detected in circulation. Bioavailability 75%
Distribution (D)	Volume of distribution is 3–6 L/kg, with extensive drug distribution into tissues	Via two-compartment model; one consists of plasma and tissues where distribution is instantaneous and the other consists of tissue where distribution is slower	Since diamorphine is considered a pro-drug for morphine, the volume of distribution of morphine is determined to approximately 1–6 L/kg	Volume of distribution of morphine is 5.31 L/kg, Bound to protein	Bound to plasma protein. Crosses placenta and breast milk	The volume distribution is 0.7–1.5 L/kg. Bound to plasma	In the range of 2.6–2.9 L/kg, has high tissue affinity. Bound to plasm protein

(Continued)

Table 8.2 (Continued)

Medication name	Codeine phosphate	Dihydrocodeine	Diamorphine hydrochloride	Morphine	Pethidine hydrochloride	Lidocaine 1%	Tramadol
Metabolism (M)	70–80% of the oral dose metabolised in the liver	In the liver by CYP 2DA into an active metabolite	Undergoes deacetylation (reverse reaction to remove the actyl group) via various esterase enzymes to generate active metabolites	Is 90% metabolised by glucuronidation by UGT2B7 and sulfation. Can be metabolised to codeine or normorphine	In the liver by hydrolysis to meperidinic acid followed by partial conjugation with glucuronic acid	Metabolised rapidly in the liver	Undergoes extensive first-pass metabolism in the liver by N- and O-demethylation and conjugation
Excretion (E)	Urinary excretion – 90% after 6 hours. Approximately 10% of the drug is unchanged	Renal elimination and urinary excretion	Via the kidney as glucuronides. About 7% via the biliary system into the faeces	70–80% excreted within 48 hours via urine, 7–10% in the faeces	Excreted in the urine. pH has a very important role as this will affect excretion	Via the kidneys with less than 5% in the unchanged form in the urine	Eliminated by the liver and the kidneys accounting for 90% of it. 10% through faeces. 30% is excreted unchanged

GI, gastrointestinal; IM, intramuscular; IV, intravenous; POM, prescription only medicine; SC, subcutaneous.

The Royal College of Midwives (RCM), in line with the WHO, states that midwives should provide women with information regarding pain relief options for labour and birth, including how analgesia works and the possibility of any side effects (RCM, 2018). It is important to emphasise that assessment of pain in labour can be challenging due to the nature of the pain and contributory factors such as psychological, emotional, social and cultural influences (Roberts et al., 2010).

Pain during the puerperium is also due to multifactorial causes, such as caesarean birth, assisted vaginal delivery, perineal pain, uterus involution or breastfeeding pain (Fahey, 2017). Controlling pain during the puerperium is vital, and analgesia should be commenced if requested; inadequate pain management postnatally could have severe consequences. New mothers may feel unable to look after themselves and their babies, which in turn could potentially affect bonding and successful establishment of breastfeeding (Deussen et al., 2020), or may contribute to postnatal depression and maternal exhaustion (East et al., 2012; Lim et al., 2020). As healthcare professionals, we advise women who are breastfeeding that analgesia does pass into the milk. However, using certain analgesics while breastfeeding may be safe, as the drug was found in the infant's body at less than 10%, and this is considered a safe option. This relative dose is established as a guide when taking analgesia and breastfeeding (Mitchell et al., 2020). If a woman is bottle feeding, analgesic advice regarding drug toxicity and safe use is meaningless, as the use of analgesia by women will not affect the infant.

Wong and Zaidi (2017) suggest that women should have a pain assessment prior to discharge from maternity units; they identified a link between pain at discharge and the need for extra support to minimise potential harm related to inappropriate use of more analgesia. Various authors, for example Boateng et al. (2019), Harris et al. (2017) and Wang et al. (2020), as well as professional bodies such as the Royal College of Obstetricians and Gynaecologists (RCOG, 2015) and the RCM (2018), recommend that women should be given information about both pharmacological and non-pharmacological analgesia. Non-pharmacological agents may include hot and cold compresses applied to the breast, comfortable positions for resting, acupuncture, music therapy and water immersion. Although this chapter's aim is not to discuss non-pharmacological analgesia methods or alternative medicines therapies in depth, the most common and most popular methods of pain relief will be mentioned.

Non-pharmacological approach to analgesia

In the UK, 57.1% of women reported that they use complementary and alternative medicine (CAM) products. However, there is a lack of evidence-based data on the safety and efficacy of these products. Therefore, it is important to understand that not all 'natural' remedies or other non-pharmacological analgesia used during pregnancy, childbirth and beyond are safe (Hwang et al., 2016). Many non-pharmacological treatments do not have statutory regulation regarding their use and women should be encouraged to assess the suitability of the practitioner performing/delivering the treatment. Women must be advised of the lack of high-quality studies into the effectiveness of complementary therapies and therefore the lack of robust evidence to support their use (Steel et al., 2015).

It should be acknowledged, however, that non-pharmacological treatments are sometimes suggested by GPs and other healthcare professionals to treat common minor disorders in pregnancy such as lower back pain or for relaxation in labour. Such treatments should only be performed by individuals who have completed additional education and training in this area. Although the National Institute for Health and Care Excellence intrapartum guideline states that pain relief strategies such as acupuncture, acupressure or hypnosis should not be offered, the guideline supports other strategies such as music or water. Women should, however, feel supported by their healthcare professionals in their choice of analgesia. Although data is limited, it is acknowledged that CAM may provide relief for women in labour even though it only has a modest effect (Arendt and Tessmer-Tuck, 2013).

Pharmacological approach to analgesia

Antenatal analgesia

Pregnant women must always be advised to speak to their midwife, GP, obstetrician or pharmacist before commencing any medication. Should analgesia be required on a regular basis, an assessment should be undertaken to exclude any adverse underlying cause for the pain. Moreover, the advice is to start with a non-pharmacological approach, progressing to pharmacological analgesia if necessary (Bisson et al., 2019).

Before 30 weeks of gestation

Paracetamol is the most frequently used analgesia in pregnancy due to its safety record. Paracetamol is effective in the treatment of mild-to-moderate pain in pregnancy before 30 weeks; although it crosses the placenta in its conjugated form, it does not appear to have an adverse effect on pregnancy outcomes or birth defects in therapeutic does (Kennedy, 2011). Non-steroidal anti-inflammatory drugs (NSAIDs) such as ibuprofen can also be used safely in pregnancy. There is conflicting information regarding the use of NSAIDs and teratogenicity in the fetus, therefore it is recommended that the lowest effective dose possible for the shortest duration is used (Bisson et al., 2019). Where moderate-to-severe pain, particularly of visceral origin, is more difficult to manage, opioids can be considered. Whilst few studies have evaluated the safety of using opioids antenatally, the UK Medicines Information service (UKMi, 2020) concluded that the use of opioids does not pose an increased risk of toxicity to the fetus. The most commonly used opioids in pregnancy are codeine, dihydrocodeine (DHC), tramadol and morphine, with codeine being the opioid of choice due to studies showing that it has no adverse effects on infant survival or congenital malformation rate (Nezvalová-Henriksen et al., 2011).

Pain experienced during pregnancy and childbirth is generally self-limiting, not persistent and requires analgesia only for a short duration (Komatsu et al., 2020).

After 30 weeks of gestation

While paracetamol is the principal drug used for pain relief throughout pregnancy, the UK Teratology Information Service (UKTIS) advises limiting analgesia for pregnant women over 30 weeks, especially NSAIDs and opioids. The most common NSAIDs used are ibuprofen, naproxen and diclofenac; limitation of their use in the third trimester is due to the potential effect on the fetus, neonatal pulmonary hypertension and premature closure of the ductus arteriosus, as well as oligohydramnios (reduced amniotic fluid) (Araujo et al., 2019). When prescribing opioids in the third trimester, the risk and severity of adverse effects in the fetus should be taken into consideration. For instance, long-term opioid analgesia in pregnancies over 30 weeks of gestation could lead to neonatal withdrawal symptoms. If used in labour, this may lead to neonatal respiratory depression (Bisson et al., 2019). Although studies on opioid analgesia in pregnancy are limited, oral or intramuscular morphine may be preferred over codeine (Babb et al., 2010).

Early labour and labour analgesia

Paracetamol is indicated for lower back pain and to alleviate pain as a result of uterine contractions. While its mechanism of action is not wholly understood, it acts predominantly by inhibiting prostaglandin synthesis in the central nervous system and peripheral action by blocking pain impulse generation (Bisson et al., 2019; EMC, 2018).

The Care Quality Commission (CQC, 2020) survey examined women's experiences of maternity care (17 151 participants) and highlighted women's preferences for pain relief once they were in established labour. The preferred analgesic was nitrous oxide (gas and air) (79%); the use of massage, hypnosis or breathing techniques was next at 34%; third was the use of epidural at 31%, followed by pethidine (or similar) accounting for over 25%. The least preferred analgesic was the use of water/birthing pool (20%).

Gas and air is a self-administered gas mixture of 50% nitrous oxide (N_2O) and 50% oxygen (O_2) and is an inhaled anaesthetic agent. It has been used since the 1880s for labour analgesia, and its discovery is attributed to the English scientist Joseph Priestley in 1772 (Broughton et al., 2020). Its analgesic effect is thought to result from the release of endogenous endorphins, dopamine and neuromodulators in the spinal cord. Nitrous oxide is inhaled and exhaled through the lungs, exhaling 99% of the unchanged gas as it does not remain in the body (Rooks, 2011). The benefit of nitrous oxide is that it is easy to use, produces rapid onset of pain relief, subsides quickly and women in labour can self-regulate its use. It has minimal side effects and a high satisfaction rate amongst women (Parsa et al., 2017).

Pethidine (hydrochloride) and diamorphine are opioid analgesics used in labour to alleviate moderate-to-severe pain (EMC, 2019). These opioids provide limited pain relief during labour and

Clinical consideration

If a woman has had an intraocular injection of gas due to retinal detachment surgery or has a severe respiratory disease such as COPD or chest trauma, the use of nitrous oxide would be contraindicated. Moreover, if a woman in labour is incapable of holding a mouthpiece due to persistent side effects (nausea, paraesthesia, dizziness, sedation), a different method of pain relief should be considered (water, paracetamol).

Episode of care

Shanice is in established labour with regular contractions for the last 4 hours and feels she cannot cope any more with the birthing pool and breathing techniques. The midwife discusses further options for analgesia with Shanice, and she decides to start using nitrous oxide. Shanice has never used it before but is keen to try. The midwife explains she needs to start using the gas at least 30 seconds before the peak of the contraction to allow for peak serum levels of nitrous oxide to coincide with the peak of the uterine contraction, therefore maximising the analgesic effect (Collins et al., 2012). Shanice is encouraged to inhale through the mouthpiece as deep as she can and exhale the gas slowly to maximise the effect. Shanice and her midwife also discuss the possible side effects before using the nitrous oxide, such as light-headedness and nausea, and how this can be minimised by stopping inhalation of the gas and breathing normally for a few minutes.

may have significant side effects for both the mother-to-be (drowsiness, nausea and vomiting) and the baby (short-term respiratory depression, drowsiness and withdrawal symptoms). Intramuscular administration of these analgesics together with an antiemetic can reduce nausea and vomiting but short-term complications (sucking and rooting reflexes (Aydin & Inal, 2016)) in the baby may arise if the woman plans to breastfeed (NICE, 2021). When providing information to women regarding the use of opioid analgesia, it should be advised that although there is negligible difference in the analgesia that diamorphine provides over pethidine, diamorphine has been found to prolong labour (Wee et al., 2014).

Pharmacological analgesia provided by an anaesthetist and monitored by midwives

Epidural

Epidural analgesia is the most effective method of pain relief during labour and childbirth. It is a nerve block technique achieved by injecting a local anaesthetic close to the nerve that transmits pain (Anim-Somuah et al., 2018). According to the CQC (2020), epidural analgesia was used considerably more when women experienced induction of labour, as women reported induction of labour to be more painful than spontaneous labour (47% of women whose labour was induced versus 19% of spontaneous labour). The NICE (2021) guideline recommends starting a test dose of 10–15 mL of 0.0625–0.1% bupivacaine with 1–2 micrograms/mL fentanyl; once an acceptable level of pain relief is established, continue analgesia until the third stage of labour and any perineal repair. Intravenous access should be secured before commencing regional analgesia and preload and a fluid infusion should be maintained throughout the epidural.

The recommended midwifery care plan after an epidural has been inserted is continuous monitoring of the fetal heartbeat with a cardiotocograph (CTG), checking the woman's blood pressure every 5 minutes for the first 15 minutes and then hourly thereafter. The level of the sensory block should also be assessed hourly. Epidurals are associated with a prolonged second stage of labour and the increased need for instrumental deliveries (NICE, 2017).

An epidural top-up typically consists of a preloaded syringe of analgesic, prescribed by the anaesthetist and administered via the epidural catheter when the woman requests further pain relief. This is different from a continuous infusion; the 'top-up' may be administered by a midwife who will assess the CTG and maternal observations following administration. The usual dosage for a 'top-up' is 10 mL of 0.1% bupivacaine + 2 micrograms/mL fentanyl (Ashagrie et al., 2020).

Combined spinal-epidural (CSE)

This approach is becoming more popular due to its quicker onset of action. It involves a single injection of mixed local anaesthetic and opioids into the subarachnoid space (spinal) and the insertion of an epidural catheter. This method of analgesia provides a rapid onset of pain relief compared with a conventional epidural and is particularly useful when women are in severe distress (Alleemudder et al., 2015). The frequency of observations and midwifery care plans should replicate those of a woman with epidural anaesthesia in situ.

Pudendal nerve block

In the event of delay in the second stage of labour (and where assisted delivery may be considered) and in the absence of epidural anaesthesia, a pudendal block may be offered; this is an effective method of pain relief providing analgesia to the vulva and anus. The obstetrician will infiltrate the trunk of the pudendal nerve with local anaesthesia, thereby inhibiting nerve transmission. The effectiveness of a pudendal nerve block is dependent on the clinician; it is not effective in the management of pain caused by uterine contractions or pain associated with the repair of lacerations, nor will it provide effective pain relief for manual exploration of the uterine cavity (Anderson, 2014). The midwife's role will be assisting the obstetrician to administer the local anaesthesia while explaining the procedure and reassuring the woman and her birth partner throughout.

Postnatal analgesia

Paracetamol should be the preferred analgesia during the puerperium, especially if the woman is breastfeeding her baby. Analgesia passes into the breast milk and assuming a normal infant breast milk intake is 150 mL/kg body weight/day, paracetamol will be proportionately present (0.6–1.5 mg/kg) if a mother ingests the recommended dose; this is well below the therapeutic dose used in infants which is 20–60 mg/kg daily (UKMi, 2020). The use of NSAIDs should be limited due to the lack of information regarding their safety around breastfeeding. However, ibuprofen and diclofenac are the NSAIDs of choice during the puerperium. Ibuprofen passes into the breast milk but at an extremely low level, therefore it is deemed safe to use while breastfeeding (Drugs and Lactation Database (LacMed), 2021).

Where stronger pain relief is required, for example following a caesarean birth, opioid analgesia should be considered. Newborns do, however, seem to be particularly sensitive to the effect of opioids and these should therefore be prescribed with caution. Codeine can cause drowsiness, depression of the central nervous system and possible death (Medicines and Healthcare products Regulatory Agency (MHRA), 2014).

Codeine was historically the analgesia of choice for pain relief in the puerperium, but according to the MHRA and EMA, its use in breastfeeding mothers is now contraindicated, following a case of morphine toxicity (an active metabolite of codeine) in a breastfeeding baby and three further fatalities in children under the age of 18. Tramadol and DHC may also be considered for use in the puerperium, but clinicians should aim for the lowest effective dosage to be given and for the shortest duration (ideally not more than three days) where mothers are breastfeeding. Treatment should be stopped if any adverse reaction or effect occurs, either to the mother or to the infant. Additionally, these opioid analgesics can be prescribed should the patient be intolerant to morphine (Bisson et al., 2019).

In the hospital setting, oral morphine (Oramorph®) is frequently used for women who have had a caesarean birth. Oramorph is compatible with breastfeeding and at therapeutic levels is unlikely to affect the infant (Joint Formulary Committee, 2021). Upon discharge, women should be advised to take paracetamol and/or ibuprofen if they require further analgesia.

Conclusion

The focus of this chapter has been largely on pharmacological analgesia used during pregnancy, labour and the puerperium, although non-pharmacological analgesia has also been considered. The importance of midwives and other healthcare providers being knowledgeable regarding the use of analgesia during pregnancy and childbirth has been highlighted.

Changes to the body's systems during pregnancy and the puerperium, and how a woman's body naturally adapts to these changes have been explored in this chapter. Moreover, the impact these changes have on the analgesia ingested and how women may need to alter the medication dosages to avoid harm to themselves, their fetuses and their infants is also framed within the chapter. Furthermore, the harm a drug can cause, depending on fetal age/development, has also been described.

Pain pathways have been described and the common drugs used in midwifery have been provided in extended tables with dosages, side effects, the four steps of pharmacokinetics and potential effects these drugs may have on breastfeeding.

Glossary

Antidote   A substance that can counteract a form of poisoning

Antipyretic   A substance that can reduce fever

Bioavailability   The rate and extent to which the active constituent of a drug is absorbed in the body through circulation

Cardiac output   The amount of blood that the heart pumps in 1 minute

Excretion   Elimination of the drug from the body, either as a metabolite (metabolised) or as an unchanged drug

Hormones   Chemical messengers produced by the endocrine system with a range of functions within the body

Neurotransmitters   Chemical messengers in the body, which signal from nerve cells to target cells, which can be muscles, nerves, glands, etc.

Organogenesis   A phase during embryonic development that starts at the end of gastrulation and continues until adulthood and encompasses the process of organ formation

Stimuli   Plural of stimulus. A stimulus is an event that elicits a sensory behavioural response in an organism

Subarachnoid space   The interval between the arachnoid membrane and the pia mater in the spine. Consists of cerebrospinal fluid, major vessels and cisterns

Toxicity   The level of damage that a drug can cause to an organism

Test yourself

Now review your learning by completing the learning activities for this chapter at www.wiley.com/go/pharmacologyformidwives.

References

Alleemudder, D.I., Kuponiyi, Y., Kuponiyi, C., McGlennan, A., Fountain, S., Kasivisvanathan, R. (2015) Analgesia for labour: an evidence-based insight for the obstetrician. *Obstetrician & Gynaecologist*, **17**(3): 147–155.

Anderson, D. (2014) Pudendal nerve block for vaginal birth. *Journal of Midwifery and Women's Health*, **59**(6): 651–659.

Anim-Somuah, M., Smyth, R.M.D., Cyna, A.M., Cuthbert, A. (2018) Epidural versus non-epidural or no analgesia for pain management in labour. *Cochrane Database of Systematic Reviews*, **5**: CD000331.

Araujo, M., Hurault-Delarue, C., Bouilhac, C. et al. (2019) Non-steroidal anti-inflammatory drug prescriptions from the 6th month of pregnancy: impact of advice from health authorities. *Fundamental and Clinical Pharmacology*, **33**(5): 581–588.

Arendt, K.W., Tessmer-Tuck, J. A. (2013) Nonpharmacologic labor analgesia. *Clinics in Perinatology*, **40**(3): 351–371.

Ashagrie, H.E., Fentie, D.Y., Kassahun, H.G. (2020) A review article on epidural analgesia for labor pain management: a systematic review. *International Journal of Surgery Open*, **24**: 100–104.

Aydin, Y., Inal, S. (2016) Effect of pethidine administered during the first stage of labor on the infants. *International Journal of Caring Sciences*, **9**(3): 914–922.

Babb, M., Koren, G., Einarson, A. (2010) Treating pain during pregnancy. *Canadian Family Physician*, **56**(1): 25–27.

Bisson, D., Newell, S., Laxton, C. (2019) Antenatal and postnatal analgesia. *British Journal of Obstetrics & Gynaecology*, **126**(59): e115–e124.

Boateng, E.A., Kumi, L.O., Diji, A.K.A. (2019) Nurses and midwives' experiences of using non-pharmacological interventions for labour pain management: a qualitative study in Ghana. *BMC Pregnancy and Childbirth*, **19**(1): 1–10.

Braz, J., Solorzano, C., Wang, X., Basbaum, A.I. (2014) Transmitting pain and itch messages: a contemporary view of the spinal cord circuits that generate gate control. *Neuron*, **82**(3): 522–536.

Broughton, K., Clark, A.G., Ray, A.P. (2020) Nitrous oxide for labor analgesia: what we know to date. *Ochsner Journal*, **20**(4): 419–421.

Care Quality Commission (2020) 2019 Survey of women's experiences of maternity care: Statistical release. www.cqc.org.uk/publications/surveys/maternity-services-survey-2019 (accessed January 2022).

Castro-Garcés, L. (2019) Analgesia en la paciente obstétrica. *Revista Mexicana de Anestesiologia*, **42**(3): 194–197.

Chen, L., Deng, H., Cui, H. et al. (2018) Inflammatory responses and inflammation-associated diseases in organs. *Oncotarget*, **9**(6): 7204–7218.

Chu, A., Ma, S., Datta, S. (2017) Analgesia in labour and delivery. *Obstetrics, Gynaecology and Reproductive Medicine*, **27**(6): 184–190.

Collins, M.R., Starr, S.A., Bishop, J.T., Baysinger, C.L. (2012) Nitrous oxide for labor analgesia: expanding analgesic options for women in the United States. *Reviews in Obstetrics & Gynecology*, **5**(3–4): e126–131.

Costantine, M.M. (2014) Physiologic and pharmacokinetic changes in pregnancy. *Frontiers in Pharmacology*, **5**: 1–5.

Deussen, A.R., Ashwood, P., Martis, R., Stewart, F., Grzeskowiak, L.E. (2020) Relief of pain due to uterine cramping/involution after birth. *Cochrane Database of Systematic Reviews*, **10**: CD004908.

Drugs and Lactation Database (2021) Ibuprofen. www.ncbi.nlm.nih.gov/books/ (accessed January 2022).

East, C.E., Sherburn, M., Nagle, C., Said, J., Forster, D. (2012) Perineal pain following childbirth: prevalence, effects on postnatal recovery and analgesia usage. *Midwifery*, **28**: 93–97.

Ebirim, L.N., Buowari, O.Y., Ghosh, S. (2012) Physical and psychological aspects of pain in obstetrics. *Pain in Perspective.* https://doi.org/10.5772/53923 (accessed January **2022**).

Electronic Medicines Compendium (2018) Paracetamol 500mg Tablets – Summary of Product Characteristics (SmPC). www.medicines.org.uk/emc/product/5164/smpc#gref (accessed January 2022).

Electronic Medicines Compendium (2019) Pethidine Hydrochloride 50mg/ml Solution for inejction. www.medicines.org.uk/emc/product/8941/smpc (accessed January 2022).

European Medicines Agency (2019) Guideline on good pharmacovigilance practices (GVP): Product or Population-Specific Considerations III: Pregnant and breastfeeding women. www.ema.europa.eu (accessed January 2022).

Fahey, J.O. (2017) Best practices in management of postpartum pain. *Journal of Perinatal and Neonatal Nursing*, **31**(2): 126–136.

Feghali, M., Venkataramanan, R., Caritis, S. (2015) Pharmacokinetics of drugs in pregnancy. *Seminars in Perinatology*, **39**(7): 512–519.

Harris, G.M.E., Wood, M., Eberhard-Gran, M., Lundqvist, C., Nordeng, H. (2017) Patterns and predictors of analgesic use in pregnancy: a longitudinal drug utilization study with special focus on women with migraine. *BMC Pregnancy and Childbirth*, **17**(1): 1–11.

Hein, A. (2018) Pain relief during labour and following obstetric and gynaecological surgery with special reference to neuroaxial morphine. https://openarchive.ki.se/xmlui/handle/10616/46194 (accessed January 2022).

Hudspith, M.J. (2016) Anatomy, physiology and pharmacology of pain. *Anaesthesia and Intensive Care Medicine*, **17**(9): 425–430.

Hwang, J.H., Kim, Y.R., Ahmed, M. et al. (2016) Use of complementary and alternative medicine in pregnancy: a cross-sectional survey on Iraqi women. *BMC Complementary and Alternative Medicine*, **16**(1): 1–7.

Illamola, S.M., Amaeze, O.U., Krepkova, L.V. et al. (2020) Use of Herbal medicine by pregnant women: what physicians need to know. *Frontiers in Pharmacology*, **10**(1483): 1–16.

John, L J., Shantakumari, N. (2015) Herbal medicines use during pregnancy: a review from the Middle East. *Oman Medical Journal*, **30**(4): 229–236.

Joint Formulary Committee (2021) Morphine. https://bnf.nice.org.uk/drug/morphine.html#breastfeeding (accessed January 2022).

Kennedy, D. (2011) Analgesics and pain relief in pregnancy and breastfeeding. *Australian Prescriber*, **34**(1): 8–10.

Kirkpatrick, D.R., McEntire, D.M., Hambsch, Z.J. et al. (2015) Therapeutic basis of clinical pain modulation. *Clinical and Translational Science*, **8**(6): 848–856.

Komatsu, R., Ando, K., Flood, P.D. (2020) Factors associated with persistent pain after childbirth: a narrative review. *British Journal of Anaesthesia*, **124**(3): e117–e130.

Labor, S., Maguire, S. (2008) The pain of labour. *Reviews in Pain*, **2**(2), 19.

Lim, G., Lasorda, K.R., Farrell, L.M., McCarthy, A.M., Facco, F., Wasan, A.D. (2020) Obstetric pain correlates with postpartum depression symptoms: a pilot prospective observational study. *BMC Pregnancy and Childbirth*, **20**(1): 1–14.

Lupattelli, A., Spigset, O., Twigg, M.J. et al. (2014) Medication use in pregnancy: a cross-sectional, multinational web-based study. *BMJ Open*, **4**(2). https://doi.org/10.1136/bmjopen-2013-004365 (accessed January 2022).

Meah, V.L., Cockcroft, J.R., Backx, K., Shave, R., Stöhr, E.J. (2016) Cardiac output and related haemodynamics during pregnancy: a series of meta-analyses. *Heart*, **102**(7): 518–526.

Medicines and Healthcare products Regulatory Agency (2014) Codeine for analgesia: restricted use in children because of reports of morphine toxicity. www.gov.uk/drug-safety-update/codeine-for-analgesia-restricted-use-in-children-because-of-reports-of-morphine-toxicity (accessed January 2022).

Melzack, R., Wall, P.D. (1965) Pain mechanisms: a new theory. *Science*, **150**(3699): 971–979.

Mitchell, J., Jones, W., Winkley, E., Kinsella, S.M. (2020) Guideline on anaesthesia and sedation in breastfeeding women 2020. *Anaesthesia*, **75**(11): 1482–1493.

Nanji, J.A., Carvalho, B. (2020) Pain management during labor and vaginal birth. *Best Practice and Research: Clinical Obstetrics and Gynaecology*, **67**: 100–112.

National Institute for Health and Care Excellence (2017) Intrapartum care for healthy women and babies. www.nice.org.uk/guidance/cg190 (accessed January 2022).

National Institute for Health and Care Exellence (2021) Pain relief in labour. https://pathways.nice.org.uk/pathways/intrapartum-care/pain-relief-in-labour (accessed January 2022).

Nezvalová-Henriksen, K., Spigset, O., Nordeng, H. (2011) Effects of codeine on pregnancy outcome: results from a large population-based cohort study. *European Journal of Clinical Pharmacology*, **67**(12): 1253–1261.

Nieuwenhuijsen, M.J., Dadvand, P., Grellier, J., Martinez, D., Vrijheid, M. (2013) Environmental risk factors of pregnancy outcomes: a summary of recent meta-analyses of epidemiological studies. *Environmental Health*, **12**(1): 1–10.

Njogu, A., Qin, S., Chen, Y., Hu, L., Luo, Y. (2021) The effects of transcutaneous electrical nerve stimulation during the first stage of labor: a randomized controlled trial. *BMC Pregnancy and Childbirth*, **21**(1): 1–8.

Nursing and Midwifery Council (2021) Practising as a midwife in the UK: An overview of midwifery regulation. www.nmc.org.uk/globalassets/sitedocuments/nmc-publications/practising-as-a-midwife-in-the-uk.pdf (accessed January 2022).

Orueta Sánchez, R., López Gil, M.J. (2011) Manejo de fármacos durante el embarazo. *Informe Terapeútico Sistema Nacional de Salud*, **35**(4): 107–113.

Osterweis, M., Kleinman, A., Mechanic, D. (eds) (1987) Pain and disability. In: *Pain and Disability: Clinical, Behavioral, and Public Policy Perspectives*. National Academies Press: Washington, DC.

Pacheco, L.D., Costantine, M.M., Hankins, G.D.V. (2013) Physiologic changes during pregnancy. In: *Mattison, D.* (ed.) Clinical Pharmacology During Pregnancy, pp. 5–15. Elsevier: St Louis.

Parsa, P., Saeedzadeh, N., Roshanaei, G., Shobeiri, F., Hakemzadeh, F. (2017) The effect of entonox on labour pain relief among nulliparous women: a randomized controlled trial. *Journal of Clinical and Diagnostic Research*, **11**(3): QC08–QC11.

Prescott, S.A., Ratté, S. (2017) Somatosensation and Pain. In: Conn, P.M. (ed.) *Conn's Translational Neuroscience*, pp. 517–539. Academic Press: New York.

Roberts, L., Gulliver, B., Fisher, J., Cloyes, K.G. (2010) The Coping With Labor Algorithm: an alternate pain assessment tool for the laboring woman. *Journal of Midwifery and Women's Health*, **55**(2): 107–116.

Rooks, J.P. (2011) Safety and risks of nitrous oxide labor analgesia: a review. *Journal of Midwifery and Women's Health*, **56**(6): 557–565.

Royal College of Midwives (2018) Midwifery care in labour guidance for all women in all settings. www.rcm.org.uk/media/2539/professionals-blue-top-guidance.pdf (accessed January 2022).

Royal College of Obstetricians and Gynaecologists (2015) Ovarian cancer. www.rcog.org.uk/globalassets/documents/patients/patient-information-leaflets/gynaecology/pi-ovarian-cancer.pdf (accessed January 2022).

Servey, J., Chang, J. (2014) Over-the-counter medications in pregnancy. *American Family Physician*, **90**(8): 548–555.

119

Shah, S., Banh, E.T., Koury, K., Bhatia, G., Nandi, R., Gulur, P. (2015) Pain management in pregnancy: multimodal approaches. https://doi.org/10.1155/2015/987483 (accessed January 2022).

Shankland, W.E. (2014) Factors that affect pain behaviour. *Journal of Craniomandibular & Sleep Practice*, **29**(2): 144–155.

Shnol, H., Paul, N., Belfer, I. (2014) Labor pain mechanisms. *International Anesthesiology Clinics*, **52**(3): 1–17.

Steel, A., Adams, J., Sibbritt, D., Broom, A. (2015) The outcomes of complementary and alternative medicine use among pregnant and birthing women: current trends and future directions. *Women's Health*, **11**(3): 309–323.

Tocher, J.M. (2011) Physiology of pain in labour. In: Mander, R. (ed.) *Pain in Childbearing and its Control: Key Issues for Midwives and Women*, 2nd edn. Wiley-Blackwell: Chichester.

UK Medicines Information (2020) Can opioids be used for pain relief during pregnancy? www.sps.nhs.uk/articles/can-opioids-be-used-for-pain-relief-during-pregnancy/ (accessed January 2022).

Virgara, R., Maher, C., Van Kessel, G. (2018) The comorbidity of low back pelvic pain and risk of depression and anxiety in pregnancy in primiparous women. *BMC Pregnancy and Childbirth*, **18**(1): 1–7.

Wang, Y., Li, H., Peng, W. et al. (2020) Non-pharmacological interventions for postpartum depression: a protocol for systematic review and network meta-analysis. *Medicine*, **99**(31): e21496.

Wee, M.Y.K., Tuckey, J.P., Thomas, P.W., Burnard, S. (2014) A comparison of intramuscular diamorphine and intramuscular pethidine for labour analgesia: a two-centre randomised blinded controlled trial. *British Journal of Obstetrics and Gynaecology*, **121**(4): 447–456.

Whitburn, L.Y., Jones, L.E., Davey, M.A., Small, R. (2014) Women's experiences of labour pain and the role of the mind: an exploratory study. *Midwifery*, **30**(9): 1029–1035.

Wong, A.M.W., Zaidi, S.T.R. (2017) Patients' understanding and use of analgesia for postnatal pain following hospital discharge. *International Journal of Clinical Pharmacy*, **39**(1): 133–138.

World Health Organization (2018) WHO recommendations: intrapartum care for a positive childbirth experience. www.who.int/reproductivehealth/publications/intrapartum-care-guidelines/en/ (accessed January 2022).

Yam, M.F., Loh, Y.C., Tan, C.S., Adam, S.K., Manan, N.A., Basir, R. (2018) General pathways of pain sensation and the major neurotransmitters involved in pain regulation. *International Journal of Molecular Sciences*, **19**(8): 2164.

Zaghw, A., Koronfel, M., Podgorski, E. et al. (2018) *Pain management for pregnant women in the opioid crisis era*. www.intechopen.com/chapters/62377 (accessed January 2022).

Chapter 9

Antibiotics and antibacterials

Amanda Waterman

University of Hertfordshire

Aim

The aim of this chapter is to develop the reader's knowledge and understanding of the common uses of antibiotics and antibacterials in obstetric and midwifery practice.

Learning outcomes

- Understand how pathogens cause infection and how antibiotic treatments can prevent and treat infection.
- Understand the classifications of antibacterial medication and be able to explain their actions and associated side-effects.
- Explore and reflect on the clinical considerations and administration of antibiotics and the impact on the woman's recovery from infection.
- Understand the midwife's role in managing antibiotic treatments and the ongoing health promotion in education supporting women undergoing antibiotic treatments and combatting antibiotic resistance.

Test your existing knowledge

- What is the difference between bacteriostatic and bactericidal treatments?
- What is the current evidence surrounding the prescribing and administration of antibiotics during pregnancy?
- What do you know about the use of prophylactic antibiotics and their effectiveness in preventing infection?
- What are the most common infections during pregnancy and what is the national guidance on how to tackle these infections?
- Which antibiotics are offered after obstetric or gynaecological surgical procedures?

Introduction

Antibiotics, described as a 'small molecule that antagonises the growth of other microbes', were first developed in 1941 by Selman Waksman, a scientist studying bacteriology in the US after the 1928

Fundamentals of Pharmacology for Midwives, First Edition. Edited by Ian Peate and Cathy Hamilton.
© 2022 John Wiley & Sons Ltd. Published 2022 by John Wiley & Sons Ltd.
Companion website: www.wiley.com/go/pharmacologyformidwives

discovery of penicillin by Alexander Fleming (Strohl et al., 2001; Clardy et al., 2009; Gaynes, 2017). The developmental period known as the Antibiotic Golden Age, from 1945 to 1990, is when most of the antibiotics we use today were originally developed from soil bacteria. Antibiotics are created through a complex process whereby living cells produce metabolites, which underpin the basis and origins of drug manufacturing (Ferro et al., 2008; Nesme et al., 2015; Mansur-Ali et al., 2018). Up until 2002, it was thought that 70 out of the 90 antibiotics originated from a natural source (Newman et al., 2003).

Antibacterial and antibiotic use in treating and preventing global bacterial infections such as pneumonia and tuberculous has seen significantly reduced mortality rates over the decades (Gattarello et al., 2014). Deaths from childbirth-related sepsis were 3 in 100 before antibiotics were used but are now less than 3 in 100 000 (Ashiru-Oredope and Hopkins, 2015). The Parliamentary Office of Science and Technology (POST, 2017) identifies infectious diseases as contributing to a significant burden to the UK's health and economic systems, causing 7% of all deaths and being responsible for a large proportion of sick days.

Terminology and differences between micro-organisms

Pathogens, such as fungi and viruses, require treatment with differently acting medications such as antifungals and antivirals respectively. These medications will not work on bacterial infections, just as antibiotics will not work on viral and fungal infections. Therefore, it is important to identify the type of infection prior to treatment with antibiotics to avoid creating bacterial and antibiotic resistance (Table 9.1).

Table 9.1   The effect of antibacterial, antifungal and antiviral medications on deactivation of the pathogen and the common medication groups and examples.

Classification	Action	Group	Example
Antibacterial	Disrupt cell wall synthesis	Beta-lactams	Benzylpenicellin
		Cephalosporins (5 generations)	Cephalexin
		Carbapenems	Imipenem
	Folate interference	Sulphonamides	Trimethoprim
			Co-trimoxazole
	Bacterial DNA inhibition	Quinolones	Ciprofloxacin
	Protein synthesis interference	Tetracyclines	Tetracycline
		Chloramphenicol	
		Aminoglycosides	Gentamycin
		Macrolides	Erythromycin
		Lincosamides	Clindamycin
Antifugal (AF)	Cell membrane damage	Polyene AF	Nystatin
		Imidazole AF	Clotrimazole
		Triazole AF	Fluconazole
Antiviral	Potential inhibition of DNA replication	Anti-HIV	Abacavir

Source: Peate & Hill (2021)/with permission of John Wiley & Sons.

Antibiotic resistance and the global impact

Antibiotic resistance has arisen over recent decades due to poor prescribing and overuse of antibiotics, such as the inappropriate use of antibiotics to treat viral and fungal infections, not completing a course of antibiotics or prescribing the incorrect minimum inhibitory concentration (MIC) or minimum bactericidal concentration (MBC) that does not equal or exceed the breakpoint at which bacteria are either inhibited in bacterial growth or destroyed. The untreated bacteria can genetically mutate or gain the ability to actively pump the medicine out of the cell, rendering the medicine ineffective and thereby creating resistance to the antibiotic (Kahlmeter, 2016). The resistant bacteria continue to multiply and pass on the resistance to neighbouring bacteria, even to those from different strains using a process called *horizontal gene transfer* and in doing so, further promoting resistance to antibacterials (Wilson et al., 2019). Resistant hospital-based infections such as *Clostridium difficile* and methicillin-resistant *Staphylococcus aureus* (MRSA) can emerge through this process and via inadequate hygiene practices of healthcare professionals can be spread further to susceptible hosts through skin-to-skin transmission (Wilson et al., 2019).

Antibiotic resistance is a global concern. In Europe, 25 000 deaths each year and 2.5 million hospital admissions occur as a result of antibiotic resistance it is estimated that a failure to address this issue will result in 10 million deaths globally by the year 2050 (Bergstrom et al., 2013; CDC, 2019). It is estimated that 70% of the world's bacteria have developed resistance to antibiotics (Public Health England (PHE), 2019b).

The World Health Organization (WHO) has reported that new resistant mechanisms in bacteria are causing difficulties in treating common infections which were previously treatable. This is resulting in delays in recovery, prolonged hospital stays and increased mortality and economic burdens on patients and their families (WHO, 2020). Therefore, the WHO has urgently requested a behavioural change in the way the medical profession prescribes antibiotics and to be more vigilant in infection preventive measures such as hand hygiene, practising safe sex and good food hygiene (WHO, 2020).

When antibiotics are no longer effective against a bacterial infection, more expensive medicines, such as intravenous immunoglobulins (IV Igs), are needed to combat the infection, adding further costs (Greer et al., 2019). Furthermore, antibiotic resistance hinders the advancement of modern medicine; for example, recovery from surgeries such as caesarean sections, organ transplants and chemotherapy are at risk without effective antibacterial treatments in preventing infections (WHO, 2020).

Clinical consideration

Here is a summary of how midwives can advise women on how to prevent and avoid common infections during pregnancy.

- Optimal nutrition: anaemia affects the immune system, so encourage an iron-rich diet and offer supplements if required. Anaemia also increases the risk of septicaemia
- Smoking cessation to minimise respiratory infections and influenza symptoms
- Personal hygiene and hand washing
- Offer vaccinations: pertussis and influenza
- Discuss foods to avoid in pregnancy that could lead to infections such as *Listeria* and *E. coli*.

Are there any other ways of preventing infections during pregnancy?
(Furber et al., 2017)

Antibacterial stewardship programme

The National Institute for Health and Care Excellence (NICE) Antibacterial Stewardship Programme offers guidance for clinicians working in all care sectors in the UK on systems and processes for the effective use of antibacterials. It provides guidance in the identification of various bacterial pathogens and the appropriate antibacterial agent to combat the infection with the minimal adverse events relating to their use, including the development of antimicrobial resistance (NICE, 2020b).

In April 2015, NHS England implemented a national programme to reduce inappropriate antibiotic prescribing. The Commissioning for Quality and Innovation (CQUIN) and the Quality Premium (QP) scheme report their progress monthly via the NHS England Antibiotic Quality Premium Monitoring Dashboard and the National Antimicrobial Stewardship Dashboard (NICE, 2015b). Alongside this, the Parliamentary Office of Science and Technology (2017) states the aim of the UK government's 5-year strategy is to identify the causative pathogen and prescribe the appropriate antibiotics and the NICE Antimicrobial Prescribing Guideline (2018) supports the need for a change in prescribing practice to slow antimicrobial resistance and prolong the effectiveness of currently available antibiotics.

Clinical consideration

How policy makers can manage antibiotic resistance (WHO, 2020)
- Ensure a robust national action plan is implemented to address antibiotic resistance
- Improve surveillance of antibiotic-resistant infections
- Strengthen policies, programmes and implementation of infection prevention and control measures
- Regulate and promote the appropriate use and disposal of medicines
- Make information available on the impact of antibiotic resistance.

For more information, visit www.who.int/news-room/fact-sheets/detail/antibiotic-resistance

Clinical consideration

How health professionals can help prevent and control the spread of pathogens and reduce antibiotic resistance (WHO, 2020)
- Adhere to infection control procedures and good hand-washing techniques
- Regularly clean the environment
- Only prescribe and dispense antibiotics when necessary, according to current guidelines
- Report antibiotic-resistant infections to surveillance teams and report through the British National Formulary (BNF) Yellow Card scheme (NICE, 2021c), which is managed by the Medicines and Healthcare products Regulatory Agency (MHRA): https://yellowcard.mhra.gov.uk/
- Follow procedures to diagnose infections and suspected antibiotic-resistance infections. A sample of the infected tissue or blood test should be sent to the laboratory for further investigation and identification, after which the correct antibiotic can be prescribed
- Inform and educate patients about correct usage of the medication and that it is only to be used as per prescription for a specific diagnosis
- Discuss with patients ways of preventing infections (for example, vaccinations, hand washing, safer sex, covering nose and mouth when sneezing).

Bacteria

A bacterium is a prokaryotic single-cell organism with a simple DNA structure that lacks a nucleus and predates the eukaryotic cells found in plants, animals and yeast by 1 billion years. In Table 9.2, bacteria are classified into the four main groups based on their appearance: cocci (spherical),

Table 9.2   Bacterial classification.

Type of bacteria	Examples of infections
Cocci (spherical)	*Staphylococcus aureus* (Gram positive)
Bacilli (rod-shaped)	*Salmonella typhimurium* (Gram negative) *Listeria monocytogenes* (Gram positive) *Mycobacterium tuberculosis*
Spirochaetes (spiral)	(Syphilis) *Treponema pallidum* (Gram negative)
Vibrio (comma shaped)	*Vibrio cholerae* (Gram negative)

Source: Anderson et al. (2012a)/with permission of John Wiley & Sons.

bacilli (rod-shaped), spirochaetes (spiral) and vibrio (comma shaped) (Vellai and Vida, 1999; Anderson et al., 2012a). Bacteria can be subdivided into gram-positive and gram-negative and mycobacteria.

Gram-positive bacteria

Gram-positive bacteria are prokaryotes composed of a single plasma membrane (monodermita), which secures the cytoplasm. The cell wall is composed of a peptidoglycan-based structure, cross-linked with a network of polysaccharide chains and lipoteichoic acids to form a robust cell wall structure to combat the increased osmotic pressure caused by the cell's higher salt content compared to its external surroundings (Desvaux et al., 2006; Anderson et al., 2012a) (Figure 9.1).

Gram-negative bacteria

Gram-negative bacteria are more complex in structure as they have two distinct membranes (diderm prokaryotes). They have a thinner cell wall composed of peptidoglycan-based proteins, which is then sandwiched by two membranes consisting of phospholipids containing lipopoly-saccharides (LPS) and porins. This extra barrier can prevent the absorption of antibacterials, which hinders the effectiveness of the treatment (Figure 9.2) (Desvaux et al., 2006; Anderson et al 2012a).

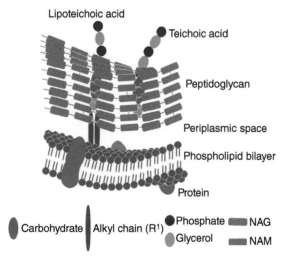

Figure 9.1   Gram-positive bacteria. Representation of the cell wall and plasma membrane.
Source: Anderson et al. (2012a)/with permission of John Wiley & Sons.

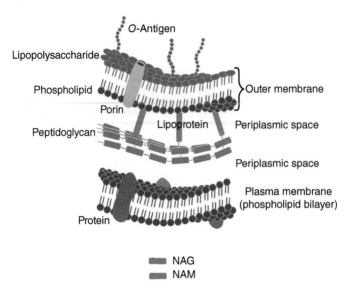

Figure 9.2 Gram-negative bacteria. Representation of the cell wall and plasma membrane. *Source*: Anderson et al. (2012a)/with permission of John Wiley & Sons.

Mycobacteria

Mycobacteria are gram-positive and have greater resistance to antibacterials due to a very strong cell wall structure made up of peptidoglycan proteins and arabinogalactan, which are then anchored to long-chain acids for strength (Figure 9.3). These are resistant to cell wall synthesis antibacterials such as the beta-lactams and cephalosporins. Mycobacteria also have the ability to survive in extreme conditions and are prevalent in the environment (Anderson et al., 2012a; Percival and Williams, 2014). This group of bacteria includes *Mycobacterium tuberculosis* (which causes tuberculosis), and *Mycobacterium leprae* (which causes leprosy).

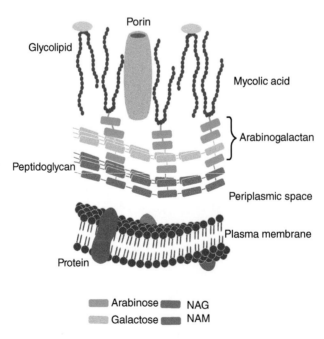

Figure 9.3 Mycobacteria. Representation of the plasma mebrane, cell wall and mycomembrane (mycolic acid layer). *Source*: Anderson et al. (2012a)/with permission of John Wiley & Sons.

Identification of bacterial classifications

Hans Christian Joachim Gram, a Danish pharmacologist, developed a staining technique to distinguish between the different subgroups of bacteria in 1884. Gram-positive bacteria were affected by the staining due to the structure of the bacterial cell envelope however, gram-negative bacteria and mycobacteria were not affected (Anderson et al., 2012a). Today, there are many different staining techniques, such as acid-fast staining to identify mycobacteria, which have a different structural cellular arrangement and do not show up with the Gram staining techniques.

Bacteria as pathogens

Bacteria are opportunist pathogens and are commonly found on human skin. They are mostly innocuous and harmless to the healthy population but they can cause illness in the immune-deficient or compromised person. The human immune response mechanisms are the innate system and the adaptive system, which work together to destroy pathogens and develop immunity. In innate immunity, the first line of defence is fast acting and on detection of the invading bacteria, dendritic cells, macrophages, neutrophils, basophils, eosinophils and mast cells are released to kill the bacteria and in doing so produce cytokines, which initiate an inflammatory response. The adaptive system responds to the action of the innate immunity mechanisms and produces T and B cells which then develop specific antigen receptors to the pathogen to continue the action of destroying the bacteria or pathogen and provide longer term immunity by forming antibodies (Alberts et al., 2002; Wilson et al., 2019). However, if the pathogen concentrations overwhelm the immune systems, this is the point at which the patient begins to present with symptoms of the infection and may feel unwell.

Bacteria can spread through food-borne pathways, such as *Salmonella* and *E. coli*, potentially causing kidney failure and death and in pregnancy have been reported to cause premature birth, miscarriage and stillbirths (RCOG, 2012; Wilson et al., 2019). Pregnant women should be advised about safety in preparation of foods and avoiding certain foods, which may contain a higher proportion of potentially pathogenic bacteria that can affect the developing fetus.

Mechanism of action of antibacterials and antibiotics

The aim of antibacterial drugs is to kill pathogenic bacteria (bactericidal action) or inhibit multiplication without affecting the host cells (bacteriostatic action). In order to achieve this effectively, it is important that the antibacterial only targets prokaryotic cells, leaving the eukaryotic cells unharmed.

Antibiotics can be divided into two groups: bactericidal and bacteriostatic (Table 9.3). Classification may vary depending on bacterial strain and bacterial minimum inhibitory concentration (MIC).

Table 9.3 Antibiotic groups.

Bactericidal	Bacteriostatic
Antibacterial or antibiotic that kills bacteria, decreasing the bacterial cell count. Irreversible cell death	Antibacterial or antibiotic which inhibits bacterial cell growth and multiplication. Bacterial cell count remains the same and awaits the immune system to destroy bacteria
Action on bacteria – disruption of cell wall or cell wall synthesis	Action on bacteria – disrupts DNA replication or metabolic functions (folate and protein inference)
Prescription – minimum bactericidal concentration (MBC) required to kill bacteria. A lower dose may result in a bacteriostatic effect	Prescription – minimum inhibitory concentration (MIC) required to inhibit bacterial growth. A higher dose may result in a bactericidal effect
Side-effects – toxic shock	Side-effects – few
Treatment – meningitis	Treatment – urinary tract infections, wounds
Example – penicillins	Example – tetracyclines and sulfonamides

Source: Pankey and Sabeth (2004); NICE (2018); Smaill and Vazquez (2019).

127

Table 9.4   Broad- and narrow-spectrum antibiotics.

Broad-spectrum antibiotics	Narrow-spectrum antibiotics
Effective against gram-positive bacteria and gram-negative bacteria.	Effective against only one type of organism that is gram-positive
Kill a variety of organisms.	Causative organisms known.
Useful if cause of infection is unknown. For example, erythromycin and doxycycline.	For example, macrolides, older penicillin (although can be broad spectrum-amoxicillin or ampicillin), and vancomycin.

Source: Peate & Hill (2021)/with permission of John Wiley & Sons.

Antibiotics are also classified as broad spectrum and narrow spectrum (Table 9.4). Generally, narrow-spectrum antibiotics are agents that treat a smaller range of bacteria and should be the first choice for non-life-threatening infections, while broad-spectrum antibiotics are agents that can treat a wide range of bacteria and are used for more serious infections.

Overuse of broad-spectrum antibiotics can create a selective advantage for bacterial resistance, as these agents indiscriminately kill both pathogenic bacteria and the normal commensal flora, leaving the patient susceptible to antibiotic-resistant harmful bacteria such as *C. difficile*. For this reason, broad-spectrum antibiotics need to be reserved for second-choice treatment when narrow-spectrum antibiotics are ineffective, as described in the Chief Medical Officer's Annual Report (Davies, 2018). It is important to refer to national and local trust guidelines when prescribing or administering drugs (British Pharmacology Association, 2021).

Disruption of cell wall synthesis

Antibacterial agents which cause cell wall synthesis disruption target the biosynthesis of peptidoglycan, the main structure of the bacterial cell wall. During formation of the cell wall, the separate units of peptidoglycans need to be cross-linked and connected through a process which occurs on the outer plasma membrane and comprises a complex sequence of catalytic enzymes that align the peptidoglycans along the peptide NAG-NAM chains (alpha), resulting in the rigid scaffolding of the cell wall.

This peptidoglycan cell wall structure is unique to bacteria, so an antibacterial agent used to disrupt the biosynthesis of peptidoglycan can have the potential for selective toxicity to the bacteria cell walls, with no injury to the host cell (eukaryotes) (Pandey and Cascella, 2021). See Figure 9.4.

Beta-lactams

Beta-lactams, such as penicillins (e.g. amoxicillin, piperacillin), are the most common broad-spectrum antibiotic used and act against gram-positive and gram-negative bacteria by disrupting cell wall synthesis, but are less effective against mycobacteria due to the different structural arrangement of the cell wall (Anderson et al., 2012b; Pandey and Cascella, 2021).

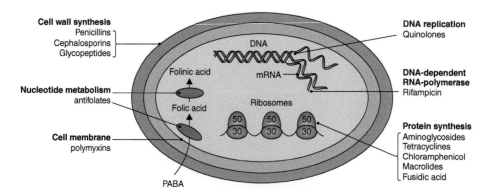

Figure 9.4   Action of antibiotic agents on different sites of the bacterial cell. *Source*: Xiu and Datta (2019)/ with permission of Elsevier.

Indications

Group B streptococcus Group B streptococcus (GBS) is the most frequent cause of severe early-onset (less than 7 days) infection in newborn infants and colonises the bowel flora of 20–40% of adults.

Common terms: group B streptococcus; GBS; GBS bacteriuria; initial antibiotic therapy (Hughes et al., 2017).

Treatment Benzylpenicillin (administered intravenously) can be offered to the woman at the onset of labour or if ruptured membranes occur at or over 18 hours (though local trust guidelines may vary). If the woman has an allergy to penicillin, an alternative should be offered based on the individuals GBS sensitivity results or local microbiological surveillance data (NICE, 2020a).

Prophylactic antibiotics can be given in order to reduce the risk of early-onset GBS infection to the newborn and offered to women who have had a previous baby with an invasive GBS infection, GBS colonisation, bacteriuria or infection in the current pregnancy (NICE, 2012).

129

Syphilis Syphilis is a sexually transmitted disease caused by a spirochaete called *Treponema pallidum* which is screened during pregnancy. Vertical transmission of the disease during pregnancy results in congenital syphilis in the newborn and without treatment in the antenatal period, the fetus may incur a permanent disability and disfiguration or be aborted (PHE, 2019a).

Treatment Penicillin is given early in pregnancy following a diagnosis of syphilis and is effective in reducing miscarriages and stillbirths (Walker, 2001).

Mastitis *Staphylococcus aureus* is the most common breastfeeding pathogen. Oral antibiotics are appropriate, where indicated, and women can continue breast feeding if they choose to (NICE, 2020a).

Treatment Flucloxacillin is the recommended treatment. If the woman is allergic to penicillin, erythromycin or clarithromycin can be prescribed (NICE, 2020a).

Contraindications and cautions

Beta-lactams are generally well tolerated but can cause hypersensitivity which increases the risk of anaphylaxis. Therefore, any woman who has a known allergy should be offered an alternative, (Miller et al., 2019; Pandey and Cascella, 2021).

When prescribing and administering beta-lactams care should be taken if the woman has any renal impairment. The woman should be informed of side-effects such as diarrhoea and superinfection for both mother and baby, which is a secondary infection such as yeast infections imposed on the original infection associated with the loss of intestinal flora caused by the actions of the antibiotic. For the developing fetus, it may cause tooth deformation and staining (Chiriac et al., 2017).

Cephalosporins

This range of antibacterials have a broad spectrum, acting on gram-negative and gram-positive micro-organisms. There are five generations of cephalosporins (Rang et al., 2019a) (Table 9.5).

Indications

Pneumonia, septicaemia, urinary tract infections, biliary tract infections, meningitis and peritonitis (NICE, 2018).

Contraindications and cautions (for all cephalosporins)

Women who have an allergy or a hypersensitivity to penicillins and beta-lactams should avoid cephalosporins and caution should be exercised if women have a mild sensitivity or report any renal or hepatic impairment.

Table 9.5 Examples of cephalosporin per generation.

Generation	Cephalosporin	
1st	Cefalexin	Usually used in gram-positive infections and in cases of staphylococci or non-enterococcal streptococci. They have limited success against gram-negative bacteria.
2nd	Cefuroxime	They act on similar strains of pathogen as the first generation with an improved spectrum of activity against gram-negative bacteria. However, they are known to be less effective against some gram-positive bacteria.
3rd	Cefotaxime	They have a broader spectrum of activity and have a greater effect on certain gram-negative aerobes.
4th	Cefepime	Indicated in the treatment of gram-positive and gram-negative bacteria.
5th	Ceftaroline fosamil	Similar in bactericidal action to third generation drugs; however, this is extended against other gram-positive pathogens which include MRSA and multidrug-resistant *Streptococcus pneumonia*. Indicated in the treatment of community-acquired pneumonia. Complicated skin, and soft-tissue infections.

Source: Modified from Burchaum and Rosenthal (2019); NICE (2019); Peate & Hill (2021)/with permission of John Wiley & Sons.

Adverse effects (for all cephalosporins)
Generally, this antibacterial group is well tolerated. The most common adverse effects with cephalosporins include nausea, vomiting and diarrhoea. Hypersensitivity reactions are seen in 10% of patients who have penicillin sensitivity and are also likely to be sensitive to cephalosporins.

Ceftriaxone can cause bleeding by interfering with the metabolism of vitamin K.

Thrombophlebitis can occur at the IV injection site or an abscess at the site of an intramuscular injection. Renal-impaired women may experience nephrological toxicity and there is also an increased risk of infection and/or superinfections due to interference with the normal flora (Pandey and Cascella, 2021).

Drug–drug interactions (for all cephalosporins)
Avoid taking with aminoglycosides as this increases the risk of nephrotoxicity or with any anticoagulants, thrombolytics, non-steroidal anti-inflammatory drugs and aspirin (and other antiplatelet drugs) as these can increase the risk of bleeding.

Carbapenems
Carbapenems have a broad spectrum of activity, including anaerobes, gram-positive and gram-negative bacteria (BNF, 2021c).

Indications
Imipenem and meropenem are active against *Pseudomonas aeruginosa* and non-MRSA and together are used to treat severe hospital-acquired infections including septicaemia, pneumonia, intra-abdominal infections, skin and soft tissue infections and complicated urinary tract infections (BNF, 2021c).

Contraindications and cautions
Side-effects of imipenem with cilastatin are similar to those of other beta-lactam antibiotics.

Monobactams
Aztreonam is effective only against aerobic gram-negative bacilli and shows no activity against gram-positive bacteria or anaerobes. It is used to treat infections, such as pneumonia and urinary

tract infections (Rang et al., 2019a). Beta-lactam and beta-lactamase inhibitor combinations (such as ceftolozane/tazobactam, ceftazidime/avibactam, meropenem/vaborbactam, imipenem/cilastatin/relebactam, aztreonam/avibactam) have been developed to combat antibiotic resistance of complicated infections, especially in intensive care units (Leone et al., 2019a, 2019b; Pandey and Cascella, 2021).

Contraindications and autions
Monobactams tend not to cause allergic reactions in penicillin-sensitive individuals (Rang et al., 2019b).

Protein synthesis interference
Proteins are vital in bacteria cell function, from enzyme activity to the formation of structural elements (Arenz and Wilson, 2016). Protein synthesis in bacterial cells occurs on the ribosomes, which are made up of the 50S and 30S subunits. Transfer RNA (tRNA) transports individual amino acids to the ribosomes. Protein synthesis occurs when the amino acids are collated by the messenger RNA (a template from the DNA) as it binds to the A position on 30S and 50S subunits and is moved along the successive codons of the subunits until the P position to group the amino acids to form larger proteins (Rang et al., 2019a) (Figure 9.4). Therefore, any disruption of these processes can interfere with protein synthesis and bacteria cell function (Arenz and Wilson, 2016).

30S antibiotic treatments – aminoglycosides
Aminoglycosides
Aminoglycosides are antibacterials which affect the 30S subunit ribosome and include gentamicin, streptomycin, neomycin, tobramycin and amikacin. They have a broad spectrum of activity and inhibit many aerobic gram-negative bacteria and some gram-positive bacteria in the presence of oxygen. These antibacterials enter bacterial cells by active transport through the polyamine transport system in the cell membrane. Once in the cell, they can disrupt protein synthesis by affecting the 30S subunit ribosome and can be enhanced by other antibacterial agents that interfere with cell wall synthesis, such as penicillins and beta-lactams (Rang et al., 2019b).

Indications (for all aminoglycosides) They are indicated in the treatment of severe infections.

Contraindications and cautions (for all aminoglycosides) The use of aminoglycosides is contraindicated in those who have experienced previous allergic reaction to aminoglycosides and patients with myasthenia gravis (requiring injectable forms of treatment). As up to 60% of the drug is expelled via the kidneys, toxic accumulation in women with renal impairment may occur rapidly based on antibacterial concentration (Rang et al., 2019b).

Aminoglycosides can cross the placenta, but do not permeate the blood–brain barrier. However, higher doses may accumulate in the pleural and joint fluid spaces. Avoid usage in the second and third trimesters as this is associated with a possible risk of auditory or vestibular damage to the fetus (Rang et al., 2019b; BNF, 2021d).

Drug–drug interactions (for all aminoglycosides) Aminoglycosides together with penicillins can be used to increase treatment efficiency, but need to be administered separately to avoid inactivation of aminoglycosides by the penicillins (BNF, 2021d).

50S antibiotic treatments – macrolides and lincoamides
Macrolides
This broad-spectrum antibacterial group inhibits bacterial protein synthesis and has a similar, but not identical antibacterial spectrum to penicillin, so can be used as an alternative for patients with a penicillin allergy. Examples of this group are erythromycin, azithromycin and clarithromycin. Erythromycin has a bacteriostatic action but can assume bactericidal properties (BNF, 2021e).

Indications Indications for the macrolides include *Campylobacter enteritis*, respiratory infections and skin infections (BNF, 2021e).

Preterm rupture of membranes is defined as the spontaneous rupture of membranes prior to 37 weeks gestation and is associated with 30–40% of preterm births. It can complicate up to 3% of pregnancies, leading to significant neonatal morbidity and mortality, and can lead to both gram-positive and gram-negative bacterial infections such as sepsis and chorioamnionitis (Wojcieszek et al., 2014).

Treatment Erythromycin for 10 days or until the woman is in established labour (Thomson, 2019; NICE, 2020a).

Contraindications and cautions (for all macrolides) Caution should be exercised for women with hepatic and renal impairment as this may alter the effect of the drug and drug excretion. As macrolides can affect the developing fetus, they should be prescribed with caution in pregnancy and for lactating women as use may increase superinfections in infants (Rang et al., 2019b).

With IV and oral administration of macrolides, there is a risk of electrolyte disturbances and a predisposition to QT prolongation, and they may exacerbate myasthenia gravis symptoms (BNF, 2021e).

Lincoamides – clindamycin and lincomycin

Lincoamides and macrolides have similar properties as they inhibit bacterial protein synthesis. Clindamycin is bacteriostatic, but it can assume bactericidal properties. It acts on most gram-positive cocci, gram-negative and gram-positive anaerobes, and gram-positive aerobes (Farrington, 2012).

Indications Clindamycin is used in staphylococcal infections, including MRSA, peritonitis, intra-abdominal sepsis and bacterial vaginosis (Farrington, 2012).

Contraindications and cautions The BNF (2021e) states that there is limited data on known harmful effects in the second and third trimesters, but to prescribe and use with caution in the first trimester. Lincoamides are transferred in breast milk and may affect the infant's gastrointestinal flora, which may cause diarrhoea, candidiasis or, antibiotic-associated colitis.

Adverse effects The most extreme effect of clindamycin is antibiotic-associated diarrhoea, which can develop several weeks after completing a course of clindamycin and is known to occur more frequently with clindamycin than other types of antibiotics (BNF, 2021e).

Drug–drug interactions Clindamycin may interact with drugs used in anaesthetic induction and surgery by increasing their effects.

Bacterial DNA inhibition and damage

DNA replication in bacteria occurs when the double helix strand of DNA separates through a series of actions by enzymes known as *helicases*, resulting in two individual DNA strands remaining in a supercoiled helix state. For replication of the DNA strand to commence, the strands need to be relaxed in order to act as a template for replication. This process is achieved through the action of enzymes called *topoisomerases*. If this process is hindered by an antibacterial agent such as quinolone, then replication of DNA is halted (Anderson et al., 2012a).

Metronidazole

Originally created as an antiprotozoal agent but active against anaerobic bacteria, metronidazole is used to treat serious infections such as sepsis. It is able to achieve high concentrations by saturating the tissues and cerebrospinal fluid. Most is excreted via the kidneys in the urine, but side-effects include dizziness, headaches and nausea and it should be avoided in pregnancy (Rang et al., 2019b).

Messenger RNA synthesis disruption

Another stage in DNA replication is the transcription process from which DNA forms ribonucleic acid (RNA) subunits, which relies on the actions of temporary proteins. Therefore, any antibacterial such as rifampicin, which can affect the action of the temporary protein, would halt the replication of bacterial DNA (Anderson et al., 2012b).

Rifampicin

Rifampicin belongs to the rifamycin group; it acts on gram-negative and gram-positive bacteria and is the most active antituberculosis agent. This antibacterial binds to the enzyme RNA polymerase and inhibits mRNA synthesis (required to synthesise larger proteins from amino acids) in prokaryote cells but not eukaryotic cells. Therefore it causes less toxicity and harm to the patient (Rang et al., 2019b).

133

Indications

Tuberculosis and legionnaire's disease (BNF, 2021a).

Contraindications and cautions

Side-effects are generally uncommon but can include skin eruptions, liver damage, jaundice, nausea, vomiting and thrombocytopenia. It is important to regularly monitor drug levels. It should be avoided in pregnancy as it can cause neonatal bleeding in the third trimester (BNF, 2021a).

Folate acid synthesis

Folate (dihydrofolic acid) is essential for synthesis of the bases purine and pyrimidine required for DNA synthesis (see Figure 9.4). Bacteria lack the protein for the uptake of folic acid from the surrounding environment and therefore rely on para-aminobenzioc acid (PABA), a metabolite that can synthesise folic acid (Anderson et al., 2012a). There are also a series of enzyme actions involved in this pathway (Bermingham and Derrick, 2002). If any antibacterial were to interfere with this cellular-level process of metabolising folic acid, then DNA replication and cell proliferation would be halted (Anderson et al., 2012a).

Sulfonamides and dihydrofolate reductase (DHFR) inhibitors

Sulfonamides are bacteriostatic, so they stop bacterial cells from multiplying but do not necessarily kill them. Sulfonamides are a structural analogue of PABA, the precursor in the synthesis of folic acid. Sulfonamides can therefore compete with PABA in binding to the PABA enzyme, thereby inhibiting the production of folic acid and halting bacterial cell formation (Rang et al., 2019b). DHFR inhibitors include trimethroprim.

Indications

Pyrimethamine is used in combination with sulfadiazine and folinic acid in the treatment of toxoplasmosis during pregnancy (BNF, 2021f).

Contraindications and cautions

Overall, sulfonamides should be avoided during pregnancy. Pyrimethamine is considered to be a potential teratogenic risk in the first trimester as it is a folate antagonist. Folate is recommended as a supplement in the first trimester as it prevents neural tube defects (NICE, 2008), therefore adequate folate supplements should be given to the woman whilst taking sulfonamides (BNF, 2021b, 2021f).

Prescribing

The Royal College of Obstetricians and Gynaecologists' review (2015) on antibiotics prescribed during pregnancy found that overall, the benefits of treating serious infections, which may contribute to improved maternal and neonatal outcomes, outweigh the potential risks caused by antibiotics and this is in accordance with current NICE guidelines to only prescribe if 'medically indicated' and to limit the overall prescribing of medications during pregnancy.

The Advisory Committee on Antimicrobial Prescribing, Resistance and Healthcare Associated Infection (APRHAI) recommends the 'Start smart – then focus' approach, which acknowledges that clinical situations may require immediate and ongoing antibiotic treatment before a formal clinical diagnosis can be made (APRHAI, 2019). Formal clinical diagnosis requires microbiological identification of the pathogen as described in the European Committee on Antimicrobial Susceptability Testing (EUCAST) guidelines for detection, through collection of infected tissue, swabs and/or blood cultures and blood tests (EUCAST, 2021a, 2021b). The approach requires that the patient is reviewed within 48–72 hours of starting a dose of antibiotics and an evaluation of available test results should be made on the effectiveness of the current treatment and suggests a change of course and a new prescription if a diagnosis has been made. This is to avoid unnecessary overuse or misuse of antibiotics and by correcting the treatment, it both results in a more effective treatment and helps in reducing further antibiotic resistance (APRHAI, 2019).

Narrow-spectrum antibiotics are the first choice in targeting and treating infections and the use of broad-spectrum antibiotics should be reserved for more serious and life-threatening infections, as overuse of broad-spectrum antibiotics can lead to detrimental disruption of the microbiome, such as the alteration of gut flora required for vitamin production and protection from pathogens that can last up to 2 years before recovery following one treatment and lead to antibiotic resistance issues (Jernberg et al., 2007).

Understanding physiological changes in pregnancy and breastfeeding when prescribing

The many physiology changes during pregnancy include the increase in hepatic metabolism, glomerular filtration rates and plasma volumes, as well as endocrine changes, such as increase in levels of prostaglandins and nitric oxide, upregulated by oestradiol to create an immunologically tolerant maternal environment to allow for fetal growth and development (NICE, 2015b; Greer et al., 2019).

A systematic review by Pariente et al. (2016) showed that pregnant women are commonly prescribed a variety of medications during pregnancy and when accompanied with changes in physiology, some of which may affect the pharmacokinetics (PK) (absorption, distribution, metabolism, excretion) of antibiotics. In the NICE *Summary of Antimicrobial Prescribing Guidance* (2020a), adjustments in dosage schedules and antibiotic treatments have been made for child-bearing women.

When considering treatment with antibiotics for pregnant or lactating women, the benefits of treatment must be balanced against risk to the fetus or infant. For example, urinary tract infections and sexually transmitted infections during pregnancy, if left untreated, could lead to adverse effects for the fetus, such as low birth weight and spontaneous abortion of the pregnancy (Bookstaver et al., 2015). Therefore, when prescribing and administering, it is important to avoid antibiotics which may have teratogenic affects, such as restricted growth and functional development of the fetus, or antibiotics which can cause possible toxic effects on fetal tissue leading to congenital abnormalities (Bookstaver et al., 2015). Some of the effects of antibiotic use in pregnancy and lactation may potentially lead to longer term effects, such as changes in gut microbiomes and asthma in children (Bookstaver et al., 2015; NICE, 2015b). Beta-lactams, metronidazole and clindamycin are considered safe to use in pregnancy but fluoroquinolones and tetracyclines are generally avoided (Bookstaver et al., 2015).

Clinical consideration

Breastfeeding

The amount of drug transferred in breast milk is rarely sufficient to produce an adverse effect on the infant. The amount of active metabolite of the antibacterial delivered to the infant is dependent on the pharmacokinetic characteristics of the mother and the efficiency of absorption, and elimination of the drug by the infant (infant pharmacokinetics) (NICE, 2020a).

However, it is important to inform parents of the benefits and risks of the treatment, including any possibility that antibacterials present in breast milk can induce a hypersensitivity reaction. This provides parents with information to make an informed decision on the treatment (NICE, 2021b).

Penicillins and cephalosporins are the drugs of choice in breastfeeding. Quinolones should be avoided whilst breastfeeding (NICE, 2020a, 2021a).

Clinical considerations

135

The effects of antibiotics on term and preterm babies

In the UK, 7.5% of all births are preterm (ONS, 2021). Preterm infants can present with a variety of health compromises, such as respiratory problems, risk of infection and brain function issues, and some will require special care (WHO, 2013).

From birth, the natural gut microbiota develops to form an intestinal barrier to pathogens and promote tolerance to foods and helps in the maturation of the immune system. Premature infants have a sparse microbiota with fewer anaerobes, compared to the healthy, full-term infant gut (Dahl et al., 2018).

Laxminarayan et al. (2016) ask clinicians to consider the use of maternal antibacterials in temporary or routine treatments for maternal indications in contrast to the unintended longer-term implications for infant health, including disruption to the microbiome, which could lead to possible chronic conditions such as paediatric obesity.

Reflection

Midwives' role

Furber et al. (2017) suggest that midwives should encourage compliance with drug regimens and advise women on the duration of treatment and any possible interactions (NICE, 2015a). Not completing the treatment may lead to any remaining bacteria being exposed to a diminished and less effective dose, thus surviving and multiplying in resistant forms (McNulty et al., 2013).

The FRAIS mnemonic by Fleming (2016) can help promote compliance and stands for:

Finish the course
Regular intervals
After, before or with food
Interactions
Side effects

Wilcock et al.'s (2019) study suggests that midwives' and nurses' knowledge in sustaining the Antimicrobial Stewardship guidance may need further support and training from the wider multidisciplinary teams, such as pharmacists.

What support is available to you in terms of training or information on antibacterial usage and Antimicrobial Stewardship?

Pharmacokinetics and pharmacodynamics

Pharmacokinetics (PK) is the study of how the body processes the medication, in other words 'what the **body** does to the drug', and is determined as the concentration of the drug in the host in relation to time (Anderson et al., 2012c). Pharmacokinetics describes drug absorption, distribution and elimination (metabolism and excretion) (Table 9.6).

Pharmacodynamics (PD) is the study of 'what the **drug** does to the body' and describes the concentration and time-dependent interactions with bacteria in the host (Anderson et al., 2012c; Fan and de Lannoy, 2014). Based on their PD, antibiotics can be divided into two categories: time-dependent bactericidal (e.g. beta-lactams, cephalosporins, vancomycin) and concentration-dependent bactericidal (e.g. aminoglycosides and fluoroquinolones) (Anderson et al., 2012c). Maximising the duration of exposure to time-dependent active antibiotics can be achieved through dose increase, prolonging the infusion time or shortening the dosing interval.

For concentration-dependent antibiotics, increased antibacterial activity is accomplished with increased drug concentration in the host. The aim is to maintain the antibiotic concentration at 2–4 times over the MIC which is described as the lowest concentration of a given antibiotic that inhibits the growth of a specific organism and whereby effects are noted in the patient (Anderson et al., 2012c). The MIC will be within the 'therapeutic range', which is considered as the safe concentration of the antibiotic in the plasma to achieve the effective therapeutic treatment and yet not exceed the therapeutic range so that it becomes toxic to the patient. Monitoring the concentration of drug in the plasma is performed via routine blood tests (Fullerton et al., 2020).

Table 9.6   Pharmacokinetics.

	Pharmacokinetics action
Absorption	How a drug is absorbed from the stomach and intestine into the body (if it is an oral drug) or via the bloodstream (i.e. IV bolus or infusion)
Distribution	How the drug becomes distributed through the body fluids and tissues, often transported in the blood by binding to proteins such as albumen, which is present in plasma, and carried to the targeted organ or tissue
Metabolism	How and to what extent a drug is metabolised by the liver through a series of enzyme actions and can be dependent on genetics and ethnicity. Inducers, such as antiepileptic medication, can increase the metabolism and the breakdown of the target drugs, meaning there will be less target drug in the plasma, resulting in a smaller effect. Inhibitors can decrease the metabolism of the target drug, which could lead to an increased amount of the target drug in the plasma, which can cause adverse effects, such as toxicity. Alcohol can also affect the metabolism of the drug
Excretion	How the drug is excreted from the body (usually via the kidneys in the urine, but can also be excreted in lungs, faeces, skin, bile, sweat and breast milk in lactating mothers). The pH of the urine can delay excretion, as well as age of the patient and kidney function

Source: Anderson et al. (2012c); Fan and de Lannoy (2014).

The importance of understanding PK and PD in managing antibiotic use

As greater understanding develops from studies on the PK and PD of antibiotics, improvements in treatment have benefited patients and women. Examples include the introduction of prolonged antibiotic infusions over classic bolus dosing in critically ill patients, patients with sepsis have achieved better outcomes, the duration of therapy is shorter and cost savings have been seen (Fullerton et al., 2020).

Antibacterial drugs are used in many different clinical contexts, including prophylactic treatments (e.g. in the perioperative period), and may be taken simultaneously with other medications, which may act as inducers or inhibitors on the target drug. 'Established' antibiotic dosing and duration of treatment for many common infections during the antenatal, intrapartum and postnatal period have been standardised through guidance offered by the Royal College of Obstetricians and Gynaecologists and the British National Formulary-NICE, which may not always best represent the individual users' PK reaction to the antibiotic treatments. Subsequently, standardised prescribing may result in overuse or the ineffective use of the antibiotic treatment in different patients, thereby contributing to antibiotic resistance (Buppasiri et al., 2014; Fullerton et al., 2020; RCOG, 2020). Therefore, it is best practice to review the antibiotic treatment plan of women and newborns on a regular basis and introduce changes to management as the clinical situation develops.

Skills in practice

- As a midwife, how do you monitor whether the antibiotic treatment is effective? How would you monitor the adverse or side-effects of the antibiotic?
- What tests could be performed to confirm whether the infection has improved and the antibiotic has been effective?
- What test would be performed to ensure the therapeutic range has not been exceeded and when would this ideally be performed?
- What signs and side-effects would you discuss with the woman?
- In the event of a side-effect or adverse effect, what processes or policies would you refer to and comply with?

New approaches to prescribing antibiotics: semi-mechanistic antibiotic PKPD modelling

In view of global concerns about antibiotic resistance and the attempt to optimise effective treatments of infections, identification of the infection needs to lead the way in which antibiotics are prescribed. PD modelling is limited due to the complexity of categorising PK extremes across the population, such as body weight (specifically, apidose tissue), gender, age and ethnicity as well as renal and hepatic function and in ensuring that the majority of the population is receiving the optimal dose-concentration-response relationship of the antibiotic treatment to effectively treat the bacterial infection, while simultaneously being mindful of the incorrect and overuse of antibiotics, which contribute to antibiotic resistance (Anderson et al., 2012a; Brill et al., 2018).

Over recent decades, the increased use of antibiotic combinations has widened the range of treatments and minimised the emergence of antibiotic resistance, as seen in the treatment of sepsis (Sullivan et al., 2020; van Belkum et al., 2019; Tamma et al., 2021). The semi-mechanistic PKPD model adopts a compartment system to examine the general characteristics of bacterial growth, drug effects and the development of bacterial resistance. Bacteria are allowed to multiply and colonise in the compartments. Each compartment represents a different stage of bacterial growth. Within each compartment, tests are carried out to clarify the kill rate or inhibition of growth using different

137

Table 9.7 Broad-spectrum antibiotics used to treat Maternal sepsis.

Antibacterial Agent	Covers	Considerations
Co-amoxiclav	Does not cover MRSA or Pseudomonas	Exposure of the fetus in utero can lead to necrotising enterocolitis in neonates
Metronidazole	Anaerobes	
Clindamycin	Most Streptococci and staphylococci, including many MRSA	Faecal excretion is predominant. As not primarily excreted via renal system, therefore not nephrotoxic.
Piperacillin–tazobactam (Tazocin) and carbapenems	Covers all except MRSA	
Gentamicin (as a single dose)	Covers all and MRSA	For normal renal function, should not pose an issue, however due to risk of nephrotoxicity, levels should be monitored before further doses.

MRSA, methicillin-resistant *Staphylococcus aureus*.
Source: Modified from RCOG (2012).

antibiotic drug concentrations. From here, an optimal antibiotic dose and concentration for the patient can be prescribed (Brill et al., 2018).

Sepsis – example of using a combination of antibiotic therapies

Sepsis, a Group A streptococcal infection, remains a major cause of maternal deaths in the UK, with 11 deaths from 2016 to 2018 relating to genital tract sepsis in pregnancy and up to 6 weeks after birth (Knight et al., 2020). Sepsis is defined as an infection accompanied with a systemic manifestation of infections. Severe sepsis can induce multiorgan dysfunction and tissue hypoperfusion and potentially lead to further complications and even death (RCOG, 2012).

Treatment

Due to the potential complications, it is vital that once sepsis is suspected, it is treated immediately with or without confirmation from microbiology. Blood cultures and other samples including throat swabs, high vaginal swabs and mid-stream urine samples may be obtained based on the clinical situation and as per local policies, prior to commencing antibiotic therapy, as subsequent results a few hours after commencing antibiotics may be uninformative. However these samples should not delay antibiotic treatment (RCOG, 2012). Administration of intravenous broad-spectrum antibiotics is recommended within 1 hour of a suspicion of severe sepsis, with or without septic shock (NICE, 2016). Table 9.7 describes the broad-spectrum antibiotics used to treat sepsis.

Episode of care

Rina is at 38 weeks gestation with her first child and is GBS positive. She attends triage, presenting with rupture of membranes, which is confirmed by the midwife on speculum examination. What is the plan of action in accordance with antibiotic therapy?

Conclusion

This chapter has provided the reader with a general overview of the use of antibacterial medication in obstetric and midwifery practice. It has highlighted the role of the midwife in treating infections and providing women with informed choice about the benefits and potential risks of antibiotic use. Applying the strategies of the Antibiotic Stewardship guidance, midwives are part of the clinical team in preventing antibiotic overuse and the emerging resistance to antibiotics.

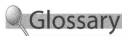# Glossary

Acid-staining technique   A staining technique using the primary stain carbol fuchsin to identify bacterial types. Cells that are 'acid fast' because of the mycolic acid in their cell wall resist decolorisation and retain the primary stain. All other cell types will be decolorised. Methylene blue is then used as a counterstain

Antifungal   Antifungal medicines are used to treat fungal infections, which most commonly affect skin, hair and nails. An example is clotrimazole

Antiviral   Antiviral drugs are used to treat viral infections. They act by killing or preventing the growth of viruses

BNF   The British National Formulary is a joint publication of the British Medical Association and the Royal Pharmaceutical Society and provides prescribers, pharmacists and other healthcare professionals with information about the use of medicines

Clostridium difficile   Also known as *C. difficile* or *C. diff*, this is a bacterium that can infect the bowel and cause diarrhoea

Fungi   Microbes that live in the air, soil, water and plants. There are also some fungi that live naturally in the human body

Mastitis   An inflammation of breast tissue which sometimes develops into an infection requiring antibiotic treatment

MRSA   Methicillin-resistant *Staphylococcus aureus* is a type of bacterium which is resistant to several widely used antibiotics. MRSA can be harder to treat than other bacterial infections

Virus   A pathogen which replicates only inside the living cells of an organism. Viruses infect all life forms, from animals to plants

Yellow Card scheme   The Yellow Card scheme run by the Medicines and Healthcare products Regulatory Agency is the UK system for collecting and monitoring information on safety concerns involving medicines and medical devices, such as suspected side-effects or adverse incidents

Test yourself

 Now review your learning by completing the learning activities for this chapter at www.wiley.com/go/pharmacologyformidwives.

Find out more

The following are common bacterial infections in pregnancy and the intrapartum and postnatal period. Identify the bacterial cause, symptoms and antibiotic or antibacterial treatments that may be used to treat the infection. Include specific considerations of pharmacokinetics or pharmacodynamics. Remember to include aspects of patient care and if these are real-life cases, please ensure no identifiable information is used in accordance with GPDR guidelines.

The condition	Comments
Lower urinary tract Infection	
Preterm rupture of membranes	
Chorioamnionitis	
Syphilis	
Sepsis	

References

Advisory Committee on Antimicrobial Prescribing, Resistance and Healthcare Associated Infection (2019) APRHAI 9th annual report. www.gov.uk/government/publications/aprhai-annual-report-2017-to-2018/aprhai-9th-annual-report (accessed January 2022).

Alberts, B., Johnson, A., Lewis, J., et al. (2002) The adaptive immune system. In: *Molecular Biology of the Cell*, 4th edn. Garland Science: New York.

Anderson, R., Groundwater, P.W., Todd, A., Worsley, A. (2012a) Introduction to micro-organisms and antibacterials chemotherapy. In: *Antibacterial Agents: Chemistry, Mode of Action, Mechanisms of Resistance and Clinical Applications*. John Wiley and Sons: New York.

Anderson, R., Groundwater, P.W., Todd, A., Worsley, A. (2012b) Agents targeting cell wall synthesis. In: *Antibacterial Agents: Chemistry, Mode of Action, Mechanisms of Resistance and Clinical Applications*. John Wiley and Sons: New York.

Anderson, R., Groundwater, P.W., Todd, A., Worsley, A. (2012c) Agents targeting protein synthesis. In: *Antibacterial Agents: Chemistry, Mode of Action, Mechanisms of Resistance and Clinical Applications*. John Wiley and Sons: New York.

Arenz, S., Wilson, D.N. (2016) Bacterial protein synthesis as a target for antibioticc inhibition. *Cold Spring Harbor Perspectives in Medicine*, **6**(9): a025361.

Ashiru-Oredope, D., Hopkins, S. (2015) Antimicrobial resistance: moving from professional engagement to public action. *Journal of Antimicrobial Chemotherapy*, **70**(11): 2927–2930.

Bergstrom, R., Wright, G.D., Brown, E.D., Cars, O. (2013) Antibiotic resistance – the need for global solutions. *Lancet Infectious Diseases*, **13**(12): 1057–1098.

Bermingham, A., Derrick, J.P. (2002) The folic acid biosynthesis pathway in bacteria: evaluation of potential for antibacterial drug discovery. *Bioessays*, **24**(7): 637–648.

BNF (2021a) Rifampicin. https://bnf.nice.org.uk/drug/rifampicin.html#indicationsAndDoses (accessed January 2022).

BNF (2021b) Sulfonamides. https://bnf.nice.org.uk/drug/sulfadiazine.html#Search?q=SULFONAMIDES (accessed January 2022).

BNF (2021c) Carbapenems. https://bnf.nice.org.uk/treatment-summary/carbapenems.html (accessed January 2022).

BNF (2021d) Aminoglycosides. https://bnf.nice.org.uk/treatment-summary/aminoglycosides.html (accessed January 2022).

BNF (2021e) Lincoamides. https://bnf.nice.org.uk/drug/clindamycin.html#pregnancy (accessed January 2022).

BNF (2021f) Pyrimethamine. https://bnf.nice.org.uk/drug/pyrimethamine.html (accessed January 2022).

Bookstaver, P.B., Bland, C.M., Griffin, B., Stover, K.R., Eiland, L.S., McLaughlin, M. (2015) A review of antibiotic use in pregnancy. *Pharmacotherapy*, **35**(11): 1052–1062.

Brill, M.J.E., Kristoffersson, A.N., Zhao, C., Nielsen, E.I., Friberg, L.E. (2018) Semi-mechanistic pharmacokinetic–pharmacodynamic modelling of antibiotic drug combinations. *Clinical Microbiology and Infection*, **24**(7): 697–706.

British Pharmacology Association (2021) Ten principles of good prescribing. www.bps.ac.uk/education-engagement/teaching-pharmacology/ten-principles-of-good-prescribing (accessed January 2022).

Buppasiri, P., Lumbiganon, P., Thinkhamrop, J., Thinkhamrop, B. (2014) Antibiotic prophylaxis for third- and fourth-degree perineal tear during vaginal birth. *Cochrane Database of Systematic Reviews*, **10**: CD005125.

Burchaum, J.R., Rosenthal, L.D. (2019) *Lehne's Pharmacology for Nursing Care*. Elsevier: St Louis.

Centers for Disease Control and Prevention (2019) Antibiotic resistance – the global threat. www.cdc.gov/globalhealth/infographics/antibiotic-resistance/antibiotic_resistance_global_threat.htm (accessed January 2022).

Chiriac, A.M., Rerkpattanapipat, T., Bousquet, P.J., Molinari, N., Demoly P. (2017) Optimal step doses for drug provocation tests to prove beta-lactam hypersensitivity. *Allergy*, **72**(4): 552–561.

Clardy, J., Fischbach, M.A., Currie, C.R. (2009) The natural history of antibiotics. *Current Biology*, **19**(11): R437–R441.

Dahl, C., Stigum, H., Valeur, J. et al. (2018) Preterm infants have distinct microbiomes not explained by mode of delivery, breastfeeding duration or antibiotic exposure. *International Journal of Epidemiology*, **47**(5): 1658–1669.

Davies, S. (2018) *Chief Medical Officer's Annual Report 2018: Better Health Within Reach*. Department of Health and Social Care: London.

Desvaux, M., Dumas, E., Chafsey, I., Hébraud, M. (2006) Protein cell surface display in Gram-positive bacteria: from single protein to macromolecular protein structure., *FEMS Microbiology Letters*, **256**(1): 1–15.

Dingsdag, S.A., Hunter, N. (2018) Metronidazole: an update on metabolism, structure–cytotoxicity and resistance mechanisms, *Journal of Antimicrobial Chemotherapy*, **73**(2): 265–279.

EUCAST (2021a) EUCAST SOPs and Guidance documents. www.eucast.org/ast_of_bacteria/guidance_documents/ (accessed January 2022).

EUCAST (2021b) EUCAST guideline for the detection of resistance mechanisms and specific resistances of clinical and/or epidemiological importance. https://eucast.org/resistance_mechanisms/#:~:text=The%20first%20version%20of%20the%20EUCAST%20guideline%20for,on%20detection%20of%20resistance%20mechanisms%20v%202.0%20%282017-07-11%29 (accessed January 2022).

Fan, J., de Lannoy, I.A.M. (2014) Pharmacokinetics. *Biochemical Pharmacology*, **87**(1): 93–120.

Farrington, M. (2012) Antibacterial Drugs. In: *Clinical Pharmacology*, 11th edn. Elsevier: St Louis.

Ferro, A., Ritter, J., Mant, T., Lewis, L. (2008) *A Textbook of Clinical Pharmacology and Therapeutics*, 5th edn. Taylor and Francis: London.

Fleming, N. (2016) Antimicrobial stewardship: the appropriate use of antibiotics. *Practice Nursing*, **27**(8): 365–370.

Fullerton, J.N., Pasqua, O.D., Likic R. (2020) Early View Model antibiotic use to improve outcomes. *British Journal of Clinical Pharmacology*, **87**(3): 738–740.

Furber, C.G., Allison, D., Hindley, C. (2017) Antimicrobial resistance, antibiotic stewardship, and the midwife's role. *British Journal of Midwifery*, **25**(11): 693–698.

Gattarello, S., Borgatta, B., Solé-Violán, J. et al., Community-Acquired Pneumonia en la Unidad de Cuidados Intensivos II Study Investigators (2014) Decrease in mortality in severe community-acquired pneumococcal pneumonia: impact of improving antibiotic strategies (2000–2013). *Chest*, **146**(1): 22–31.

Gaynes, R. (2017) The discovery of penicillin – new insights after more than 75 years of clinical use. *Emerging Infectious Diseases*, **23**(5): 849–853.

Greer, O., Shah, N.M., Johnson, M.R. (2019) Maternal sepsis update: current management and controversies. *Obstetrician and Gynaecologist*, **22**(1): 44–45.

Hughes, R.G., Brocklehurst, B., Steer, P.J., Heath, P., Stenson, B.M. (2017) Prevention of onset neonatal group B streptococcal disease. *British Journal of Obstetrics and Gynaecology*, **124**: 280–305.

Jernberg, C., Lofmark, S., Edlund, C., Jansson, J.K. (2007) Long-term ecological impacts of antibiotic administration on the human intestinal microbiota. *ISME Journal*, **1**(1): 56–66.

Kahlmeter, G. (2016) What is antibiotic resistance? *Pharmaceutical Technology Europe*, **28**(5): 8.

Knight, M., Bunch, K., Tuffnell, D., et al. on behalf of MBRRACE-UK (2020) *Saving Lives, Improving Mothers' Care. Lessons learned to inform maternity care from the UK and Ireland Confidential Enquiries into Maternal Deaths and Morbidity 2016–18*. National Perinatal Epidemiology Unit: Oxford.

Laxminarayan, R., Duse, A., Wattal, C. et al. (2016) Exploring the contribution of maternal antibiotics and breastfeeding to development of the infant microbiome and pediatric obesity. *Seminars in Fetal and Neonatal Medicine*, **21**(6): 406–409.

Leone, S., Damiani, G., Pezone, I. et al. (2019a) New antimicrobial options for the management of complicated intra-abdominal infections. *European Journal of Clinical Microbiology and Infectious Diseases*, **38**(5): 819–827.

Leone, S., Cascella, M., Pezone, I., Fiore, M. (2019b) New antibiotics for the treatment of serious infections in intensive care unit patients. *Current Medical Research and Opinion*, **35**(8): 1331–1334.

Mansur-Ali, S., Siddiqui, R., Khan, N.A. (2018) Antimicrobial discovery from natural and unusual sources. *Journal of Pharmacy and Pharmacology*, **70**(10): 1287–1300.

McNulty, C.A.M., Nichols, T., French, D.P., Joshi, P., Butler, C.C. (2013) Expectations for consultations and antibiotics for respiratory tract infection in primary care: the RTI clinical iceberg. *British Journal of General Practice*, **63**(612): 429–436.

Miller, R.L., Shtessel, M., Robinson, L.B., Banerji, A. (2019) Advances in drug allergy, urticaria, angioedema, and anaphylaxis in 2018. *Journal of Allergy and Clinical Immunology*, **144**(2): 381–392.

National Institute for Health and Care Excellence (2008) Maternal and child nutrition (updated 2014). www.nice.org.uk/guidance/ph11/chapter/4-recommendations#folic-acid-2 (accessed January 2022).

National Institute for Health and Care Excellence (2012) Neonatal infection (early onset): antibiotics for prevention and treatment. www.nice.org.uk/guidance/cg149/chapter/1-Guidance#intrapartum-antibiotics-2 (accessed January 2022).

National Institute for Health and Care Excellence (2015a) Antimicrobial stewardship: systems and processes for effective antimicrobial medicine use. www.nice.org.uk/guidance/ng15/chapter/What-is-this-guideline-about-and-who-is-it-for (accessed January 2022).

National Institute for Health and Care Excellence (2015b) Antimicrobial stewardship: prescribing antibiotics. www.nice.org.uk/advice/ktt9/resources/antibiotic-prescribing-especially-broad-spectrum-antibiotics-1632178559941 (accessed January 2022).

National Institute for Health and Care Excellence (2016) Sepsis: recognition, diagnosis and early management. www.nice.org.uk/guidance/ng51/chapter/Recommendations#antibiotic-treatment-in-people-with-suspected-sepsis (accessed January 2022).

141

National Institute for Health and Care Excellence (2018) Urinary tract infection (lower): antimicrobial prescribing NICE guideline. www.nice.org.uk/guidance/ng109/chapter/summary-of-the-evidence#choice-of-antibiotic-2 (accessed January 2022).

National Institute for Health and Care Excellence (2019) Joint Formulary www.JointFormulary.org/products/JointFormulary-online/ (accessed January 2022).

National Institute for Health and Care Excellence (2020a) Summary of antimicrobial prescribing guidance – managing common infections. www.nice.org.uk/Media/Default/About/what-we-do/NICE-guidance/antimicrobial%20guidance/summary-antimicrobial-prescribing-guidance.pdf (accessed January 2022).

National Institute for Health and Care Excellence (2020b) Antimicrobial Stewardship. *www.nice.org.uk/guidance/health-protection/communicable-diseases/antimicrobial-stewardship on Dec 10 2020* (accessed January 2022).

National Institute for Health and Care Excellence (2021a) Prescribing in pregnancy. https://bnf.nice.org.uk/guidance/prescribing-in-pregnancy.html (accessed January 2022).

National Institute for Health and Care Excellence (2021b) Prescribing in breast-feeding. https://bnf.nice.org.uk/guidance/prescribing-in-breast-feeding.html (accessed January 2022).

National Institute for Health and Care Excellence (2021c) Adverse reactions to drugs: Yellow Card scheme. https://bnf.nice.org.uk/guidance/adverse-reactions-to-drugs.html (accessed January 2022).

Nesme, J., Simonet, P. (2015) The soil resistome: a critical review on antibiotic resistance origins, ecology and dissemination potential in telluric bacteria. *Environmental Microbiology*, **17**(4): 913–930.

Newman, D.J., Cragg, G.M., Snader, K.M. (2003) Natural products as sources of new drugs over the period 1981–2002. *Journal of Natural Products*, **66**: 1022.

Office for National Statistics (2021) Provisional births in England and Wales: 2020. www.ons.gov.uk/peoplepopulationandcommunity/birthsdeathsandmarriages/livebirths/articles/provisionalbirthsinenglandandwales/2020 (accessed January 2022).

Pandey, N., Cascella, M. (2021) *Beta Lactam Antibiotics*. StatPearls: Treasure Island.

Pankey, G.A., Sabath, L.D. (2004) Clinical relevance of bacteriostatic versus bactericidal mechanisms of action in the treatment of gram-positive bacterial infections. *Clinical Infectious Diseases*, **38**(6): 864–870.

Pariente, G., Leibson, T., Carls, A., Adams-Webber, T., Ito, S., Koren, G. (2016) Pregnancy-associated changes in pharmacokinetics: a systematic review. *PLoS Medicine*, **13**(11): e1002160.

Parliamentary Office of Science and Technology (2017) UK trends in infectious disease. https://researchbriefings.files.parliament.uk/documents/POST-PN-0545/POST-PN-0545.pdf (accessed January 2022).

Peate, I., Hill, B. (2021) *Fundamentals of Pharmacology for Nursing and Healthcare Students*. Wiley: Chichester.

Percival, S., Williamson, D.L. (2014) Mycobacterium. In: *Microbiology of Waterborne Diseases*, 2nd edn, pp.177–207. Academic Press: London.

Public Health England (2019a) *Addressing the Increase in Syphilis in England: PHE Action Plan*. PHE Publications: London.

Public Health England (2019b) Syphilis: surveillance, data and management. www.gov.uk/government/collections/syphilis-surveillance-data-and-management (accessed January 2022).

Rang, H.P., Ritter, J.M., Flower, R.J., Henderson, G. (2019a) Basic principles of antibacterial chemotherapy. In: *Rang and Dale's Pharmacology*, 9th edn. Elsevier Churchill Livingstone: Edinburgh.

Rang, H.P., Ritter, J.M., Flower, R.J., Henderson, G. (2019b) Drugs used for treatment of infections and cancers. In: *Rang and Dale's Pharmacology,* 9th edn. Elsevier Churchill Livingstone: Edinburgh.

Royal College of Obstetricians and Gynaecologists (2012) Bacterial sepsis in pregnancy. www.rcog.org.uk/globalassets/documents/guidelines/gtg_64a.pdf (accessed January 2022).

Royal College of Obstetricians and Gynaecologists (2015) RCOG statement on the use of antibiotics in pregnancy and the relative risk of neurological disorders. www.rcog.org.uk/en/news/rcog-statement-on-the-use-of-antibiotics-in-pregnancy-and-the-relative-risk-of-neurological-disorders/ (accessed January 2022).

Royal College of Obstetricians and Gynaecologists (2017) Group B streptococcal disease, early-onset. www.rcog.org.uk/en/guidelines-research-services/guidelines/gtg36/ (accessed January 2022).

Royal College of Obstetricians and Gynaecologists (2020) Perineal wound breakdown. www.rcog.org.uk/en/patients/tears/perineal-wound-dehiscence/ (accessed January 2022).

Smaill, F.M., Vazquez, J.C. (2019) Antibiotics for asymptomatic bacteriuria in pregnancy. *Cochrane Database of Systematic Reviews*, **11**: CD000490.

Strohl, W.R., Woodruff, H.B., Monaghan, R.L., Hendlin, D., Mochales I ., Demain, A.L. (2001) The history of natural products research at Merck & Co. *Inc SIM News*, **51**: 5–19.

Sullivan, G.J., Delgado, N.N., Maharjan, R., Cain, A.K. (2020) How antibiotics work together: molecular mechanisms behind combination therapy. *Current Opinion in Microbiology*, **57**: 31–40.

Tamma, P.D., Cosgrove, S.E., Maragakis, L.L. (2021) Combination therapy for treatment of infections with gram-negative bacteria. *Clinical Microbiology Reviews*, **25**: 450–470.

Thomson, A.J. (2019) Care of women presenting with suspected preterm prelabour rupture of membranes from 24+0 weeks of gestation. *British Journal of Obstetrics and Gynaecology*, **126**(9): e152–e166.

Uzlikova, M., Nohynkova, E.(2014) The effect of metronidazole on the cell cycle and DNA in metronidazole-susceptible and -resistant Giardia cell lines. *Molecular and Biochemical Parasitology*, **198**(2): 75–81.

van Belkum, A., Bachmann, T.T., Lüdke, G. et al. (2019) Developmental roadmap for antimicrobial susceptibility testing systems. *Nature Reviews Microbiology*, **17**: 51–62.

Vellai, T., Vida, G. (1999) The origin of eukaryotes: the difference between prokaryotic and eukaryotic cells. *Biological Sciences*, **266**(1428): 1571–1577.

Walker, G.J.A. (2001) Antibiotics for syphilis diagnosed during pregnancy. *Cochrane Database of Systematic Reviews*, **3**: CD001143.

Wilcock, M., Powell, N., Underwood, F. (2019) Antimicrobial stewardship and the hospital nurse and midwife: how do they perceive their role? *European Journal of Hospital Pharmacy*, **26**: 89–92.

Wilson, B.A., Winkler, M., Ho, B.T. (2019) *Bacterial Pathogenesis: A Molecular Approach*. ASM Press: Newark.

Wojcieszek, A.M., Stock, O.M., Flenady, V.(2014) Antibiotics for prelabour rupture of membranes at or near term. *Cochrane Database of Systematic Reviews*, **10**: CD001807.

World Health Organization (2013) Newborn health: challenges facing preterm babies. www.who.int/news-room/q-a-detail/newborn-health-challenges-facing-preterm-babies (accessed January 2022).

World Health Organization (2020) Antibiotics resistance. www.who.int/news-room/fact-sheets/detail/antibiotic-resistance (accessed January 2022).

Xiu, P., Datta, S. (2019) *Pharmacology*, 5th edn. Elsevier: London.

143

Further reading

National Institute for Health and Care Excellence (2018) Antimicrobial Stewardship. www.nice.org.uk/guidance/ng15 (accessed January 2022).

National Institute for Health and Care Excellence (2019) Joint formulary. https://JointFormulary.nice.org.uk/ (accessed January 2022).

National Institute for Health and Care Excellence (2019) NICE guidelines. www.nice.org.uk/guidance (accessed January 2022).

World Health Organization (2015) Global action plan on antimicrobial resistance. www.who.int/ antimicrobial-resistance/publications/global-action-plan/en (accessed January 2022).

World Health Organization (2018) Factsheet on antimicrobial resistance. www.who.int/antimicrobial-resistance/en (accessed January 2022).

World Health Organization (2018) Factsheet on antibiotic resistance. www.who.int/en/newsroom/fact-sheets/detail/antibiotic-resistance (accessed January 2022).

Part 3

Medications used during pregnancy and childbirth

Chapter 10

Medications used in labour

Chin Swain

University of Hertfordshire, Hatfield, UK

Aim

This chapter aims to introduce the reader to the midwife's role in the use of medications in induction of labour, regional block analgesia and key issues surrounding the function of medication used.

Learning outcomes

After reading this chapter, the reader will be able to:
- Discuss the role of the midwife in association with medicines management
- Understand the contraindications and side-effects of these medications
- Discuss the administration route and dosages of medications
- Understand the role of the Code (NMC, 2018) and professional duties.

Test your existing knowledge

- List the medications used for induction of labour.
- These medications are administered via which route?
- Outline the midwife's role in caring for a woman undergoing induction of labour.
- How would you measure the effectiveness of an epidural?
- What frequency of monitoring of the level of epidural block must be carried out after an epidural top-up?

Introduction

Induction of labour is one of the most frequently performed obstetric procedures in the world. Induction of labour (IOL) is defined as an artificial initiation of labour (National Collaborating Centre for Women's and Children's Health, 2008) and rates vary widely from 6.8–33% in Europe to 24.5% in the United States (Marconi et al., 2019). Rates of IOL in the UK have increased from 29.4% in 2016–17 to 31.6% in 2017–18 (NHS, 2021). Findings from the Care Quality Commission (CQC) survey of women's experiences of maternity care found that as a consequence of IOL, women are more likely to have stronger analgesia such as epidural and assisted delivery (CQC, 2020). Midwives are in a

Fundamentals of Pharmacology for Midwives, First Edition. Edited by Ian Peate and Cathy Hamilton.
© 2022 John Wiley & Sons Ltd. Published 2022 by John Wiley & Sons Ltd.
Companion website: www.wiley.com/go/pharmacologyformidwives

unique position as they are the main carer for many complex cases such as intrauterine growth retardation, multiple pregnancies so they need to be equipped with the skills and knowledge to carry out the care required to keep both mother and baby safe.

Induction of labour is considered when the benefits outweigh maternal and/or fetal risks of waiting for a spontaneous labour, for example, for cases such as pre-eclampsia or severe fetal growth restriction. IOL should be carried out with informed consent and the reason for the induction, including risks, benefits and methods used, must be clearly explained to the person. IOL can be divided into two categories: low and high risk. Cases such as pregnancy beyond 41 weeks with no other complications are considered low risk whereas high-risk IOL cases have significant risk to mother and/or fetus, such as pre-eclampsia, unstable lie and intrauterine growth restriction (IUGR). As well as IOL, labour can be augmented for slow progress or labour dystocia.

Indications for induction of labour

- Post maturity
- Concerns about fetal well-being
- Intrauterine growth retardation
- Prolonged rupture of membranes
- Pre-eclampsia
- Multiple pregnancies
- Fetal death
- Fetal anomaly not compatible with life
- Maternal request – psychological/social reasons; the mother must be fully counselled regarding the implications of the request

Contraindications for induction of labour

- No informed consent
- Transverse lie
- Cord prolapse
- Placenta previa
- Malposition or compound presentation

Clinical consideration

Effective communication between the midwife and the woman in labour is essential. It should be supported by evidence-based written information tailored to the needs of the woman. Any information given to the woman regarding treatment options should be culturally appropriate. This information should be accessible to women, their partners and families; it should also take into consideration any additional physical needs, cognitive disabilities and inability to speak or read English (NICE, 2008).

Uterotonic drugs

Uterine stimulants (uterotonics or oxytocics) are medications given to cause a woman's uterus to contract or to increase the frequency and intensity of contractions. The three uterotonic drugs most commonly used are oxytocics, such as Syntocinon®, and prostaglandins and ergot alkaloids. Uterotonic drugs may be given intramuscularly (IM), intravenously (IV) and as a gel, tablet or suppository (Prevention of Postpartum Haemorrhage Initiative (POPPHI), 2008).

Methods of induction

Uterotonic drugs can be used to induce labour (start labour) and as part of the labour induction process. Uterotonics such as prostaglandins are commonly used to induce labour, and this is usually followed with Syntocinon in the form of an infusion to continue the labour process.

Prostaglandins

There are several methods of IOL but vaginal PGE_2 is the preferred method, unless there is a specific clinical reason for not using it, such as risk of uterine hyperstimulation. Prostaglandins are a prescription only medication and can be administered as a gel, tablet or controlled-release pessary. It should be inserted into the posterior fornix, avoiding administration into the cervical canal because this may cause hyperstimulation. The main complication associated with prostaglandin administration is uterine hyperstimulation with or without fetal compromise (Bartholomew et al., 2017). Prostin E2® vaginal gel is available in doses of 1 mg or 2 mg. Caution should be exercised in the administration of Prostin E2 vaginal gel for IOL in patients with:

- asthma or a history of asthma
- epilepsy or a history of epilepsy
- glaucoma or raised intraocular pressure
- compromised cardiovascular, hepatic or renal function
- hypertension.

149

Method of administration of vaginal PGE2

1. Collect the prescription chart and prescribed medication.
2. Prepare the PGE_2, for example Prostin E2 vaginal gel – check the name, dose, expiry date of the medication and always adhere to local policy and procedure.
3. Ensure you have sterile gloves and lubricant.
4. Wash hands and put on an apron.
5. Explain the procedure to the woman and obtain consent.
6. Ensure you have analgesia available such as Entonox for the woman to use, if necessary, as the procedure can be uncomfortable.
7. Abdominal palpation is carried out to determine the presentation, position and station of the fetus. An electronic trace of the fetal heart is carried out to ensure the fetus's well-being for 30 minutes before the administration of Prostin.
8. Perform the 5 Rights for medication administration.
9. Position the woman on her back. The midwife will perform a vaginal examination to check for dilation, presentation and station of the presenting part. This must be done sensitively and carefully.
10. For Prostin E_2 vaginal tablet – secure the tablet between the index and middle fingers of the examination hand. Insert lubricated fingers gently into the vagina in a downwards and backwards direction along the posterior vaginal wall. The tablet is inserted into the posterior fornix.
11. For Prostin gel – this comes with a syringe applicator. Locate the posterior fornix as above and gently guide the syringe applicator along the examining fingers; squirt the gel into the posterior fornix.
12. For Propess® – this needs to be placed cross-wise, high in the posterior fornix. To do this, place the Propess between the index and middle fingers, enter the vagina and locate the posterior fornix. Manoeuvre the Propess into a transverse position, remove your fingers and be careful not to pull the retrieval tape out.
13. The woman remains in a semi-recumbent position for the next 30 minutes; an electronic trace of the fetal heart is carried out for 30 minutes post insertion to monitor the fetus's well-being.
14. Explain your findings and inform the woman of the signs and symptoms to report to the midwife, e.g. vaginal bleeding, rupture of membranes or if the Propess falls out.
15. Ensure the call bell is within easy reach.
16. Safely dispose of used equipment.
17. Wash hands.
18. Document your actions in the notes.

See also Chapter 4 in relation to the management of medications.

Clinical consideration

In a primigravida with unfavourable induction features (Bishop score of 4 or less; Table 10.1), an initial dose of 2 mg should be administered vaginally. In other cases (multiparous women), an initial dose of 1 mg should be administered vaginally. In both groups, a second dose of 1 mg or 2 mg may be administered after 6 hours as follows:1 mg should be used where uterine activity is insufficient for satisfactory progress of labour or 2 mg may be used where the response to the initial dose has been minimal (NICE, 2017). In any medication administration, it is imperative that the midwife adheres to the 5 Rights of medication administration.

The Bishop score is a group of measurements achieved by performing a vaginal examination, and is based on the station, dilation, effacement (or length), position and consistency of the cervix; a score of 8 or more generally indicates that the cervix is 'ripe' or 'favourable'. When there is a high chance of spontaneous labour or response to interventions made to induce labour, the fetal heart should be assessed and recorded, and a normal fetal heart rate pattern should be confirmed using electronic fetal monitoring (NICE, 2021b).

Table 10.1 Bishop score.

Source	Dilation (cm)	Position of cervix	Effacement (%)	Station (−3 to +3)	Cervical consistency
0	Closed	Posterior	0–30	−3	Firm
1	1–2	Mid position	40–50	−2	Medium
2	3–4	Anterior	60–70	−1, 0	Soft
3	5–6	–	80	+1, +2	–

Source: Wormer et al. (2021)/StatPearls Publishing LLC/CC BY 4.0.

Oxytocin

Oxytocin is a uterotonic drug widely used in labour. It has many uses, such as inducing labour (after prostaglandins), augmenting labour, active management of the third stage of labour, and managing emergency haemorrhage (see Chapter 23). It has a short half-life of approximately 3–5 minutes and can be used as an infusion to maintain contractions (Gallos et al., 2019). When used intramuscularly, the latent phase lasts 2–5 minutes but the uterine activity can last 2–3 hours. The types of oxytocin frequently found in maternity units are Syntocinon 10 IU/mL ampoules and Syntometrine® given by intramuscular injection (Table 10.2).

Effect on the body

Oxytocin is synthetic and obtained by chemical synthesis; it is identical to the natural hormone stored in the posterior pituitary and released into the systemic circulation in response to suckling and labour. Oxytocin stimulates the smooth muscle of the uterus, more powerfully towards the end of pregnancy, during labour and immediately postpartum. Oxytocin elicits rhythmic contractions in the upper segment of the uterus, similar in frequency, force and duration to those observed during labour. Being synthetic, the oxytocin in Syntometrine does not contain vasopressin, but even in its pure form, oxytocin possesses some weak intrinsic vasopressin-like antidiuretic activity.

Storage

These drugs are usually stored between 2 °C and 8 °C in the drug fridge in clinical areas. However, it can be stored safely up to 30 °C for 3 months but must then be discarded. This is usually the case for community midwives where they carry a variety of drugs in their car for home births.

Table 10.2   Commonly used medications.

Medication	Legal classification	Midwives' exemption list	Route	Indication
Prostin	POM	No	Vaginal gel, pessary or tablets	Medication for IOL
Syntocinon	POM	Yes	IV/IM	Tocolytic to expedite third stage of labour when Syntometrine is contraindicated. Also used for control of postpartum bleeding
Syntometrine	POM	Yes	IM	Tocolytic to expedite the third stage of labou.
Terbutaline	POM	No	IM or subcutaneous	To delay or stop contractions

IM, intramuscular; IOL, induction of labour; IV, intravenous; POM, prescription only medication.

151

Indications and dose

Induction of labour

Oxytocin can be used to induce labour (starting labour) or as part of the labour process. Oxytocin is usually used after the administration of prostaglandins to continue the induction labour process. It is administered as an intravenous (IV) infusion via a variable-speed infusion pump. An example of an infusion for IOL is 5 IU of Syntocinon added to 500 mL of sodium chloride or normal saline 0.9% or 500 mL of 5% dextrose solution. The solution must be mixed well by inverting the bag several times. The rate of infusion will be determined by local guidance.

Augmentation of labour

Labour progress is measured by cervical dilation, the descent of the presenting part and the strength and length of contractions (NICE, 2017). Actively managing labour by increasing contractions may reduce the need for instrumental delivery or caesarean section. A delay in labour is diagnosed when cervical dilation is less than 2 cm in 4 hours or there is a delay in descent and rotation of the baby's head and a reduction in the strength, duration and frequency of uterine contractions. This is more common amongst nulliparous than multiparous women (WHO, 2014). When a delay is diagnosed, the midwife will discuss these findings with the labourer and the obstetric team. A plan to augment (speed up) the labour would be discussed. If the membranes are still intact, an amniotomy would be offered, after an explanation of the procedure and advice that it will shorten the labour by about an hour but may increase the strength and pain of contractions (NICE, 2017). A vaginal examination should be carried out 2 hours post amniotomy to monitor progress.

The preparation of drugs for augmentation of labour is similar to that of IOL.

Role of the midwife

Any induction or augmentation of labour will need to be discussed with the woman to ensure she fully understands the process. The obstetric team will be involved with the care and management of induced or augmented labour along with the midwife. They should discuss the reason for induction, when, where and how the induction will be carried out, arrangements for pain relief, the risks and benefits of induction, alternative options if the woman chooses not to have IOL and what the options would be if the induction is not successful (NICE, 2021a). Ideally, the woman would be allowed time to discuss the information with her partner (if appropriate) before coming to a decision.

The midwife can support this process by encouraging the woman to ask questions and think of her options and support the woman in whatever decision she makes. The woman's obstetric history would also be carefully scrutinised for any high-risk factors such as previous caesarean section or low-lying placenta.

Before induction of labour, engagement of the presenting part is assessed by abdominal palpation. A preliminary vaginal examination is carried out to check for any umbilical cord presentation, findings from the Bishop score should be assessed and recorded, and a normal fetal heart rate pattern should be confirmed using electronic fetal monitoring. The midwife should inform the labourer that oxytocin will increase the frequency and strength of contractions and that its use will mean that the baby must be monitored continuously along with considerations for analgesia. The frequency, strength and duration of contractions and the fetal heart rate must be carefully monitored throughout the infusion by continuous electronic monitoring, usually by cardiotocograph (CTG). Further observations required include vital signs and monitoring of pain by the midwife. The midwife will palpate the contractions to ascertain strength and length while simultaneously monitoring fetal well-being, such as heart rate and colour of the liquor.

Once an adequate level of uterine activity is attained, aiming for 3–4 contractions every 10 minutes, the infusion rate is maintained or reduced if necessary (NICE, 2017). Amniotomy is usually carried out before starting a Syntocinon infusion.

Syntocinon

The labouring woman will need to be cannulated for access for the infusion of Syntocinon (Box 10.1). Typically, at this point, the midwife would also obtain a sample of blood for full blood count and group and save. This is to avoid the need to obtain any blood samples if there is an indication for further intervention such as a caesarean section at a later stage. Continuous monitoring of the fetal heart rate is also commenced 30 minutes before starting the Syntocinon solution to ensure fetal well-being.

Box 10.1 Syntocinon

Indications	Antepartum use for induction of labour for medical reasons. Postpartum use to stimulate contraction following delivery
Dose and frequency	Antepartum dose 5 IU of Syntocinon added to 500 mL of physiological electrolyte solution such as sodium chloride 0.9%. Example infusion rate is 1–4 milliunits/minute, gradually increasing every 20 minutes until 3–4 contractions are attained
Interactions (examples relevant in pregnancy)	Syntocinon must not be administered within 6 hours after vaginal prostaglandins have been given
Side-effects	Arrhythmias, headache, nausea and vomiting
Absorption (A)	Plasma levels of oxytocin following intravenous infusion at 4 milliunits/minute at term are 2–5 microunits/mL
Distribution (D)	Plasma protein binding is negligible for oxytocin; it crosses the placenta. Oxytocin can be found in small quantities in breast milk
Metabolism (M)	The plasma half-life of oxytocin ranges from 3 to 20 minutes. It is excreted in urine

Syntocinon infusion must be carefully titrated when used for inducing or augmenting labour. The dosage and rate will depend on local policy and procedure. Where fluid restrictions are necessary, such as pre-eclampsia for IOL, an alternative dose of Syntocinon is infused. An example of a smaller quantity of infusion: dilute 5 IU of Syntocinon in 49 mL of normal saline (sodium chloride 0.9%) solution. Use a 50 mL syringe for this infusion. The infusion would be administered via an infusion pump connected to the labourer. The infusion rate would be 4 mL/h for primiparous or 2 mL/h for multiparous labourers. The infusion rate would increase incrementally until an adequate level of uterine activity is attained, aiming for 3–4 contractions every 10 minutes, lasting for approximately 60 seconds. Once this is achieved, the rate of Syntocinon can be maintained until delivery of the baby.

During the induction, women should be informed of the availability of pain relief options (also see Chapter 8), as IOL often makes the contractions stronger and more painful for the woman. In the event of uterine hyperstimulation and/or fetal distress, the infusion must be discontinued immediately and help summoned. The Syntocinon infusion would be discontinued after the birth of the baby.

Clinical consideration

Any additive added to an intravenous infusion must be clearly labelled; refer to local trust guidelines. The label usually indicates name, hospital number, drug added, dosage, date and time.

153

Syntocinon infusion must not be administered within 6 hours of the administration of vaginal prostaglandins as this may cause hyperstimulation. Because oxytocin has a slight antidiuretic effect, its prolonged IV administration at high doses in conjunction with large volumes of fluid, as may be the case in the management of postpartum haemorrhage, may cause water intoxication associated with hyponatraemia. The combined antidiuretic effect of oxytocin and the IV fluid administration may cause fluid overload, leading to acute pulmonary oedema without hyponatraemia. To avoid these rare complications, the following precautions must be observed whenever high doses of oxytocin are administered over a long time.

- An electrolyte-containing diluent must be used (not dextrose).
- The volume of infused fluid should be kept low (by infusing oxytocin at a higher concentration than recommended for the induction or enhancement of labour at term).
- Fluid intake by mouth must be restricted.
- A fluid balance chart must be kept.
- Serum electrolytes must be measured when electrolyte imbalance is suspected (EMC, 2021).

The midwife must be alert to the symptoms of water intoxication: headache, nausea, vomiting, lethargy, drowsiness, unconsciousness and convulsions.

Syntocinon for management of the third stage

The third stage of labour is the time from the birth of the baby to the expulsion of the placenta and membranes (NICE, 2017). Active management includes administering an oxytocin medication, delayed clamping and cutting of the umbilical cord, and controlled cord traction (CCT) after the signs of separation of the placenta are evident. Active management of the third stage is recommended to reduce the risk of blood loss or postpartum haemorrhage (PPH) and the need for blood transfusion (NICE, 2017).

In active management, a uterotonic is used to reduce the risk of blood loss. Common drugs used for this purpose are Syntocinon and Syntometrine. Syntocinon is preferred because it has fewer side-effects than Syntometrine. It is recommended that Syntocinon 10 IU/mL be given IM at the delivery of the anterior shoulder of the baby or soon after the delivery of the baby and before the cord is clamped and cut. This would have been discussed by the midwife with the woman to gain consent during the first stage of labour.

Side-effects of Syntocinon include:

- arrhythmias
- headaches
- nausea and vomiting.

Syntometrine

Syntometrine can also be used to actively manage the third stage of labour (Box 10.2). It consists of 500 micrograms of ergometrine maleate and 5 units of oxytocin per 1 mL. This is administered by IM injection at delivery of the baby's anterior shoulder or soon after. The effects of Syntometrine are quickly felt, resulting in the expulsion of the placenta within 2.5 minutes, which is normally separated by the first strong uterine contraction and should be assisted by CCT. Syntometrine is not recommended where elevated blood pressure is diagnosed, such as pre-eclampsia, hypertension, severe cardiac disorders and hepatic or renal impairment. Common side-effects from Syntometrine are:

- arrhythmias
- headache
- nausea, vomiting.

Box 10.2   Syntometrine

Indications	Active management of the third stage; to prevent or treat postpartum haemorrhage
Dose and frequency	For active management of the third stage: intramuscular injection of 1 mL after delivery of the anterior shoulder or immediately after the delivery of the baby. Expulsion of the placenta should be assisted by controlled cord traction
Interactions (examples relevant in pregnancy)	Syntometrine may enhance the effects of prostaglandins and vice versa
Side-effects	Headache, nausea and vomiting
Absorption (A)	Quickly absorbed from the intramuscular injection site
Distribution (D)	Ergometrine is known to cross the placenta and its clearance from the fetus is slow. Ergometrine is also excreted in breast milk and may reduce milk secretion
Metabolism (M)	The plasma half-life of ergometrine ranges from 30 to 120 minutes. It can be detected up to 8 hours in urine

Clinical consideration

In 2007, NICE guidance changed from recommending Syntometrine for active management of the third stage to Syntocinon 10 IU. This was recommended for low-risk labours. There were concerns about a perceived increase in major postpartum haemorrhages; however, studies by Rogers et al. (2013a, 2013b) and Hofmeyr et al. (2015) found no statistically significant increase in estimated blood loss (EBL) above 1000 mL.

Clinical consideration

Controlled cord traction (CCT) is performed during active management of the third stage of labour. The third stage of labour starts with the delivery of the fetus and ends when the placenta is delivered (Hutchinson, 2021). Once the baby is delivered with the administration of an oxytocic medication, the midwife performs CCT when the uterus is felt to contract; traction is applied to the umbilical cord with counterpressure applied suprapubically on the uterus until the placenta delivers (Hofmeyr et al., 2015).

In breech presentation and other abnormal fetal presentations, Syntometrine should not be given before delivery of the baby is completed, and in multiple births not before the last baby has been delivered (EMC, 2021).

Terbutaline or terbutaline sulfate

Terbutaline (Bricanyl®) is usually used to reduce or stop contractions, in cases of premature labour or overstimulation of the uterus by oxytocin infusion. 'Tocolysis' is when women are given medication to reduce the strength or frequency of contractions, or both. There is concern that uterine tachysystole may reduce fetal oxygenation by interrupting maternal blood flow to the placenta during contractions. The use of a tocolytic drug to relax the uterine muscles and reduce or stop contractions may improve blood flow and therefore improve the baby's well-being (Leathersich et al., 2018). Babies who are deprived of oxygen can develop cerebral palsy, organ damage or death. For women who have unexpectedly gone into premature labour between 22 and 37 weeks gestation, terbutaline would provide a short delay in the early delivery of the baby (EMC, 2021) and this would be via an intravenous infusion.

Terbutaline can also be given for hyperstimulation of the uterus. Hyperstimulation of the uterus is diagnosed when there are five contractions every 10 minutes for 20 minutes and uterine hypersystole/hypertonicity is diagnosed when a contraction lasts at least 2 minutes (National Collaborating Centre for Women's and Children's Health, 2008).

The dose of terbutaline is 0.25 mg administered by subcutaneous injection. One contraindication to use of terbutaline is sensitivity to the medication and/or pregnancy below 22 weeks. Monitoring of blood pressure, maternal and fetal heart rate, electrolyte and fluid balance is important when using terbutaline.

Special warnings and precautions

Bricanyl should be used with caution in tocolysis and supervision of cardiorespiratory function and ECG monitoring should be performed throughout treatment (EMC, 2021).

The following monitoring measures must be constantly applied to the mother and, when feasible/appropriate, to the fetus.

- *Blood pressure*: maternal blood pressure may fall slightly during infusion, the effect being greater on diastolic than on systolic pressure. Falls in diastolic pressure are usually within the range of 10–20 mmHg. The effect of infusion on fetal heart rate is less marked but increases of up to 20 beats per minute may occur.
- *Maternal heart rate*: increases in maternal heart rate of the order of 20–50 beats per minute usually accompany infusion of beta-agonists. The maternal pulse rate must be monitored and the need to control such increases by dose reduction or drug withdrawal should be evaluated on a case-by-case basis. Generally, maternal pulse rate must not be allowed to exceed a steady rate of 120 beats per minute (EMC, 2021).
- Electrocardiogram (ECG) where necessary.
- Electrolyte and fluid balance to monitor for pulmonary oedema.
- *Glucose and lactate levels with regard to women with diabetes*: during treatment of preterm labour, when high doses of Bricanyl are used, mothers with diabetes may develop hyperglycaemia and lactacidosis. In these cases, glucose and acid–base balance should be carefully monitored.
- *Potassium levels*: beta-agonists are associated with a decrease in serum potassium which increases the risk of arrhythmias.

Skills in practice

The midwife must carefully monitor contractions when oxytocics are used as hyperstimulation of the uterus can be dangerous to the fetus. If hyperstimulation is suspected, the oxytocic infusion must be stopped immediately and the labourer placed into the left lateral position whilst help is summoned. If indicated, terbutaline may be prescribed and administered as a 0.25 mg subcutaneous injection. Do not forget to explain to the labourer and any birthing partners present the reasons for the emergency and seek consent where appropriate.

Epidural

An epidural aims to block pain signals travelling from the spine to the brain, making the birth more comfortable. Epidural (regional) anaesthesia is an invasive procedure carried out by an anaesthetist. An anaesthetic drug (an opioid) is injected into the space between the spine called the epidural space. The epidural space is filled with fluid and surrounds the spinal cord. Spinal nerves carry pain signals from the body to the brain. The anaesthetic drug numbs these nerves, blocking the pain signals. This effectively relieves pain, whilst making it possible for the labourer to be awake during the labour experience.

The procedure is carried out in an aseptic manner using equipment from an epidural pack. During the labour, the medication is injected into the lumbar area, which, if working effectively, numbs the lower part of the body and hence the painful contractions. Most labourers who have an epidural feel little or no pain.

An example of opioid solution used for epidural is bupivacaine 10–15 mlL concentration of 0.0625–0.1% or equivalent with 1.0 –2.0 micrograms/mL fentanyl (Silva & Halpern, 2010; NICE, 2017.

Common side-effects of epidurals include the following (Anim-Somuah et al., 2018):

- *Low blood pressure*: in about 14 out of 100 women, the epidural causes blood pressure to drop, which can lead to dizziness or nausea.
- *Fever*: epidurals cause fever in about 23 out of 100 women. By comparison, this is only the case in about 7 out of 100 women who use another type of pain management.
- *Problems urinating*: an epidural can interfere with the sensation of urination, therefore the labourer can be catheterised to avoid distension of the bladder.

If a labouring woman is contemplating epidural analgesia, she must be made aware of the risks and benefits and the implications, including the arrangements and time involved for transfer of care to an obstetric unit if she is at home or in a midwifery-led birthing unit. An epidural is only available in obstetric units and is a more effective form of pain relief when compared to opioids. It is not associated with long-term backache, or with longer first stage of labour or increased risk of caesarean birth (NICE, 2017).

An intravenous infusion is commenced before siting the epidural to ensure intravenous access is available should the woman's blood pressure fall rapidly and fluid replacement is required. Epidural is associated with a longer second stage of labour and an increase in vaginal instrumental birth (NICE, 2017).

Preparation of the labourer for epidural

The procedure is carried out with the labourer in a sitting position or lying on her left side (Figure 10.1). After a careful explanation of the procedure, including the risks and benefits, the anaesthetist must gain the appropriate consent. The labourer is usually in an open-back gown to allow ease of access to the back and spine. Intravenous access would have been established before the epidural procedure. It is good practice to monitor the fetal heart rate for 30 minutes before the epidural procedure to obtain a baseline of fetal well-being (NICE, 2017).

The labourer is made comfortable sitting at the edge of the bed with her legs resting on a small stool. A pillow is usually given to the labourer to hug, which gives her more comfort for the forthcoming procedure. Continuous monitoring of the fetal heart must be established in this position. The labourer is encouraged to flex her spine to increase the space between the vertebrae. The skin is cleansed with an antiseptic solution and a Touhy needle is inserted into the spine between the second and third lumbar vertebrae into the epidural space (see Figure 10.1). A fine tube (catheter) is inserted along the length of the needle to guide the tube to its resting position. The labourer must remain still at this stage to avoid the Touhy needle puncturing the meninges and causing a dural tap (Bartholomew, 2017). The needle is then withdrawn, and the catheter is secured by tape once the anaesthetist is satisfied it is in the correct position. The woman is then made comfortable. The catheter is left in situ to allow access, initial administration and topping up of the analgesia. Epidural can be administered continuously (basal infusion) or via patient-controlled epidural analgesia (PCEA).

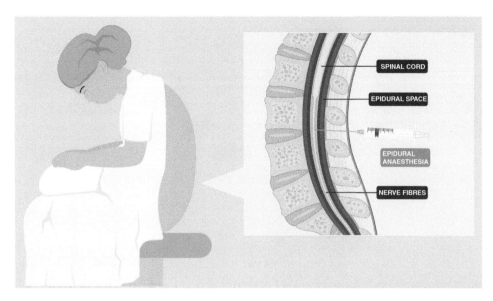

Figure 10.1 Spinal anaesthesia.

Role of the midwife during epidural

Throughout the procedure, the midwife should support the labourer and her birthing partner physically and psychologically. The midwife is responsible for the ongoing care of the woman receiving epidural analgesia (Figure 10.2). Where facilities are available, epidural administration can be controlled by the labourer via a pump and monitored by the midwife. The labourer's blood pressure must be monitored closely, at 5-minute intervals for 15 minutes after the initial dose and after every top-up (NICE, 2017). The labourer should be pain free for 30 minutes after each admin-istration of local anaesthetic or opioid solution; the anaesthetist should be recalled if this does not occur (NICE, 2017). The labourer can adopt an upright position that is comfortable for the duration of the labour.

The level of block can be assessed by using dermatome assessment with an approved cold spray (Bartholomew, 2017). The sensation of the cold spray is first tested on an area that is not affected by the epidural, such as the labourer's arm, and the sensation is then compared with the level of the block on the abdomen. The desired level is between T10 and L1. The level of the block must be assessed hourly to ensure it has not risen; if it rises, this may cause difficulty in breathing for the woman and if left unmonitored could lead to respiratory arrest or signs of dura puncture headache, which must be reported to the anaesthetist. The initial sign that the level of the epidural block is rising is a tingling tongue with rapid deterioration of the patient; the midwife must act quickly by stopping the epidural infusion, summoning help and preparing for resuscitation (Bartholomew, 2017).

Other complications of an epidural are numbness or tingling in the legs, hypotension, dura puncture and consequent headache, loss of bladder control and toxicity leading to cardiac arrest. A dura puncture is a leakage of spinal fluid from the dura layer created by the epidural procedure. If too much fluid is lost, it can cause severe headaches that may last a few days. This occurs in 1 in 100 labourers who have an epidural.

Mobility is usually impaired with an epidural, and it is the midwife's role to ensure the labourer's position is changed regularly to avoid pressure area issues. However, the epidural can be set to a lower dose that allows the labourer to mobilise during labour. Mobilising is thought to make the birth easier but studies have found that this is not the case (Informed Health, 2018).

The level of the epidural block is measured by the midwife intermittently throughout labour, as the degree of block will change. It is also important to measure motor block in both legs, since the

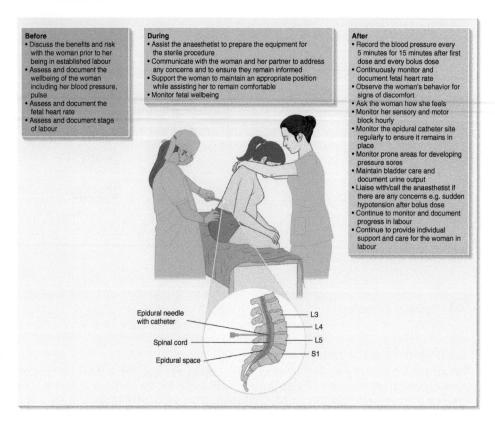

Before
- Discuss the benefits and risk with the woman prior to her being in established labour
- Assess and document the wellbeing of the woman including her blood pressure, pulse
- Assess and document the fetal heart rate
- Assess and document stage of labour

During
- Assist the anaesthetist to prepare the equipment for the sterile procedure
- Communicate with the woman and her partner to address any concerns and to ensure they remain informed
- Support the woman to maintain an appropriate position while assisting her to remain comfortable
- Monitor fetal wellbeing

After
- Record the blood pressure every 5 minutes for 15 minutes after first dose and every bolus dose
- Continuously monitor and document fetal heart rate
- Observe the woman's behavior for signs of discomfort
- Ask the woman how she feels
- Monitor her sensory and motor block hourly
- Monitor the epidural catheter site regularly to ensure it remains in place
- Monitor prone areas for developing pressure sores
- Maintain bladder care and document urine output
- Liaise with/call the anaesthetist if there are any concerns e.g. sudden hypotension after bolus dose
- Continue to monitor and document progress in labour
- Continue to provide individual support and care for the woman in labour

Epidural needle with catheter — L3
L4
Spinal cord — L5
S1
Epidural space

Figure 10.2   The role of the midwife in supporting a woman who chooses an epidural to cope with her labour.

block maybe asymmetrical. The midwife will monitor the level of the motor block using the Bromage scale (Anaesthesia UK, 2017). This scale is commonly used to assess the motor movement of the labourer after an epidural has been sited. The category of movement is divided into grades, where in grade one the labourer is able to move her legs freely, grade two in where the labourer is able to flex her knees and move her feet freely, grade three is where the labourer is unable to flex her knees but can move her feet and grade four is where the labourer is unable to flex her knees or move her feet (Anaesthesia UK, 2017).

The midwife must ensure the fetal heart is continuously monitored after the epidural procedure. Some labourers may still feel the urge to push in the second stage but many will require the assistance of a midwife to guide them on when to do this. The midwife does this by palpating for contractions and preparing the labourer to push simultaneously, using the strength of the contractions to expel the fetus.

After delivery of the baby, the epidural catheter is removed by aseptic technique. The area is covered by a small plaster and the actions recorded in the notes.

Spinal anaesthesia

Spinal anaesthesia works the same way as epidurals. With spinal anaesthesia, the medication is injected into an area of the spine called the subarachnoid space. The effect of this is total numbness of the lower half of the labourer's body, rendering the person immobile. Spinal anaesthesia works very quickly and is sometimes used in situations where it is too late to have an epidural, such as caesarean section (Informed Health, 2018).

Documentation

The midwife must ensure that any administration of medication is documented according to Nursing and Midwifery Council (NMC, 2018) and local policy. To do this, the front of the drug chart or electronic patient record or notes for medication must have the patient's name, date of birth, hospital number and any allergies. For each administration, the following should be recorded in the notes.

- Date
- Drug
- Dose
- Route
- Time

This should then be signed by the person who administered the drug. If the drug is given by a student, the student should sign for the administration, and this must be countersigned by the supervising midwife.

Conclusion

The midwife's priority is to ensure that care always focuses on the needs, views, preferences and decisions of the woman and the newborn infant's needs. Therefore, it is imperative that midwives have the necessary skills and knowledge to carry out care and administer medications safely.

This chapter has summarised the primary medications used within the process of labour with an aim to prepare the reader for the skills and knowledge needed for complex midwifery care.

Find out more

The following are a list of scenarios where medication may need to be administered by a midwife. Take some time and write notes about each scenario and what information you may require to aid you in your decision making. Think about the medications that may be used and be specific about the pharmacokinetics and pharmacodynamics. Remember to include aspects of care. If you are making notes about people you have offered care and support to, you must ensure that you have adhered to the rules of confidentiality (NMC, 2018).

The scenario	Your notes
Discuss the IOL process and medication used for this	
Discuss the steps that need to be considered if a woman declines IOL	
What monitoring is required for epidural management?	
What are the precautions required when caring for a labouring woman with an epidural?	
What is the role of the midwife in gaining informed consent for administration of medication during labour?	

159

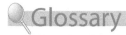 Glossary

Active management of third stage   An oxytocic injection to facilitate placental separation plus manual delivery of placenta by controlled cord traction

Amniotomy   Artificial rupture of the membranes to initiate or speed up labour

Anaesthesia   State in which whole or part of the body is insensible to pain or sensation

Analgesia   Pain relief without loss of consciousness

Antenatal   Before birth

Antidiuretic   Pertaining to or causing suppression of urinary secretion

Arrhythmia   Abnormal heart rhythm

Augmention of labour   A process in which the progress of labour is enhanced by amniotomy or administration of an infusion of oxytocin

Beta-agonists   Also known as beta-adrenergics, are medications that reduce blood pressure

Bishop score   A group of measurements achieved by performing a vaginal examination, based on the station, dilation, effacement (or length), position and consistency of the cervix; a score of 8 or more generally indicates that the cervix is 'ripe' or 'favourable'

Breech   Initial presentation of the fetal buttocks or feet ('footling breech') in the birth canal

Bromage scale   Commonly used tool to assess motor movement of the labourer after an epidural has been sited

Caesarean section   Operative delivery of the fetus through an abdominal incision

Cardiotocography (CTG)   Electronic monitoring of the fetal heart rate

Compound presentation   Labour complication, when more than one part of the fetus presents, e.g. head and hand

Controlled cord traction   Method of delivery by placing the ulnar border of the hand in the suprapubic region, pushing the contracted uterus upwards (guarding); the other hand gains firm hold of the cord and exerts gentle traction to deliver the placenta and membranes

Cord prolapse   Umbilical cord prolapse is where the umbilical cord slips past the presenting part after the rupture of membranes; the cord can protrude past the cervix

Dural tap   Occurs occasionally during siting of an epidural anaesthetic; the needle being introduced punctures the dura mater, causing a leak in cerebrospinal fluid

Electrocardiogram   See cardiotocograph

Epidural   An analgesic procedure; a thin catheter is inserted into the lower back (epidural space) by an anaesthetist to inject analgesic drugs for labour

Hypertension   High blood pressure

Hypotension   Low blood pressure

Induction of labour   Artificial initiation of labour

Infusion   Introducing fluid to the body

Instrumental delivery   Vaginal birth by instruments, e.g. forceps, Ventouse

Intramuscular injection   An injection into the muscle

Intrauterine growth restriction   Growth of the fetus that is less than normal

Malposition   Cephalic presentation other than normal, well-flexed anterior position, e.g. occipitoposterior

Multiparous   A woman who has given birth to more than one baby

Multiple pregnancy   Pregnancy with more than one fetus

Nulliparous   A woman who has never given birth

Opioid   A powerful habit-forming analgesic, narcotic drug, e.g. pethidine

Oxytocin   A hormone released naturally from the pituitary gland that stimulates the contraction of the uterus during labour and facilitates ejection of milk from the breast during nursing. It can be made artificially and is used therapeutically to induce or augment labour

Placenta previa   Placenta located in the lower segment of the uterus

Pre-eclampsia A disorder specific to pregnancy. It is usually of rapid onset and characterised by raised blood pressure, excess protein in the urine, headache, puffiness of the tissues and visual disturbance. It may lead to convulsions. The cause is still not completely understood

Prolonged rupture of membranes Rupture of the membranes before the onset of labour

Prostaglandin Any member of a group of hormone-like substances that mediate a wide range of physiological functions, such as contraction of smooth muscle

Third stage of labour From the birth of the baby to the separation of the placenta

Tocolysis The use of short-acting uterine relaxants such as terbutaline, in the management of uterine hyperstimulation

Transverse lie Longitudinal fetal axis lying across the maternal uterus

Unstable lie Continual alteration of the fetal lie after 36 weeks of gestation

Uterine hyperstimulation Overactivity of the uterus as a result of induction of labour

Test yourself

Now review your learning by completing the learning activities for this chapter at www.wiley.com/go/pharmacologyformidwives.

References

Anaesthesia UK (2017) www.frca.co.uk/article.aspx?articleid=100316 (accessed January 2022).

Anim-Somuah, M., Smyth, R., Cyna, A., Cuthbert, A. (2018) Epidural versus non-epidural or no analgesia for pain management in labour. Cochrane Database of Systematic Reviews, **5**: CD000331.

Bartholomew, C.M. (2017) Supporting choices in reducing pain and fear during labour. In: Macdonald, S., Magill-Cuerden, J., Mayes, M. (eds) *Mayes' Midwifery*. Baillière Tindall Elsevier: Edinburgh.

Care Quality Commission (2020) *2019 survey of women's experiences of maternity care*. www.cqc.org.uk/sites/default/files/20200128_mat19_statisticalrelease.pdf (accessed January 2022).

Electronic Medicines Compendium (2021) www.medicines.org.uk/emc/ (accessed January 2022).

Gallos, I., Williams, H., Price, M. et al. (2019) Uterotonic drugs to prevent postpartum haemorrhage: a network meta-analysis. *Health Technology Assessment*, **23**.9: Chapter 1.

Hofmeyr, G.J., Mshweshwe, N.T., Gülmezoglu, A.M. (2015) Controlled cord traction for the third stage of labour. *Cochrane Database of Systematic Reviews*, **1**(1): CD008020.

Hutchison, J., Mahdy, H., Hutchison, J. (2021) *Stages of Labor*. StatPearls: Treasure Island.

Informed Health.org (2018) *Pregnancy and Birth: Epidurals and painkillers for labor pain relief*. Institute for Quality and Efficiency in Health Care: Cologne.

Leathersich, S.J., Vongel, J.P., Tran, T., Hofmeyr, G. (2018) Medications for reducing contractions during labour for excessively strong/frequent contractions or when the unborn baby is thought to be distressed. *Cochrane Database of Systematic Reviews*, **7**: CD009770.

Marconi, A.M. (2019) Recent advances in the induction of labor. *F1000Research*, **8**: 1829.

National Collaborating Centre for Women's and Children's Health (2008) *Induction of Labour*. RCOG Press: London.

National Institute for Health and Care Excellence (2008) *Complications of induction of labour*. www.ncbi.nlm.nih.gov/books/NBK53624/ (accessed January 2022).

National Institute for Health and Care Excellence (2017) *Intrapartum care for healthy women and babies (CG190)*. www.nice.org.uk/guidance/cg190/resources/intrapartum-care-for-healthy-women-and-babies-pdf-35109866447557 (accessed January 2022).

National Institute for Health and Care Excellence (2021a). *BNF*. https://bnf.nice.org.uk/ (accessed January 2022).

National Institute for Health and Care Excellence (2021b) *Induction of labour overview*. http://pathways.nice.org.uk/pathways/induction-of-labour (accessed January 2022).

NHS (2021) *Maternity statistics, England 2017–18*. https://digital.nhs.uk/data-and-information/publications/statistical/nhs-maternity-statistics/2017-18 (accessed January 2022).

Nursing and Midwifery Council (2018) *The Code: Professional standards of practice and behaviour for nurses, midwives and nursing associates*. www.nmc.org.uk/globalassets/sitedocuments/nmc-publications/revised-new-nmc-code.pdf (accessed January 2022).

POPPHI (2008) *Fact sheets: Uterotonic drugs for the prevention and treatment of postpartum hemorrhage.* PATH: Seattle.

Rogers, C., Villar, R., Pisal, P., Yearley, C. (2013a) Effects of syntocinoin use in active management of third stage labour. *British Journal of Midwifery*, **19**(6).

Rogers, C., Harman, J., Selo-Ojeme, D. (2013b) The management of the third stage of labour – a national survey of current practice. *British Journal of Midwifery*, **20**(12).

Silva, M., Halpern, S.H. (2010) Epidural analgesia for labor: current techniques. *Local and Regional Anaesthesia*, **3**: 143–153.

World Health Organization (2014) *WHO recommendations for augmentation of labour.* https://apps.who.int/iris/bitstream/handle/10665/112825/9789241507363_eng.pdf;jsessionid=772D417593A33FBE6E5E75556AAF807D?sequence=1 (accessed January 2022).

Wormer, K.C., Bauer, A., Williford, A.E. (2021) *Bishop Score.* StatPearls: Treasure Island.

Chapter 11

Medications and the cardiovascular system

Carl Clare

University of Hertfordshire, Hatfield, UK

Aim

The aim of this chapter is to provide the reader with an introduction to drugs used in the management of disorders of the cardiovascular system

Learning outcomes

After reading this chapter the reader will:
- Understand the use of antiarrhythmic drugs in the management of atrial tachycardias
- Be able to discuss the variety of fibrinolytic drugs and their uses
- Be able to justify the use of anticoagulants in the management of cardiovascular disease in pregnancy
- Be able to explain the signs and symptoms of digoxin toxicity.

Test your existing knowledge

- Is amiodarone a useful drug in the management of arrhythmias in pregnancy?
- What are the uses of beta-blockers in the management of cardiovascular disease in pregnancy?
- What anticoagulants are available for the pregnant woman with a mechanical heart valve?
- What options are available for the management of bradyarrhythmia in pregnancy?
- What drugs are available for the management of hyperlipidaemia in pregnant women?

Introduction

The management of cardiovascular disorders in maternity can be separated into three types.

- Disorders of the cardiovascular system already present preconception and continuing throughout the pregnancy. This includes cardiovascular disorders present in the general population such

Fundamentals of Pharmacology for Midwives, First Edition. Edited by Ian Peate and Cathy Hamilton.
© 2022 John Wiley & Sons Ltd. Published 2022 by John Wiley & Sons Ltd.
Companion website: www.wiley.com/go/pharmacologyformidwives

as hypertension, coronary heart disease, cardiomyopathy, cardiac arrhythmias, heart valve disorders, congenital heart disease and so on.

- Disorders that develop during the pregnancy. Cardiovascular disorders that can develop in pregnancy include hormonally activated accessory pathways leading to atrial arrhythmias, myocardial infarction, pulmonary embolism, hypertension and so on.
- Disorders that develop post partum. Cardiovascular disorders post partum include cardiomyopathy, heart failure, hypertension, clotting disorders such as pulmonary embolism and so on.

As the management of cardiovascular disorders is often complicated and dependent on a number of factors, this chapter will be structured to review the variety of drugs used in common cardiovascular disorders and the pregnant woman. Those wishing to review the full range of potential disorders present during the maternal journey and their medical or surgical management are recommended to access the 2018 ESC Guidelines for the management of cardiovascular diseases during pregnancy (Regitz-Zagrosek et al., 2018).

Some medications are used for a variety of conditions (for instance, beta-blockers can be used in the management of heart failure, cardiomyopathy, valve disease or hypertension) and this will be detailed where necessary. With each drug, the recommendations for use will be discussed, general care considerations noted and any particular consideration for the use in pregnancy will be made explicit. Explicit guidance will not be given as to the doses of drugs, as the most up-to-date guidance on this can be found in the British National Formulary.

Cardiac disease and pregnancy

Cardiac disease complicating pregnancy is on the rise in general care. Incidence remains low at 1–4% of pregnancies, though this increases when hypertension is taken into account (Ramlakhan et al., 2020). However, despite low incidence, cardiovascular disease is a leading cause of maternal mortality. A variety of causative factors have been suggested for this increase in incidence, including increasing maternal age, increased cardiovascular risk factors in the general population (including obesity, hypertension and diabetes) and the successful management of congenital heart disease in women of child-bearing age (Halpern et al., 2019). The most commonly used cardiovascular medications in maternity care are beta-blockers, platelet aggregation inhibitors and diuretic agents but it should be noted that these are only the most commonly used drugs and consideration should be given to a wide variety of cardiovascular drugs in order to ensure that midwives are fully informed when encountering such drugs in their everyday practice.

The use of medications in pregnancy often focuses on the effect on the fetus and whilst many drugs are considered to be safe for use in the pregnant woman, there are certain drugs where there is a definite contraindication or the evidence base for safety is limited. Where necessary, this will be made explicit. In cases where the evidence base for the drug is poor or equivocal, the use of the drug will be a partnership decision between the medical staff in charge of the patient, who will review the risks and benefits of the medication, and the pregnant woman who makes the ultimate decision (assuming there is capacity). The role of the midwife in these situations is to help the pregnant woman, and any significant other, understand the information that has been presented to them, clarifying terminology and requesting further information where necessary. This is especially true when discussing medications used in the management of cardiovascular disorders as both the disorders and the medications used are uncommon.

It is important that the midwife does not get drawn into making the decision for the woman, nor engage in speculation about what they would do in the woman's situation as this would be an abuse of professional status and a potential cause for complaint if complications arise.

Physiological changes in pregnancy and the effects on cardiovascular disease presentation and management

Healthy women can adapt to the complex physiological changes in pregnancy without significant consequences. However, in women with underlying cardiac conditions, the changes may unmask a previously unknown condition or exacerbate a known condition.

Table 11.1   Physiological changes in pregnancy and effects on concentration, kinetics and dosing.

Physiological change	Effect on drug concentration and kinetics	Potential effect on drug dosage
Progressive increase in plasma volume (up to 50%)	Haemodilution	Higher loading dose required
Decreased plasma protein levels	Decreased protein-bound drug concentration. Increased free/unbound drug concentration	Potential increase in drug toxicity at the beginning of drug loading. Increase in dose frequency but no increase in total daily dose
Increased renal blood flow	Increased drug clearance	May require increased total daily dosage
Blood flow to the liver may increase or remain stable	Potential for increased drug clearance in drugs with hepatic clearance or increased drug availability in drugs with first-pass liver metabolism	May require increased total daily dosage in the case of increased clearance or changes in dosage frequency in those drugs with first-pass liver metabolism

During pregnancy, oestrogen activates the renin-angiotensin-aldosterone system (RAAS), increasing plasma volume and promoting sodium and water retention.

When considering the use of any drug in maternal care, there are a number of factors that must be considered, and these are summarised in Table 11.1.

In addition to those changes noted above, consideration should be given to the gastrointestinal effects of pregnancy. In pregnancy, decreased motility in the small bowel, nausea and vomiting, and the use of antacids and iron supplements all decrease the bioavailability of drugs. Despite these changes, several studies have shown there is no difference in bioavailability of cardiac drugs (Halpern et al., 2019).

With the potential variety of effects on drug concentration and clearance when prescribing medication, the altered pharmacokinetics during pregnancy should be considered in addition to fetal safety, and regular serum measurements can be beneficial because drug concentrations can change.

Antiarrhythmic drugs

Maternal palpitations and cardiac arrhythmias may increase in pregnancy. The primary mechanisms for this are increased dilation of the heart chambers and the effects of progesterone and oestrogen, especially in increasing adrenergic responses (Roberts et al., 2019).

Palpitations are a common complaint in pregnancy but only a few women reporting palpitations will have significant cardiac arrhythmias. Palpitations are defined as an unpleasant awareness of the heartbeat, including feelings of the heartbeat being rapid, forceful or irregular and may be described as a 'pounding' heartbeat or the heart 'skipping' a beat. Around 50% of women investigated for palpitations are found to have ventricular ectopics (also known as ventricular premature beats or premature ventricular contractions) or non-sustained arrhythmias and are not considered problematic though reassurance and counselling may be of value.

When considering the differential diagnosis between palpitations and arrhythmias, one of the most valuable tools can be a thorough history taking. There are a number of signs and symptoms that can be suggestive of a benign versus malignant arrhythmia (Table 11.2). Despite the changes in maternal blood volume, these changes can increase the perception of 'normal' palpitations.

Further aspects of patient history associated with palpitations that are suggestive of a malignant arrhythmia include shortness of breath, fainting, and chest pain, all being suggestive of a loss of blood pressure related to the arrhythmia.

Table 11.2   History taking and arrhythmias.

History	Comment
Onset and end of palpitations	Sudden onset and end may suggest a malignant arrhythmia
	A gradual onset and end may suggest a normal change in heart rate
Time of onset	Onset at rest is more suggestive of a malignant arrhythmia
	Onset with exertion is more suggestive of a normal change in heart rate
Associated symptoms	Syncope (fainting) is often associated with malignant arrhythmias
Did the symptoms predate the pregnancy?	Symptoms predating the pregnancy are more likely to be suggestive of malignant arrhythmias
Drug use	Illicit drug use can be a provoking factor for arrhythmias. The use of substances such as nicotine or caffeine can provoke palpitations unrelated to arrhythmias
Personal or family history of heart disease	Arrhythmias are much more likely in the presence of structural heart disease

Source: Modified from Roberts et al. (2019).

Cardiac arrhythmias can be split into two main categories: tachyarrhythmias and bradyarrhythmias.

Clinical consideration

Cardiac monitoring

Any pregnant woman developing a new-onset cardiac arrhythmia should be considered for cardiac monitoring in the short term. Women with haemodynamically unstable arrhythmias should be continually monitored as the risk of deterioration is high. Where a haemodynamically unstable mother should be cared for is a matter of local policy but consideration should be given to transfer to a high-dependency unit or cardiac care unit until the rhythm is stabilised.

Tachyarrhythmias

An increase in maternal heart rate is a normal change in the later stages of pregnancy and may be noticed by the woman as palpitations, especially when lying in bed.

The definition and pathophysiology of tachyarrhythmias are complicated and include the presence or absence of structural heart disease as a predisposing factor. This level of analysis is beyond the scope of this chapter but a brief overview will be given of a few of the more common arrhythmias.

Supraventricular arrhythmias are the most common form of tachyarrhythmia. These are arrhythmias that originate from above the ventricle and can arise from any part of the atria or atrioventricular bundle. Depending on the definition, some sources exclude atrial fibrillation and atrial flutter from the definition of supraventricular arrhythmias

One of the most common supraventricular arrhythmias is an atrioventricular nodal re-entrant tachycardia (AVNRT). This is an arrhythmia caused by the re-entry of electrical activity from the ventricle to the atria via the atrial tissue around the atrioventricular bundle and node. Otherwise, an accessory pathway may be present (Figure 11.1) leading to an atrioventricular re-entrant tachycardia (AVRT).

Atrial fibrillation and atrial flutter are arrhythmias that are contained within the tissues of the atria and do not involve any re-entrant pathway from the ventricle. Atrial fibrillation is a disorganised atrial arrhythmia involving multiple ectopic foci (Figure 11.2) and leading to an irregular heart rhythm; in the case of atrial fibrillation, the ECG will show an absence of atrial activity ('p' waves).

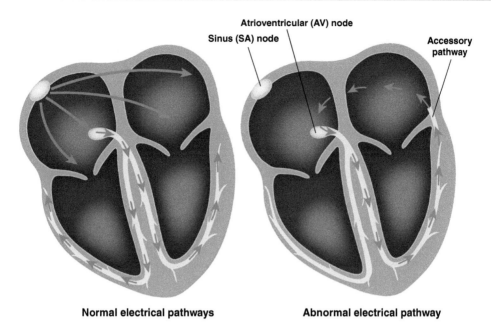

Normal electrical pathways   **Abnormal electrical pathway**

Figure 11.1   Accessory pathway causing a re-entrant tachycardia.
Source: Tom Lück/Wikimedia Commons/CC BY 3.0. https://commons.wikimedia.org/wiki/File:WPW.jpeg.

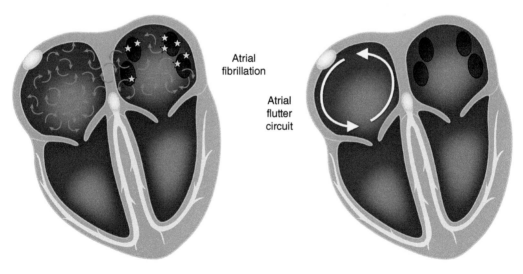

Figure 11.2   Atrial fibrillation.   Figure 11.3   Atrial flutter.

Atrial flutter is a more organised atrial rhythm associated with an internal (atrial) re-entry circuit (Figure 11.3) and a 'saw tooth' atrial trace on the ECG.

Thromboembolic risk in atrial fibrillation and atrial flutter during pregnancy is considered to be low and thus anticoagulation is often not required (Kugamoorthy and Spears, 2020). However, risk assessment for thromboembolic risk would be carried out using standard risk tools such as CHADS2 (Chan et al., 2020).

Ventricular tachyarrhythmias can be broadly broken down into two major categories: ventricular tachycardia and ventricular fibrillation. Ventricular fibrillation is a cardiac arrest arrhythmia and should be dealt with using standard Advanced Life Support protocols regardless of trimester

(Resuscitation Council (UK), 2021). Ventricular tachycardia is a ventricular rate of 100 beats per minute or greater without associated atrial activity. As a rhythm, it can be well tolerated but untreated it can deteriorate into a physiologically unstable rhythm and even ventricular fibrillation. As with supraventricular tachycardias, ventricular tachycardias can be constant or paroxysmal. Treatment options will depend on the incidence, frequency and duration of the tachycardia as well as associated symptoms (such as syncope, chest pain or shortness of breath).

Treatment of tachyarrhythmias

In the presence of a physiologically unstable supraventricular tachycardia, treatment options are (Vaidya et al., 2020) as follows.

- Valsava manoeuvres
- Administration of adenosine by increasing bolus dose
- DC electrical cardioversion
- Pharmacological cardioversion or stabilisation

Neither the Valsalva manoeuvre nor the use of adenosine is indicated in the presence of identified atrial fibrillation or atrial flutter and as such, both these rhythms will only be treated by electrical cardioversion or pharmacological cardioversion.

Clinical consideration

Valsalva manoeuvres

Officially, the Valsalva manoeuvre is a forced expiration against a closed glottis. However, this is extremely difficult to explain to an expectant mother so several approaches have been developed to induce the effect of a Valsalva manoeuvre in women, including the use of an ice-cold cloth on the back of the neck. However, the lack of availability of ice-cold cloths and the relative unpleasantness of this method mean it is very rare in adults. One of the most common methods of inducing a Valsalva manoeuvre is to ask the patient to blow out the plunger of a clean 20 mL syringe by blowing into the open end of the syringe. The effort of the patient can be seen by the presence of facial flushing, engorged neck veins and visible strain.

It is important to note that the Valsalva manoeuvre is associated with increased intraocular pressure and thus it is contraindicated in women with retinopathy or intraocular lens implantation.

The use of the Valsalva manoeuvre creates a physiologically complex response in the cardiovascular system with the clinically useful outcome that it may terminate supraventricular tachycardias (Pstras et al., 2017). The Valsalva manoeuvre is normally considered as the first option as it is considered to be very safe and offers no risk to mother or fetus.

Adenosine is a purine nucleoside base normally associated with the molecule adenosine triphosphate (ATP). Pharmacologically, it has value in that it acts on the tissues of the atrioventricular node, leading to a significantly prolonged conduction time. The aim of adenosine administration is to terminate any re-entry tachycardia by effectively blocking one of the electrical pathways in the circuit. Adenosine has no value in the treatment of atrial fibrillation or atrial tachycardia and should be used with extreme caution in any patient with Wolff–Parkinson–White syndrome and a fast ventricular rate due to atrial fibrillation. Adenosine has a very short half-life and thus any side-effects are transient, usually lasting much less than a minute (Gupta et al., 2021). However, the side-effects are very unpleasant and sometimes distressing; they include:

- dizziness
- flushing
- difficulty breathing
- chest tightness
- flushing
- blurred vision.

Thus, counselling the woman before adenosine administration is essential to help prevent unnecessary fear and distress. Adenosine is contraindicated in patients with asthma as it may precipitate bronchospasm. Adenosine is considered safe in pregnancy with no known placental transfer, but the potential risks of its use in breast feeding are currently unknown (Kugamoorthy and Spears, 2020).

Electrical cardioversion is known to be safe at all stages of pregnancy (Djakpo and Quan, 2019) but consideration must be given to the choice of anaesthetic agent and the need for anticoagulation. In women without structural heart disease, anticoagulation will not normally be required but risk assessment should be undertaken (as noted earlier). In women with known structural heart disease, the onset of the supraventricular tachycardia (SVT) will dictate the need for prior anticoagulation. If the onset of SVT is within 24–48 hours of cardioversion, or the woman is haemodynamically unstable, anticoagulation will be commenced immediately after cardioversion. If the onset of SVT is beyond 48 hours (and the woman is haemodynamically stable), then it is recommended that she undergoes transoesophageal echocardiogram to exclude an intracardiac thrombus, or anticoagulation is commenced at least 3 weeks prior to cardioversion (Kugamoorthy and Spears, 2020). Following cardioversion, all women with structural heart disease should have 4 weeks anticoagulation therapy.

169

Clinical consideration

DC electrical cardioversion

Electrical cardioversion is the attempted termination of a tachyarrhythmia by the use of direct current electrical shock through the thoracic cavity. Cardioversion is known to be safe for the fetus as the shock travels through the thoracic cavity and not the abdominal cavity.

Cardioversion requires the woman to be anaesthetised as it is very painful and thus, in most healthcare organisations, it is performed in theatre recovery with an anaesthetist managing sedation and the woman's airway.

The electrical shock is delivered in synchrony with the 'R' wave of the ECG to prevent the delivery of the shock on the 'T' wave of the ECG, which may precipitate ventricular fibrillation. The shock is delivered with a standard defibrillator and defibrillation pads and most defibrillator manufacturers recommend the addition of three-lead monitoring of the heart via the defibrillator as well as the defibrillation pads to ensure accurate synchronisation.

The full procedure for electrical cardioversion by synchronised shock is beyond the scope of this text but can be found in your local policies and procedures, the Resuscitation Council (UK) Advanced Life Support manual (2021) or a number of cardiology texts.

Pharmacological cardioversion or stabilisation of SVT is the last option for the pregnant woman experiencing SVT as the risks of side-effects and complications (such as bradycardia) are high. If all other mechanisms have failed, it is a necessity in some mothers.

The first-line pharmacological treatment in non-pregnant women is the antiarrhythmic drug amiodarone. However, amiodarone is generally contraindicated in pregnancy (except for very short-term use) as it is associated with intrauterine growth retardation, congenital goitre and thyroid disorders. Intravenous administration of a calcium channel blocker, such as verapamil or diltiazem, is considered to be a safe and effective method of terminating acute SVT (but must not be used in the presence of ventricular dysfunction). Though long-term use is relatively common, there is limited data as to the effects of verapamil on the fetus (reports to date have shown no fetal effects) and diltiazem should not be used in the first trimester as it has been associated with skeletal malformation in animal studies (Kugamoorthy and Spears, 2020).

In the woman with atrial fibrillation or atrial flutter and associated rapid heart rate that is resistant to cardioversion, rate control by the use of beta-blockers (such as labetalol or bisoprolol) is recommended as first-line therapy, with the potential addition of digoxin for improved rate control (Roberts et al., 2019). Beta-blockers are generally considered safe for use at all stages in pregnancy but fetal growth should be monitored as there is a potential relationship to intrauterine growth retardation, although it is considered that the benefits outweigh the risks (Roberts et al., 2019). Digoxin is an extremely safe drug for use in pregnancy unless toxic levels develop. Due to the alterations in plasma volume and renal blood flow in pregnancy and the risk of toxicity, serum levels should be monitored regularly (Kaye et al., 2019).

Clinical Consideration

Digoxin toxicity

Digoxin toxicity can be extremely dangerous as it can cause high serum potassium levels leading to arrhythmia or cardiac arrest. Digoxin toxicity is detected by serum drug level measurement by laboratory analysis, but common signs of toxicity can be noted in clinical practice, including (Ibrahim, 2019):

- nausea and vomiting
- increased respiration rate
- bradycardia
- headache
- malaise
- drowsiness
- dizziness
- abdominal pain
- hallucinations
- confusion.

Notable cardiac effects are bradycardia, prolonged P-R interval and the characteristic down-sloping ST segment ('reverse tick') on the ECG trace.

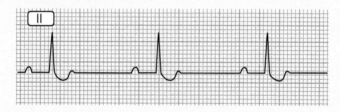

Prolonged P-R interval and down sloping ST segment.

Episode of care

New-onset palpitations

Jennifer is a 32-year-old woman who has been admitted to the antenatal ward at 26 weeks pregnant with palpitations. Three-lead monitoring and then 12-lead ECG show an irregularly irregular heart rhythm with no obvious 'p' waves. Jennifer reports that the palpitations commenced 3 days ago and she saw her GP today who referred her to the obstetric consultant outpatient clinic for urgent review. Following ECG analysis, Jennifer was admitted to the antenatal ward for further care. An urgent referral to the cardiology team was made.

Jennifer's NEWS 2 score is noted below.

Physiological parameter	3	2	1	0	1	2	3
Respiration rate				18			
Oxygen saturation %				96			
Air or oxygen				Air			

Physiological parameter	3	2	1	0	1	2	3
Temperature °C				37			
Systolic BP mmHg				130			
Heart rate						130	
Level of consciousness				A			
Score	0	0	0	0	0	2	0
Total	2						

Take time to reflect on this case study and then consider the following.

1. Jennifer's heart rate has increased. What do you think is happening and why? Consider the role of atrial fibrillation and heart rate.
2. What is the potential role of Valsalva manoeuvres and adenosine in the management of Jennifer's arrhythmia?
3. What treatment options might be recommended to treat the new-onset atrial fibrillation?
4. Given Jennifer's NEWS2 score of 2, what is the recommended escalation action according to your local organisational policy?
5. What is the role of anticoagulation in Jennifer's case?

171

Jennifer was admitted to the ward and commenced on three-lead monitoring whilst a cardiology referral was undertaken. As Jennifer has no history of heart disease, diabetes or thrombotic disease, the CHADS2 score was 0 and thus the risk of thrombus was very low. As the onset of the palpitations was more than 48 hours earlier, Jennifer underwent transoesophageal echocardiography to rule out any atrial thrombus. The next day, the transoesophageal echocardiography was reported as clear and Jennifer underwent successful DC cardioversion in theatre. With no evidence of structural heart disease, it was decided there was no need for anticoagulation and Jennifer was discharged home with instructions to return to the antenatal ward if the palpitations returned.

The treatment of ventricular tachycardia follows a similar protocol to the treatment of SVT in that treatment is partially dictated by whether the rhythm is haemodynamically stable or unstable. Ventricular tachycardia can be a cardiac arrest rhythm and the first consideration is whether the woman is conscious and has a pulse. In the presence of a cardiac arrest rhythm standard Advanced Life Support protocols are followed.

Skills in practice

Placing defibrillation pads

Defibrillation pads are used to facilitate cardioversion and defibrillation; some allow ECG monitoring and external cardiac pacing.

It is important when placing the DC pads for shocking that the manufacturer's instructions are followed and local policy and procedure are adhered to.

The packet containing the gel pads must not have been opened otherwise the pads may have dried out.

The pads are for single patient use but can be used for multiple shocks; the pads protect the skin from being burnt.

There must be good contact between the pad and the skin (the skin needs to be dry and clean). This enhances adherence and decreases the chance of arcing/burns.

It is important that the pad is not in contact with any other equipment, for example, ECG dots, GTN pads, lines and cables.

Arcing (electricity travelling through the air directly between electrodes which can result in explosive noises, burns and impaired delivery of current) is a potential complication as are:

- electrical injury to bystanders
- risk of explosion if oxygen flow continues during shock delivery
- skin burns from repeated shocks
- myocardial injury and postdefibrillation dysrhythmias and 'stunning'
- skeletal muscle injury
- thoracic vertebral fractures.

In the event of a pulsed ventricular tachycardia but with associated haemodynamic instability (systolic blood pressure lower than 90 mmHg) or other signs of instability (dizziness, chest pain, shortness of breath) then immediate electrical cardioversion is advocated as per the treatment of an unstable SVT (Roberts et al., 2019). In women with known structural heart disease, ventricular tachycardia is considered to be very dangerous and associated with the risk of sudden death, and immediate cardioversion should be considered. Pharmacological control of ventricular tachycardia may include short-term (emergency) use of amiodarone, but beta-blockade is generally considered the first-line choice.

Bradyarrhythmias

Bradyarrhythmias, in most women, are a heart rate less than 60 beats per minute though in athletes the resting heart rate may be below 60 beats per minute normally. Bradyarrhythmias are uncommon in pregnancy and are often well tolerated. The treatment of symptomatic bradyarrhythmias is normally the institution of pacing (Roberts et al., 2019). Consideration should be given to the potential cause of the bradyarrhythmia, including antiarrhythmic drugs and doses altered or administration ceased.

Antihypertensive drugs

Hypertensive disorders are present in 5–10% of pregnancies (Ying et al., 2018) and include pre-eclampsia, pre-existing hypertension and gestational hypertension. Hypertension in pregnancy is defined as a blood pressure equal to or greater than 140/90 mmHg, with a blood pressure of over 160/110 mmHg being considered severe hypertension requiring admission to hospital (NICE, 2019). Current European Society of Cardiology (ESC) guidelines recommend treating hypertension above 150/90 mmHg or 140/90 mmHg in cases of gestational hypertension (Regitz-Zagrosek et al., 2018). Unfortunately, the use of antihypertensive agents does not seem to reduce the risk of pre-eclampsia (Ying et al., 2018).

Clinical consideration

Antihypertensive drugs and fetal circulation

As the placenta does not appear to autoregulate the blood flow to the fetus, extreme care should be taken to avoid overtreatment as maternal hypotension will lead to fetal distress.

When treating maternal hypertension, NICE guidelines on regular blood pressure readings, urine dipstick analysis for proteinuria, blood tests and fetal monitoring should be followed (NICE, 2019).

The first-line antihypertensive drugs in maternal hypertension are labetalol, nifedipine if labetalol is contraindicated and methyldopa if neither labetalol nor nifedipine is suitable (NICE, 2019). In hypertensive emergencies, intravenous labetalol is recommended and sodium nitroprusside should be avoided due to the potential for cyanide poisoning if administered incorrectly (Ying et al., 2018).

Clinical consideration

ACE inhibitors

Angiotensin converting enzyme (ACE) inhibitors and angiotensin receptor blockers (ARBs) are common drugs used in the treatment of hypertension in the general population. However, there is sufficient evidence to show that they can cause significant fetal and neonatal problems and they are thus contraindicated for use in pregnancy. NICE (2019) suggests that women who are already taking ACE inhibitors or ARBs should be counselled that their continued use may cause fetal abnormalities and they should cease taking these drugs as soon as possible (but only once an agreed alternative drug regime has been agreed with medical staff).

173

Labetalol is a selective alpha, beta-1 and beta-2 receptor blocker used as the first-line drug for both acute and chronic hypertension in pregnancy. As when commencing any new drug, the woman should be counselled that labetalol does carry a risk of certain side-effects, such as fetal hypoglycaemia, intrauterine growth retardation and fetal bradycardia. However, it is not associated with any fetal abnormalities and several studies have shown it to be more effective than nifedipine in reducing maternal blood pressure (Prasanthi and Jyothsna, 2020). Labetalol is contraindicated in women with asthma or diabetes. The most common side-effects of labetalol that may lead to non-compliance include dizziness, excessive lethargy and headaches but the woman should contact her healthcare provider before stopping labetalol therapy.

Nifedipine is a calcium channel blocker with no known effects on fetal growth and is not associated with any fetal abnormalities. Some brands of nifedipine are contraindicated in pregnancy by the manufacturer in the product summary so it is important to check the individual preparation for details (NICE, 2019). Nifedipine is generally well tolerated but is contraindicated in women with liver failure or unstable angina. Due to the potential for increased liver metabolism, more frequent dosing intervals or higher doses of nifedipine should be considered. Methyldopa is not known to be harmful in pregnancy but has a limited antihypertensive action and a short half-life (Hoeltzenbein et al., 2017). It is generally recommended that diuretics are not used in pregnancy (NICE, 2019) but if a diuretic is necessary then furosemide is the most commonly used of all the diuretics in pregnancy and spironolactone is contraindicated. It should be noted that furosemide is associated with neonatal jaundice and thrombocytopenia (Regitz-Zagrosek et al., 2018).

Of all maternal deaths globally, pre-eclampsia and eclampsia are directly associated with 10–15% of cases (van Doorn et al., 2021). Whilst the treatment of pre-eclampsia and eclampsia is based on the use of antihypertensive drugs, they have not been shown to prevent these disorders. There is clear evidence for the use of aspirin from 12 weeks gestation to birth to help prevent both pre-eclampsia and eclampsia (van Doorn et al., 2021). Current NICE guidance (2019) suggests a daily dose of 75–150 mg of aspirin from 12 weeks gestation until birth.

Fibrinolytics

Pregnancy is associated with an increase in clotting factors, a decrease in antithrombotic protein activity and a decrease in thrombolytic activity and these changes are thought to be linked to the higher rate of thrombotic disorders in pregnancy (Sousa-Gomes et al., 2019). The majority of thromboembolic events in pregnancy are venous in nature (deep vein thrombosis [DVT], pulmonary embolism and cerebro-vascular events [CVE or stroke]) whereas myocardial infarction is very rare (Bloria et al., 2020). In the non-pregnant woman, the use of a fibrinolytic agent (otherwise known as a thrombolytic agent) is common and uncontentious whereas in the pregnant woman a lot of fear exists around their use, with discussion of placental haemorrhage, haemorrhagic events and fetal death.

It is unlikely that any fibrinolytic agent crosses the placental barrier as their molecular weight is too great. However, in a recent systematic review of case reports in 141 women given fibrinolytics in pregnancy, there were four maternal deaths (none associated with the administration of fibrinolytic drugs), 12 major bleeding episodes, two fetal deaths (probably associated with maternal complications) and nine miscarriages (Sousa-Gomes et al., 2019). Unfortunately, the review is, by necessity, only based on case reviews as any form of controlled trial would be unethical and thus a greater range of data is required for certainty (Blondon et al., 2021). However, with the often fatal outcome of untreated thromboembolic events, fibrinolytic drugs should be administered in the absence of other treatment methodologies (such as surgical embolectomy) and are only recommended in the presence of severe hypotension or shock.

There are a small number of fibrinolytic agents available for the treatment of thromboembolic disorders and the exact indication for each drug is noted in Table 11.3.

The treatment of all thromboembolic disorders is time critical as the prevention of blood flow to tissues leads to infarction and necrosis of the affected area.

Anticoagulants

Anticoagulants can be used for the prevention or treatment of thromboembolism in pregnancy. Unlike fibrinolytics which are recommended for use in acute thromboembolic events associated with shock or infarction of at-risk organs (such as the brain or heart), anticoagulants are recommended for treatment of lower risk thromboembolic events such as DVT (Regitz-Zagrosek et al., 2018). Current data suggests that in untreated women with risk factors, the incidence of venous thromboembolism (VTE) varies between 2.4% and 12.2%, in comparison with 0–5.5% in patients who receive treatment (Regitz-Zagrosek et al., 2018).

The most common anticoagulant used in the prevention or treatment of VTE is low molecular weight heparin (LMWH). LMWH is relatively easy to administer and women can be taught to self-administer the drug from a prefilled syringe with relative ease. LMWH is considered superior for longer term use in that it carries a lower risk of osteoporotic fracture and has less associated bone density loss than unfractionated heparin (UFH) (Regitz-Zagrosek et al., 2018). LMWH is relatively safe and, as with any drug in pregnancy, its use is based on a risk–benefit analysis. LMWH has a 0.5% risk of antepartum bleeding and a 1% risk of postpartum haemorrhage when used in the prevention of VTE. When used at treatment dosing levels, there is a 1.5% risk of antepartum bleeding and a 2% risk of postpartum haemorrhage (Lu et al., 2017).

The newest class of anticoagulants is direct oral anticoagulants (DOAC) for the treatment or prevention of clotting in atrial fibrillation, DVT and pulmonary embolism. As the use of LMWH may not provide adequate anticoagulation levels due to a lack of dosing guidelines, there is increasing

Table 11.3 Fibrinolytic agents and their indications for use.

Fibrinolytic agent	Bolus or infusion	Approved for management of high-risk pulmonary embolism?	Approved for management of myocardial infarction?	Approved for management of acute stroke?
Urokinase	Infusion	Yes	Yes	No
Streptokinase	Infusion	Yes	Yes	No
Alteplase (recombinant tissue plasminogen activator – rt-PA)	Infusion	Yes	Yes	Yes
Tenecteplase	Bolus	No	Yes	No

interest in DOACs. Though DOACs are well tolerated in non-pregnant women and are considered to be preferable for patients due to the oral preparation (as opposed to the injection-based LMWH), there is limited data as to their safety in pregnancy. The limited data currently available regarding DOACs suggests that they are potentially unsafe for use in pregnancy. A recent systematic review of current studies of the use of DOACs in pregnancy (Lameijer et al., 2018) shows there is little data available as DOACs were normally terminated within 2 months of the discovery of pregnancy. The data that is available suggests that DOACs are not safe for use in pregnancy; for instance, rivaroxaban was associated with a 4% rate of fetal abnormalities and DOACs in general are possibly associated with an increased rate of miscarriage.

Clinical consideration

Mechanical heart valves

The most common mechanical heart valves are used to replace the mitral valve or the aortic valve. Historically, these valves were manufactured from metal and surgical-grade plastic and are associated with increased thrombus formation. Recently, there has been an increase in the use of valves coated in endothelium to reduce coagulation or the implantation of natural valves from specially grown pigs. However, mechanical valves remain common and even valves coated in endothelium still require some level of anticoagulation.

The risk of thromboembolism associated with mechanical heart valves is greatly increased in pregnancy and anticoagulation remains essential. The standard anticoagulant for use in the patient with a mechanical heart valve is warfarin. However, warfarin crosses the placental barrier and is associated with significant fetal abnormalities (especially if administered in the first trimester); in later stages of pregnancy, it is associated with fetal intracranial haemorrhage and has been linked to fetal death at all stages of pregnancy (Lewey et al., 2021). Studies have suggested that the fetal effects of warfarin are dose dependent and not as prevalent at lower doses (less than 5 mg per day) though this has not been shown by all studies. Therefore, the continuation of warfarin in pregnancy is dose dependent and the decision must be made in full consultation with the woman. Women who refuse to continue with warfarin therapy in pregnancy (or are unable to continue) should be managed with LMWH by subcutaneous injection. Women who are transferred to anticoagulation by LMWH should be aware that the current evidence is not clear on the required dosage and blood assay of anti-Xa levels will be required on a regular basis. At present, there is no guidance to add low-dose aspirin to the anticoagulation regimen in European guidelines.

Planned delivery is essential in the management of the woman with a mechanical heart valve and it is recommended that she is admitted to hospital prior to delivery and transferred onto unfractionated heparin for anticoagulation control as dose adjustment is easier and serum levels are quicker to respond. If labour begins before the planned change in anticoagulation regime then caesarean section is recommended (Regitz-Zagrosek et al., 2018).

Cardiomyopathy

Whilst this chapter has focused on the classes of drugs that may be used in pregnancy, there are two conditions that merit individual attention: cardiomyopathy and heart failure.

Cardiomyopathy is a congenital or acquired disorder of the heart muscle and can be split into four types.

Dilated cardiomyopathy

Dilated cardiomyopathy (DCM) can be primary or secondary to myocarditis (inflammation of the heart muscle), the use of alcohol or other toxins, endocrine and autoimmune disorders, and nutritional factors. Dilated cardiomyopathy is associated with adverse outcomes in pregnancy and in women with poor left ventricular function or poor exercise tolerance, pregnancy is not advised. In those with preserved ejection fraction, pregnancy may continue but if left ventricular function deteriorates then the pregnancy may need to be terminated (Bloria et al., 2020). Women with DCM will often be treated before pregnancy with ACE inhibitors or ARBs and these should be stopped before conception. Beta-blockade should be continued, and fluid management should be restricted to the use of furosemide.

Hypertrophic cardiomyopathy

In hypertrophic cardiomyopathy (HCM), the heart muscle becomes thicker and stiffer, often reducing left ventricular size. Pregnancy is normally well tolerated by women with HCM. Regular monitoring is important in patients with HCM as the left atrium will often become dilated, and the patient is at risk of atrial fibrillation and thrombus development. In the event of atrial fibrillation developing, the restoration of normal sinus rhythm is essential as blood pressure will often be significantly affected. Beta-blockade should be continued if present or instituted in the development of resistant atrial fibrillation with a fast ventricular rate to reduce heart rate (Regitz-Zagrosek et al., 2018).

Restrictive cardiomyopathy

The restrictive cardiomyopathies are a heterogeneous group of diseases, the most common of which is cardiac amyloidosis (Adityawati et al., 2021). Amyloidosis is poorly tolerated in pregnancy and is associated with miscarriage, stillbirth, intrauterine growth restriction and preterm birth. Therefore, it is normally advised that pregnancy is terminated. However, if pregnancy continues, management is similar to other cardiomyopathies, though digoxin should be avoided in amyloidosis as it binds to the amyloid infiltrates, increasing the risk of digoxin toxicity (Adityawati et al., 2021).

Episode of care

New onset of shortness of breath and fatigue

Giselle is a 27-year-old woman who gave birth to her first child 1 week ago. She was recently reviewed at home by her community midwife who noted that Giselle seemed to be short of breath (especially when lying down) and constantly fatigued. A full set of vital signs were taken, and a history of the present condition showed that Giselle developed these symptoms gradually over the last 2 days.

Vital sign	Observation	Normal
Temperature	36.5 °C	36.0–37.9 °C range
Pulse	110 beats per minute	60–100 beats per minute
Respiration	20 breaths per minute	12–20 breaths per minute
Blood pressure	96/65 mmHg	100–139 mmHg (systolic) range
O₂ saturations	94% on air	94–98%

Giselle's NEWS 2 score is noted below

Physiological parameter	3	2	1	0	1	2	3
Respiration rate				20			
Oxygen saturation %			94				
Air or oxygen				Air			
Temperature °C				36.5			

176

Physiological parameter	3	2	1	0	1	2	3
Systolic BP mmHg		96					
Heart rate					110		
Level of consciousness				A			
Score	0	2	1	0	1	0	0
Total	**4**						

Take time to reflect on this case study and then consider the following.

1. What is the potential diagnosis for Giselle's sudden deterioration?
2. What tests are required to confirm the diagnosis?
3. What treatment options might be recommended to treat the new-onset heart failure both immediately and ongoing?
4. Given Giselle's NEWS2 score of 4, what is the recommended escalation action according to your organisational policy?
5. What medications (including anticoagulants) are likely to be prescribed and why?

Following review, Giselle was admitted to the cardiology ward and an echocardiogram showed reduced left ventricular function and left ventricular dilation. Chest x-ray showed pulmonary oedema. Giselle was placed on oxygen via facemask and attached to a heart monitor to observe for potential arrhythmias.

As Giselle had made the choice not to breast feed, the medication commenced included ACE inhibitors, warfarin and bromocriptine. Giselle was advised that she would need to attend hospital for regular echocardiograms to monitor the progress of the disease and she would need to have weekly blood tests (INR) to monitor the anticoagulant effects of the warfarin and ensure optimal levels.

Peripartum cardiomyopathy

The aetiology of peripartum cardiomyopathy (PPCM) is unknown but its development is associated with significant morbidity and mortality (Bloria et al., 2020). Most cases present in the first week post delivery. Risk factors for PPCM include multiparity, African ethnicity, smoking, diabetes, pre-eclampsia, malnutrition and older age pregnancy (Regitz-Zagrosek et al., 2018). PPCM is normally associated with left ventricular dilation (and possibly right ventricular dilation) leading to the signs and symptoms of heart failure

- Pulmonary oedema with associated reduction in oxygen levels
- Hypotension
- Shortness of breath, especially when resting or lying down (orthopnoea)
- Cough
- Water retention (causing swelling in the ankles and abdomen)
- Palpitations (a change in the heart rate or rhythm that the person may become aware of, particularly tachycardia)
- Extreme fatigue
- Finding it hard to exercise or be active

Diagnosis of PPCM is based on the timing of presentation, the absence of any previous heart failure and the presence of ventricular dysfunction on echocardiogram. Management of PPCM depends on when it is diagnosed. During pregnancy, standard therapy will include beta-blockers, furosemide, digoxin and LMWH. Post delivery, management can include commencing ACE inhibitors and anti-

177

coagulation with warfarin. Further treatment includes the insertion of an automated implantable cardioverter defibrillator (AICD) for arrhythmia management where necessary. Bromocriptine (a dopamine receptor agonist) stops lactation and is associated with enhanced postpartum recovery (Regitz- Zagrosek et al., 2018).

Hyperlipidaemia

Dyslipidaemia is associated with adverse maternal outcomes, such as hypertensive disease, gestational diabetes and preterm birth. Unfortunately, the optimal management of dyslipidaemia in pregnancy is still unknown as statins are contraindicated in pregnancy (Tummala et al., 2021).

Breast feeding

Whilst this chapter has focused on the use of cardiovascular drugs in pregnancy, guidance should be given on the use of drugs in breast feeding. Most drugs that can be used in pregnancy can be used during breast feeding, with the exception of methyldopa which is associated with an increased rate of postpartum depression. Angiotensin receptor blockers and amiodarone remain contraindicated in breast feeding as they can be found in high levels in breast milk.

Conclusion

This chapter has discussed the drugs used in the management of cardiovascular disorders in pregnancy. The different classes of drugs have been reviewed and recommendations explored in accordance with recognised guidelines. It should be noted that the American Heart Association guidelines differ in part from those of the European Society for Cardiology and the National Institute for Health and Care Excellence and it is important to access the correct guidelines when exploring guidance for cardiovascular drugs. The variety of cardiac arrhythmias present in pregnancy have been explored but detailed exploration of the diagnosis and pathophysiology of these arrhythmias is beyond the scope of this chapter and those interested in advanced rhythm interpretation are advised to access texts dedicated to ECG interpretation. Finally, a brief discussion was presented regarding the management of cardiomyopathy in pregnancy.

Find out more

The following are a list of conditions associated with the cardiovascular system. Take some time and write notes about each of the conditions. Think about the medications that may be used in order to treat these conditions and be specific about the pharmacokinetics and pharmacodynamics. Remember to include aspects of patient care. If you are making notes about people you have offered care and support to, you must ensure that you have adhered to the rules of confidentiality.

The condition	Your notes
Atrial fibrillation	
Postpartum cardiomyopathy	
Pulmonary embolism	
Myocardial infarction	
Hyperlipidaemia	

Glossary

Aorta   Main artery leading from the left ventricle

Aortic valve   Valve that lies between the left ventricle and the aorta

Arterial   Pertaining to the arteries

Atria   Upper chambers of the heart (singular, atrium)

Atrial fibrillation   Heart condition that causes an irregular and often abnormally fast heart rate

Atrial flutter   When the atria beat regularly, but much faster than usual

Atrioventricular bundle   Bundle of conductive nerve fibres that transmit action potentials from the AV node to the ventricular conduction system. Otherwise known as the bundle of His

Atrioventricular node   Otherwise known as the AV node. Specialised area of cardiac cells located just above the point where the right atrium and right ventricle meet

Atrioventricular valve   Collective name for the two valves that lie between the atria and the ventricles (bicuspid and tricuspid)

Beta-blockers   A class of drugs which prevent stimulation of the beta-adrenergic receptors, used to control heart rhythm, treat angina and reduce high blood pressure

Bicuspid valve   The atrioventricular valve that lies between the left atrium and the left ventricle. Also known as the mitral valve

Bundle of His   See Atrioventricular bundle

Calcium channel blocker   A drug that blocks the entry of calcium into the muscle cells of the heart and the arteries

Echocardiogram   Ultrasound imaging of the heart and valves

Hypertension   High blood pressure

Hypotension   Low blood pressure

INR   International normalised ratio. A measurement of clotting used in the management of warfarin

Mitral valve   See Bicuspid valve

Myocardium   Muscle layer of the heart

Orthopnoea   Shortness of breath when lying down

Pulmonary valve   Valve that lies between the right ventricle and the pulmonary circulation

Purkinje fibres   Specialised conductive fibres that rapidly transport action potentials through the ventricle walls

Semilunar valves   The valves that lie between the ventricles and the pulmonary or systemic circulation (aortic valve and pulmonary valve)

Sinoatrial node   Otherwise known as the SA node. Specialised area of cardiac cells located in the upper part of the right atrium, usually referred to as the pacemaker of the heart

Stroke volume   The amount of blood ejected by a ventricle in one beat

Systemic circulation   The circulatory system of the body (excluding the lungs)

Systole   The contraction of a heart chamber (atrium or ventricle)

Tricuspid valve   The atrioventricular valve that lies between the right atrium and ventricle

Venous   Pertaining to the veins

Ventricles   The large lower chambers of the heart

Test yourself

Now review your learning by completing the learning activities for this chapter at www.wiley.com/go/pharmacologyformidwives.

References

Adityawati, A.A.D., Rahimah, A.F., Martini, H., Tjahjono, C.T. (2021) Cardiomyopathy in pregnancy: a review of the literature. *Heart Science Journal*, **2**(1): 15–24.

Blondon, M., de Tejada, B.M., Glauser, F., Righini, M., Robert-Ebadi, H. (2021) Management of high-risk pulmonary embolism in pregnancy. *Thrombosis Research*, **204**: 57–65.

Bloria, S.D., Bajaj, R., Luthra, A., Chauhan, R. (2020) Managing heart disease in pregnancy. *EMJ*, **5**(1): 58–66.

Chan, A., Wolfe, D.S., Zaidi, A.N. (2020). Pregnancy and congenital heart disease: a brief review of risk assessment and management. *Clinical Obstetrics and Gynecology*, **63**(4): 836–851.

Djakpo, D.K., Quan, W.Z. (2019) Cardioversion for atrial fibrillation during pregnancy. *International Journal of Medical Reviews and Case Reports*, **3**(6): 322–326.

Gupta, A., Lokhandwala, Y., Rai, N., Malviya, A. (2021) Adenosine – a drug with myriad utility in the diagnosis and treatment of arrhythmias. *Journal of Arrhythmia*, **37**(1): 103–112.

Halpern, D.G., Weinberg, C.R., Pinnelas, R. et al. (2019) Use of medication for cardiovascular disease during pregnancy. JACC state-of-the-art review. Journal of the American College of Cardiology, **73**(4): 457–476.

Hoeltzenbein, M., Beck, E., Fietz, A.K. et al. (2017) Pregnancy outcome after first trimester use of methyldopa: a prospective cohort study. *Hypertension*, **70**(1): 201–208.

Ibrahim, N.A.M. (2019) An up-to-date review of digoxin toxicity and its management. *International Journal of Research in Pharmacy and Pharmaceutical Sciences*, **4**(3): 59–64.

Kaye, A.B., Bhakta, A., Moseley, A.D. et al. (2019) Review of cardiovascular drugs in pregnancy. *Journal of Women's Health*, **28**(5): 686–697.

Kugamoorthy, P., Spears, D.A. (2020) Management of tachyarrhythmias in pregnancy – a review. *Obstetric Medicine*, **13**(4): 159–173.

Lameijer, H., Aalberts, J.J., van Veldhuisen, D.J., Meijer, K., Pieper, P.G. (2018) Efficacy and safety of direct oral anticoagulants during pregnancy: a systematic literature review. *Thrombosis Research*, **169**: 123-127.

Lewey, J., Andrade, L., Levine, L.D. (2021) Valvular heart disease in pregnancy. *Cardiology Clinics*, **39**(1): 151–161.

Lu, E., Shatzel, J.J., Salati, J., DeLoughery, T.G. (2017) The safety of low-molecular-weight heparin during and after pregnancy. *Obstetrical & Gynecological Survey*, **72**(12): 721–729.

National Institute for Health and Care Excellence (2019) *NG133 Hypertension in Pregnancy: diagnosis and management*. NICE: London.

Prasanthi, P.S.L.K., Jyothsna, T.H. (2020) Comparision of efficacy of labetalol vs nifedipine in pregnancy induced hypertension. *International Journal of Clinical Obstetrics and Gynaecology*, **4**(1): 275–278.

Pstras, L., Thomaseth, K., Waniewski, J., Balzani, I., Bellavere, F. (2017) Mathematical modelling of cardiovascular response to the Valsalva manoeuvre. *Mathematical Medicine and Biology*, **34**(2): 261–292.

Ramlakhan, K.P., Johnson, M.R., Roos-Hesselink, J.W. (2020) Pregnancy and cardiovascular disease. *Nature Reviews Cardiology*, **17**(11): 718–731.

Regitz-Zagrosek, V., Roos-Hesselink, J.W., Bauersachs, J. et al. (2018) 2018 ESC guidelines for the management of cardiovascular diseases during pregnancy: the Task Force for the Management of Cardiovascular Diseases During Pregnancy of the European Society of Cardiology (ESC). *European Heart Journal*, **39**(34): 3165–3241.

Resuscitation Council (UK) (2021) Advanced Life Support Manual 8th Edition. Resuscitation Council (UK)

Roberts, A., Mechery, J., Mechery, A., Clarke, B., Vause, S. (2019) Management of palpitations and cardiac arrhythmias in pregnancy. *Obstetrician & Gynaecologist*, **21**(4): 263–270.

Sousa Gomes, M., Guimarães, M., Montenegro, N. (2019) Thrombolysis in pregnancy: a literature review. *Journal of Maternal-Fetal & Neonatal Medicine*, **32**(14): 2418–2428.

Tummala, L.S., Agrawal, A., Lundberg, G. (2021) Management considerations for lipid disorders during pregnancy. *Current Treatment Options in Cardiovascular Medicine*, **23**(7): 1–12.

Vaidya, V.R., Mehra, N.S., Sugrue, A.M., Asirvatham, S.J. (2020) Supraventricular tachycardia in pregnancy. In: Malik, M. (ed.) *Sex and Cardiac Electrophysiology*, pp. 671–679. Academic Press: New York.

Van Doorn, R., Mukhtarova, N., Flyke, I.P. et al. (2021) Dose of aspirin to prevent preterm preeclampsia in women with moderate or high-risk factors: a systematic review and meta-analysis. *PLoS One*, **16**(3): e0247782.

Ying, W., Catov, J.M., Ouyang, P. (2018) Hypertensive disorders of pregnancy and future maternal cardiovascular risk. *Journal of the American Heart Association*, **7**(17): e009382.

Further reading

Cardiomyopathy Society (UK) is a national charity dedicated to the support of patients with cardiomyopathy and has a section on resources for healthcare professionals. www.cardiomyopathy.org/

European Society of Cardiology: Cardiovascular Diseases during Pregnancy Guidelines. Note, the British Cardiovascular Society is a member group of the European Society and thus the European guidelines are used in the UK. www.escardio.org/Guidelines/Clinical-Practice-Guidelines/Cardiovascular-Diseases-during-Pregnancy-Management-of

NICE Guidance on Hypertension in Pregnancy (NG133). www.nice.org.uk/guidance/ng133

Chapter 12

Medications and the renal system

Sam Bassett

King's College, London, UK

Aim

The aim of this chapter is to introduce the reader to some of the common renal complications seen within maternity care, and to introduce and explore the pharmacological therapies used in their management. The associated pharmacodynamics and pharmacokinetics will also be explored.

Learning outcomes

After reading this chapter, the reader will have:
- Gained an understanding of key renal physiology and how pregnancy alters this physiology
- Explored the common renal complications seen within childbirth
- Looked at the side-effects of common renal pharmacotherapy used in pregnancy and how this should be considered when counselling a woman to reach an informed decision regarding her evidence-based care.
- Explored the current evidence base behind the key recommendations introduced within this chapter.

Test your existing knowledge

- Describe the principal functions of the renal system and its main components
- Describe two normal physiological changes seen within pregnancy and explain how these may affect the renal system
- Name three medical conditions commonly seen within maternity care that can affect the renal system
- Which analgesic commonly used within the postnatal period has a large adverse effect on the kidneys?

Fundamentals of Pharmacology for Midwives, First Edition. Edited by Ian Peate and Cathy Hamilton.
© 2022 John Wiley & Sons Ltd. Published 2022 by John Wiley & Sons Ltd.
Companion website: www.wiley.com/go/pharmacologyformidwives

Introduction

Renal disease encompasses a wide range of reduced kidney functions due to an acute or chronic insult to the kidney. Aa a general umbrella term, this can include acute kidney injury (AKI), chronic kidney disease (CKD) and end-stage renal disease (ESRD), the latter being relatively rare in pregnancy. This chapter will describe AKI and CKD and introduce the most common pregnancy-related causes of both, exploring how pregnancy may affect the course of their development as well as the pharmacology used in their treatment.

Anatomy and physiology of the renal tract

To understand safe medicines management and pharmacology for women with renal complications in pregnancy, first it is important to have a fundamental understanding of renal physiology and in particular the target sites used for the application of appropriate pharmacotherapy.

Comprising the kidneys, ureters, urinary bladder and urethra, the renal system receives its blood supply via the two renal arteries, arising directly from the abdominal aorta (Figure 12.1). With around 25% of cardiac output delivered to the kidneys each minute, this is more than any other tissue in the body. Supplied by the autonomic system, the kidneys have a rich supply of sympathetic fibres and lesser parasympathetic fibres facilitating vasoconstriction, reduced blood flow, reduced glomerular filtration rate (GFR) and the release of renin from the juxtaglomerular apparatus. In addition, some sensory nerve fibres allow the perception of pain usually from distension of the renal capsule arising from complications such as bleeding, inflammation or obstruction from renal calculi, with ischaemia also causing pain on occasion (Rankin, 2017).

The main function of the kidneys is the maintenance of homeostasis, through various excretory, regulatory and metabolic mechanisms. For example, they regulate fluid, electrolyte and acid–base balance through glomerular filtration, selective tubular absorption and tubular secretion of water, sodium, potassium, calcium, phosphate and hydrogen and bicarbonate ions. Most of this occurs within the nephrons which are composed of the Bowman's capsule, glomerulus, proximal convoluted tubule, loop of Henle, distal convoluted tubule and collecting ducts (Figure 12.2) Approximately 180 L of plasma is filtered daily, with 99% of filtrate reabsorbed by the nephrons, leading to around 1.5 L of urine being produced on average daily providing excretion of metabolic waste such as urea and creatinine.

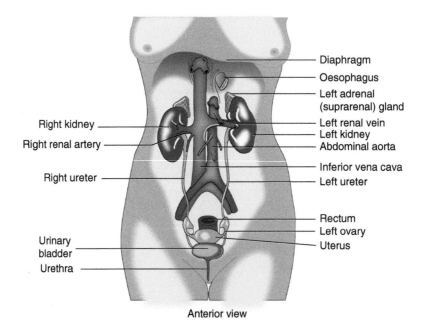

Anterior view

Figure 12.1   Urinary system. *Source*: Peate (2017)/with permission of John Wiley & Sons.

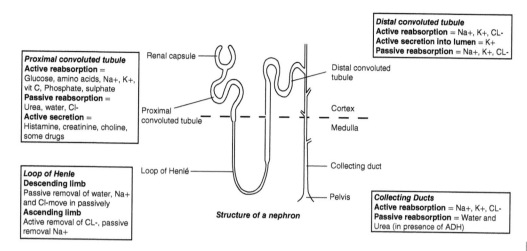

Proximal convoluted tubule
Active reabsorption =
Glucose, amino acids, Na+, K+,
vit C, Phosphate, sulphate
Passive reabsorption =
Urea, water, Cl-
Active secretion =
Histamine, creatinine, choline,
some drugs

Distal convoluted tubule
Active reabsorption = Na+, K+, CL-
Active secretion into lumen = K+
Passive reabsorption = Na+, K+, CL-

Loop of Henle
Descending limb
Passive removal of water, Na+
and Cl-move in passively
Ascending limb
Active removal of CL-, passive
removal Na+

Collecting Ducts
Active reabsorption = Na+, K+, CL-
Passive reabsorption = Water and
Urea (in presence of ADH)

Renal capsule
Proximal convoluted tubule
Loop of Henlé
Distal convoluted tubule
Cortex
Medulla
Collecting duct
Pelvis

Structure of a nephron

Figure 12.2   Reabsorption and secretion in the nephron.

183

In addition, the kidneys have an endocrine function in the secretion of hormones such as erythropoietin, involved in red cell production, and renin, which has a role in blood pressure regulation. Conversion of vitamin D into an active form also occurs in the kidney, which has a role in the regulation of calcium and phosphate, prostaglandin synthesis, in part protecting the renal system from profound vasoconstriction. Lastly, the kidneys have a role in glucose homeostasis through gluconeogenesis and reabsorption of glucose (Diamond-Fox and Gatehouse, 2021).

Physiological changes to the renal system during pregnancy

Significant haemodynamic changes occur during the duration of a normal healthy pregnancy to accommodate and nourish the developing fetus. Blood volume increases by around 1.5 litres, usually peaking at around 34 weeks gestation. This results in haemodilution with the 50% increase in plasma volume not matched by the 30% increase in red blood cells. The increase in plasma volume also causes a decreased oncotic pressure in the glomeruli and a subsequent rise in glomerular filtration rate (GFR).

Although the increase in blood flow results in an increase in cardiac output (CO = SV × HR), this is not matched by an increase in blood pressure as at the same time there is a 40% fall in systemic vascular resistance (SVR) in pregnancy. This fall in SVR is brought about by an increase in vasodilators, such as relaxin and nitric oxide, as well as a relative resistance to vasoconstrictors such as angiotensin II. As a result, blood pressure (BP) usually falls in pregnancy, reaching a nadir at around 20 weeks gestation. Vascular resistance in both afferent and efferent renal arterioles also decreases, allowing glomerular hydrostatic pressure to remain stable despite a rise in renal plasma flow estimated to be around 60–80% (Gonzalez Suarez et al., 2019).

The combination of increased renal vasodilation and increased renal plasma flow causes the GFR to rise by around 50% with the resulting hyperfiltration leading to a physiological reduction in serum creatinine and urea. In addition, urine protein excretion over a 24-hour urine collection increases, meaning the thresholds in pregnancy are set at a higher level, with a 24-hour urine being 300 mg/day (usual <150 mg/day). Or as is now more commonly used in pregnancy, due to it being a much faster test with high sensitivity and specificity, a urine protein:creatinine ratio (PCR) at a threshold of 30 mg/mmol. Whilst commonly attributed to hyperfiltration, it is worth noting that changes to glomerular permeability are also thought to play a part in the increase in proteinuria (Gonzalez Suarez et al., 2019). As such, it is important to note that investigative values considered normal outside pregnancy may be abnormal in pregnancy (Table 12.1).

Table 12.1 Physiological changes in common indices of renal function during healthy pregnancy. Values are mean (SD).

Measure	Stage of pregnancy			
	Before pregnancy	First trimester	Second trimester	Third trimester
Effective renal plasma flow (mL/min)	480 (72)	841 (144)	891 (279)	771 (175)
Glomerular filtration rate (mL/min) measured by 24 h creatinine clearance	105 (24)	162 (19)	174 (24)	165 (22)
Serum creatinine (µmol/L)	73 (10)	60 (8)	54 (10)	64 (9)
Plasma urea (mmol/L)	4.3 (0.8)	3.5 (0.7)	3.3 (0.8)	3.1 (0.7)

Source: Adapted from Williams & Davison (2008).

The increase in renal blood flow leads to a significant increase in kidney volume, weight and size, with bladder capacity increasing by term up to around 1000 mL from the usual 300–600 mL outside pregnancy. In addition, progesterone dilates the ureters, renal pelves and calyces, leading to a physiological pregnancy hydronephrosis in around 80% of women. The resulting urinary stasis in the dilated collecting system then predisposes pregnant women with asymptomatic bacteriuria to pyelonephritis (Rasmussen and Nielson, 1988).

There are also changes to the tubular handling of wastes and nutrients, with the reabsorption of glucose in the proximal and collecting tubule being less effective. As a result, around 90% of women with normal blood glucose will excrete 1–10 g of glucose a day, meaning that if a woman has had a particularly high-sugar diet that day, this is often evident on urinalysis with further follow-up and/or investigations warranted to exclude pathology (Soma-Pillay et al., 2016).

Common renal conditions in pregnancy
Urinary tract infection

On occasion, the presence of bacteria in a urine sample will be detected in an individual who has no signs or symptoms of a urinary tract infection (UTI), known as asymptomatic bacteriuria. Defined as bacteriuria with >100 000 organisms/mL of urine in a clean catch, a negative urinalysis for protein is not a reliable indicator. As UTI is thought to affect around 2–15% of pregnant women, it is particularly important that women are screened antenatally at booking for asymptomatic bacteriuria via means of a urine culture, as if left untreated up to 40% of women will develop a symptomatic UTI and 30% acute pyelonephritis, with associations of low birthweight and preterm birth (Smaill and Vazquez, 2019).

At least 50% of women at some time in their lives will experience a UTI, with around 10% of these developing in pregnancy. In part, this is due to the pressure of the gravid uterus on the renal system and the relaxing effects of progesterone leading to dilation, urinary stasis and vesicourethral reflux. However, pregnancy is a state of relative immunocompromise and intrapartum interventions such as repeated urinary catheterisations and changes to bladder sensitivity and bladder overdistension in the postpartum period may also play a part in the frequency of UTIs seen.

Management should be prompt treatment with oral antibiotics using agents known to be safe in pregnancy (Table 12.2). In addition, any woman with known reflux nephropathy, congenital anomalies of the kidneys and urinary tract (CAKUT), chronic kidney disease (CKD) taking immunosuppressive therapy or a history of recurrent UTI should be offered antibiotic prophylaxis during pregnancy after a single UTI, including asymptomatic bacteriuria (Wiles et al., 2019).

Table 12.2   Common drugs used in the treatment of a lower UTI in pregnancy with choice based recent culture and susceptibility results.

Drug name	Dosage	Notes	Absorption, distribution, metabolism, excretion (ADME)
Nitrofurantoin	50 mg 4 times a day, or 100 mg (modified release) twice daily for 7 days	First choice recommended antibiotic	**A** = readily absorbed from gastrointestinal tract, mainly in small intestine **D** = widely into most body fluids, can cross placenta **M** = 2/3rds by the liver, small fraction reduced to aminofurantoin **E** = rapidly via bile and urine (appears in urine within 30 min). Small amounts excreted in breast milk
		Not recommended at term because it may produce neonatal haemolysis	
Cefalexin	500 mg twice daily, or 250 mg 6-hourly, for 7 days	Recommended as second choice antibiotic if symptoms do not improve on first choice after 48 h or first choice is not suitable	**A** = upper intestine **D** = widely to body fluids and tissues; can cross placenta **M** = not metabolised in body **E** = over 90% by urine after 6 h – risk of toxicity with impaired renal function. Small amounts excreted in breast milk
Amoxicillin	250–500 mg taken 3 times a day		**A** = rapidly absorbed from gastrointestinal tract **D** = readily in most body tissues and fluids **M** = <30% by liver, 60% of oral dose excreted unchanged in urine **E** = in urine within 6–8 h; small amounts excreted in breast milk
Cefalexin	250 mg once daily	Used in continuous prophylaxis	As above
Trimethoprim	200 mg twice daily	Off prescription use so seek specialist advice Has an antifolate effect so usually avoided: • in 1st trimester due to its associated with neural tube defects • if a woman is folate deficient or taking a folate antagonist • or has been treated with trimethoprim in the past year. If given in first trimester, administer with 5 mg daily of folic acid	**A** = rapidly through gastrointestinal tract **D** = widely to body fluids and tissues; can cross placenta **M** = 10–20% in liver, 80% of oral dose excreted unchanged in urine **E** = 50–60% in urine within 24 h, faeces 4%, small amounts excreted in breast milk

Source: Adapted from NICE (2018).

185

Acute kidney injury

Acute kidney injury (AKI) is defined as an abrupt, often within hours, decrease in kidney function. It can arise from injury involving structural damage or, more commonly in pregnancy, from impairment resulting in loss of function. Defined by a rapid increase in serum creatinine, decrease in urine output or both, it is estimated to occur in around 10–15% of patients admitted to hospital, rising to 50% if intensive care is required (Ronco, 2019). Whilst many cases should be reversible, data from large observational and epidemiological studies is now suggesting a strong link between AKI and subsequent CKD or even in the worse scenario ESRD (See et al., 2019).

In pregnancy, the physiological change to the renal system complicates the usual international consensus definitions of AKI (Table 12.3). As such, serum creatinine (sCr) values must be interpreted within the context of pregnancy. For example, a 'normal' laboratory value for sCr in women (52.2–91.9 μmol/L) could mask renal impairment in pregnancy and any at a level of above 77 μmol/l should be considered as diagnostic of kidney injury (Wiles et al., 2019).

The cause of AKI varies geographically according to available resources. In developing countries, the main cause is severe sepsis from septic abortion whilst in developing countries it tends to be from hypertensive disorders of pregnancy and haemorrhage (Gonzalez Suarez et al., 2019). Within the UK, AKI is thought to complicate around 1.4% of obstetric admissions and is increasingly attributed to more than one aetiology, for example postpartum haemorrhage and the use of non-steroidal anti-inflammatory drugs (NSAIDS) (Table 12.4) (Mihalache et al., 2012).

Fundamental to the management and treatment of AKI is the maintenance of renal perfusion. However, the physiological changes of pregnancy mean that women compensate much longer for hypovolaemia and hypotension. Therefore, they typically present with signs much later than expected, with over 40% of cases of AKI thought to be unrecognised by the clinical team, highlighting a need for better diagnosis and management of AKI within the obstetric population (Wiles and Banerjee, 2016).

The clinical approach to management should include fluid status assessment, medication review, consideration of fluid replacement, thorough diagnostic work-up including appropriate investigative tests (haematological and biochemical monitoring, ultrasound) and early involvement of a nephrologist if no response to initial management. Dosages for medication such as antibiotics, anticoagulants, insulin and opiates may need adjustment if the glomerular filtration rate is below 30 mL/min/1.73 m^2.

Table 12.3   Definition and staging of AKI.

Stage	Serum creatinine	Urine output
1	1.5–1.9 times baseline Or ≥0.3 mg/dL (≥26.5 μmol/L) increase	<0.5 mL/kg/h for 6–12 hours
2	2.0–2.9 times baseline	<0.5 mL/kg/h for ≥12 hours
3	3.0 times baseline Or ≥4.0 mg/dL (≥353.6 μmol/L) Or Initiation of renal replacement therapy (RRT) Or In patients <18 years a decrease in eGFR to <35 mL/min per 1.73m^2	<0.3 mL/kg/h for ≥24 hours Or Anuria for ≥12 hours

AKI is defined as any of the following

- Increase in sCr by ≥0.3 mg/dL(≥26.5 μmol/L) within 48 hours; or
- Increase in 1.5 times baseline, which is known or presumed to have occurred within the prior 7 days; or
- Urine volume <0.5 mL/kg/h for 6 hours

Source: Kidney Disease Improving Global Outcomes (KDIGO, 2012a).

Table 12.4 Common causes of acute kidney injury in pregnancy.

Gestation	Diagnosis
First trimester	• Hyperemesis gravidarum • Septic abortion/miscarriage • Acute urinary retention
Second and third trimesters	• Pre-eclampsia and HELLP • Ureteral obstruction • Placental abruption • Acute fatty liver of pregnancy • Microangiopathic haemolytic anaemia (TTP/HUS)
Peripartum	• Chorioamnionitis • Postpartum haemorrhage • Ureteric injury • NSAIDs
At any time	• Urosepsis • Lupus nephritis • Glomerulonephritis • Interstitial nephritis • Renal stone disease • Intravascular volume depletion, i.e. sepsis from any cause, vomiting, DKA

DKA, diabetic ketoacidosis; HELLP, haemolysis, elevated liver enzymes and low platelets; HUS, haemolytic uraemic syndrome; NSAIDs, non-steroidal anti-inflammatory drugs; TTP, thrombotic thrombocytopenic purpura.
Source: Aadapted from Wiles and Banerjee (2016).

Chronic kidney disease

Chronic kidney disease (CKD) often presents silently both clinically and biochemically until renal impairment is advanced. As such, symptoms are often absent until the GFR rate declines to less than 25% of normal, with more than 50% of renal function lost before serum creatinine (sCr) rises above 120 µmol/l (Williams and Davison, 2008). Worldwide rates of CKD are estimated to be around 5–15% attributed mainly to diabetes, glomerular nephritis, pyelonephritis, polycystic kidney and hypertension, with cases increasing in line with age (UK Renal Registry, 2021).

Chronic kidney disease is classified into five stages according to the level of renal function (Table 12.5) and is thought to affect 3% of pregnant women in developing countries (Piccoli et al., 2018). In England, this equates to around 15–20 000 pregnancies per year, with figures only predicted to rise further due to increasing maternal age and obesity (Wiles et al., 2019).

Table 12.5 Stages of CKD.

Stage	Description	Estimated GFR (mL/min/1.73 m²)
1	Kidney damage with normal or raised GFR	≥90
2	Kidney damage with mildly low GFR	60–89
3	Moderately low GFR	30–59
4	Severely low GFR	15–29
5	Kidney failure	<15

GFR, glomerular filtration rate.
Source: Adapted from KDIGO (2012b).

Table 12.6   An outline of monitoring required for women with CKD during pregnancy.

Measure	Monitoring details
Urine	Every 4–6 weeks check for: • UTI – commence prophylactic antibiotics after one urinary tract infection • Proteinuria – quantification should be by protein:creatinine ratio (μPCR) or albumin:creatinine ratio (μACR); 24-h urine collection is not required. • If in nephrotic range (μPCR >300 mg/mmol or μACR>250 mg/mmol) commence thromboprophylaxis with low weight molecular heparin and continue post partum unless there is a specific contraindication • If haematuria perform microscopy for red cell casts, which can suggest active renal parenchymal (functioning part of kidney) disease. Normal red cell morphology suggests urological pathology – seek urological advice
Blood pressure (BP)	Check BP regularly dependent on control. Aim for 135/85 mmHg or less If already on antihypertensives continue unless systolic BP is consistently <110 mmHg or diastolic BP consistently <70 mmHg, or there is symptomatic hypotension
Renal function	eGFR is not valid for use in pregnancy so renal function should be assessed by serum creatinine concentrations. Assess more frequently for stages 3–5 and in second half of pregnancy
Full blood count (FBC)	Check haemoglobin and, dependent on serum ferritin, commence iron and/or erythropoietin to keep levels at 100–110 g/L
Ultrasound (USS) of renal tract	Perform baseline renal USS at booking for pelvicalyceal (renal pelvis major and minor calyces) dimensions. Repeat if maternal symptoms suggest an obstruction

eGFR, estimated glomerular filtration rate; UTI, urinary tract infection.
Source: Adapted from Wiles et al. (2019).

Although CKD can be diagnosed for the first time in pregnancy, it is important to bear in mind the silent nature of the disease which means it could have been an underlying condition for several years. When present in pregnancy, CKD can increase adverse maternal and fetal outcomes including pre-eclampsia, fetal growth restriction, preterm delivery, increased caesarean delivery, increased neonatal unit admission and accelerated loss of maternal renal function. Therefore, known cases require early referral to an obstetrician, nephrologist or expert physician to plan antenatal monitoring with the woman (Table 12.6), with the most important aspect being the management of any related CKD signs and symptoms rather than the type of kidney disease.

Whilst many women with CKD can have reduced fertility, unintended pregnancies do occur. As such, advice on safe and effective contraception is recommended for all women of reproductive age with CKD, with progesterone-only methods advised, including the progesterone-only pill, implant, intrauterine system and emergency contraceptive all recommended (Wiles et al., 2019). For those planning a pregnancy, preconception counselling is crucial to achieve the best potential pregnancy outcome (Table 12.7), with women fully aware of the risks to their long-term renal function and to the fetus (Table 12.8). Preconceptionally, folic acid 400 μg is recommended as usual up to 12 weeks gestation as well as the commencement of low-dose aspirin (75–150 mg/day) in early pregnancy to reduce the risk of pre-eclampsia and improve perinatal outcome.

Electrolyte disorders

The renal system has an integral role in the maintenance of homeostasis, controlling fluid, electrolyte and acid–base balance. Renal complications may disrupt all these processes, and this section will explore this further and identify how pharmacotherapy may be utilised in the subsequent management and treatment.

Fluid balance refers to the distribution of body fluid within the intracellular (interstitial) and extracellular (intravascular) compartments. Electrolytes are substances that, when dissolved in water, dissociate into positively and negatively charged ions. Operating in both extracellular and

Table 12.7 Recommended pre-pregnancy counselling for optimisation of maternal and neonatal outcomes in women with CKD.

Aim	Medication
• Stabilising disease activity in advance of pregnancy with the aim for minimised doses of pregnancy-appropriate medications	• If vitamin D deficient, prescribe supplementation in pregnancy • Discontinue non-calcium-based phosphate binders
• Optimising blood pressure control (<140 mmHg) on pregnancy-appropriate medication	• Labetalol, nifedipine, methyldopa all safe to use in pregnancy
• Optimising glycaemic control in women with diabetes mellitus	• Metformin can be used in women with a pre-pregnancy eGFR>30 mL/min/1.73 m^2 and stable renal function during pregnancy
• Minimising risk of exposure to teratogenic medications	• Women taking ACE inhibitors should have a plan for discontinuation/conversion • Angiotensin receptor antagonists should be discontinued in advance of pregnancy • If women have been exposed to teratogenic drugs in the first trimester, refer to a specialist fetal medicine unit
• Making a treatment plan in the event of hyperemesis or disease exacerbation/relapse during pregnancy	

Source: Adapted from Wiles et al. (2019).

intracellular fluid compartments, electrolytes in total need to balance to achieve a neutral electrical charge. Therefore, not surprisingly, several pairs of oppositely charged ions are so closely linked that a problem with one ion causes a problem with the other, i.e. sodium and chloride, calcium and phosphorus. Likewise, if a body requires a particular ion, it must swap a similarly charged ion in order to maintain neutrality, i.e. sodium could be retained by the kidneys to the detriment of potassium.

Total body water is regulated within a narrow range, through alteration of sodium and water content (Peate, 2017). The sodium–potassium pumps (Na+-K+) drive sodium from the tubular cells into the blood, and this creates a lower concentration gradient within the cell. Sodium and water then move from the tubular infiltrate into the cell via various channels or co-transporters, according to the permeability of the cell membrane and the concentration gradient (Diamond-Fox and Gatehouse, 2021).

Inappropriate renal handling of sodium may occur due to a primary renal problem or an abnormality in the volume regulation mechanism. The most common issue seen in pregnancy is severe hyponatraemia, which can arise from a variety of complications including pre-eclampsia (inadequate sodium excretion usually from renal failure), peripartum dilution (due to a woman taking on more fluid of low sodium content than she can excrete), the antidiuretic effect of oxytocin (synthetic and/or endogenous) and desmopressin (can lead to renal water retention). Primary treatments used in the management of hyponatraemic patients usually rely on the use of intravenous sodium-containing fluids and fluid restriction and diuretics. However, conditions such as pre-eclampsia can complicate fluid administration and the use of loop diuretics such as furosemide is best avoided in pregnancy unless the benefits outweigh the risks which will be discussed in more depth later (Sandhu et al., 2010). Hypernatremia is fortunately relatively rare in pregnancy but has been noted in extreme cases of hyperemesis gravidarum complicated by diabetes insipidus.

Potassium is integral to the maintenance of an electrochemical gradient across the cell membrane, and the ability of nerves and muscle to create an action potential. Hypokalaemia and hyperkalaemia are life-threatening, causing cardiac dysrhythmias and potentially cardiac arrest, and the

Table 12.8 Estimated effects of pre-pregnancy renal function on pregnancy outcome and maternal renal function.

Mean (SD) pre-pregnancy serum creatinine value (μmol/L)	Effects on pregnancy outcome (%)					Loss of >25% renal function		
	Fetal growth restriction	Preterm delivery	Pre-eclampsia	Perinatal deaths	During pregnancy	Persists postpartum	End-stage renal failure after 1 year
<125	25	30	22	1	2	0	0
125–180	40	60	40	5	40	20	2
>180	65	>90	60	10	70	50	35
On dialysis	>90	>90	75	50[a]	N/A	N/A	N/A

[a]If conceived on dialysis, 50% of infants survive; if conceived before introduction of dialysis, this rises to 75% of infants surviving.

Source: Williams and Davison (2008).

kidneys and adrenal glands are vital in the maintenance of potassium homoeostasis. Within the nephron, most of the potassium is reabsorbed prior to the collecting duct, and excretion of potassium occurs in this segment through several mechanisms. The sodium–potassium pumps and potassium channels in the cell membranes of the collecting duct are affected by the extracellular potassium concentration, the release of aldosterone, the pH, flow rates within the collecting duct, filtrate sodium concentration and intracellular magnesium.

In pregnancy, hyperkalaemia is usually associated with AKI/CKD, tissue injury, diabetes, infection or dehydration, while hypokalaemia is usually associated with potassium deficiency, hyperaldosteronism and gastrointestinal disorders that cause fluid loss, the most noticeable being hyperemesis gravidarum.

Calcium and phosphate are closely linked and essential to the maintenance of bone density and regulated by one of several mechanisms including gut reabsorption, bone reabsorption and renal handling. Calcium is regulated by the thyroid gland and when levels fall, parathyroid hormone (PTH) stimulates bone reabsorption (release of calcium and phosphate from bone) and increases vitamin D synthesis, renal phosphate excretion and renal calcium reabsorption. Vitamin D is synthesised within the kidney, increasing phosphate and calcium levels via reabsorption through the gut, bones and renal tubules. In pregnancy, extra active vitamin D is produced by the placenta, meaning levels circulate at twice non-gravid levels. However, at the same time parathyroid hormone levels are halved and there is a physiological hypercalciuria (excess calcium in the urine) as well as increased fetal requirements, which all combine to keep plasma calcium levels unchanged. As such, pharmacotherapy to maintain normal calcium and phosphate levels in pregnancy is rarely needed and hyperparathyroidism rarely occurs (Lightstone, 2007).

Acid–base balance, and so pH, is controlled by the respiratory, buffer and renal systems. By regulating carbon dioxide (respiratory) and bicarbonate (renal), the pH may be normalised when acidosis or alkalosis occurs. Under normal circumstances, the kidneys excrete excess hydrogen ions (H+) or acid through increased synthesis of the Na+H+ exchangers or H+ ATPase pump, reabsorb bicarbonate via the Na+HCO3– co-transporters and produce more ammonium salts (NH4+) for excretion. In pregnancy, it is important to note that increased alveolar ventilation causes a respiratory alkalosis to which the kidneys respond by increasing bicarbonaturia (abnormally increased concentration of hydrogen carbonate in the urine) and a compensatory metabolic acidosis.

In renal disease, the kidneys are unable to perform these processes effectively and so metabolic acidosis can occur, causing hyperkalaemia, due to H+ moving into cells and driving K+ out, with eventual worsening renal bone disease due to the loss of carbonate buffers in an acidic environment. RRT may be used to correct severe metabolic acidosis in both the acute and chronic settings of renal failure.

Specific conditions and their management

Hypertension

The mainstay of treatment for hypertension and/or renal disease in the general adult population tends to focus on inhibitors of the renin-angiotensin-aldosterone system such as angiotensin-converting enzyme (ACE) inhibitors and angiotensin II receptor blockers (ARBs) (Table 12.9). However, these are contraindicated in pregnancy due to teratogenic effects, with discontinuation recommended before conception or within 2 days of notification of pregnancy (NICE, 2019). The neonatal mortality rate is also as high as 25%, with any surviving children showing an increased risk of renal function impairment and childhood and adolescent hypertension (Maynard and Thadhani, 2009).

Other medications commonly used in the control of hypertension include diuretics. Similarly, thiazide or thiazide-like diuretics have been associated with an increased risk of congenital abnormalities and neonatal complications if taken in pregnancy so alternatives should be sought (NICE, 2019). Loop diuretics, especially furosemide, are also not recommended in pregnancy or when breast feeding unless the benefit to the mother outweighs the risk to the fetus due to the potential risk of neonatal hyperbilirubinaemia and suppression of lactation. Circumstances where they may be considered include the treatment of pulmonary hypertension, severe hypertension in the presence of chronic kidney disease or congestive heart failure (Ghamen and Movahed, 2008).

191

Table 12.9 Antihypertensives recommended for use in pregnancy.

Type of drug	Drug	Comment	Absorption, distribution, metabolism, excretion (ADME)
Combined alpha/beta-blocker	Labetalol (oral or intravenous)	• Recommended as first-line treatment by NICE (2019) • Not for long-term use in pregnancy as beta-blockers can affect fetal growth	**A** = rapidly in gastrointestinal tract **D** = some CNS penetration; crosses placenta **M** = rapidly in liver, 85% first-pass hepatic metabolism **E** = 55–60% in urine, 12–27% in faeces, small amounts in breast milk
Calcium channel blocker	Nifedipine (oral) Amlodipine (oral)	• First choice for African/Caribbean family origin • Use if woman has used successfully in the past	**A** = rapidly in gastrointestinal tract **D** = 92–98% bound to plasma proteins **M** = liver **E** = 60–80% in urine, rest in faeces
Alpha-blocker	Methyldopa (oral)	• Most studied antihypertensive in pregnancy; good track record • Side-effects depression, sedation, postural hypertension	**A** = 25% from gastrointestinal tract (range 8–62%) **D** = lipid soluble **M** = liver **E** = 70% urine, 30% faeces
Vasodilator	Hydralazine (intravenous)	• Rapid drop in BP. Consider using up to 500 mL crystalloid before or simultaneously with administration in the antenatal period	**A** = rapidly in gastrointestinal tract **D** = rapid **M** = liver **E** = metabolites in urine

BP, blood pressure; CNS, central nervous system.
Source: Adapted from NICE (2019).

Pre-eclampsia

Pre-eclampsia is a complex medical disorder thought to be responsible for over 500 000 fetal and neonatal deaths and over 70 000 maternal deaths worldwide each year (Brown et al., 2018). Renal dysfunction associated with pre-eclampsia is well documented and can include severe endothelial dysfunction in the glomerulus, changes in expression of podocyte-(specialised epithelial cells in Bowman's capsule that cover the outer surface of the glomerular capillaries) associated proteins and possibly even podocyte injury and loss, resulting in significant proteinuria, impaired glomerular filtration, AKI and in severe cases CKD (Craici et al., 2014). Research is still ongoing but current epidemiological studies appear to strongly imply that a history of pre-eclampsia (particularly early preterm) greatly increases the risk of CKD, hypertensive kidney disease and glomerular and proteinuric disease later in life (Kristensen et al., 2019). This is of particular note when the recurrence of pre-eclampsia in a subsequent pregnancy is around 16%, rising to 33% if the birth was preterm at 28–34 weeks gestation.

While pre-eclampsia only leads to AKI in around 1% of women in pregnancy, due to the incidence of pre-eclampsia this makes it the most common cause, with AKI often used as a marker of severity (Prakash and Ganiger, 2017). Fluid management is key in pre-eclampsia, but the oliguria often seen does not imply volume depletion. Women are hypovolaemic, with fluid displaced into the tissues due to endothelial damage, meaning that any intravenous hydration needs to be carefully managed, with women often fluid restricted to 80 mL/h to avoid any associated pulmonary oedema or increased maternal mortality. It is also important to note here that a degree of oliguria before the physiological postpartum diuresis at 36–48 hours is a relatively common phenomenon and should not be aggressively managed. If necessary, invasive monitoring should be utilised to guide complex fluid management (Wiles and Banerjee, 2016).

HELLP syndrome

HELLP syndrome is a combination of **H**aemolysis, **E**levated **L**iver enzymes and **L**ow **P**latelets, thought to be a variation of pre-eclampsia. However, the incidence of renal impairment is much higher with HELLP, with AKI affecting around 3–15% of cases, increasing further if associated with abruption, disseminated intravascular coagulation, sepsis, haemorrhage or intrauterine death (Prakash and Ganiger, 2017). Therefore, AKI in the context of HELLP can worsen prognosis, leading in some cases to the need for temporary renal replacement therapy, usually in the form of haemodialysis. Fortunately, unless there is underlying CKD, most will recover haematological and biochemical markers by 48 hours as well as renal function (August, 2013).

Lupus nephritis

In pregnancy there are also several changes to the maternal innate and adaptive immune systems, mainly to establish fetal tolerance. All of these can have an important impact on the behaviour of autoimmune diseases, which is a common cause of reduced renal function in young women due to a complex interaction of hormonal, genetic and epigenetic factors (Table 12.10). Autoimmune diseases such as systemic lupus erythematosus (SLE), rheumatoid arthritis (RA) and systemic scleroderma (SS) are all characterised by systemic inflammation leading to target organ dysfunction, including the kidney.

While RA and SS are known to affect women mainly aged 45–55 and 50–60, SLE is known to disproportionally affect women in their reproductive years. It is thought to arise from a complex interplay of number and genetic variants on the X chromosome, the role of oestrogen on the disease, and interferon proteins that help regulate the activity of the immune system. SLE affects the kidneys in around 50% of cases, including inflammation, glomerular, interstitial and vascular lesions in the kidney, resulting in what is known as lupus nephritis (Piccoli et al., 2018).

Therefore, kidney disease remains integral to any pre-pregnancy counselling with previous kidney involvement and low levels of complement C4 (associated with autoimmune diseases), both indicating a high risk of active nephritis occurring in pregnancy (Buyon et al., 2017). The need for optimal disease control with appropriately safe medications during pregnancy should also be explained (Table 12.11). Thyroid function should also be assessed as it is associated with poorer pregnancy outcome in SLE (Stagnaro-Green et al., 2011). If women have hyperparathyroidism and are on calcimimetics, such as cinacalcet, it is worth noting that these will need to be discontinued due to the high risk of maternal and fetal complications, including hyperemesis, nephrolithiasis, recurrent urinary tract infection, pre-eclampsia and pancreatitis. Fetal complications include spontaneous abortion, stillbirth and perinatal death and a 30–50% incidence rate of neonatal tetany and are probably due to suppression of the neonatal parathyroid gland, which in rare cases could be permanent (Bashir et al., 2019).

Table 12.10   Sex differences in the incidence and severity of autoimmune diseases.

Peak incidence	Systemic lupus erythematosus	Rheumatoid arthritis	Systemic scleroderma
Female/male ratio	Peak 15:1 Total 9:1	Peak 4:1 After age 60 1:1	Peak 14:1 Total 3:1
Influence of oestrogen: • High levels • Low levels	Negative Unknown	Positive Negative	Unknown Negative

Source: Piccoli et al. (2018)/Springer Nature/CC BY 4.0.

Table 12.11   Medications safe for use during pregnancy in systemic lupus erythematosus (SLE).

Drugs	Effects during pregnancy	Recommendations	Absorption, distribution, metabolism, excretion (ADME)
Anticoagulants • Low molecular weight heparin	Mainstay of treatment for APS. In addition women with glomerular disease may experience increasing proteinuria, commonly reaching nephrotic-range values which is associated with increased risk of VTE	Indicated for all women with SLE and APS and a history of venous thrombotic events (VTE/s) or those who, although they do not have a history of VTE, meet the obstetric criteria for APS, such as 3 or more pregnancy losses or a late pregnancy loss	**A** = rapidly when given SC **D** = protein bound; does not cross placenta **M** = rapidly in liver **E** = non-saturable renal. Unlikely to have any clinical effect in breast milk
Antimalarials Hydroxychloroquine	Historically used to treat malaria; known to help treat some symptoms of SLE Discontinuation has been associated with increased lupus activity and flares, requiring higher steroid doses to control symptoms No known risk of teratogenicity	Continue throughout pregnancy	**A** = rapidly from gastrointestinal tract **D** = protein bound in plasma **M** = liver **E** = 16–21% unchanged drug in urine, 5% sloughed off in skin, 24–25% in faeces
Corticosteroids • Glucocorticoids, i.e. prednisolone, pulse methyl prednisolone • Fluorinated compounds, i.e. betamethasone, dexamethasone	High doses can lead to higher maternal complications, i.e. gestational diabetes, cleft lip and palate, premature rupture of membranes Some associations with impaired child neurophysiological development	Use lowest doses possible of glucocorticoids; pulse therapy can be used for acute flares Limit fluorinated compounds to one course for fetal lung maturation	**A** = rapidly via gastrointestinal tract **D** = serum proteins **M** = liver **E** = 90% urine
Immunosuppressants (recommended) • Azathioprine • Calcineurin inhibitors – Ciclosporin Tacrolimus	Animal studies have shown evidence of teratogenicity but no controlled data in humans	Potential benefits are likely to outweigh risks. Limit dosages. Low levels found in breast milk Recommended concentrations of calcineurin inhibitors are checked throughout pregnancy and immediately postpartum, as blood concentrations change Avoid medications that interfere with calcineurin inhibitor metabolism, i.e. erythromycin, clarithromycin	**A** = gastrointestinal tract but highly variable as to rate **D** = serum proteins **M** = liver **E** = urine

(Continued)

194

Table 12.11   (Continued)

Drugs	Effects during pregnancy	Recommendations	Absorption, distribution, metabolism, excretion (ADME)
Immunosuppressants (contraindicated in pregnancy and breast feeding) • Cyclophosphamide • Mycophenolate mofetil • Methotrexate (unknown risk) • Rituximab	Fetal malformations, higher rates of pregnancy loss Teratogenic (cleft lip palate, ear abnormalities), higher rate of pregnancy loss Transient fetal B-cell depletion, unknown long-term outcomes	May need fertility preservation with cyclophosphamide 3-month interval before conception advised to facilitate transfer to a pregnancy-safe alternative and ensure stable disease/kidney function	As above

APS, antiphospholipid syndrome; FBC, full blood count; LFT, liver function tests; SC, subcutaneous.

195

Immunoglobulin A nephropathy

Nephropathy is a general term for the deterioration of kidney function. Immunoglobulin A (IgA) nephropathy, also known as Berger disease, occurs when the antibody IgA builds up in the kidneys. The resulting inflammation damages the glomeruli of the kidney and its ability to filter waste. Largely diagnosed in the 20–30 year age group, by default it has the potential to affect women of child-bearing age. While current available evidence suggests that pregnancy itself does not increase the risk of adverse renal events, any pre-existing hypertension, a baseline GFR <60 mL/min/1.73 m² or proteinuria (μPCR >300 mg/mmol or μACR >250 mg/mmol) can significantly increase the risk for kidney disease progression (Lui et al., 2016).

Regarding medication, most patients with mild, stable or slow progressive IgA nephropathy do not receive immunosuppressive therapy but if prescribed, as before these will need review and transfer to pregnancy-safe alternatives ideally preconceptionally or as soon as pregnancy is confirmed. Similarly, treatment with ACE inhibitors or ARBs will also require review. If immunosuppression is needed for more active disease, steroids such as prednisolone can be used.

Diabetic nephropathy

Diabetic nephropathy is the name given to kidney damage caused by diabetes, either type 1 or 2, characterised by gradual development of hypertension, albuminuria and loss of GFR. Around 40% of diabetics will eventually develop nephropathy, often linked with increasing age, although it can be prevented or delayed with optimal control of blood glucose and BP levels. As such, it is less commonly seen in pregnancy and is thought to affect around 6% of pregnant women. Like other glomerular diseases, the risk of adverse pregnancy outcomes is related to the level of renal function pre-pregnancy.

While ACE inhibitors and ARBs are contraindicated as usual in pregnancy, 3–6 months of therapy before conceiving may in fact offer a certain degree of renal protection. Likewise, tighter glycaemic control pre-pregnancy for at least 6 months is associated with improved outcomes, with the aim for an HbA1C <6.5%. Insulin remains the mainstay of therapy although metformin is considered safe to use in pregnancy in women with a pre-pregnancy eGFR >30 mL/min/1.73 m² and stable renal function during pregnancy.

Thrombotic microangiopathy: haemolytic uraemic syndrome and thrombotic thrombocytopenic purpura

Haemolytic uraemic syndrome (HUS) consists of a triad of microangiopathic haemolytic anaemia, thrombocytopenia and acute renal failure resulting from uncontrolled complement activation. There are two types of HUS, the first of which mainly occurs in children due to Shiga toxin-producing

Escherichia coli (STEC), causing 90% of cases. The second mainly occurs in adults and is known as atypical HUS (aHUS) and is due to abnormalities in the alternative complement regulatory pathway, resulting in endothelial damage and microvascular thrombosis.

As such, aHUS may be triggered by any process that activates the alternative complement regulatory pathway. Pregnancy is a prime example of this, with a retrospective study reporting that 86% of women with pregnancy-associated HUS have a detectable complement gene mutation leading to uncontrolled activation, 79% presenting post partum when placental expression of complement regulatory proteins is lost (Fakhouri et al., 2010). The same study also illustrated that these women were at increased risk of fetal loss and pre-eclampsia, with 62% reaching end-stage renal disease (ESRD) by 1 month post partum and 76% by their last follow-up.

Pregnancy-associated thrombotic thrombocytopenic purpura (TTP) microangiopathy is relatively rare, occurring in 1 in 25 000 pregnancies (Matthews et al., 1990). Historically, it was divided into two different phenotypes: TTP with predominantly neurological symptoms and HUS with predominantly renal dysfunction. Both have considerable overlap but a better understanding of the underlying pathophysiology has led to more accurate diagnosis, meaning that when either is suspected, plasma exchange should be started while awaiting ADAMTS13 activity results. The ADAMTS13 protein breaks down the von Willebrand factor which induces the formation of a platelet plug. When deficient, this leads to an accumulation of thrombi in the microcirculation, leading to TTP. If ADAMTS13 activity is normal, then the diagnosis is most likely to be aHUS and treatment with eculizumab (a humanised monoclonal IgG2/4 antibody targeting C5) can be initiated (Wiles and Banerjee, 2016). Although pregnancy data on eculizumab remains limited, comparable drugs have been used without teratogenic effects and it has been shown to reduce mortality, so the benefits are thought to outweigh the risks (Stefanovic, 2019).

Kidney transplant recipients

Kidney Disease: Improving Global Outcomes (KDIGO, 2009) currently recommend that women wait for at least 1 year post transplant to conceive. The rationale behind this is that transplantation improves fertility and the risk of pregnancy complications, i.e. pre-eclampsia and preterm delivery. In addition, pregnancy is a known sensitising event resulting in the formation of anti-HLA antibodies, making the identification of a suitable donor more complex. Evidence of efficient renal function with no significant hypertension or proteinuria, no evidence of graft rejection and limited drug therapy are all indicators of increased prognosis for a successful pregnancy.

Preconception counselling is key as immunosuppressants such as mycophenolate mofetil (MMF) and enteric-coated mycophenolate sodium (EC-MPS), both widely used in the field of transplantation, should be discontinued or replaced with a combination of azathioprine tacrolimus/ciclosporine and prednisolone, ideally at least 3 months before conception. Other immunosuppressant drugs, such as the MTORi (mammalian target of rapamycin inhibitors) sirolimus and everolimus, are also contraindicated due to insufficient safety data (Wiles et al., 2019).

Drugs

Drug-induced disease is responsible for around 60–70% of acute interstitial nephritis and kidney injury, so prompt diagnosis and discontinuation of the causative agent are key, as patients can ultimately develop CKD (Perazella and Markowitz, 2010). Drugs associated with interstitial nephritis include penicillins, cephalosporins, proton pump inhibitors and H2 receptor antagonists. Within the postpartum period, the most prescribed nephrotoxic drug is non-steroidal anti-inflammatories (NSAIDs).

Non-steroidal anti-inflammatories

Non-steroidal anti-inflammatory drugs, often used as postpartum analgesia, are contraindicated in AKI and CKD due to the known adverse effects on the kidney (Table 12.12) (Schneider et al., 2006). Whilst the risk of AKI remains rare, equating to around 0.5–1% of patients taking NSAIDs, the increased frequency of usage in postnatal protocols could potentially equate to a large number of women. Therefore, NSAIDs are contraindicated in women with renal factors such as volume depletion, pre-existing CKD or antenatal and/or peripartum AKI. Risk of AKI should also be considered when using NSAIDs in conjunction with nephrotoxic drugs such as gentamicin. Another important contraindication to NSAIDs is pre-eclampsia. The pharmacodynamic effects of NSAIDs in the kidney

Table 12.12   Renal adverse effects of NSAIDs.

Renal complication	Mechanism(s)
Acute kidney injury	• Inhibition of vasodilatory prostaglandins leading to decreased renal blood flow • Drug reaction leading to interstitial nephritis • Vasoconstriction and resulting hypoxia leading to papillary necrosis
Hyperkalaemia	• Inhibition of prostaglandin-mediated potassium excretion • Renal tubular acidosis type IV
Hypertension and fluid retention	• Increased sodium co-transport in ascending loop of Henle
Glomerulopathy	• Exact cause unknown; thought to arise from an inflammatory reaction leading to lymphokine production and proteinuria

Source: Based on Wiles and Banerjee (2016).

Table 12.13   Pharmacokinetics of commonly used NSAIDs.

Drug	Dosage (mg/day)	Half-life (h)	Renal clearance (%)
Ibuprofen	1200–3200	2	45-79
Diclofenac	100–150	2	65
Naproxen	500–1000	12-17	95
Indomethacin	75–100	4.5	60
Ketoprofen	200–300	2.1	80
Fenoprofen	800–3200	3	Predominantly clearance of metabolites
Celecoxib	200	11	27
Etoricoxib	60	22	75
Meloxicam	7.5–15	15–20	50

Source: Based on Coxib Collaboration (2013).

include sodium retention, hypertension and fluid overload, all of which are found in pre-eclampsia. As such, NSAIDs have the potential to exacerbate the pre-eclamptic state, meaning that even in the context of normal renal function they should be avoided.

If NSAIDs are considered for use in pregnancy, comparative data on the most 'renal-friendly' NSAIDs is limited. The most common method of excretion of NSAIDs is through the renal system (Table 12.13). As such, any impairment to renal function as a result of AKI or CKD will impair excretion of NSAIDs and lead to a higher effective dose and exacerbation of toxicity. Naproxen has been shown to have the highest risk of AKI (Coxib Collaboration, 2013).

Episode of care

Lucy is a 38-year-old G4P2 African woman who booked at 11 weeks of pregnancy. Obstetric notes show two previous early terminations of pregnancy, two previous spontaneous vaginal deliveries, the first at term in 2015, the second at 35 weeks gestation in 2018. Lucy was diagnosed and treated for postnatal depression after both births. Past medical and family history nil to note.

This pregnancy, Lucy is noted to be well supported by partner and family. Folic acid was commenced at 6 weeks of pregnancy. Routine antenatal screening bloods show Lucy is Rhesus negative with all results showing nothing abnormal detected.

Day 1 = 28 + 4 weeks gestation

Admitted to labour ward at 23.00 with history of reduced fetal movements, Blood pressure (BP) on admission 150/95 mmHg, urinalysis +1 protein, no history of headaches or flashing lights seen but complaint of right upper quadrant pain. Facial oedema noted.

Working differential diagnosis of potential pre-eclampsia.

Plan

Commence continuous fetal monitoring.
- Commence nifedipine to lower BP.
- Administer betamethasone for maturation of fetal lungs.
- Administer magnesium sulfate (MgSO$_4$) infusion for fetal neuroprotection and prophylactically to prevent eclamptic seizures.
- Send midstream urine for microscopy and culture and test for PCr.
- Take bloods for full blood count (FBC), liver (ALT and/or AST) and renal function (urea & sCr), and group and save (G&S).

Blood results

Haemoglobin (Hb) = 130 g/L (normal range 115–165 g/L)
- Platelets (PLT) = 100×10^9/L (normal range 150–450×10^9/L)
- White blood cells (WBC) = 25.64×10^9/L (normal 4.5–11×10^9/L)
- Alanine aminotransferase (ALT) = 45 U/L (normal 2–25 U/L)
- Serum creatinine (sCr) = 200 μmol/l (normal 50–120 μmol/L, in third trimester = 64 μmol/L)
- Plasma urea = 6.8 mmol/L (normal 2.5–7.0 mmol/L, in third trimester = 3.1 mmol/L)

Urine

- PCr = 80 mg/mmol (threshold in pregnancy 30 mg/mmol)

Although haemoglobin is within normal range, this is often lower in pregnancy so could be indicative of haemoconcentration, which is commonly found within pre-eclampsia. Needs to be compared to previous antenatal blood test results to place in context. Low platelets and increased WBC indicate inflammatory response which is associated with pre-eclampsia. Raised ALT illustrates impaired liver function and raised sCr and plasma urea impaired kidney function. On digital urinalysis, the protein:creatinine ratio is also raised, illustrating significant proteinuria. When combined, all these results point towards a diagnosis of pre-eclampsia.

Pharmacotherapy

- *Management of hypertension*: blood pressure control is key in the management of pre-eclampsia to prevent morbidity or mortality for both mother and baby. Antihypertensives should be administered and titrated to keep diastolic near to 90 mmHg as too low a BP may compromise placental perfusion further. In this case oral nifedipine has been chosen due to Lucy's ethnicity.
- *Prevention of seizures*: in cases of severe hypertension or severe pre-eclampsia, prophylactic MgSO$_4$ should be administered as it is associated with a 50–67% reduction of seizures and maternal death. Prematurity is a known risk factor for the rapid development of severe pre-eclampsia, making the timely administration of MgSO$_4$ imperative in this case. In addition, MgSO$_4$ also has a role in fetal neuroprotection and tocolysis, which in this case will only be beneficial. However, as discussed earlier in this chapter, pre-eclampsia is associated with AKI and magnesium is almost exclusively excreted in the urine, with 90% of the dose excreted during the first 24 hours after intravenous infusion. Magnesium toxicity can include nausea and vomiting, confusion, muscle weakness, respiratory depression, arrhythmias and myocardial weakness. However, routine serum magnesium levels are not required unless there is oliguria, urea >10 mmol/L or an ALT >250 iu/L and women on MgSO$_4$ should be monitored hourly for level of consciousness, respiratory rate, oxygen saturations, patellar reflexes and continuous ECG.

- *Fluid management*: the endothelial dysfunction associated with pre-eclampsia results in a fluid shift into the tissues and a resulting hypovolaemia. As such, the use of diuretics is usually avoided as they deplete the intravascular volume further. The only time they may be considered is if fluid overload is suspected due to amount infused and/or falling oxygen saturations. Such cases will require a fluid challenge and/or the administration of furosemide with oxygen, with careful monitoring of electrolytes at least every 6 hours.
- *Consideration of other medication in conjunction with AKI*: an important contraindication to NSAIDs is pre-eclampsia. The pharmacodynamic effects of NSAIDs in the kidney include sodium retention, hypertension and fluid overload, all of which are found in pre-eclampsia. As such, NSAIDs have the potential to exacerbate the pre-eclamptic state, meaning even in the context of normal renal function they should be avoided.

Conclusion

As a midwifery student, you will undoubtedly be involved in the care of a number of women with one or multiple types of renal disorders, especially if you work within a tertiary referral centre. As discussed in this chapter, these disorders can be very complex, often interlinked with other co-morbidities such as pre-eclampsia and diabetes. Despite interventions, conditions such as AKI continue to rise so it is imperative that all healthcare professionals involved in their care have a sound understanding of the pathophysiological, pharmacological and evidence base that underpins safe quality care. This chapter has provided the foundation for this understanding but once qualified, this can only grow with the concept of life-long learning underpinning continuing research into this all too important area.

Find out more

The following is a list of conditions associated with the renal tract. Take some time and write notes about each of the conditions. Think about the medications that may be used to treat these conditions and be specific about the pharmacokinetics and pharmacodynamics. Remember to include aspects of patient care. If you are making notes about people you have offered care and support to, you must ensure that you have adhered to the rules of confidentiality.

The condition	Your notes
Metabolic acidosis	
Hyperemesis gravidarum	
Postpartum haemorrhage	
Pre-eclampsia	
Urinary retention postnatal	

Glossary

Afferent   Conducting or conducted inwards or towards something. The opposite of *efferent*

Bacteriuria   The presence of bacteria in the urine

Cortex   An outer layer of an organ or body part such as a kidney

Distal   Situated away from the centre of the body or from the point of attachment. The opposite of *proximal*

Efferent   Directed away from a central organ or section. The opposite of *afferent*

Haemoconcentration   Thickening of the blood from loss of plasma or water

Haemodialysis   A way of replacing some of the functions of the kidney, if the kidneys have failed, by using a machine to filter and clean the blood

Haemodilution   Increase in the volume of plasma in relation to red blood cells; reduced concentration of red blood cells in the circulation

Homeostasis   Mechanisms that maintain a stable internal environment despite changes present in the external environment

Lesion   A region in an organ or tissue which has suffered damage through injury or disease

Medulla   The inner region of an organ or tissue, especially when it is distinct from the outer region or cortex

Microangiopathy   Any defect of very small blood vessels, usually capillaries

Nephropathy   An abnormal state of the kidney

Proximal   Situated nearer to the centre of the body or the point of attachment. The opposite of *distal*

Purpura   A haemorrhagic disease characterised by extravasation of blood into the tissues, under the skin and through the mucous membranes, producing spontaneous bruises and petechiae (small   haemorrhagic spots) on the skin

Urosepsis   A type of sepsis caused by an infection in the urinary tract

Test yourself

Now review your learning by completing the learning activities for this chapter at www.wiley.com/go/pharmacologyformidwives.

References

August, P. (2013) Preeclampsia: a "nephrocentric" view. *Advances in Chronic Kidney Disease*, **20**(3): 280–286.

Bashir, M., Mokhtar, M., Baager, K., Jayyousi, A., Naem, E. (2019) A case of hyperthyroidism treated with cinacalcet during pregnancy. *AACE Case Reports*, **5**(1): e40–e43.

Brown, M., Magee, L., Kenny, L. et al. (2018) The hypertensive disorders of pregnancy: ISSHP classification, diagnosis & management recommendations for international practice. *Pregnancy Hypertension*, **13**: 291–310.

Buyon, J.P., Kim, M.Y., Guerra, M.M. et al. (2017) Kidney outcomes and risk factors for nephritis (flare/de novo) in a multiethnic cohort of pregnant patients with lupus. *Clinical Journal of the American Society of Nephrology*, **12**(6): 940–946.

Coxib and traditional NSAID Trialists' (CNT) Collaboration, Bhala, N., Emberson, J., Merhi, A. et al. (2013) Vascular and upper gastrointestinal effects of non-steroidal anti-inflammatory drugs: meta-analyses of individual participant data from randomised trials. *Lancet*, **382**(9894): 769–779.

Craic, I., Wagner, S., Weissgerber, T., Grande, J., Garovic, V. (2014) Advances in the pathophysiology of pre-eclampsia and related podocyte injury. *Kidney International*, **86**: 275–285.

Diamond-Fox, S., Gatehouse, A. (2021) Medications and the renal system. In: Peate, I., Hill, B. (eds) *Fundamentals of Pharmacology for Nursing and Healthcare Students*. Wiley Blackwell: Oxford.

Fakhouri, F., Roumenina, L., Provot, F. et al. (2010) Pregnancy-associated hemolytic uremic syndrome revisited in the era of complement gene mutations. *Journal of the American Society of Nephrology*, **21**(5): 859–867.

Ghnem, F., Movahed, A. (2008) Use of antihypertensive drugs during pregnancy and lactation. *Cardiovascular Drug Reviews*, **26**(1): 38–49.

Gonzalez Suarez, M., Kattah, A., Grande, J., Garovic, V. (2019) Renal disorders in pregnancy: core curriculum 2019. *American Journal of Kdney Disease*, **73**(1): 119–130.

KDIGO (2009) Clinical practice guideline for the care of kidney transplant recipients: a summary. https://kdigo.org/wp-content/uploads/2017/02/KITxpGL_summary.pdf (accessed January 2022).

KDIGO (2012a) Clinical practice guideline for acute kidney injury. https://kdigo.org/wp-content/uploads/2016/10/KDIGO-2012-AKI-Guideline-English.pdf (accessed January 2022).

KDIGO (2012b) Clinical practice guideline for the evaluation and management of chronic kidney disease. https://kdigo.org/wp-content/uploads/2017/02/KDIGO_2012_CKD_GL.pdf (accessed January 2022).

Kristensen, J.H., Basit, S., Wohlfahrt, J., Damholt, M.B., Boyd, H.A. (2019) Pre-eclampsia and risk of later kidney disease: nationwide cohort study. *BMJ* **365**: l1516.

Lightstone, L. (2007) *Renal disease and pregnancy. Medicine*, **35**: 524–528.

Liu, Y., Ma, X., Zheng, J., Liu, X., Yan, T. (2016) A systematic review and meta-analysis of kidney and pregnancy outcomes in IgA nephropathy. *American Journal of Nephrology*, **44**(3): 187–193.

Matthews, J.H., Benjamin, S., Gill, D.S., Smith, N.A. (1990) Pregnancy-associated thrombocytopenia: definition, incidence and natural history. *Acta Haematologica*, **84**(1): 24–29.

Maynard, S.E., Thadhani, R. (2009) Pregnancy and the kidney. *Journal of the American Society of Nephrology*, **20**(1): 14–22.

Mihalache, A., Ateka, O., Palma-Reis, I., Harding, K., Nelson-Piercy, C., Banerjee, A. (2012) Acute kidney injury in pregnancy: experience from a large tertiary care referral centre. *Journal of the American Society of Nephrology*, **23**: SA-PO076

National Institute for Health and Care Excellence (2018) Urinary tract infection (lower): antimicrobial prescribing (NG109). www.nice.org.uk/guidance/ng109/resources/urinary-tract-infection-lower-antimicrobial-prescribing-pdf-66141546350533 (accessed January 2022).

National Institute for Health and Care Excellence (2019) Hypertension in pregnancy: diagnosis and management (NG133). www.nice.org.uk/guidance/ng133/resources/hypertension-in-pregnancy-diagnosis-and-management-pdf-66141717671365 (accessed January 2022).

Peate, I. (ed.) (2017) Fluid and electrolyte balance and associated disorders. In: *Fundamentals of Applied Pathophysiology: An Essential Guide for Nursing and Healthcare Students*, pp. 506–533. Wiley: Chichester.

Perazella, M., Markowitz, G. (2010) Drug-induced acute interstitial nephritis. *Nature Reviews Nephrology*, **6**: 461–470.

Piccoli, G., Arukhaimi, M., Zhi-Hong, L., Zakharova, E., Levin, A. (2018) What we do and do not know about women and kidney disease: questions unanswered and questions unquestioned: reflection on World Kidney Day and International Woman's Day. *Nephrology*, **23**: 199–209.

Prakash, J., Ganiger, V.C. (2017) Acute kidney injury in pregnancy-specific disorders. *Indian Journal of Nephrology*, **27**(4): 258–270.

Rankin, J. (2017) *Physiology in Childbearing: with anatomy and related biosciences*, 4th edn. Elsevier: London.

Rasmussen, P., Nielson, F. (1988) Hydronephrosis during pregnancy: a literature survey. *European Journal of Obstetrics and Gynecology and Reproductive Biology*, **27**(3): 249–259.

Ronco, C. (2019) Acute kidney injury. *Lancet*, **394**(10212): 1949–1964.

Sandhu, G., Ramaiyah, S., Chan, G., Meisels, I. (2010) Pathophysiology and management of preeclampsia-associated severe hyponatraemia. *American Journal of Kidney Diseases*, **155**(3): 599–603.

Schneider, V., Lévesque, L., Zhang, B., Hutchinson, T., Brophy, J. (2006) Association of selective and conventional nonsteroidal antiinflammatory drugs with acute renal failure: a population-based, nested case-control analysis. *American Journal of Epidemiology*, **164**(9): 881–889.

See, E., Jayasinghe, K., Glassford, N., Polkingorne, K., Toussaint, N., Bellamo, R. (2019) Long-term associated risk of adverse outcomes after acute kidney injury: a systematic review and meta analysis of cohort studies using consensus definitions of exposure. Clinical Investigation, **95**(1): 160–172.

Smaill, F., Vazquez, J. (2019) Antibiotics for asymptomatic bacteriuria in pregnancy. *Cochrane Database of Systematic Reviews*, **11**: CD000490.

Soma-Pillay, P., Nelson-Piercy, C., Tolppanen, H., Mebazaa, A., Tolppanen, H., Mebazaa, A. (2016) Physiological changes in pregnancy. *Cardiovascular Journal of Africa*, **27**(2): 89–94.

Stagnaro-Green, A., Akhter, E., Yim, C., Davies, T.F., Magder, L., Petri ,M. (2011) Thyroid disease in pregnant women with systemic lupus erythematosus: increased preterm delivery. *Lupus*, **20**: 690–699.

Stefanovic, V. (2019) The extended use of eculizumab in pregnancy and complement activation-associated diseases affecting maternal, fetal and neonatal kidneys – the future is now? *Journal of Clinical Medicine*, **8**(3): 407.

UK Renal Registry (2021) 23rd Annual report – data to 31-12/2019. https://ukkidney.org/audit-research/annual-report (accessed January 2022).

Wiles, K., Banerjee, A. (2016) Acute kidney injury in pregnancy and the use of non-steroidal ani-inflammatory drugs. *Obstetrician and Gynaecologist*, **18**: 127–135.

Wiles, K., Chappell, L., Clark, K. et al. (2019) Clinical practice guideline on pregnancy and renal disease. *BMC Nephrology*, **20**: 401.

Williams, D., Davison, J. (2008) Chronic kidney disease in pregnancy. *BMJ*, **336**(7637): 211–215.

Chapter 13

Medications and diabetes

Carl Clare and Celia Wildeman

University of Hertfordshire, Hatfield, UK

Aim

The aim of this chapter is to provide the reader with an introduction to pharmacology associated with drugs used in the management of diabetes in women who are pregnant.

Learning outcomes

After reading this chapter the reader will:
- Understand the types of diabetes that may be encountered in the care of the pregnant woman
- Be able to discuss the drugs used in the management of non-insulin-dependent diabetes mellitus (NIDDM)
- Be able to discuss the types of insulin available for the management of insulin-dependent diabetes mellitus (IDDM)
- Be able to explain the drug management of gestational diabetes.

Test your existing knowledge

- What three hormones are released by the pancreas?
- Type 1 diabetes normally develops at what time in life?
- Do women have to report gestational diabetes to the Driver and Vehicle Licensing Agency (DVLA)?
- Which oral hypoglycaemics are contraindicated in pregnancy?
- What is the difference between hyperosmolar hyperglycaemic state (HHS) and diabetic ketoacidosis (DKA)?

Introduction

Estimates suggest that each year, up to 5% of women who become pregnant in the UK either have pre-existing diabetes or develop gestational diabetes during their pregnancy (Hugason-Briem, 2018). Diabetes is broken down into three main categories: type 1 diabetes mellitus (T1D), type 2 diabetes mellitus (T2D) and gestational diabetes mellitus (GDM). Traditionally, type 1 diabetes was known as insulin-dependent diabetes and type 2 diabetes as non-insulin-dependent diabetes. However, these

Fundamentals of Pharmacology for Midwives, First Edition. Edited by Ian Peate and Cathy Hamilton.

categories are slowly being eroded as the use of insulin increases in the management of type 2 diabetes and therefore this chapter will use the 'type' classification of diabetes which is based on the pathophysiology of the disease, as opposed to the 'insulin dependence' categorisation that is based on treatment. Gestational diabetes is specific to pregnancy and as such is classified as its own category.

This chapter reviews the three types of diabetes and their management, including the typical medications used for control. It should be noted that the management of diabetes, regardless of type, is not restricted to medication use and therefore discussion will be presented regarding the lifestyle modifications required for the woman with diabetes in pregnancy.

Physiology

In order to understand the pathophysiology of diabetes, it is essential that the role of the pancreas in the control of blood glucose levels is explored.

The pancreas

The pancreas is an elongated organ situated next to the first part of the small intestine (Figure 13.1). The pancreas is composed of two different types of tissue; the largest part of the pancreas is made up of exocrine tissues (tissues that produce hormones that are secreted into a duct). This tissue produces and secretes a fluid rich with digestive enzymes into the small intestine to aid digestion. Distributed throughout the exocrine tissues are multiple clusters of cells known as islets of Langerhans (islets) which contain endocrine cells (cells that secrete hormones into the bloodstream). Each islet has three major cell types. each of which produces a different hormone.

- Alpha cells which secrete glucagon.
- Beta cells which secrete insulin.
- Delta cells which secrete somatostatin.

This chapter discusses alpha cells and beta cells. The role of delta cells and somatostatin is not integral to the management of blood glucose and will not be discussed.

Insulin

The main action of insulin is well known; it reduces the blood glucose levels in the blood.

- With the exception of the brain and the liver (which do not use insulin), insulin facilitates the passage of glucose into muscle, adipose tissue and several other tissues.
- Insulin promotes the storage of glucose (as glycogen) in the tissues of the liver.

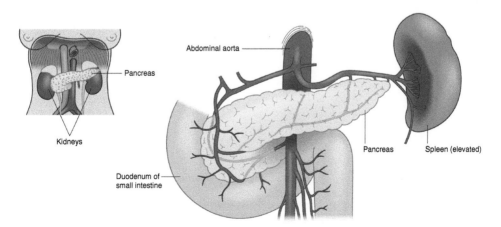

Figure 13.1   The pancreas. *Source*: Peate (2014)/with permission of John Wiley & Sons.

Furthermore, insulin has an effect on protein and mineral metabolism, as well as lipid metabolism. For instance, when the levels of stored glycogen in the liver rise to approximately 5% of the total liver mass, further glycogen creation is suppressed and glucose is diverted into fatty acid and triglyceride production. These fatty acids and triglycerides are then stored in the tissues.

The main stimulus for insulin creation and secretion is the rise in blood glucose levels, although a rise in the levels of amino acids and fatty acids in the blood is also known to stimulate insulin secretion. As with many endocrine systems, insulin synthesis and secretion is controlled by a negative feedback loop (Figure 13.2); as blood glucose levels fall, there is a corresponding fall in the production and secretion of insulin. Enzymes that break down glycogen become active, leading to an increase in the levels of glucose in the blood.

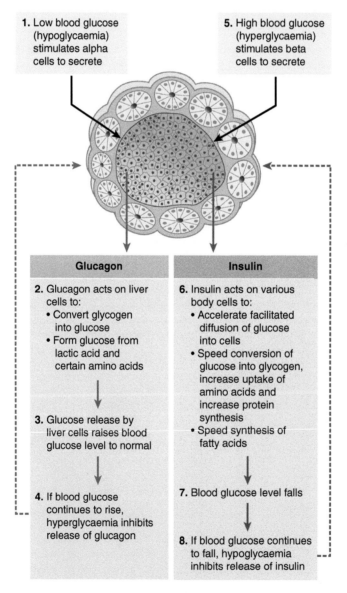

Figure 13.2   The negative feedback control of insulin (red arrows) and glucagon (blue arrows) production. *Source*: Peate (2014)/with permission of John Wiley & Sons.

Glucagon

Glucagon has the opposite effect to insulin and thus plays an important role in maintaining normal blood glucose levels. The effect of glucagon is to increase blood glucose levels by:

- stimulating the breakdown of the glycogen stored in the liver to create glucose
- activating the creation of glucose in the liver.

The production and secretion of glucagon is stimulated in response to a reduction in blood glucose concentrations (see Figure 13.2). Whilst glucagon production and secretion appear to be controlled by a negative feedback loop, it is unknown whether a decrease in glucagon release is a direct effect of the increasing blood glucose levels or a response to rising levels of insulin.

Pathophysiology

There are three types of diabetes related to glycaemic control (diabetes insipidus is not included as it is a completely different disorder).

Type 1 diabetes

Type 1 diabetes develops most commonly in childhood or early adulthood and comprises about 15% of the total incidence of diabetes in the UK; however, the rate of type 1 diabetes is increasing, particularly in children less than 5 years of age (Buzzetti et al., 2020). Type 1 diabetes is typically linked to the autoimmune destruction of the beta cells of the pancreas and is therefore associated with a severe reduction in, or complete loss of, insulin production (Atkinson et al., 2014).

Type 2 diabetes

Type 2 diabetes is the most common form of diabetes and is generally considered to develop in patients over the age of 40 years; however, the rates of juvenile-onset type 2 diabetes are rising (Val-aiyapathi et al., 2020). Type 2 diabetes is characterised by the development of resistance to the effects of insulin in the tissues (especially body fat and skeletal muscles) and the continued production and release of glucose by the liver. These tissues are unable to respond effectively to insulin and absorb glucose from the blood. Recent developments suggest that beta cell dysfunction is already present in patients at risk of type 2 diabetes, especially those with a family history of diabetes, and this may be the underlying factor in many cases. Furthermore, the impact of environmental factors (such as dietary intake and type of diet) is almost certainly a factor in the increase of type 2 diabetes (Kahn et al., 2014).

Regardless of the primary cause, an increasing blood glucose level results. The ensuing high blood levels of glucose lead to toxic damage of the beta cells, further reducing the production of insulin in an ongoing vicious circle. Insulin production is rarely completely stopped in type 2 diabetes. Risk factors for type 2 diabetes include being overweight, lack of exercise, genetic inheritance and increasing age. Genetic predisposition to type 2 diabetes appears to be especially strong in people from South Asian or Afro-Caribbean backgrounds (Goff, 2019).

Gestational diabetes

Gestational diabetes is the most common medical disorder in pregnancy (Saravanan, 2020) though the actual cause is not known. Traditionally, GDM was defined as any level of glucose intolerance first diagnosed in pregnancy but it was recognised that many women were entering pregnancy with previously undiagnosed type 2 diabetes and so the diagnostic criterion is now glucose intolerance first diagnosed after the first trimester (usually at 24–28 weeks) (American Diabetes Association, 2021).

Signs and symptoms

The signs and symptoms of diabetes are common to all forms of diabetes and are mostly related to the high blood glucose levels and include:

- passing urine more often than usual, especially at night
- increased thirst

- extreme tiredness
- unexplained weight loss (usually only in type 1 diabetes)
- genital itching or regular episodes of thrush
- slow healing of cuts and wounds
- blurred vision
- increased blood glucose
- glucose in the urine
- ketones in the urine.

In all forms of diabetes, the increased blood glucose leads to excretion of glucose in the urine. The glucose has an osmotic effect, drawing water into the renal tubules and increasing urine production. The increased excretion of glucose in the urine leads to water depletion and increased thirst.

In type 1 diabetes, and occasionally in advanced type 2, the inability of the cells to utilise glucose leads to the use of fats and amino acids as the primary fuel source in the cells, leading to weight loss and the production of ketones as a by-product. Ketones are strong acids which are passed into the urine. As the ketones are negatively charged, there is usually a simultaneous excretion of positively charged sodium and potassium ions, leading to electrolyte imbalance and abdominal pain.

Diagnosis and investigations

The rapid onset of type 1 diabetes means that patients rarely remain undiagnosed for long. Many patients will present to their GP due to their symptoms; however, in some cases, the onset is so rapid or is precipitated by an acute illness that the patient develops diabetic ketoacidosis (DKA) and is admitted to hospital as an emergency.

Type 2 diabetes is more insidious in onset and many patients will remain unaware of the fact they have diabetes for years before they are diagnosed, by which point they may have developed complications.

The diagnosis of type 1 diabetes is based on the presence of the classic symptoms of high blood glucose on fingerprick test, weight loss, thirst and increased urine output. Formal diagnosis can then be confirmed by laboratory blood glucose measurement.

Type 2 diabetes is often diagnosed after opportunistic screening or as a chance finding while being treated for another condition. Current guidance is focused on identifying people at risk of developing type 2 diabetes and encouraging them to have a risk assessment and risk identification (NICE, 2020a). NICE recommends the following strategy.

1. Identify those at risk and either administer a validated risk assessment tool or encourage those potentially at risk to self-administer a risk assessment tool such as the one found on the Diabetes UK website: https://riskscore.diabetes.org.uk/start.
2. Those found to have high risk scores should be offered formal blood tests, such as HbA1c, fasting blood glucose or glucose tolerance test.
3. Those found to be at risk but who have not developed diabetes should be offered guidance on managing risk, such as healthy eating, losing weight and exercise. Guidance on recommendations can be found on the NICE website at www.nice.org.uk/guidance/ph38/chapter/Recommendations.

Testing for gestational diabetes

Assessment for the risk of gestational diabetes should be offered to women with risk factors. At the booking appointment, check for the following risk factors (NICE, 2020b):

- BMI above 30 kg/m^2
- previous macrosomic baby weighing 4.5 kg or more
- previous gestational diabetes
- family history of diabetes (first-degree relative with diabetes)
- an ethnicity with a high prevalence of diabetes.

Or offer testing if urine glucose testing shows:

- +2 glucose on one occasion or
- +1 glucose on two occasions.

For women who have had gestational diabetes in a previous pregnancy, offer:

- early self-monitoring of blood glucose, or
- a 75 g 2-hour oral glucose tolerance test (OGTT) as soon as possible after booking (whether in the first or second trimester), and a further 75 g 2-hour OGTT at 24–28 weeks if the results of the first OGTT are normal.

For women with any of the other risk factors for gestational diabetes, offer a 75 g 2-hour OGTT at 24–28 weeks.
Diagnose gestational diabetes if the woman has either:

- a fasting plasma glucose level of 5.6 mmol/L or above, or
- a plasma glucose level of 7.8 mmol/L or above after a 2-hour oral glucose load.

Following a diagnosis of gestational diabetes:

- offer a review with the joint diabetes and antenatal clinic within 1 week
- tell their primary healthcare team.

Clinical consideration

Diabetes is associated with significant mental health problems. Adults have been shown to suffer from a specialised form of anxiety known as diabetes distress which is related to the stress of the daily management of diabetes. Diabetes distress is associated with increased adverse outcomes in diabetes (Sachar et al., 2020).

Clinical consideration

Oral glucose tolerance test

Preparation

- Prepare the glucose solution in advance. Glucose dissolves better in warm water but is more palatable when cold. On the day before the test, dissolve 75 grams of anhydrous glucose (82.5 grams of glucose monohydrate, obtainable preweighed from pharmacy) in warm water and store in a fridge overnight.
- The patient must be fasted from midnight (sips of water only.)

Procedure

- Check patient identity.
- Check that the patient has fasted from midnight.
- Perform venepuncture, taking 2 mL of blood; test a small sample using a near patient glucose testing meter. Other baseline bloods should be taken if requested by referring clinician.
- Place the remainder of the blood sample into a glucose collection tube and label with patient identification, date and **"0"** minutes in time on sample.
- If the result on the glucose meter is greater than or equal to 11 mmol/L, send the blood sample urgently to laboratory. If it is confirmed by biochemistry to be above 11 mmol/L, there is no need to continue test, and the patient can go home.

- If the result is less than 11 mmol/L on meter, give the patient the glucose solution to drink (within 10 minutes).
- Collect a further blood sample for glucose measurement 2 hours after the glucose solution has been drunk. Label with patient details, date and time of sample (**120** minutes).
- Send samples all together with request form to laboratory.

Episode of care

Joanne is a 24-year-old woman. She is attending her second appointment at the hospital antenatal clinic. Joanne is now 24 weeks pregnant with her first baby. A routine urine specimen with a dipstick revealed two pluses (++) of glucose in her urine. This means that her urine sample is positive for glucose. She has no other presenting symptoms. She has informed you that there is a family history of diabetes mellitus. You added this information to her medical history as you noticed that it was not previously entered. She is also overweight with a body mass index of 30 kg/m². All your findings are recorded in the antenatal care notes and she is referred to the obstetrician who refers her to have an oral glucose tolerance test (OGTT). This confirms that she has gestational diabetes mellitus (GDM)

Advising and supporting pregnant women are key aspects of the midwife's role (NMC, 2019). It is therefore important to advise Joanne, among other things, how to care for her feet to prevent serious complications of diabetes. This might not be something she thinks is relevant to her as a young woman. However, foot care is essential as diabetes can be dangerous to feet due to its ability to cause nerve damage. This can result in the loss of feeling in the feet and blood flow can also be reduced, making it harder to heal an injury or resist infection. Suggest the following to Joanne.

Be gentle when bathing your feet and carefully dry between the toes.

- Moisturise your feet but not between the toes which could result in a fungal infection.
- Cut toe nails carefully. Cut them straight across and file the edges.
- Never treat corns or calluses yourself.
- Wear clean dry socks, changing them daily.
- Wear socks in bed if feet get cold. Never use heating pad or hot water bottle.
- Shake out your shoes and feel inside before wearing.
- Keep your feet warm and dry and wear warm socks and shoes in winter.
- Consider using an antiperspirant on the sole of your feet. This is useful if you have excessive sweating of the feet, for example with body temperature rising in pregnancy.
- Never walk barefoot – even at home.
- Consider using a magnifying hand mirror to examine the soles of the feet for signs of injury or infection.
- Take care of your diabetes – keep blood glucose levels under control.
- Do not smoke.
- Get periodic foot examinations .

Source: Adapted from Tidy (2020).

Treatment of diabetes

The treatment of type 1 diabetes is based on the replacement of insulin by the subcutaneous injection of insulin. Insulin is well known for its effect in reducing the blood glucose levels. It does this by:

- facilitating the entry of glucose into muscle, adipose tissue and several other tissues. Note that the brain and the liver do not require insulin to facilitate the uptake of glucose
- stimulating the liver to store glucose in the form of glycogen.

As well as its effects on glucose, insulin is known to have an effect on protein, lipid and mineral metabolism but these are of secondary importance in the clinical use of insulin. Insulin is excreted via the renal system.

There are several forms of insulin, but they are all classified by:

* how soon the insulin starts working (onset)
* when the insulin works the hardest (peak time)
* how long the insulin lasts in the body (duration).

All insulin preparations are presented in the formulation of 100 international units (iu) per milliliter (mL). The exact dose is individual and varies with trimester. Women with pre-existing diabetes will often have a higher insulin requirement than pre-pregnancy in the first weeks of pregnancy which drops somewhere in the 10th to 16th week of pregnancy and then, in weeks 20–24, reduced skeletal muscle uptake of glucose leads to higher maternal glucose levels, providing more glucose to the growing fetus (Murphy et al., 2018).

Insulin dose adjustments are further complicated by the pharmacokinetics of insulin. There is a slower time to peak plasma concentration of insulin and more day-to-day variability in insulin pharmacokinetics in late pregnancy. While fast-acting insulin analogues (such as aspart, Humalog®) should normally be injected at least 15 min before eating, the significantly slower absorption in late pregnancy means that premeal injections are administered earlier. For many pregnant women, this means injecting 30–60 minutes before eating in late pregnancy.

The variety of insulin activity curves can be seen in Figure 13.3. The decision about which insulin to choose is based on an individual's lifestyle, the physician's preference and experience, and the person's blood glucose levels as measured over a period of time.

* *Basal insulin*: an intermediate- or long-acting insulin, that is usually injected once a day (often at bedtime) and used to keep blood glucose levels stable during periods of fasting (e.g. between meals or while sleeping).
* *Prandial insulin*: short- or rapid-acting insulin injected at mealtimes to control postprandial (post-meal) glucose levels.
* *Premixed insulin*: premixed solutions that contain two types of insulin (e.g. a prandial and a basal insulin).

Common insulin preparations are shown in Box 13.1.

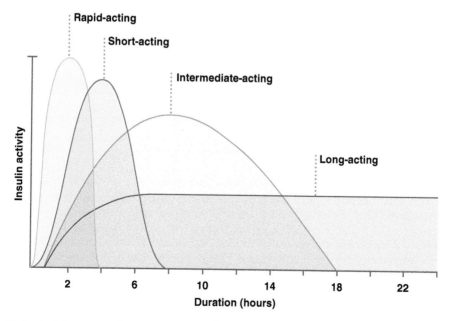

Figure 13.3   Activity curves of different types of insulin. *Source*: Type 2 Diabetes: Insulin Therapy, May 3, 2021. Accessed from https://tools.cep.health/tool/type-2-diabetes-insulin-therapy

Box 13.1   Common insulin preparations

- Humalog: a very rapid-acting insulin, which usually begins working within 15 minute.
- Lantus®: a long-acting analogue insulin
- Levemir®: a long-acting analogue insulin. Tends to have a slightly shorter duration than Lantus, is often taken twice daily
- NovoRapid®: the active ingredient is insulin aspart. When injected, it is very fast-acting. Novorapid begins working after 10–20 minutes and lasts for between 3 and 5 hours
- Humulin®: short-acting, intermediate acting and premixed Humulin insulins are available
- Insuman®: comes in several different forms. Insuman basal is an intermediate-acting insulin with the active ingredient isophane insulin
- Insulatard®: comes in preloaded pens, penfill cartridges and vials based around the active ingredient human isophane insulin

Clinical consideration

Insulin storage
In the hospital setting, insulin is often stored in the fridge (check your local policy for insulin storage procedures). However, it must be noted that cold insulin is known to increase the pain of the injection and also decreases insulin absorption, so for patient comfort and insulin efficacy, it is advisable to take the insulin out of the refrigerator a minimum of 1 hour prior to injection.

Insulin pens
Patients should be advised not to store opened insulin pens in the fridge. Unopened pen cartridges are stored in a fridge, but once inserted into an insulin pen, the pen should be kept out of the fridge. The insulin can be stored at room temperature for 28 days (International Diabetes Federation, nd) but should be kept in a closed container to minimise temperature changes.

Premixed insulins
When the woman (or healthcare professional) is going to administer a cloudy, or premixed, insulin, it is important that the pen or vial is gently rotated end over end 20 times (not shaken), otherwise the insulin may not be mixed correctly. Research has shown that patients are often confused about this technique, and the actual mixing of insulin by patients has a large variation that may affect glycaemic control.

Injection sites
The most common injection sites are the thighs, the abdomen (above and below the umbilicus), the upper arms and the buttocks. However, it has been observed that patients will repeatedly inject into the abdomen below the umbilicus as this is an easy area to access when clothed. Repeated use of the same injection sites can lead to the development of lipohypertrophy (fatty lumps) that are not only unsightly but can affect insulin absorption at the injection site. It has been shown that the rotation of injection site at every injection reduces the risk of lipohypertrophy. Thus, it is recommended that at every clinic appointment, time is taken to remind patients to rotate the site of injection and that healthcare staff carry out a skin assessment to assess for the development of lipohypertrophy (Deeb et al., 2019).

Dietary advice

Dietary advice for all type 1 diabetic patients should include:

- discussion of the hyperglycaemic effects of different foods and ensuring adequate insulin to cover this
- types, timing and number of snacks taken between meals and at bedtime
- healthy eating to reduce arterial risk
- if the person wants it, information on:
  - effects of alcohol-containing drinks on blood glucose and calorie intake
  - use of high-calorie and high-sugar 'treats'
  - use of foods with a high glycaemic index.

Patients with type 1 diabetes will also require education on the recognition and management of hypoglycaemia (often called 'hypos').

The treatment of type 2 diabetes will depend on the severity of the condition. Treatment will always include dietary adjustments (healthy diet with reduced fat and sugar) and lifestyle changes (such as exercise and losing weight if required), and in some patients with type 2 diabetes this will be enough to maintain normal blood glucose levels. Dietary advice for patients with type 2 diabetes includes:

- include high-fibre, low-glycaemic index sources of carbohydrate
- include low-fat dairy products and oily fish
- control the intake of foods containing saturated fats and *trans*-fatty acids
- avoid the use of foods marketed specifically for people with diabetes as they often contain fructose as a substitute for sucrose. Fructose still affects blood glucose levels.

However, women with type 2 diabetes may also require oral medication. Drugs for type 2 diabetes generally have one of three potential actions:

- reducing the amount of glucose released by the liver
- increasing the cells' ability to utilise insulin (decreasing insulin resistance)
- promoting the production of insulin by the pancreas.

Self-monitoring of type 2 diabetes is occasionally advised, and the patient will need to be educated in the use of capillary blood measurement of glucose. More commonly, the primary care provider will monitor the HbA1c (long-term blood glucose measurement) every 2–6 months.

General advice

Patients with all types of diabetes will require advice on the following.

- *Regular physical activity*: however, strenuous exercise can reduce blood glucose levels and people with type 1 diabetes will need to monitor blood glucose levels and adjust insulin doses accordingly. Exercise regimens should be agreed with appropriate healthcare staff.
- *Stopping smoking*: smoking is a risk for anybody, but diabetic patients have an increased risk of cardiovascular disease, which is compounded by smoking.
- Monitoring cholesterol levels and managing cholesterol intake.
- Reducing salt in the diet.
- Weight loss, if required. Weight loss improves diabetic control in all types of diabetes.

Newly diagnosed patients will require education regarding self-injection and insulin doses. This should be reviewed and skills reassessed with the patient regularly. Patients should be advised regarding the storage of insulin and the rotation of injection sites.

People with newly diagnosed type 1 diabetes should be offered a structured programme of education delivered by a qualified health professional and the opportunity for education and information should be offered on a regular basis (NICE, 2020a).

Care of the woman during pregnancy in the presence of pre-existing diabetes

Preconception care of the woman with diabetes

Providing information, advice and support to the woman with diabetes preconception ensures a more positive experience of pregnancy and enables the woman to feel in control during her pregnancy. Women with diabetes who plan on becoming pregnant should be informed that if they have good glycaemic control before becoming pregnant and throughout their pregnancy then the risk of miscarriage, congenital malformation, stillbirth and neonatal death is reduced but cannot be eliminated (NICE, 2020b). Therefore, the use of contraception is strongly advised until good glycaemic control is maintained and confirmed (by HbA1c levels). To that aim, women with diabetes who plan on pregnancy should be offered regular HbA1c testing (up to monthly). Women with a BMI greater than 27 kg/m^2 should be advised on weight loss before pregnancy.

Women with diabetes who are planning on becoming pregnant will require information on how diabetes affects pregnancy and pregnancy affects diabetes. Information should include (NICE, 2020b):

- the role of diet, body weight and exercise in glycaemic control
- the risks of hypoglycaemia during pregnancy and the fact that awareness of hypoglycaemia is often impaired during pregnancy
- how nausea and vomiting in pregnancy can affect blood glucose control
- the increased risk of having a baby who is large for gestational age
- the need for diabetic retinopathy assessment before and during pregnancy
- the need for diabetic nephropathy assessment before pregnancy
- the importance of blood glucose control during labour and birth
- the need for early feeding of the baby, to reduce the risk of neonatal hypoglycaemia
- the possibility that the baby may have health problems in the first 28 days, that may lead to the need for admission to a neonatal unit
- the increased risk of the baby developing obesity and diabetes in later life.

With the exception of metformin hydrochloride, the majority of oral hypoglycaemics are currently contraindicated in pregnancy and should be stopped when pregnancy is planned (or unplanned pregnancy is discovered) and insulin therapy instituted.

Metformin is an oral hypoglycaemic that mostly acts to increase peripheral utilisation of glucose and decrease gluconeogenesis (the production of glucose by the breakdown of substrates such as amino acids). However, it is only active in the presence of insulin and thus is only of use if some pancreatic insulin production remains (Hyer et al., 2018).

Metformin is normally presented in 500 mg tablets and the standard dose is 500 mg three times a day (each dose to be taken with food). However, it should be noted that multiple preparations are available (such as modified release, liquid preparation and oral metformin powder) and that different strengths are available, including doses up to 1 gram per tablet. If metformin treatment is instituted (a rare occurrence in pregnancy) then it is commenced at 500 mg once a day for 1 week, increased to twice a day for 1 week until finally reaching three times a day. The maximum dose is 2 grams per day. Metformin is excreted by the renal system and there is evidence of increased speed of clearance in pregnancy related to increased active renal transport (Liao et al., 2020).

Episode of care

Neelam is a 22-year-old woman who is 12 weeks pregnant. At her antenatal booking appointment, she presents with a medical history of diabetes mellitus since the age of 14 years. She is dependent on insulin medication and this has controlled her diabetes well. Neelam complains of nausea and vomiting in the mornings and at times during the day. This has caused her difficulties with eating and drinking. The midwife is concerned as Neelam is taking insulin to control her blood glucose and this means that not eating or drinking adequately can result in hypoglycaemia. This can also affect the well-being of the developing fetus.

Nausea and vomiting, particularly during early pregnancy, occurs in approximately 80% of pregnant women (RCOG, 2016). However, if a woman also has diabetes, management of the condition must be monitored carefully. She should be advised about the signs and symptoms of hypoglycaemia and the actions to take if she is concerned that she may be developing hypoglycaemia.

Neelam should be advised to test her fasting blood glucose, 1 hour before a meal and at bedtime. Her fasting blood glucose level before a meal should be 5.3 mmol/L, 1 hour after meals it should be 7.8 mmol/L and 2 hours after a meal it should be 6.4 mmol/L. Ideally, Neelam should try to maintain her capillary plasma glucose at 4 mmol/L (NICE, 2020b).

Additionally, she should be advised to:

always have a fast-acting form of glucose available (for example, dextrose tablets or glucose-containing drinks)

- eat small amounts often – meals that are high in carbohydrate and low in fat, such as potato, rice and pasta, are easier to tolerate, as are plain biscuits and crackers
- avoid any food or smells that trigger symptoms
- avoid foods with high fat content
- if symptoms do not settle, she should be advised to contact her GP who will prescribe anti-sickness medication, that is safe to take in pregnancy.

213

DVLA rules on driving with diabetes

If treated with insulin, the client will need to tell the DVLA if:

- their insulin treatment lasts (or will last) over 3 months
- they had gestational diabetes and their insulin treatment lasts over 3 months after the birth
- they get disabling hypoglycaemia (low blood glucose) or a medical professional has told the woman that she is at risk of developing it.

Diabetes treated by tablet: the client should discuss the need to report her condition to the DVLA with the team caring for her.

Diabetes treated by diet: there is no requirement to inform the DVLA.

Care of the woman with gestational diabetes

- Explain to women with GDM that good blood glucose control throughout pregnancy will reduce the risk of:
  - fetal macrosomia
  - trauma during birth (for her and her baby)
  - induction of labour and/or caesarean section
  - neonatal hypoglycaemia
  - perinatal death.
- Explain that treatment will include changes in diet and exercise and could involve medicines.
- Teach women with gestational diabetes how to self-monitor their blood glucose.
- When women are diagnosed with gestational diabetes, offer advice about changes in diet and exercise.
  - Advise women with GDM to eat a healthy diet during pregnancy, and to switch from high to low glycaemic index food.
  - Refer all women with gestational diabetes to a dietitian.

- Advise women with gestational diabetes to exercise regularly (for example, walking for 30 minutes after a meal).
- For women with gestational diabetes who have a fasting plasma glucose level below 7 mmol/L at diagnosis, offer a trial of diet and exercise changes.
  - If blood glucose targets are not met with diet and exercise changes within 1–2 weeks, offer metformin. If metformin is contraindicated or unacceptable to the woman, offer insulin.
  - If blood glucose targets are not met with diet and exercise changes plus metformin, offer insulin as well.
- For women with GDM who have a fasting plasma glucose level of 7 mmol/L or above at diagnosis, offer:
  - immediate treatment with insulin, with or without metformin, and
  - diet and exercise changes.
- For women with gestational diabetes who have a fasting plasma glucose level of between 6.0 and 6.9 mmol/L and complications such as macrosomia or hydramnios, consider:
  - immediate treatment with insulin, with or without metformin, and
  - diet and exercise changes.

214

Blood glucose monitoring in diabetes

Women who were diagnosed with type 1 diabetes before pregnancy will be aware of the process of monitoring blood glucose; women newly diagnosed with GDM or type 1 diabetes during pregnancy will require teaching on the use of intermittent blood glucose meters for the testing of blood glucose levels (see Skills in practice box). Pregnant women with type 1 diabetes should be advised to test their blood glucose premeal, 1 hour postmeal and at bedtime. Pregnant women with type 2 diabetes or gestational diabetes who are on a multiple daily insulin injection regimen should be advised to test their blood glucose premeal, 1 hour postmeal and at bedtime. Women with type 2 diabetes or GDM who are managing their diabetes with diet alone, with oral medications or single-dose intermediate-acting (or long-acting) insulin should test their premeal and 1 hour postmeal blood glucose levels.

Generally, urine testing for glucose in a pregnant woman with known diabetes (of any type) is not recommended as it lacks sensitivity and changes in blood glucose are only reflected after a prolonged period of time.

Skills in practice

Undertaking point-of-care (capillary) blood glucose testing

Ensuring a woman diagnosed with new-onset or gestational diabetes is educated as to the correct procedure for capillary blood glucose testing is essential to good care.

- Ensure the woman washes and dries her hands prior to testing as sugar or hand cream on the skin can affect the result. Alcohol wipes and hand gel should not be used as they can also affect the reading.
- Turn on the glucose meter.
- Insert the test strip.
- 'Load' the lancet to prepare it for use (always use a new lancet).
- Remove the cover of the lancet and hold it firmly to the side of the finger.
- Prick the finger – the anticipation of the coming prick may cause hesitancy or flinching. It is important that the woman holds the lancet against the skin to ensure proper entry, otherwise the capillary will not be punctured and the pricking will need to be repeated (Figure 13.4).
- Gently squeeze the finger to produce a drop of blood (avoid squeezing too tightly).
- Place the drop of blood on to the test strip (Figure 13.5).
- The test strip may use a capillary action using a tube in the end of the strip, in which case, present the blood to the opening so it can draw up the blood.

- Ensure a sufficient sample has been collected (depending on the system used).
- Use a piece of gauze to stop the bleeding.
- Read the value.
- Dispose of the lancet in a sharps bin.
- Dispose of all other clinical waste safely.
- Record the results (Peate, 2021a).

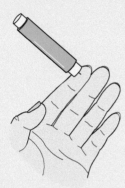

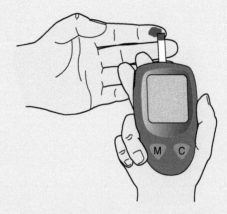

Figure 13.4   **Finger prick.**
Source: Peate (2021a)/with
permission of John Wiley & Sons.

Figure 13.5   **Dropping blood onto the test strip.**
Source: Peate (2021a)/with permission of John Wiley & Sons.

Clinical consideration

Variables that may affect blood glucose monitoring by fingerprick testing

The procedure for undertaking point-of-care testing (fingerprick testing) is explained in detail in the Skills in practice box. However, there a number of factors that may affect point-of-care testing as detailed below.

Preanalysis factors
- Arterial versus capillary blood samples – arterial samples can give different results to capillary samples and should not be used.
- Inadequate cleaning of the testing instrument – always clean according to manufacturer's instructions.
- Incorrect quality control or testing procedures – always ensure quality control is undertaken.
- Sweat or body temperature extremes – sweat can dilute the blood sample. Body temperature extremes can alter capillary blood flow in the extremities.
- Systolic blood pressure less than 80 mmHg – low systolic blood pressure reduces blood flow to the fingertips; thus, capillary blood at the fingertips may not reflect the actual blood glucose in the central circulation.

Analytical factors
- Extremes of glucose – most testing machines can only read glucose levels within a certain range. Check the manufacturer's handbook for information.
- Improper technique.
- Incorrect match between glucose monitor calibration and test strip calibration.

Postanalytical factors
- Data entry errors.

Most common errors
Audit of errors in blood glucose monitoring shows the four most common errors to be:

- inadequate cleaning
- poor-quality control procedures
- improper technique
- incorrect match between calibration of machine and test strip calibration (Peate, 2021a).

For women with type 1 diabetes, offer continuous glucose monitoring (CGM) to help them meet their pregnancy blood glucose targets and improve neonatal outcomes. For a description of continuous glucose monitoring, see Box 13.2. For women who do not have type 1 diabetes but are treated with insulin, consider CGM if they are prone to severe hypoglycaemia or have unstable blood glucose levels (NICE, 2020b).

The advantages of CGM include the following.

- The user can see trends – when their glucose levels are starting to rise or drop – so action can be taken earlier.
- The user will not need to do so many fingerprick checks.
- It can help improve HbA1c levels as insulin doses can be tailored more carefully.
- It can help reduce hypoglycaemias as the user can see a downward trend before the hypoglycaemia occurs.
- The user can set the system to alarm at high and low levels.

Blood ketone monitoring in diabetes

Pregnant women with type 1 diabetes should be offered a blood ketone testing meter and be advised to test for ketones in the blood and seek urgent medical help if they become hyperglycaemic or unwell. Advise women with type 2 diabetes to seek urgent medical help if they develop hyperglycaemia or become unwell. If any pregnant woman with diabetes presents with hyperglycaemia or is unwell, test immediately for blood ketones.

Any pregnant woman presenting with hyperglycaemia and suspected diabetic ketoacidosis or hyperosmolar hyperglycaemic state should be urgently admitted to level 2 critical care.

HbA1c

HbA1c levels measure the average blood glucose levels over the course of the previous weeks/months and thus show historical blood glucose levels. NICE (2020b) states that professionals caring for a pregnant woman should measure the HbA1c level:

- at the booking appointment for all pregnant women with pre-existing diabetes. The level of risk for the pregnancy for women with pre-existing diabetes increases when the HbA1c level is above 48 mmol/mmol (6.5%)
- when women are diagnosed with GDM, to identify those who may have pre-existing type 2 diabetes (HbA1c will be raised in the existence of type 2 diabetes).

Box 13.2   Continuous glucose monitoring

Continuous glucose monitoring is a system that measures the glucose in the interstitial fluid rather than the blood and therefore there is always a slight lag in results showing the increase in glucose following a meal.

CGM systems consist of:

- a sensor that sits just underneath the skin and measures the glucose levels
- a transmitter attached to the sensor which sends the glucose levels to a display device
- a display device that shows the glucose level.

Diabetic emergencies

Hypoglycaemia

Hypoglycaemia is a potentially life-threatening condition characterised by a low blood glucose. The patient will present with:

- hunger
- nervousness and shakiness
- perspiration
- dizziness or light-headedness
- sleepiness
- confusion
- difficulty speaking
- feelings of anxiety or weakness.

If possible, the woman should be encouraged to eat glucose (in the form of jam or chocolate, for example) or glucose paste (such as GlucoGel®) should be rubbed into the gums. The glucose will be short-acting and must be followed with a longer-acting carbohydrate (such as brown bread) if the patient is able to eat safely.

Semi-conscious and unconscious patients will require the administration of glucagon or intravenous glucose. Women with diabetes should be advised to always carry a form of rapidly digested glucose with them (such as glucose tablets or a chocolate bar). NICE (2020b) also suggests that women with type 2 diabetes should be offered glucagon injection and both they and their family taught how to administer it.

Glucagon is the counter-regulatory hormone to insulin which acts by promoting the release of hepatic glucose. Glucagon is normally secreted in response to hypoglycaemia but in women with diabetes, this mechanism is mostly absent and thus hypoglycaemia will continue unchecked. At present, glucagon can only be administered by injection (usually subcutaneous or intramuscular but it can be given intravenously) and the standard adult dose is 1 mg. Glucagon for emergency use is usually presented as an injection kit containing a syringe prefilled with solvent and a vial of powder (1 mg of glucagon) for reconstitution. A prefilled emergency syringe (similar to an EpiPen®) has been developed in the USA but is not authorised for use in the UK. The action of glucagon is normally within 10 minutes of administration.

Note: glucagon given as an emergency treatment is exempt from normal prescription only medicine restrictions in the UK (British National Formulary, 2021).

Hyperosmolar hyperglycaemic state and diabetic ketoacidosis

Hyperosmolar hyperglycaemic state (HHS) is commonly associated with type 2 diabetes. The onset is usually over days to weeks, and it may be the first indication that the woman is suffering from type 2 diabetes. HHS is characterised by a very high blood glucose (>33.3 mmol/L and often over 50 mmol/L), dehydration and confusion, but the absence of significant levels of ketones and therefore no acidaemia (reduced blood pH). Dehydration occurs due to excessive urine output, and low blood levels of sodium and potassium are common.

Diabetic ketoacidosis is associated with type 1 diabetes and has a rapid onset (normally less than 24 hours). Patients present with hyperglycaemia (but usually not greater than 40 mmol/L due to the rapid onset of DKA), ketosis (ketones in the blood), acidaemia (reduced blood pH), dehydration and reduced blood levels of sodium and potassium. The characteristic 'pear drop' or 'acetone' smell to the breath of a patient with DKA is produced by the excess of ketones in the blood.

The management of both HHS and DKA is similar and is aimed at replacing the lost fluid, reducing the blood glucose and correcting electrolyte imbalances. Large amounts of intravenous fluids are given (typically 1–1.5 L in the first hour), and potassium is usually added to subsequent fluids after the initial rapid fluid resuscitation. Low-dose intravenous insulin is commenced to slowly reduce the blood glucose, and the patient is closely monitored, including regular assessment of vital signs, blood glucose and electrolytes (Peate, 2021b).

217

Diabetes and birth

Preterm labour

Diabetes should not be considered a contraindication to tocolysis or steroids. However, avoid beta-mimetics for tocolysis. Women using insulin for diabetes during pregnancy who receive steroids (for fetal lung maturation) should be offered additional insulin and monitoring of blood glucose due to the potential for increased blood glucose from steroid administration.

Timing of birth

NICE (2020b) provides the following advice.

- Pregnant women with type 1 or type 2 diabetes and no other complications should be advised to have an elective birth by induced labour or caesarean section, between 37 weeks and 38 weeks plus 6 days of pregnancy.
- Consider elective birth before 37 weeks for women with type 1 or type 2 diabetes who have metabolic or other maternal or fetal complications.
- Women with gestational diabetes should be advised to give birth no later than 40 weeks plus 6 days.
- Consider elective birth before 40 weeks plus 6 days for women with gestational diabetes who have maternal or fetal complications.
- For pregnant women with diabetes who have a macrosomic fetus, explain the risks and benefits of vaginal birth, induction of labour and caesarean section.

During birth

Monitor blood glucose every hour during labour and birth for women with diabetes, or every half hour during general anaesthesia. Aim to maintain blood glucose between 4 mmol/L and 7 mmol/L. Consider intravenous dextrose and intravenous variable rate insulin infusion from the onset of established labour for women with type 1 diabetes.

Stop all oral antidiabetic medications in patients with GDM; consider insulin infusion if required (hyperglycaemia above 7 mmol/L on two consecutive blood glucose readings). Continue monitoring blood glucose premeal and 1 hour postmeal for up to 24 hours to capture pre-existing diabetes, new-onset diabetes and avoid hypoglycaemia (Joint British Diabetes Societies for In Patient Care (JBDS-IP), 2017).

Neonatal care

Women with diabetes should be advised to give birth in hospitals where advanced neonatal resuscitation skills are available 24 hours a day (NICE, 2020b). Unless there are complications that require the baby to be admitted to intensive or special care, babies can stay with their mothers. Carry out blood glucose testing routinely at 2–4 hours after birth in babies of women with diabetes and do not transfer babies to community care until:

- they are at least 24 hours old, and
- you are satisfied that the baby is maintaining blood glucose levels and is feeding well.

Postnatal care

Women with pre-existing diabetes treated by insulin should reduce their insulin dose immediately after birth and monitor their blood glucose levels to find the appropriate dose of insulin going forward. Explain to women with diabetes treated by insulin that there is an increased risk of hypoglycaemia in the postnatal period (especially when breast feeding), and they should have a meal or snack before feeds or available during feeds (NICE, 2020b). Women with pre-existing type 2 diabetes can resume or continue metformin immediately after birth, including when breast feeding. However, other oral blood glucose-lowering therapies should be avoided if breast feeding.

218

Women with pre-existing diabetes should be referred to their usual diabetic care team following discharge. Women with GDM should be tested to exclude ongoing hyperglycaemia. If hyperglycaemia has resolved, offer lifestyle advice and a further fasting glucose test at the 6 weeks follow-up. Remind the mother of the potential of gestational diabetes in further pregnancies and the advisability of testing if they become pregnant again.

Women with a fasting plasma glucose level between 6.0 mmol/L and 6.9 mmol/L (or a HbA1c of 5.7% and 6.4%) should be advised that they are at high risk of developing type 2 diabetes and given appropriate advice on preventing it. If the fasting plasma glucose level is 7.0 mmol/L or above, the woman should be advised that she is likely to have type 2 diabetes and be offered a further test to confirm this. If the woman has a HbA1c of 6.5% or above, then advise her that she has type 2 diabetes and refer for further care.

Conclusion

Diabetes may present in any of three types:

- type 1 diabetes mellitus
- type 2 diabetes mellitus
- gestational diabetes mellitus.

All women with diabetes should be given advice on lifestyle and diet regardless of the type of diabetes they present with. Despite recent research, national guidelines recommend that, with the exception of metformin and insulin, all antidiabetic drugs are contraindicated in pregnancy. Good glycaemic control is essential to both maternal and fetal health before and during pregnancy. Delivery of the baby should normally be undertaken in the hospital setting as the risk of complications requires the availability of neonatal resuscitation skills. Postnatal diabetes care will depend on the presence of hyperglycaemia post partum.

Find out more

The following are a list of conditions associated with diabetes. Take some time and write notes about each of the conditions. Think about the medications that may be used in order to treat these conditions and be specific about the pharmacokinetics and pharmacodynamics. Remember to include aspects of patient care. If you are making notes about people you have offered care and support to, you must ensure that you have adhered to the rules of confidentiality.

The condition	Your notes
Hypoglycaemia	
Hyperosmolar hyperglycaemic state	
Diabetic ketoacidosis	
Lipohypertrophy	
Fetal macrosomia	

Glossary

Carbohydrate   A group of compounds (including starches and sugars) that are a major food source

Electrolytes   A group of chemical elements or compounds that includes sodium, potassium, calcium, chloride and bicarbonate

Exocrine gland   A gland that secretes its products into an external space

Fatty acids   Dietary fats that have broken down into elements that can be absorbed into the blood

Gland   Refers to any organ in the body that secretes substances not related to its own internal functioning

Glycogen   A carbohydrate (complex sugar) made from glucose

Hormone   Chemical substance released into the blood by the endocrine system and which has a physiological control over the function of cells or organs other than those that created it

Hyperglycaemia   High blood levels of glucose

Hypoglycaemia   Low blood levels of glucose

Insulin resistance   A condition where the usual body reaction to insulin is reduced

Lipids   Group of organic compounds, including the fats, oils, waxes, sterols and triglycerides

Opportunistic screening   Testing a patient for particular diseases or conditions when they are accessing healthcare for other reasons

Osmotic   Movement of water through a semi-permeable barrier from an area of low concentration of a chemical to an area of high concentration of a chemical

Triglycerides   A form of fatty acid having three fatty acid components

Test yourself

Now review your learning by completing the learning activities for this chapter at www.wiley.com/go/pharmacologyformidwives.

References

American Diabetes Association (2021) 2. Classification and diagnosis of diabetes: Standards of Medical Care in Diabetes – 2021. *Diabetes Care*, **44**(suppl 1), S15–S33.

Atkinson, M.A., Eisenbarth, G.S., Michels, A.W. (2014) Type 1 diabetes. *Lancet*, **383**(9911): 69–82.

British National Formulary (2021) Glucagon. https://bnf.nice.org.uk/drug/glucagon.html#directionsForAdministration (accessed January 2022).

Buzzetti, R., Zampetti, S., Pozzilli, P. (2020) Impact of obesity on the increasing incidence of type 1 diabetes. *Diabetes, Obesity and Metabolism*, **22**(7): 1009–1013.

Deeb, A., Abdelrahman, L., Tomy, M. et al. (2019) Impact of insulin injection and infusion routines on lipohypertrophy and glycemic control in children and adults with diabetes. *Diabetes Therapy*, **10**(1): 259–267.

Hyer, S., Balani, J., Shehata, H. (2018) Metformin in pregnancy: mechanisms and clinical applications. *International Journal of Molecular Sciences*, **19**(7): 1954.

Goff, L.M. (2019) Ethnicity and type 2 diabetes in the UK. *Diabetic Medicine*, **36**(8): 927–938.

Hugason-Briem, J. (2018) *Diabetes Care in Pregnancy*. Diabetes Care Trust (ABCD): Solihull.

International Diabetes Federation (IDF) (nd) Storage of insulin. https://idf.org/images/IDF_Europe/Storage_of_Insulin_-_IDF_Europe_Awareness_Paper_-_FINAL.pdf (accessed January 2022).

Joint British Diabetes Societies for In Patient Care (JBDS-IP) (2017) Management of glycaemic control in pregnant women with diabetes on obstetric wards and delivery units. www.diabetologists-abcd.org.uk/JBDS/JBDS_Pregnancy_201017.pdf (accessed January 2022).

Kahn, S.E., Cooper, M.E., Del Prato, S. (2014) Pathophysiology and treatment of type 2 diabetes: perspectives on the past, present, and future. *Lancet*, **383**(9922) : 1068–1083.

Liao, M.Z., Nichols, S.K.F., Ahmed, M. et al. (2020) Effects of pregnancy on the pharmacokinetics of metformin. *Drug Metabolism and Disposition*, **48**(4): 264–271.

Murphy, H.R., Bell, R., Dornhorst, A., Forde, R., Lewis-Barned, N. (2018). Pregnancy in diabetes: challenges and opportunities for improving pregnancy outcomes. *Diabetic Medicine*, **35**(3): 292–299.

National Institute for Health and Care Excellence (2020a) *Type 1 Diabetes in Adults: Diagnosis and Management*. NICE Guideline NG17. NICE: London.

National Institute for Health and Care Excellence (2020b) *Diabetes in Pregnancy: Management from Preconception to the Postnatal Period*. NICE Guideline NG3. NICE: London.

Nursing and Midwifery Council (2019) *Standards of Proficiency for Midwives*. NMC: London.

Peate, I. (ed.) (2014). *Nursing Practice*. John Wiley & Sons: Chichester.

Peate, I. (ed.) (2021a) *The Nursing Associate's Handbook of Clinical Skills*. John Wiley & Sons: Chichester.

Peate, I. (ed.). (2021b). *Fundamentals of Applied Pathophysiology: An Essential Guide for Nursing and Healthcare Students*. John Wiley & Sons: Chichester.

Royal College of Obstetricians and Gynaecologists (2016) Pregnancy sickness (nausea and vomiting of pregnancy and hyperemesis gravidarum). www.rcog.org.uk/en/patients/patient-leaflets/pregnancy-sickness/ (accessed January 2022).

Sachar, A., Willis, T., Basudev, N. (2020) Mental health in diabetes: can't afford to address the service gaps or can't afford not to? *British Journal of General Practice*, **70**(690): 6–7.

Saravanan, P., Magee, L.A., Banerjee, A. et al. for the Maternal Medicine Clinical Study Group (2020) Gestational diabetes: opportunities for improving maternal and child health. *Lancet Diabetes & Endocrinology*, **8**(9): 793–800.

Tidy, C. (2020) *Diabetes Foot Care and Foot Ulcers*. Egton Medical Information: Leeds.

Valaiyapathi, B., Gower, B., Ashraf, A.P. (2020) Pathophysiology of type 2 diabetes in children and adolescents. *Current Diabetes Reviews*, **16**(3): 220–229.

Further reading

Diabetes UK is the leading diabetes charity in the UK and their website contains much information for people with all types of diabetes: www.diabetes.org.uk/

Gestational Diabetes UK is a website specifically for pregnant women with gestational diabetes mellitus: www.gestationaldiabetes.co.uk/

Both NICE guidelines listed in the references above are standard documents for diabetes care in adults and in pregnancy.

Chapter 14

Medications and respiration

Helen McIntyre

University of Leicester, Leicester, UK

Aim

The aim of this chapter is to provide a pharmacological overview of respiratory conditions which may be pre-existing in women and exacerbated when pregnant and perinatal or occurring during pregnancy and requiring additional support.

Learning outcomes

After reading this chapter, the reader will be able to:
- Identify and explain the associated pharmacology for maternal and fetal health in the following: asthma, chronic obstructive pulmonary disease (COPD), tuberculosis, influenza, pneumonia, COVID-19, pertussis, pulmonary embolism, cystic fibrosis, human immunodeficiency virus
- Consider key assessments of the respiratory system which guide pharmacological treatments
- Consider medicinal management and mechanisms
- Explore the role of the student midwife in medicines administration and reviews of holistic management in these women.

Test your existing knowledge

- What changes in the respiratory system would you not expect to see in pregnancy?
- What lung disease is the most prevalent in the UK?
- Describe the clinical manifestations of asthma.
- Discuss the pharmacokinetics and pharmacodynamics associated with one of the following: beclometasone dipropionate, salbutamol, formoterol and ipratropium bromide.
- What do you understand by chronic obstructive pulmonary disease?

Introduction

Globally, respiratory disease is in the top five causes of mortality (WHO, 2017), with asthma and COPD due to smoking being key causes. However, tuberculosis, pertussis, pneumonia, influenza, lung carcinoma, pulmonary embolism, cystic fibrosis and now COVID-19 are contributory. The

---

Fundamentals of Pharmacology for Midwives, First Edition. Edited by Ian Peate and Cathy Hamilton.
© 2022 John Wiley & Sons Ltd. Published 2022 by John Wiley & Sons Ltd.
Companion website: www.wiley.com/go/pharmacologyformidwives

application to midwifery further highlights changes over time when considering morbidity and mortality within the UK. The Mothers and Babies: Reducing Risk through Audits and Confidential Enquiries across the UK (MBRRACE) 2015–18 triennial report (Knight et al., 2020) identified 10 directly related respiratory maternal deaths: six due to asthma and four in women with cystic fibrosis; 34 survived a pulmonary embolism (Goodacre et al., 2019). In contrast to the women who died, these 34 women 'were on average younger, more likely to be having their second or subsequent pregnancy, to be white European and employed, and less likely to be overweight or obese with fewer who smoked. Around half (53%) had a pre-existing medical or mental health problem compared with 73% (159/217) of women who died' (p.38).

In pregnancy, the respiratory rate is not changed but progesterone causes hyperventilation by term. The free ribs are splayed, particularly at the end of pregnancy as the diaphragm is raised which decreases the expiratory and residual volumes. The altered immune system may make a vulnerable individual more prone to respiratory infections.

Asthma

Episodes of care are presented at the start of each section, with the conclusion at the end.

Episode of care

Elizabeth is pregnant for the first time and knows that her asthma will be exacerbated during the summer months. It is April and she is due her 20-week ultrasound scan.

As the student midwife caring for Elizabeth, what further information may you want to ascertain and what advise would you give her?

The incidence of asthma in the UK is 5.4 million (NICE, 2021a). Asthma is characterised by reversible obstruction of the airways causing breathlessness with an associated cough or wheeze and tightness of the chest (British Thoracic Society/Scottish Intercollegiate Guidelines Network (BTS/SIGN), 2019). Usually chronic in nature, it can become acute and severe, causing a status asthmaticus. The usual bronchoconstriction is exacerbated by inflammatory changes to the mucosa leading to increased mucus, shedding of cells and swelling of respiratory tissue. There is a familial incidence but environmental factors act as triggers, including dust mite allergens, pollens, foods, drugs, smoking, cold air and exercise.

Pathology of asthma

An increase in the thickness of the smooth muscle is noted in airways of asthmatics which reduces the lumen diameter. Further bronchoconstriction occurs as an immune response to an allergen mediated by immunoglobulin E (IgE).

Figure 14.1 shows the differences in the airway lumen between a healthy airway, a chronic asthmatic and an acute asthmatic event.

IgE triggers the release of inflammatory substances such as histamine, bradykinin, prostaglandins and thromboxane A and further chemotactic factors including aggregating eosinophils, neutrophils, T lymphocytes and platelets. The normal defence mechanisms of inflammation and mucus production are impeded by the activity of eosinophils which increase the shedding of epithelial cells and prevent the normal ability of cilia to move debris toward the pharynx.

Pregnancy

Between 8% and 13% of pregnant women have pre-existing asthma and numbers are increasing (Murphy, 2015). Mehita et al. (2015) noted that a third of women had improved symptoms, a third had no change in symptoms and a third had exacerbated symptoms. However, being asthmatic does make the pregnant woman more susceptible to chest infections. The mechanism by which asthma affects pregnancy is not clear but preterm births, low-birthweight babies and additional

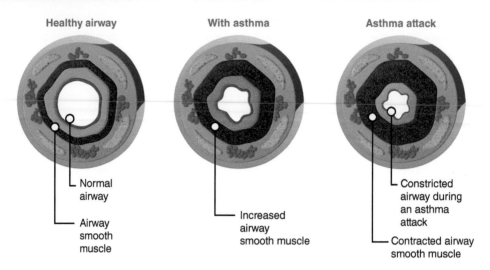

Healthy airway   With asthma   Asthma attack

Normal
airway

Airway
smooth
muscle

Increased
airway
smooth muscle

Constricted
airway during
an asthma
attack

Contracted airway
smooth muscle

Figure 14.1 Altered airway lumen in asthmatics.

224

support for pre-eclampsia are more frequent (Scullion and Holmes, 2013). Obstetric complications due to dyspnoea include pulmonary embolism (discussed later in the chapter). Anxiety exacerbates the symptoms of asthma so care provision needs to be calm and consideration should be given to relaxation or yoga techniques in the long term.

Pharmacological management

The main medicines used are bronchodilators and anti-inflammatory agents, commonly referred to as relievers and preventers.

Bronchodilators come in short- and long-acting beta-2-adrenergic agonists and work by relaxing the smooth muscle of the airways. Salbutamol is short-acting and often used as required in an aerosol or nebuliser. The maximum effect occurs within 30 minutes, lasting for 4–6 hours. Salmeterol and formoterol are long-acting up to 12 hours so are prescribed twice daily. The key side-effects are tremor and tachycardia.

Theophylline, a methylxanthine, acts as a bronchodilator and anti-inflammatory. It has a short half-life and is often used in emergency acute asthma. Erythromycin and ciprofloxacin should be avoided as the method of excretion uses the same liver enzyme, cytochrome P450, risking theophylline accumulation. Its narrow therapeutic range and index lead to numerous side-effects such as overalertness and sleep interference, raised heart rate and blood pressure and indigestion.

Another group of bronchodilators activate the parasympathetic nervous system by blocking muscarinic receptors. Ipratropium is used as an aerosol or nebuliser, taking effect after 45 minutes and lasting for 3–5 hours.

Corticosteroids act as anti-inflammatories and immunosuppressants, the most common being beclometasone dipropionate. When inhaled, corticosteroids prevent the release of arachidonic acid which reduces the production of prostaglandins and leukotrienes. When taken regularly, they reduce the frequency of 'reliever' bronchodilators but can take a number of weeks for the effect to be noticeable. Local side-effects include sore throat and oral candidiasis. Leukotriene receptor antagonists are effectively used with montelukast, a group of drugs which act as a bronchodilator and anti-inflammatory.

Treatment guidelines would include:

- bronchodilator inhaler only
- bronchodilator inhaler and corticosteroid inhaler
- oral theophylline

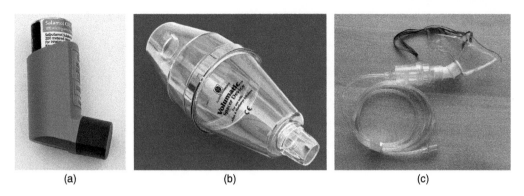

    (a)   (b)   (c)

Figure 14.2 Inhaler, spacer and nebuliser. *Source*: Peate & Hill (2021)/with permission of John Wiley & Sons.

- leukotriene antagonist
- steroid tablets
- avoid ergometrine and syntometrine for third-stage management
- avoid the use of non-steroidal anti-inflammatory analgesia.

Figure 14.2 shows an inhaler, spacer and nebuliser.

For a step-by-step guide on how to use inhalers, go to: www.nationalasthma.org.au/living-with-asthma/how-to-videos/how-to-use-a-standard-mdi-and-spacer.

Table 14.1 identifies the absorption, distribution, metabolism and excretion (ADME) of key asthma medicines and their normal adult dosage.

Episode of care

In pregnancy, women should be advised to continue using their medication as previously instructed but seek midwifery/medical support when symptomatic or suspecting a chest infection.

Extra information includes: frequency and nature of exacerbations, regular medication requirements and any additional medications presently available to Elizabeth.

Chronic obstructive pulmonary disease

Chronic obstructive pulmonary disease (COPD) covers a range of pulmonary diseases which have irreversible tissue damage including bronchitis (inflammation of the bronchioles) and emphysema (inflammation of the alveoli) (Tharpe et al., 2016).

Episode of care

Sharon is G3P2 and booking at 10 weeks gestation, with previous preterm births and small for gestational age babies. During the appointment, it becomes clear that Sharon has been a smoker since she was 16 years old and is now 23.

As the student midwife booking Sharon, what would be your actions and advice for the antenatal, intrapartum and postnatal periods?

Table 14.1   ADME of common medicines used in the treatment of asthma.

Medicine	Absorption	Distribution	Metabolism	Excretion
Salbutamol	Bronchodilator through inhalation (100–200 micrograms <4x per day or 2.5–5 mg when nebulised), oral or intravenous (IV) (3–20 micrograms per minute – adjust to maintain a normal heart rate)	Maximum effect at 30 minutes, lasting for 4–6 hours Beta-antagonist enabling relaxation of local muscle, stabilises mast cells, reducing inflammatory response and increases ciliary activity, clearing mucus	Predominantly in the liver	After oral inhalation, 80–100% of dose is excreted via the kidney, whilst the 10% may be eliminated in faeces. After oral administration, 75% of dose is excreted in urine as metabolites, while 4% may be found in faeces. Completely excreted by 72 hours
Salmeterol or Formoterol	Long-acting bronchodilator (LABA) through inhalation, oral, IV. Inhalation: Salmeterol – 50 micrograms BD Formoterol – 6–12 micrograms, 1–2 times per day	Long acting up to 12 hours. Beta-antagonist enabling relaxation of the local muscle, stabilises the mast cells, reducing inflammatory response and the increasing ciliary activity, clearing mucus	Predominantly in the liver	Salmeterol is over 57% excreted in faeces, 20% in urine and 5% unchanged with similar data on Formoterol
Theophyllin/ Aminophylline (caution in pregnancy)	Fast-acting bronchodilator usually used IV in emergencies. Aminophylline 5 mg/kg stat then 500–700 micrograms/kg/h	Local muscle relaxant and respiratory centre in the brain	Predominantly in the liver	Large percentage is excreted via the kidney unchanged, remainder via the faeces
Ipratropium bromide	Bronchodilator through inhalation – aerosol 20–40 migrograms 3–4 times per day or nebuliser 250–500 micrograms 3–4 times per day, oral, IV	Maximum effect at 45 minutes lasting for 3–6 hours. Muscarinic inhibitor preventing the production of mucus	Liver and gastrointestinal tract	57% excreted via faeces and the remainder in urine. Completely excreted by 72 hours
Beclometasone dipropionate	Inhaled corticosteroid which is anti-inflammatory and immune-suppressive. 200–400 micrograms twice daily up to a maximum of 800 micrograms twice daily	Lung and gut assumed to contribute 36% and 26% to systemic exposure, respectively, when inhaled	Metabolised in the gut, lungs and liver	Excreted via the gut and liver

Source: BNF (2021); go.drugbank.com.

The World Health Organization (WHO) reported that more than 3 million people died due to COPD in 2015 – 5% percent of all deaths worldwide. About 90% of those deaths took place in low- or middle-income regions. Smoking is linked to up to 86% of all COPD deaths in the UK (British Lung Foundation, 2016). Of the pregnant population, 10.6% are smoking at the time of their baby's birth (ONS, 2019). Regional and demographic variations exist.

Key symptoms of COPD are a persistent productive (mucus) cough, shortness of breath, wheeze, chest tightness and repeated chest infections.

Pathology of COPD

The cause of COPD is long-term exposure to lung irritants such as tobacco smoke, passive smoking, air pollution, workplace and environmental factors. The most common first sign is a productive cough which becomes increasingly persistent with concomitant breathlessness and wheeze on minor exertion. Bacterial or viral infections exacerbate the chronic symptoms, requiring appropriate pharmacological management.

Figure 14.3 identifies the differences between healthy alveoli and those with symptoms of COPD.

Pregnancy

The mortality and morbidity resulting from tobacco smoking affect the woman and her fetus or newborn. This occurs through the reduction in oxygen and nutrients being transferred to the fetus via the placenta but also the transfer of carcinogenic additives in cigarettes which circulate through the maternal bloodstream (NICE, 2008, 2010).

Table 14.2 lists the maternal and fetal/newborn impact of cigarette smoke.

Due to the severe consequences of women continuing to smoke through pregnancy, every effort is made to support them and their families to quit (NICE, 2021b). Although 50% of pregnant smokers will attempt to quit (Cooper et al., 2014), community norms can make it more challenging. Cooper et al. (2017) note that up to 22% of pregnant women will be smokers which increases with reducing income and age. UK CCG data records the number of women still smoking at birth, which has seen a decline from 13.7% in 2010–11 to 10.4% in 2019–20 and 9.5% in 2020–21.The current national ambition, to achieve a level of 6% or less by 2022, is unlikely to be reached by most regions (NHS Digital, 2018).

227

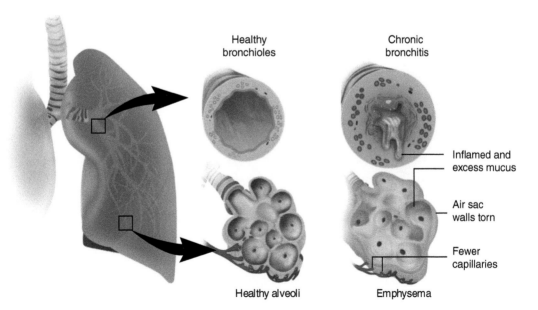

Figure 14.3   Changes in alveoli due to COPD.

Table 14.2   Consequences of smoking to mother and fetus/newborn.

Maternal impact of smoking	Fetal/newborn impact of a smoking environment
Miscarriage	Stillbirth (1/3 attributed to smoking)
Ectopic pregnancy	Fetal facial/palate abnormalities
Antepartum haemorrhage/placental abruption	Small for gestational age occurs with carbon monoxide readings over 5 ppm
Pre-eclampsia	Preterm birth
	Sudden infant death syndrome (SIDS)
Male infertility	Asthma, ear and chest infections, pneumonia
	Behaviour problems, attention deficit hyperactivity disorder (ADHD)

Source: Based on Royal College of Physicians (2018).

228

Women have routine carbon monoxide screening at every antenatal appointment, information about smoking cessation (Royal College of Physicians (RCP), 2018), referral to specialists and guidance on the use of nicotine replacement patches and e-cigarettes. A 12-week plan including support with replacement behavioural activities is successful in four out of five women who succeed in quitting for 28 days (Royal College of Obstetricians and Gynaecologists (RCOG), 2015). Serial fetal growth and umbilical Doppler ultrasound scans are recommended from 26–28 weeks gestation until birth (NHS England, 2019).

Post birth, the risks to the newborn continue through passive smoking by any member of the family. Therefore, smoke-free areas are recommended wherever the newborn will be sleeping or awake, including public places such as pubs, to reduce the risk of sudden infant death syndrome (SIDS). The newborn should not be handled within 30 minutes of a smoke by any individual (Baby Sleep Information Source (BASIS), 2021; Lullaby Trust, 2021).

Pharmacological management of COPD

Due to the chronic nature of COPD, bronchodilators and muscarinic antagonists used are long-acting, so last for 12–24 hours rather than 4–6 hours, which appears to lower the rate of exacerbation. The newest long-acting beta-2 agonist (LABA) is indacaterol which acts for 24 hours. Patients need to be advised to report any side-effects such as palpitations and tremor. Glycopyrronium is a long-acting muscarinic antagonist (LAMA) providing 24-hour relief. These drugs are also available in a combined preparation.

Nicotine replacement therapy can be used to reduce smoking or enable quitting. Numerous routes of administration are available, with patches, inhalation and gum.

Nicotine is absorbed through the skin using nicotine patches, available in 16-hour and 24-hour preparations, in a range of strengths. Peak plasma levels are reached within 8–10 hours. The 24-hour preparation may be suitable for people who experience strong cravings for cigarettes on waking. Some patches are translucent and may be preferred as they are more discrete.

Inhaled nicotine 'vaping' is absorbed through the buccal mucosa. When used like a cigarette, on average it delivers 1 mg in 80 puffs, and 2 mg of nicotine is released during 20 minutes of intensive use. Each 15 mg cartridge can be used for approximately eight 5-minute sessions, with each cartridge lasting for approximately 40 minutes of intense use.

Nicotine chewing gum is absorbed through the buccal mucosa, with peak plasma concentrations after 20–30 minutes. Available in different flavours and strengths, one piece of gum lasts for about 30 minutes. Gum is difficult to use with dentures and may damage them.

Table 14.3 provides the ADME of key medicines used in the treatment of COPD.

Table 14.3   Common treatments for COPD.

Medicine	Absorption	Distribution	Metabolism	Excretion
Indacaterol	Rapid absorption when given IV. Inhalation 150–300 micrograms daily	Beta-antagonist enabling relaxation of local muscle	Limited metabolic breakdown	Majority of excretion is via the faeces
Glycopyrronium	Rapid absorption when given IV and an elimination half-life of approximately 50 minutes. Inhalation 50 micrograms daily	Muscarinic inhibitor preventing the production of mucus	Conversion to glycopyrrolate in the kidneys	Excretion via urine. It becomes severely impaired in patients with renal failure
Alternatives to tobacco smoking				
Nicotine patch	16 and 24 hours through the buccal mucosa	Peak plasma levels in 8–10 hours	The major site of metabolism is the kidneys	The major site of elimination for nicotine and its metabolites is in urine. Approximately 10% of nicotine and 10% of cotinine are excreted unmetabolised in the urine, although the process is pH dependent
Nicotine inhalator	Through the buccal mucosa	Peak plasma levels in 20 minutes		
Nicotine gum	Through the buccal mucosa	Peak plasma levels in 20–30 minutes		

Source: BNF (2021); go.drugbank.com.

Episode of care

Conclusion

Antenatally: carbon monoxide monitoring at each visit. Offer smoking cessation support and involve the family as appropriate. Consider alternatives to tobacco smoking. Vigilant monitoring of fetal growth and signs of concern such as altered fetal movements.

Intrapartum: in preparation, consider relaxation methods for analgesia: yoga, hypnobirthing and acupressure. Provide alternatives for smoking such as patches if not already in place. Managing a potentially compromised fetus during labour and birth.

Postnatally: SIDS prevention advice including smoke-free zones at home and in public, sleeping arrangements, handling of the baby by smokers. Breast feeding should be recommended.

Tuberculosis

Tuberculosis (TB) is a bacterial infection caused by *Mycobacterium tuberculosis* which is spread through respiratory droplets and therefore exacerbated in densely populated communities of poor housing and recent migrants (Rankin, 2017; Miele et al., 2020).

Episode of care

Zaneb has recently arrived in the UK from Pakistan to join her husband and is 32 weeks pregnant with their first baby. When she meets the midwife, she complains of a persistent productive cough, breathlessness and night sweats.

As the student midwife caring for Zaneb, what would you be suspecting and what is your advice?

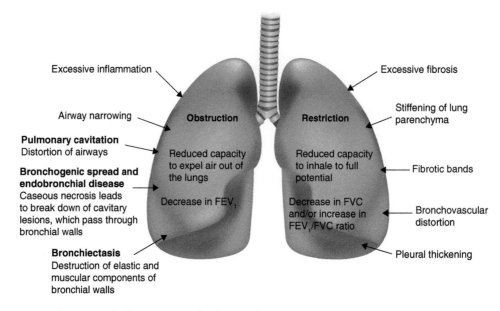

Figure 14.4   Changes in the lungs as a result of a TB infection.
FEV, forced expiratory volume; FEV1, in the first second; FVC, forced vital capacity.

Figure 14.4 identifies the effect of a TB infection on the lungs.

Key symptoms of TB are a chronic cough, blood-stained sputum, weight loss, night sweats/fever, chest pain and shortness of breath.

Pathology of TB

Long-term infection causes scarring on the lungs, noted on x-ray, and anaemia. Bacterial growth can occur in any part of the body, including the brain and kidneys, prior to respiratory symptoms being identified. The TB Mantoux test is diagnostic. Multiresistant TB is proving to be an increasing challenge in relation to effective treatment and reduced spread.

Pregnancy

Poor oxygenation reduces the effective transfer of oxygen to the fetus and ultimately its ability to metabolise and adequately grow. In utero and birth transfer of the bacteria to the fetus or newborn may occur. Treatment of active TB is important in pregnancy though treating latent TB may be delayed (Miele et al., 2020).

Table 14.4 details the pharmacological management of TB.

Table 14.4 Pharmacological management of TB.

Medicine	Absorption	Distribution	Metabolism	Excretion
Isoniazid	Rapidly absorbed orally when the individual has fasted, usually first thing in the morning. Food delays and decreases the extent of absorption. Orally ~300 mg daily for 6 months	Maximum concentration at 1–2 hours in serum, cerebrospinal fluid. Plasma half-life in adults is 1–4 hours	Metabolised in the liver via acetylation into acetylhydrazine. Two forms of the enzyme are responsible for acetylation, so some patients metabolise the drug more quickly than others	About 75% of a dose is excreted in urine as unchanged drug and metabolites in 24 hours; some drug is excreted in saliva, sputum, faeces and breast milk
Vitamin B6 (e.g., Pyridoxine 2 gms during the day)	Water soluble so rapidly absorbed in the jejunum through diffusion	Transported through plasma protein binding to albumin	In the liver	Excretion is via the urine
Rifampicin	Antimycobacterial, rapidly absorbed from the intestine and the absorption rate increases with time. Orally ~ 600–900 mg 3 times per week for 6 months	80% transported in blood bound to plasma proteins, mainly albumin	In the liver	Metabolised products are excreted in faeces, unmetabolised via urine
Ethambutol	Up to 80% absorption orally with a 3.5 hour half-life. Orally ~ 15 mg/kg daily for 2 months	Bound to protein in plasma	In the liver	Ethambutol is 50% eliminated in the urine as the unmetabolised parent compound and 8–15% as inactive metabolites. The remainder via faeces
Bacille Calmette-Guerin (BCG) vaccine	Intradermal injection Adult – 0.1 mL injected into the deltoid muscle. Child 1–11 months – 0.05 mL injected into the deltoid muscle	When challenged, immunised individual has a rapid increase in CD4 and CD8 T cells		

Source: BNF (2021); go.drugbank.com.

Episode of care

Conclusion

A referral to the GP/obstetrician is required for management of immediate relief of symptoms.

Mantoux test, sputum sample and chest x-ray to confirm the diagnosis of TB as appropriate. Vigilant monitoring of the fetus to ensure adequate growth and normal fetal movements.

Treatment of TB for the mother, vaccination of the baby and immediate family following the birth as required.

Influenza

Influenza (flu) is a potentially serious disease caused by two main groups of influenza virus: A and B. Influenza can make the person feel miserable. Fever, cough, shaking chills, body aches and extreme weakness are common symptoms. The flu vaccination has been found to be safe in pregnancy and advisable (NHS, 2021).

The inactivated influenza virus vaccine (IIV) is usually administered intramuscularly, 0.5 mL per one dose (BNF, 2021); intradermal vaccines are also available. Protection usually occurs within 10–14 days of administration. Postvaccine antibody titres are generally high enough in healthy young adults and children to provide resistance against infection by specifically targeted strains found in the vaccine as well as related strains. The duration of immunity imparted by the influenza vaccine generally lasts 6–12 months.

All pregnant women in the UK are offered and advised to have the flu vaccine prophylactically leading up to the winter months.

Pneumonia and COVID-19

Episode of care

Selena is 24 weeks pregnant with her first baby and is living in a multigenerational household. She contacts the maternity assessment unit (MAU) for advice on the following symptoms: persistent cough with recent onset, fever, lethargy, altered fetal movements.

What will your action be as the student midwife receiving this call?

What subsequent advice may be provided following the birth?

Pneumonia

Pneumonia is swelling (inflammation) of the tissue in one or both lungs. It is usually caused by a bacterial infection but it can also be caused by a virus, such as coronavirus (COVID-19) and influenza. The symptoms of pneumonia can develop suddenly over 24–48 hours, or they may come on more slowly over several days.

Figure 14.5 shows the differences between influenza and COVID-19.

Key symptoms of pneumonia include a cough, which may be dry or produce thick yellow, green, brown or blood-stained mucus (phlegm), difficulty breathing – breathing may be rapid and shallow and the woman may feel breathless, even when resting, rapid heartbeat, high temperature, feeling generally unwell, sweating and shivering, loss of appetite and chest pain which gets worse when breathing or coughing.

Less common symptoms of pneumonia include haemoptysis, headaches, fatigue, feeling or being sick, wheezing, joint and muscle pain and feeling confused or disorientated, particularly in elderly people.

Mild pneumonia can usually be treated at home with rest, a course of antibiotics (if it is likely to be caused by a bacterial infection) and drinking plenty of fluids. More severe cases may need hospital treatment.

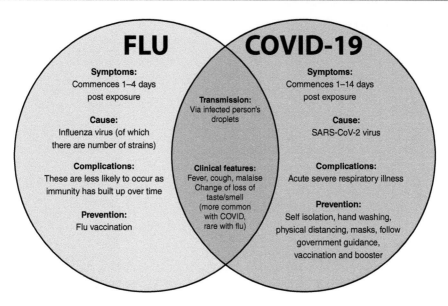

Figure 14.5 Differences between flu and COVID-19.

233

As a general guide, after:

- 1 week – high temperature should have gone
- 4 weeks – chest pain and mucus production should have substantially reduced
- 6 weeks – cough and breathlessness should have substantially reduced
- 3 months – most symptoms should have resolved, but the woman may still feel very tired (fatigue)
- 6 months – most people will feel back to normal.

The following antibiotics could be considered as treatment for pneumonia.

- Penicillins, including amoxicillin, ampicillin.
- Cephalosporins, including cefaclor, cephalexin.

Both these groups of beta-lactam antibiotics act as bactericides of Gram negatives by breaking down the cell wall of the bacterium, thereby preventing its effective development and replication.

- Erythromycin.
- Clindamycin.

Both these macrolides prevent protein synthesis in the bacterium by binding to the 50s ribosome unit to prevent its replication. Erythromycin is often used when there is a known allergy to penicillin or the bacterium is Gram positive.

Some antibiotics are known to be teratogenic and should be avoided entirely during pregnancy. These include streptomycin and kanamycin (which may cause hearing loss) and tetracycline (which can lead to weakening, hypoplasia and discoloration of long bones and teeth in the fetus). Please refer to Chapter 9 for further detail on the mechanism of antibiotic action.

Table 14.5 identifies key antibiotics used in the care of pneumonia.

COVID-19

Care of pregnant women during the COVID-19 (RCOG, 2021; UNICEF BFI, 2021) pandemic covered:
- self-isolation to avoid contracting the disease
- vaccination once it was deemed safe to offer the variety of vaccines following trials which were extrapolated to pregnancy or
- prevention of spread once suspected or known to be infected and treatment when symptomatic and confirmed.

Table 14.5   Antibiotics used in pneumonia.

Medicine	Absorption	Distribution	Metabolism	Excretion
Penicillin	The half-life of amoxicillin is 61.3 minutes. Oral amoxicillin – 500 mg, 8 hourly	Detectable serum levels are observed up to 8 hours after an orally administered dose of amoxicillin	Poorly metabolised in the liver	Approximately 60% of an orally administered dose of amoxicillin is excreted in the urine within 6–8 hours
Cephalosporins	Serum half-life of 1–2 hours. Cephalexin orally 250 mg every 6 hours	Most body fluids and tissues	In the kidneys	Excreted by the kidneys
Erythromycin	Readily absorbed orally but has a short half-life of 1.4 hours. Orally – 250–500 mg 4 times per day	Erythromycin has a low volume of distribution	Mostly metabolised in the liver	Some excretion in the kidneys
Clindamycin	Average half-life is 2.4 hours. Orally 150–300 mg every 6 hours	Most body fluids and tissues	In the liver	10% in urine and 3.6% in faeces; remainder is excreted as bioinactive metabolites

Source: BNF (2021); go.drugbank.com.

Vaccinations include those manufactured by Pfizer, Astra-Zeneca, Moderna and Johnson and Johnson. Symptomatic relief of fever was advised with paracetamol and more severe cases needed steroids.

Pulmonary embolism

Pulmonary embolism (PE) occurred in 34 pregnancies reported in the MBRRACE report (Knight et al., 2020). The reported incidence despite better treatment and survival is suggestive of implications due to raised BMI, ethnicity and co-morbidities.

Pulmonary emboli usually occur from a detached mobile part of deep venous thrombosis which travels to the lungs and occludes a blood vessel. This causes poor perfusion and then poor ventilation, leading to reduced surfactant production, collapse of the alveoli and hypoxaemia (Marshall and Raynor, 2020).

Assessment would include monitoring of oxygen saturation, arterial blood gases, ECG, chest x-ray, CT scan and potential VQ scan following consent due to the exposure to radioisotopes. Immediate treatment with low molecular weight heparin (LMWH) would be commenced before further anticoagulation therapy. LMWH such as enoxaparin sodium extends the clotting time.

Table 14.6 identifies the most frequently used LMWH in preventing PE.

Episode of care

There are two major concerns with Selena, the first being her symptoms of a respiratory infection and secondly the condition of her baby due to altered fetal movements which will need a face-to-face review. Selena will need an immediate lateral flow test with a subsequent polymerase chain reaction (PCR) test for a definitive diagnosis.

Selena will be admitted to the Maternity Assessment Unit (MAU) wearing a mask and using hand sanitiser. Full personal protective equipment will be required by staff, single room isolation, no relatives and care provided assuming COVID-19 positive.

Given a satisfactory/reassuring assessment of the altered fetal movements, Selena would be returned home with guidance on management of her symptoms such as paracetamol for her fever, antibiotics and drinking plenty. Isolation from the intergenerational family and full COVID-19 testing of all members in the home. Should her symptoms deteriorate, she would need to seek further advice through 111 or the MAU.

Post birth she should still be advised to get to know her baby, care for her baby and breastfeed her baby. Minimal vertical transfer has been noted either in pregnancy or breastfeeding.

Episode of care

Conclusion
Nihal has a BMI of 35, is a grand multip and diagnosed with gestational diabetes in this pregnancy. At 30 weeks she complains of acute chest pain, breathlessness, coughing blood and feeling hot.

Given Nihal's symptoms, what may you suspect and what would your management be?

Table 14.6   Low molecular weight heparin used in preventing PE.

Medicine	Absorption	Distribution	Metabolism	Excretion
Enoxaparin sodium	Nearly 100% via subcutaneous route – over 90 kg 100 mg ×2 daily	Via the bloodstream	Due to the cascade of effects resulting from enoxaparin binding, thrombin is unable to convert fibrinogen to fibrin and form a clot	Via the kidneys

Source: BNF (2021).

Episode of care

Conclusion
The acuteness of the chest pain is suggestive of a larger pulmonary embolism, therefore this is a medical emergency and urgent referral and admission to the hospital are required.

Assessment and treatment would be as above. Continued self-administration of twice-daily LMWH into the postnatal period, increased fluids and exercise with a strong recommendation to eat healthily during pregnancy and aim to sustainably lose weight postnatally.

Cystic fibrosis

There are three key papers that chart the course of pregnancy care in women with cystic fibrosis (CF) (Edenborough et al., 2008; Koon et al., 2018; Ashcroft et al., 2020). Cystic fibrosis is an autosomal recessive disorder which is screened for in babies at 5 days of age through the newborn blood spot heel prick test. This has improved the outcomes and survival rates of women of child-bearing age. Despite potential challenges, fertility can now be realised through natural or assisted methods. A multidisciplinary approach is required, including medical and nursing specialists, nutritionists, physiotherapists, genetic counsellors and discussions about the care of a healthy baby who may be more energetic than its mother or whose CF condition may deteriorate, needing end-of-life care.

Antenatal women with CF will often develop gestational diabetes and experience recurrent chest infections. Preterm births and small for gestational age babies are correlations of lung function and nutritional status (Ashcroft et al., 2020). Postnatally, anxiety and postnatal depression should be monitored (Edenborough et al., 2008). Koon et al. (2018) reviewed medicine combinations and their suitability for pregnant and lactating women.

Human immunodeficiency virus

Complications of the human immunodeficiency virus (HIV) affecting the lungs are pneumonia and tuberculosis. However, most women in the UK who become pregnant have a satisfactory and stable blood pathology. For further details on management, see the RCOG Green Top guidelines (2010): www.rcog.org.uk/en/guidelines-research-services/guidelines/gtg39/ or British HIV Association guidelines (2019): www.bhiva.org/pregnancy-guidelines.

Find out more

The following is a list of conditions associated with the respiratory system. Write short notes on each condition and consider the medications that may be used to treat them. Be specific about the pharmacokinetics and pharmacodynamics. If you are making notes about specific women to whom you have offered care, please ensure that you adhere to the NMC Code (2018) regarding confidentiality.

The condition	Your notes
Asthma	
COPD	
Tuberculosis	
Pertussis	
COVID-19	
Pulmonary embolism	
Cystic fibrosis	

Glossary

Bronchoconstriction   A tightening of smooth muscle surrounding the bronchi and bronchioles with consequent wheezing and shortness of breath

Chronic obstructive pulmonary disease   The name for a group of lung conditions that cause breathing difficulties

Co-morbidities   The simultaneous presence of two or more diseases or medical conditions in a patient

Hypoxaemia   This condition occurs when levels of oxygen in the blood are lower than normal

Immunoglobulins   Proteins (globulins) in the body that act as antibodies

Intradermal injection   Injections that are delivered into the **dermis,**   or the skin layer underneath the epidermis

Mantoux test   A test that is widely used for latent TB. It involves injecting a small amount of a substance called PPD tuberculin into the skin of the forearm. It is also called the tuberculin skin test (TST)

Polymerase chain reaction test   A PCR test is a method widely used to rapidly make millions to billions of copies (complete copies or partial copies) of a specific DNA sample, allowing scientists to take a very small sample of DNA and amplify it (or a part of it) to a large enough amount so they are able to study it in detail

Surfactant   An agent that decreases the surface tension between two media

Teratogens   Substances that may produce physical or functional defects in the embryo or fetus after the pregnant woman is exposed to the substance

Test yourself

Now review your learning by completing the learning activities for this chapter at www.wiley.com/go/pharmacologyformidwives**.**

References

Ashcroft, A., Chapman, SJ., Mackillop, L. (2020) The outcome of pregnancy in women with cystic fibrosis: a UK population-based descriptive study. *British Journal of Obstetrics Gynaecology*, **127**: 1696–1703.

Baby Sleep Information Source (BASIS) (2021) www.basisonline.org.uk/ (accessed February 2022).

British Lung Foundation (2016) *Policy position statement: admissions for conditions attributable to smoking in 2016/17*. British Lung Foundation: London.

British National Formulary (2021) https://bnf.nice.org.uk/(accessed February 2022).

British Thoracic Society (2019). BTS/SIGN British guideline on the management of asthma. www.brit-thoracic.org.uk/quality-improvement/guidelines/asthma/ (accessed February 2022).

Cooper, S., Taggar, J., Lewis, S. et al. (2014) Effect of nicotine patches in pregnancy on infant and maternal outcomes at 2 years: follow-up from the randomised, double-blind, placebo-controlled SNAP trial. *Lancet*, **2**: 728–737.

Cooper, S., Orton, S., Leonardi-Bee, J. et al. (2017) Smoking and quit attempts during pregnancy and postpartum: a longitudinal UK cohort. *BMJ Open*, **7**: e018746.

Edenborough, F.P., Borgod, G., Knoopf, C. et al. (2008) Guidelines for the management of pregnancy in women with cystic fibrosis. *Journal of Cystic Fibrosis*, **7**: S2–S32.

Goodacre, S., Horspool, K., Nelson-Piercy, C. et al. (2019) The DiPEP study: an observational study of the diagnostic accuracy of clinical assessment, D-dimer and chest x-ray for suspected pulmonary embolism in pregnancy and postpartum. *British Journal Obstetrics and Gynaecology*, **126**: 383–392.

Knight, M., Bunch, K., Tuffnell, D. et al. on behalf of MBRRACE-UK (2020) Saving Lives, Improving Mothers' Care – Lessons learned to inform maternity care from the UK and Ireland Confidential Enquiries into Maternal Deaths and Morbidity 2016–18. www.npeu.ox.ac.uk/assets/downloads/mbrrace-uk/reports/maternal-report-2020/MBRRACE-UK_Maternal_Report_Dec_2020_v10_ONLINE_VERSION_1404.pdf (accessed February 2022).

Kroon, M., Akkerman-Nijland, A.M., Rottier, B.L., Koppelman, G.L., Akkerman, O.W., Touw, D.J. (2018) Drugs during pregnancy and breast feeding in women diagnosed with cystic fibrosis – an update. *Journal of Cystic Fibrosis*, **17**: 17–25.

Lullaby Trust (2021) Safer sleep for babies. www.lullabytrust.org.uk/safer-sleep-advice/ (accessed February 2022).

Marshall, J.E., Raynor, D.M. (2020) *Myles Textbook for Midwives*, 17th edn. Elsevier: London.

Mehita, N., Chen, K., Hardy, E. et al. (2015) Respiratory disease in pregnancy. *Best Practice and Research in Obstetrics and Gynaecology*, **29**: 598–611.

Miele, K., Morris, S.B., Tepper, N.K. (2020) Tuberculosis in pregnancy. *Obstetrics and Gynaecology*, **135**(6): 1444–1453.

Murphy, V.E. (2015) Managing asthma in pregnancy. *Breathe*, **11**: 258–267.

National Institute for Health and Care Excellence (2008) Antenatal care for uncomplicated pregnancies. www.nice.org.uk/guidance/cg62 (accessed February 2022).

National Institute for Health and Care Excellence (2010) Smoking: stopping in pregnancy and after childbirth. www.nice.org.uk/guidance/ph26 (accessed February 2022).

National Institute for Health and Care Excellence (2021a) Asthma: diagnosis, monitoring and chronic asthma management. nice.org.uk/guidance/ng80 (accessed February 2022).

National Institute for Health and Care Excellence (2021b) Nicotine replacement therapy. https://cks.nice.org.uk/topics/smoking-cessation/prescribing-information/nicotine-replacement-therapy-nrt/ (accessed February 2022).

NHS (2021) The flu jab in pregnancy. www.evidence.nhs.uk/search?ps=50&q=flu+vaccine+pregnancy (accessed February 2022).

NHS Digital (2018) Statistics on women's smoking status at time of delivery: England. https://digital.nhs.uk/data-and-information/publications/statistical/statistics-on-women-s-smoking-status-at-time-of-delivery-england (accessed February 2022).

NHS England (2019) Saving babies' lives version two: a care bundle for reducing perinatal mortality. www.england.nhs.uk/publication/ saving-babies-lives-version-two-a-care-bundle-for-reducingperinatal-mortality (accessed February 2022).

Nursing and Midwifery Council (2018) The Code: Professional standards of practice and behaviour for nurses, midwives and nursing associates. www.nmc.org.uk/globalassets/sitedocuments/nmc-publications/nmc-code.pdf (accessed February 2022).

Office for National Statistics (2019) Smoking in pregnancy. www.ons.gov.uk (accessed February 2022).

Peate, I., Hill, B. (2021) *Fundamentals of Pharmacology for Nursing and Healthcare Students*. Wiley: Chichester.

Rankin, J. (2017) *Physiology in Childbearing*. Elsevier: London.

Royal College of Obstetricians and Gynaecologists (2015) Smoking and pregnancy. www.rcog.org.uk/en/patients/patient-leaflets/smoking-and-pregnancy/ (accessed February 2022).

Royal College of Obstetricians and Gynaecologists (2021) Coronavirus infections in pregnancy. www.rcog.org.uk/en/guidelines-research-services/guidelines/coronavirus-pregnancy/covid-19-virus-infection-and-pregnancy/ (accessed February 2022).

Royal College of Physicians (2018) Hiding in plain sight: treating tobacco dependency in the NHS. www.rcplondon.ac.uk/ projects/outputs/hiding-plain-sight-treating-tobacco-dependencynhs (accessed February 2022).

Scullion, J., Holmes, S. (2013) Allergic rhinitis and asthma. www.independentnurse.co.uk/clinical-article/allergic-rhinitis-and-asthma/63488/ (accessed February 2022).

Tharpe, N.L., Farley, C.L., Jordan, R.G, (2016) *Clinical Practice Guidelines for Midwifery and Women's Health*. Jones and Bartlett Learning: Burlington.

UNICEF BFI (2021) Supporting babies, mothers and families during the coronavirus (Covid-19) outbreak. www.unicef.org.uk/babyfriendly/covid-19/ (accessed February 2022).

World Health Organization (2017) Maternal mortality: Levels and trends 2000 to 2017. www.who.int/reproductivehealth/publications/maternalmortality-2000-2017 (accessed February 2022).

Chapter 15

Medicines and the gastrointestinal system

Debbie Gurney

University of Hertfordshire, Hatfield, UK

Aim

The aim of this chapter is to provide an overview of gastrointestinal changes that occur during pregnancy and an introduction to resulting gastrointestinal conditions and the pharmacological interventions used in their management.

Learning outcomes

After reading this chapter, the reader will:
- Be able to relate the signs and symptoms of common gastrointestinal disorders of pregnancy to their underlying physiology and pathophysiology
- Demonstrate an understanding of gastrointestinal disorders of pregnancy, including their causes and clinical presentation
- Understand pharmacological treatment options for gastrointestinal disorders of pregnancy
- Understand the pharmacokinetics and pharmacodynamics of gastrointestinal medicines used in pregnancy.

Test your existing knowledge

- Describe the constituent parts and main functions of the gastrointestinal tract.
- What are the common routes for the administration of gastrointestinal medications?
- Write down the names of the hormones that influence gastrointestinal conditions in pregnancy.
- Write down the common gastrointestinal disorders you have seen in your practice.
- How is gastric acidity managed during labour where you are on placement?

Introduction

The gastrointestinal (GI) tract is a continuous hollow tube, that extends from the mouth to the anus (Figure 15.1). It comprises the oesophagus, stomach, small and large intestines and the rectum. The

Fundamentals of Pharmacology for Midwives, First Edition. Edited by Ian Peate and Cathy Hamilton.
© 2022 John Wiley & Sons Ltd. Published 2022 by John Wiley & Sons Ltd.
Companion website: www.wiley.com/go/pharmacologyformidwives

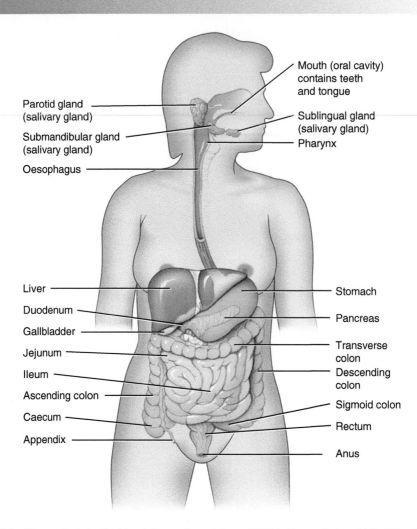

Figure 15.1 The gastrointestinal tract. *Source*: Peate & Evans (2020)/with permission of John Wiley & Sons.

hepatobiliary system is also an essential component of the GI tract. Its functions include digestion and absorption, protection and immunity, extraction of nutrients and energy and excretion of waste matter. It is controlled by enteric nerves as well as the autonomic (involuntary) part of the central nervous system.

During pregnancy, the physiological adaptations made by the body alter the functioning of the GI tract. These changes occur in response to endocrine changes as well as physical changes as organs are displaced as the fetus grows. This chapter will focus on conditions of the GI tract and their underlying physiological and pathophysiological changes, specifically, nausea and vomiting and heartburn, constipation, irritable bowel syndrome (IBS) and diarrhoea. Information is also given on anorectal conditions. Each section will be presented with an overview of the gastrointestinal condition and the medications that are commonly used in its management.

Nausea and vomiting in pregnancy
Physiology

Nausea and vomiting in pregnancy (NVP) affects up to 80% of pregnant women (Royal College of Obstetricians and Gynaecologists (RCOG), 2016). For the majority of women, it occurs in the first trimester and is mild in nature. However, Koren et al. (2014) point out that for around 25% of women it continues into the second trimester and in 5% of cases to the third trimester. The pathophysiology of NVP is not well understood but Jarvis and Nelson-Piercy (2011) suggested that the cause is likely to be a combination of endocrine, gastrointestinal, psychosocial and environmental factors. A reduction in oesophageal pressure and delayed gastric emptying occurs as a result of smooth muscle relaxation, mediated by progesterone (Jarvis and Nelson-Piercy, 2011). In addition, rising levels of beta human chorionic gonadotropin (B-HCG) in the first trimester are thought to cause NVP and very high levels of B-HCG, such as in cases of multiple pregnancy and trophoblastic disease, can result in more severe NVP (RCOG, 2016).

Clinical consideration

Red flag signs: nausea and vomiting in pregnancy
- Impairment of renal function
- Severe electrolyte disturbance
- Cognitive impairment
- Indication of suicide ideation

Hyperemesis gravidarum

241

Hyperemesis gravidarum (HG) is the severe form of NVP and affects 0.3–3.6% of pregnant women (RCOG, 2016). HG is associated with dehydration, electrolyte imbalance, vitamin deficiencies, weight loss and profound psychosocial consequences; it is the leading cause of admission to hospital in the first trimester

Clinical consideration

The severity of NVP should be assessed using an objective tool, such as the Pregnancy-Unique Quantification of Emesis (PUQE) (Bharj and Daniels, 2017).

Management

Psychological support should be given to women with NVP, such as reassurance that it is not harmful to the fetus and that it is likely to diminish as the pregnancy progresses (Jarvis and Nelson-Piercy, 2011), along with advice relating to diet and oral hydration and antiemetic medication (RCOG, 2016).

Antiemetic medications are the mainstay of treatment for NVP (RCOG, 2016) but the frequency, dose and route of administration should be determined by the severity of the NVP. Clinical history, examination and investigations should be undertaken to exclude other pathological causes. Mild-to-moderate NVP should be managed in the community with oral antiemetics in the majority of cases (RCOG, 2016).

Antiemetic medications prescribed to treat NVP include antihistamines (H1 receptor antagonists), selective 5-hydroxytryptamine receptor antagonists (5-HT3), dopamine D2 antagonists or a combination of these (Jarvis and Nelson-Piercy, 2011).

Clinical consideration

Antiemetic medications should only be prescribed once the aetiology of the vomiting is known, as they may mask symptoms and delay diagnosis. In some situations, antiemetics may be unnecessary and potentially harmful, particularly in cases where there is a treatable cause for the vomiting, for example, in cases of diabetic ketoacidosis (DKA) (Joint Formulary Committee, 2020).

First-line treatments for NVP

H1 receptor antagonists, specifically cyclizine, are recommended as one of the first-line treatments for NVP and HG (Dean et al., 2018; Electronic Medicines Compendium, 2018). Cyclizine is a histamine H1 receptor antagonist of the piperazine class which is characterised by a reduced likelihood of drowsiness. It has both anticholinergic and antiemetic properties. The exact mechanism by which cyclizine prevents or reduces both nausea and vomiting due to various causes is unknown. Cyclizine is known to increase lower oesophageal sphincter tone and reduces the sensitivity of the labyrinthine apparatus. It is thought that it may inhibit the part of the midbrain known collectively as the emetic centre. Cyclizine produces its antiemetic effect within 2 hours and lasts for approximately 4 hours.

H1-blockers are well absorbed from the GI tract. Following oral administration, effects develop within 30 minutes, are maximal within 1–2 hours and last, for cyclizine, for 4–6 hours. In healthy adult volunteers, the administration of a single oral dose of 50 mg cyclizine resulted in a peak plasma concentration of approximately 70 ng/mL occurring at about 2 hours after drug administration. The plasma elimination half-life was approximately 20 hours.

The N-demethylated derivative norcyclizine has been identified as a metabolite of cyclizine. Norcyclizine has little antihistaminic (H1) activity compared to cyclizine. It is widely distributed throughout the tissues and has a plasma elimination half-life of approximately 20 hours. After a single dose of 50 mg norcyclizine given to a single adult volunteer, urine collected over the following 24 hours contained less than 1% of the total dose administered.

Prochlorperazine and chlorpromazine are also recommended first-line treatments and belong to a class of medicines known as phenothiazines. They are dopamine (D2) antagonists and may also be prescribed as antipsychotics (RCOG, 2016).

The pharmacodynamic properties of chlorpromazine include depressant actions on the central nervous system (CNS), with alpha-adrenergic blocking and anticholinergic activities. It inhibits dopamine and prolactin release inhibitory factor, thus stimulating the release of prolactin. It increases the turnover of dopamine in the brain and has antiemetic, antipruritic, serotonin-blocking and weak antihistamine properties and slight ganglion blocking activity. It inhibits the heat regulating centre in the brain and is analgesic and can relax skeletal muscle.

Due to its action on the autonomic nervous system, it causes vasodilation, hypotension and tachycardia. Salivary and gastric secretions are reduced.

The pharmacokinetic properties of chlorpromazine demonstrate that it is readily absorbed in the GI tract. It is subject to first-pass metabolism in the gut wall. It is extensively metabolised in the liver and excreted in the urine and faeces. The plasma half-life is only a few hours, but it has a prolonged terminal elimination phase of up to about 3 weeks. Chlorpromazine is extensively bound to plasma proteins. It may possibly affect the control of diabetes or the action of anticoagulants. Antacids can impair absorption. Tea and coffee may prevent absorption by causing insoluble precipitates.

Clinical consideration

The first-pass effect is a phenomenon in which a drug is metabolised at a specific location in the body that results in a reduced concentration of the active drug reaching its site of action or the systemic circulation. The first-pass effect is often associated with the liver, as this is a major site of drug metabolism. However, the effect can also occur in the lungs, vasculature, GI tract and other metabolically active tissues in the body. This effect can be augmented by various factors such as plasma protein concentrations, enzymatic activity and gastrointestinal motility. The extent to which a patient may experience the first-pass effect varies from person to person, and this must be taken into consideration when determining appropriate dosing. If the first-pass effect is exceptionally prominent in a patient, the drug may require administration via a different route to bypass the first-pass effect (Herman and Santos, 2020).

Second-line treatments for NVP

Second-line antiemetics include the dopamine antagonists metoclopramide and domperidone (RCOG, 2016). Metoclopramide is a similar medicine to phenothiazines. It is considered very effective in the treatment of NVP as it acts directly on the GI tract but has been associated with extrapyramidal side-effects (Dean et al., 2018) such as tremor and slurred speech. Dopamine has been associated with an increased risk of cardiac abnormalities (Bhakta and Goel, 2017). The mechanism of action of metoclopramide is associated with parasympathetic nervous control of the upper GI tract where it has the effect of promoting normal peristaltic action.

Pharmacokinetic properties of metoclopramide include metabolism in the liver and the principal route of elimination is via the kidneys. The clearance of metoclopramide can be reduced by up to 70% in patients with severe renal impairment, while the plasma elimination half-life is increased.

The 5-HT3 receptor antagonist ondansetron has shown benefits in patients with persistent and severe NVP. However, studies have identified a small increase in the risk of cleft lip or palate in babies born to women who used oral ondansetron in the first trimester of pregnancy (Joint Formulary Committee, 2020).

Third-line treatments for NVP

Third-line options include either oral or intravenous corticosteroids. The antiemetic effect of corticosteroids is not well understood and is thought to enhance the effect of other antiemetics when used in combination (Dean et al., 2018). Bhakta and Goel (2017) pointed out that regardless of which antiemetics are recommended, the woman should be counselled as to the risks and benefits of treatment before proceeding. If the woman fails to respond to a single agent, combinations of agents should be used, as they have varying mechanisms and synergistic effects.

Table 15.1 gives an overview of the absorption, distribution, metabolism and excretion for various antiemetics.

243

Heartburn

Pathophysiology

Heartburn, or gastro-oesophageal reflux disease (GORD), is experienced by up to 80% of pregnant women and is described as a burning sensation in the throat or behind the sternum; it may also be associated with a bitter taste in the mouth as stomach acid is regurgitated into the throat or mouth (Bharj and Daniels, 2017). The competence of the lower oesophageal sphincter is affected by high levels of progesterone in pregnancy, making regurgitation more likely. In addition, from the beginning of the second trimester, the sphincter is displaced and the stomach is distorted, leading to a worsening of symptoms as the pregnancy progresses (Coad and Dunstall, 2011). Meteerattanapipat and Phupong (2017) suggested that atypical gastric emptying and reduced gut motility may also contribute to GORD.

Management

Non-pharmacological treatments

The aim of management of GORD is to provide relief of symptoms. Dietary and lifestyle advice should be given to pregnant women experiencing symptoms of GORD relating to maintaining a healthy weight as well as the avoidance of alcohol, caffeine and smoking as these are known to be gastric irritants and may worsen GORD (NICE, 2019). Referral should be offered to smoking cessation or weight management services if available. Smaller, more frequent meals and ensuring a 3–4-hour interval between meal consumption and lying down can help to alleviate symptoms of GORD. Sleeping in a propped-up position or raising the head of the bed 10–15 degrees can also lessen the impact of the condition (Bharj and Daniels, 2017). Where lifestyle and dietary alterations have not been effective, antacids may be considered.

Pharmacological treatments

Over-the-counter (OTC) antacids are safe to use in pregnancy and may also be prescribed by the GP or obstetrician. NICE (2017) recommends alginate-based antacids, such as Gaviscon Advance, as first-line treatment as the preparation is an oral suspension and the mechanism of action is not

Table 15.1   Absorption, distribution, metabolism and excretion of antiemetics.

Drug	Cyclizine	Metoclopramide	Ondansetron
Absorption	H1 blockers are well absorbed from the GI tract. Following oral administration effects develop within 30 minutes, are maximal within 1–2 hours and last, for cyclizine, for 4–6 hours	Metoclopramide is rapidly absorbed in the gastrointestinal tract with an absorption rate of about 84%. The bioavailability of the oral preparation is reported to be about 40.7%, but can range from 30% to 100%	Following oral administration, ondansetron is passively and completely absorbed from the gastrointestinal tract and undergoes first-pass metabolism. Bioavailability, following oral administration, is slightly enhanced by the presence of food but unaffected by antacids
Distribution	In healthy adult volunteers the administration of a single oral dose of 50 mg cyclizine resulted in a peak plasma concentration of approximately 70 ng/mL occurring at about 2 hours after drug administration. The plasma elimination half-life was approximately 20 hours	The volume of distribution of metoclopramide is approximately 3.5 L/kg. This implies a high level of tissue distribution. Metoclopramide crosses the placental barrier and can cause extrapyramidal symptoms in the fetus	The volume of distribution of ondansetron has been recorded as being approximately 160 L. Ondansetron is cleared from the systemic circulation predominantly by hepatic metabolism through multiple enzymatic pathways
Metabolism	Cyclizine is metabolised to its N-demethylated derivative, norcyclizine, which has little antihistaminic (H1) activity compared to cyclizine	Metabolism varies according to the individual. This drug is metabolised by cytochrome P450 enzymes in the liver	Ondansetron is cleared from the systemic circulation predominantly by hepatic metabolism through multiple enzymatic pathways. Following oral or IV administration, ondansetron is extensively metabolised and excreted in the urine and faeces
Excretion	After a single dose of 50 mg cyclizine given to a single adult male volunteer, urine collected over the following 24 hours contained less than 1% of the total dose administered	An average of 18–22% of a 10–20 mg dose was recovered as free drug within 3 days of administration	Less than 5% of the absorbed dose is excreted unchanged in the urine

Source: medicines.org.uk.

dependent upon absorption into the systemic circulation. Upon ingestion, the suspension reacts with gastric acid to rapidly form a raft of alginic acid gel with a near-neutral pH which floats on the stomach contents, effectively preventing gastro-oesophageal reflux for up to 4 hours and protecting the oesophagus from acid, pepsin and bile (Medicines.org, 2021).

Other antacids are based on magnesium, calcium and aluminium formulations. NICE (2017) advises that antacids containing magnesium can have a laxative effect and calcium-based antacids are associated with constipation. All antacids may affect the absorption of other medicines and may need to be taken at different times.

If these measures do not improve the condition, medications can be prescribed to treat heartburn in pregnancy, including proton pump inhibitors (PPIs). The PPI recommended for use in pregnancy is omeprazole. NICE (2017) states that the dosage should be the smallest effective dose to control symptoms, usually 10–20 mg once daily. Absorption of omeprazole takes place in the small intestine and is rapid, with peak plasma levels occurring approximately 1–2 hours after ingestion. Concomitant intake of food does not influence bioavailability; systemic bioavailability from a single oral dose of omeprazole is approximately 40%. After repeated daily administration, bioavailability increases to about 60%.

Distribution of omeprazole is 97% plasma protein bound. Omeprazole is completely metabolised by the cytochrome P450 system (CYP). (Cytochrome P450 is a superfamily of enzymes responsible for the bioactivation of medicines to more reactive intermediates. They are primarily found in liver cells but also located in cells throughout the body.)

The plasma elimination half-life of omeprazole is usually shorter than 1 hour both after single and repeated oral once-daily dosing. Omeprazole is eliminated from plasma between doses with no tendency for accumulation during once-daily administration. Almost 80% of an oral dose of omeprazole is excreted as metabolites in the urine, the remainder in the faeces, primarily originating from bile secretion.

Caution is advised for women with vitamin B12 deficiency, as omeprazole may reduce vitamin B12 absorption. Adverse effects of omeprazole include nausea, vomiting, constipation and diarrhoea. It is recommended for short-term use but as the cause of GORD in pregnancy is usually associated with normal physiological changes, the symptoms are expected to resolve following birth.

Current national guidance from NICE (2017) also recommends the use of H2 receptor antagonists to treat GORD by reducing gastric acid output. The H2 receptor antagonist recommended for use in pregnancy is ranitidine. It has been in use for many years, although its use in pregnancy has never been licensed. Ranitidine was withdrawn worldwide in late 2019 after it was found to have been contaminated with low levels of a carcinogenic called N-nitrosodimethylamine. The resulting shortage in this medicine led to an increase in the use of omeprazole despite ranitidine remaining part of national guidance at this time.

Controlling gastric acidity in labour

General anaesthesia carries a small risk of regurgitation and aspiration of stomach contents into the lungs. This can cause severe morbidity and, rarely, mortality, particularly if the contents of the stomach are acidic (Gyte and Richens, 2006). Women in normal labour may occasionally require general anaesthesia if labour becomes abnormal, for example if a caesarean section becomes necessary. As previously described, in late pregnancy, the stomach is displaced upwards by the gravid uterus, increasing intragastric pressure. With delayed gastric emptying at the onset of labour, a reduction in oesophageal sphincter tone and physiological oedema of the pharynx and larynx, intubation can be difficult in pregnant women if a general anaesthetic (GA) becomes necessary (Delgado et al., 2020). This risk can be further increased with the administration of parenteral opioids.

Table 15.2 gives an overview of absorption, distribution, metabolism and excretion for ranitidine and omeprazole.

In cases assessed as low risk, antacids or H2 antagonists are not indicated (NICE, 2014). When women in labour are assessed as at high risk of maternal or fetal complications that may require general anaesthesia, for example in cases of previous caesarean section or the use of IV oxytocin, women are frequently encouraged to consume only clear fluids and prophylactic oral ranitidine, or omeprazole is routinely administered to reduce stomach acid and decrease the risk of aspiration of gastric contents if a GA becomes necessary.

Episode of care

Tanya is a 30-year-old low-risk multigravida, pregnant with her third baby. She has attended the midwife-led clinic for her routine 34-week appointment. She reports that she has been feeling nausea as well as a burning sensation in her chest, particularly at night and after she has eaten a large meal.

The midwife checks Tanya's blood pressure, which is 100/60 mmHg, and undertakes urinalysis, which reveals no proteinuria or other abnormalities. The midwife asks Tanya if she has experienced headaches, oedema or visual disturbances in recent weeks, which Tanya denies. Her maternity notes show that her previous babies were born under midwifery-led care and she has no history of hypertension or pre-eclampsia. Having assessed Tanya's medical and obstetric history and ruled out other potential causes for her symptoms, the midwife diagnoses gastro-oesophageal reflux disease and advises Tanya that it is very common in the third trimester of pregnancy due to hormonal changes and the pressure of the baby growing in the uterus, but there are lifestyle and dietary changes that Tanya can make to prevent worsening and improve her symptoms.

The midwife advises Tanya to:

- eat a healthy diet and drink around 2 litres of fluid per day
- maintain her activity levels but not to commence vigorous exercise if she has not done so before
- try to find ways to relax and avoid stress and anxiety as this can exacerbate GORD symptoms
- avoid getting very full when she eats, as smaller, more frequent meals are less likely to cause the symptoms of GORD that she has been experiencing
- eat in an upright sitting position
- avoid eating very late or lying down within 3 hours following eating
- avoid smoking, alcohol, caffeine, very creamy, fatty or spicy foods as these can exacerbate GORD symptoms
- sleep with her head and shoulders propped up with pillows or raise the head of her bed by 10–20 cm.

The midwife advises Tanya that if these measures do not help, she can discuss her symptoms with a pharmacist who may advise over-the-counter antacids or alginates.

The midwife also advises Tanya to contact a midwife or her GP if she has persistent abdominal pain, is vomiting or her GORD symptoms do not improve so that further assessment and treatment with medication can be considered.

Table 15.2   Absorption, distribution, metabolism and excretion for ranitidine and omeprazole.

Drug	Ranitidine	Omeprazole
Absorption	Maximum plasma concentrations (300–550 ng/mL) occurred after 1–3 hours. Two distinct peaks or plateaux in the absorption phase result from reabsorption of drug excreted into the intestine. The absolute bioavailability of ranitidine is 50–60% and plasma concentrations increase proportionally with increasing dose up to 300 mg	Omeprazole is acid labile and is therefore administered orally as enteric-coated granules in hard-gelatin capsules. Absorption of omeprazole is rapid, with peak plasma levels occurring 1–2 hours after the dose. Absorption of omeprazole takes place in the small intestine and is usually completed within 3–6 hours. Concomitant intake of food has no influence on bioavailability. The systemic availability (bioavailability) from a single oral dose of omeprazole is approximately 40%. After repeated once-daily administration, bioavailability increases to about 60%
Distribution	Ranitidine is not extensively bound to plasma proteins (15%), but exhibits a large volume of distribution ranging from 96 to 142 L	The volume of distribution in healthy subjects is approximately 0.3 L/kg body weight. Omeprazole is 97% protein bound
Metabolism	Ranitidine is not extensively metabolised. The fraction of the dose recovered as metabolites is similar after both oral and IV dosing and includes 6% of the dose in urine as the N-oxide, 2% as the S-oxide, 2% as desmethylranitidine and 1–2% as the furoic acid analogue	Omeprazole is completely metabolised by the cytochrome P450 system (CYP). The major part of metabolism is dependent on the polymorphically expressed CYP 2C19 responsible for the formation of hydroxyomeprazole, the major metabolite in plasma

Table 15.2 (continued)

Drug	Ranitidine	Omeprazole
Excretion	Plasma concentrations decline biexponentially, with a terminal half-life of 2–3 hours. The major route of elimination is renal. After IV administration of 150 mg 3H-ranitidine, 98% of the dose was recovered, including 5% in faeces and 93% in urine. Less than 3% of the dose is excreted in bile. Renal clearance is approximately 500 mL/min, which exceeds glomerular filtration	The plasma elimination half-life of omeprazole is usually shorter than 1 hour after both single and repeated oral once-daily dosing. Omeprazole is completely eliminated from plasma between doses with no tendency for accumulation during once-daily administration. Almost 80% of an oral dose of omeprazole is excreted as metabolites in the urine, the remainder in the faeces, primarily originating from bile secretion

Source: medicines.org.uk.

Constipation

Constipation is defined as difficulty passing stool or a reduction in the frequency of bowel movements, in the absence of an underlying cause (Moriarty and Irving, 1992). The prevalence of constipation varies significantly and is reported as 11–44% (Rungsiprakarn et al., 2015). Excessive straining, discomfort, hard or lumpy stools, infrequency and a feeling of incomplete evacuation are all characteristics of constipation, and it is common in pregnancy as dietary changes and a reduction in physical activity are more likely (Rungsiprakarn et al., 2015). In addition, tone and motility of the gut are decreased under the influence of increased levels of progesterone, resulting in an increase in gut transit time. Relaxation of the colon also leads to increased water absorption and this frequently causes constipation. Constipation that predates the pregnancy may become worse as the pregnancy progresses, and the compressing effects of the growing uterus can also lead to a worsening of symptoms. Iron supplementation, low oral fluid intake and maternal anxiety also affect the severity of constipation (Rungsiprakarn et al., 2015).

Constipation is associated with a reduction in quality of life due to discomfort and a negative body image. It can also be a predisposing factor for haemorrhoids (Bharj and Daniels, 2017).

Management
Non-pharmacological treatments

Information should be given to women relating to increasing their oral fluid intake and eating a diet that is high in fibre. NICE (2020) also recommends giving advice to increase physical activity levels to prevent constipation in pregnancy. Bran and wheat fibre supplements can be useful in the management of constipation in pregnancy (Joint Formulary Committee, 2020). If dietary and lifestyle changes are ineffective or do not lead to an adequate improvement in symptoms, an oral laxative should be offered for short-term symptom relief.

Pharmacological treatments

The choice and dose of laxative offered are dependent upon the symptoms, severity, response to treatment and preferences of the pregnant woman. There are many laxative medications available, but not all are suitable during pregnancy.

- It is recommended that a bulk-forming laxative is offered as the first-line treatment. The typical bulk-forming laxative offered in pregnancy is ispaghula husk, Fybogel oral solution . Bulk-forming laxatives relieve constipation by increasing faecal mass to stimulate peristalsis. The onset of their action is up to 72 hours. Adequate oral fluid intake of approximately 2 litres per day should be maintained to avoid oesophageal or intestinal obstruction. Side-effects of ispaghula husk include abdominal distension and allergic reactions, including rhinitis and skin reactions.
- If stools remain hard, add or switch to an osmotic laxative. Generally, the osmotic laxative chosen in pregnancy is lactulose. Omotic laxatives act by increasing the amount of water in the large

intestine, either by retaining the fluid they are administered with or drawing fluid into the bowel from the body. The onset of action can be up to 48 hours, and there may be undesirable effects associated with its use, including abdominal pain, diarrhoea, nausea and flatulence.

- If stools are soft but there is difficulty in passing them, or a feeling of incomplete emptying of the bowel, a short course of a stimulant laxative may be commenced. Stimulant laxatives, such as senna and bisacodyl, increase gut motility. They are the least often prescribed laxative in pregnancy and should be used with caution as they have been known to stimulate uterine contractions. They are usually prescribed when conservative measures and other types of laxatives have been unsuccessful. Caution is advised if prescribed to breast-feeding mothers, as these types of stimulant laxatives can be excreted in breast milk (Verghese et al., 2015).
- In cases where there is still an inadequate response to treatment, glycerol suppositories may be considered. Faecal softeners, such as glycerol, act by decreasing surface tension and increasing penetration of intestinal fluid into the faecal mass. Glycerol suppositories have softening properties and may promote a bowel movement by lubricating and softening the stool.

Skills in practice

Administration of medicines per rectum (PR)

Preparation and equipment
The midwife should understand the anatomy of the rectum before administering PR medications. All equipment should be available and within reach, including:

- prescription
- prescribed medication (warmed enema or suppositories – checking expiry date)
- water-based lubricant
- clean trolley or tray
- personal protective equipment – non-sterile gloves, disposable apron
- clinical waste bag
- disposable incontinence pad
- clean bed sheet.

Procedure
- Confirm the woman's identity against her medication chart and ID bracelet.
- Explain the procedure to the woman to gain informed consent.
- Ask the woman to remove her underwear and assume a left lateral position, with both knees flexed and the right knee higher than the left. Provide privacy and maintain dignity.
- Place the disposable incontinence pad under the buttocks and cover the woman with the bed sheet.
- Wash and dry hands thoroughly.
- Put on the plastic apron and non-sterile gloves.
- Apply lubricant to the suppositories.
- Lift the sheet, exposing the only the buttocks.
- Gently lift the right buttock, inspecting the anal area for any abnormalities such as warts, haemorrhoids or fissures.
- Ask the woman to take a deep breath as this relaxes the sphincter.
- Communicate continuously, keeping in mind that the woman is facing away from you.
  - *Laxative suppositories*. Insert the suppository tapered end first (2–4 cm); laxative suppositories should be placed between the faeces and the rectal wall.
  - *Systemic suppositories*. Insert the suppository as per the manufacturer's instructions. The suppository should be in contact with the rectal wall.
  - *Enemas*. Ensure the enema is warmed to body temperature with the excess air expelled and the tubing lubricated. Insert the enema tubing (2–4 cm) and slowly advance. Squeeze the container until empty and then remove.

- Gently clean the woman with gauze or tissues, assist into a comfortable position and cover to maintain dignity.
- Encourage the woman to retain the suppositories or enema for at least 10–20 minutes.
- Ensure she has access to call bell, toilet or bedpan.
- Dispose of equipment in accordance with local guidelines.
- Wash hands.
- Document administration and effect and take appropriate action

Source: Johnson and Taylor, 2016.

Irritable bowel syndrome

Irritable bowel syndrome (IBS) is a relapsing, chronic, often lifelong disorder of the GI tract, with no identifiable biochemical or structural cause. Usual clinical features of IBS include abdominal pain, which may be related to changes in the frequency or form of stool. The abdominal pain may also be related to bloating and defaecation (NICE, 2020). Globally, IBS is thought to affect 5–20% of the general population, with women affected more than men. It is most often diagnosed between the ages of 20 and 30 years and the prevalence reduces with increasing age (NICE, 2020). The Rome IV criteria are frequently used to classify IBS into subtypes by identification of the prominent stool type.

249

- Diarrhoea predominant (IBS-D) – the most common subtype.
- Constipation predominant (IBS-C).
- Mixed, fluctuating between diarrhoea and constipation (IBS-M).
- Unclassified (IBS-U).

Moosavi et al. (2021) highlighted that research studies and guidelines relating to IBS in pregnancy are scarce, despite women of child-bearing age commonly being affected and that ovarian hormone changes may contribute to GI symptoms in pregnancy (About IBS, 2014).

Management

Multidisciplinary treatment of pregnant women with IBS is essential and the emphasis should be on education and dietary modifications. Pharmacological treatments that are considered safe in pregnancy can be utilised judiciously (Moosavi et al., 2021). However, concerns relating to lack of formal clinical trial data, adverse effects and the potential impact on fetal development lead many women to avoid or limit the use of drug therapies in pregnancy (About IBS, 2014).

Non-pharmacological treatments

- Education
- Relaxation therapy
- Cognitive behavioural therapy
- Regular physical activity

Dietary changes

- Increased dietary fibre for those with inadequate fibre intake (IBS-C).
- Reduction of insoluble fibre in diarrhoea-predominant IBS (IBS-D) such as wholemeal bread, high-fibre cereals and whole grains such as brown rice.
- Reduction of gas-producing foods to reduce abdominal discomfort.
- Reduction in caffeine, alcohol and carbonated drinks that can exacerbate symptoms.
- Adequate oral fluid intake – recommended amount is 2 litres per day.

Pharmacological treatments

Bulk-forming laxatives for the treatment of IBS-C – ispaghula husk also known as psyllium (see constipation treatments).

Antispasmodic medications

Antispasmodic medications can be classified as antimuscarinics and smooth muscle relaxants. Antimuscarinics (formerly called anticholinergics) such as hyoscine butylbromide (Buscopan®) reduce gut motility and are known to cross the placenta (Moosavi et al., 2021). They are generally avoided in pregnancy, but may be prescribed in cases where the benefit outweighs the risks.

Peppermint oil is a calcium channel antagonist that can cause smooth muscle relaxation. It also has anti-inflammatory antagonist properties that may alter gut sensitivity (Moosavi et al., 2021). Peppermint oil has been shown to significantly reduce abdominal pain, discomfort and IBS severity and in a large epidemiological study was not associated with low birthweight when used in the second and third trimesters. The side-effects of peppermint oil include heartburn, nausea and peppermint breath and taste (Moosavi et al., 2021).

Diarrhoea

IBS-D in the non-pregnant population is often managed with antidiarrhoeal medications such as loperamide (Imodium®), an opioid receptor antagonist that inhibits peristalsis. Studies have shown that it improves the consistency and decreases the frequency of stool, but does not alleviate abdominal discomfort, bloating and pain. Studies into its use in pregnancy are limited and suggest that it carries an increased risk of placenta praevia and caesarean section as well as congenital malformations such as hypospadias in babies (Moosavi et al., 2021). Avoidance of loperamide is recommended in pregnancy due to lack of information (Joint Formulary Committee, 2020).

Anorectal conditions

Anorectal conditions in pregnancy and the early postnatal period are common, affecting around 30–50% of women who are pregnant (Poskus et al., 2014). Symptoms frequently experienced include pain and discomfort, burning, anorectal itching, bleeding, mucous discharge and painful protrusions at the anus. The causes are most frequently identified as haemorrhoids or anal fissures. Anorectal conditions are uncommon in the first trimester, affecting only around 2% of pregnant women, and are most common in the third trimester and the immediate postnatal period (Poskus et al., 2014).

Perianal conditions in pregnancy are largely transient and mild. The aim of treatment for perianal conditions in pregnancy is to minimise symptoms, particularly pain relief. Corrective treatment is usually deferred until after the birth because once levels of circulating hormones return to normal, many symptoms will improve or resolve spontaneously (Bharj and Daniels, 2017).

Haemorrhoids

Haemorrhoids are defined as inflamed and swollen veins located around the anus and lower rectum. They are classified as:

- external haemorrhoids – which form under the skin around the anus
- internal haemorrhoids – which form in the lining of the anus and lower rectum.

The aetiology of haemorrhoids is, like many changes seen in pregnancy, thought to originate from the high levels of progesterone, leading to relaxation of the smooth muscle walls of veins. This is combined with increased intra-abdominal pressure from the gravid uterus and changes in the tone and position of the pelvic floor and sphincters (Bharj and Daniels, 2017). In addition to the physiological changes that increase the likelihood of haemorrhoids in pregnancy, BMI greater than 25 m², family or personal history of perianal disorders, constipation and multiparity were also shown to increase the risk (Poskus et al., 2014).

Anal fissures

An anal fissure is a small tear or ulcer that develops in the anal mucosa. The most common cause is constipation, when the stool is large or hard and causes trauma to the tissue. Anal fissure was identified as the most prevalent perianal condition in the second trimester in a study by Ferdinade et al. (2018).

Management

Non-pharmacological treatment

Constipation is known to be a significant cause of haemorrhoids in pregnancy and should be managed and treated as outlined previously. Women may be given advice about how to prevent and ease the discomfort of haemorrhoids, including avoiding standing for long periods, taking regular exercise to improve circulation, avoiding straining when passing a stool and using moist rather than dry toilet tissue for comfort.

Pharmacological treatment

If non-pharmacological treatments are ineffective, topical preparations with zinc oxide and bismuth, for example Anusol® or Germoloids® cream or ointment, may be used. Although these are widely available in supermarkets and pharmacies, it is recommended that products for pregnant women containing local anaesthetics or corticosteroids are prescribed by a clinician and only used if it is deemed that the benefit outweighs the risk (Joint Formulary Committee, 2020).

Creams and ointments, such as Anusol or Germoloids, are indicated for relief of symptoms in uncomplicated internal and external haemorrhoids and provide antiseptic, astringent and emollient properties. In addition to lidocaine hydrochloride, other ingredients include balsam of Peru, soft yellow paraffin, anhydrous lanolin, methyl salicylate, propylene glycol and menthol crystals.

Topical treatments containing local anaesthetics may be prescribed in cases where quality of life is being negatively affected by the condition. In such cases, caution must be exercised as local anaesthetics can be readily absorbed through the rectal mucosa and cause sensitisation of the anal skin. Lidocaine is the preferred topical anaesthetic as cinchocaine, tetracaine and pramocaine are more irritant (NICE, 2016). Treatments containing local anaesthetic should be limited in their duration of treatment as well as frequency of application.

Haemorrhoid treatments may also contain corticosteroids, such as Anusol Plus HC which includes lidocaine and hydrocortisone 2.5% and is available over the counter. However, prescription-only treatments containing more potent steroids, such as Scheriproct® ointment which is a combination of cinchocaine and prednisolone 0.2%, may be prescribed, but only in cases where quality of life is being negatively affected by the condition. Topical haemorrhoid treatments containing corticosteroids should only be prescribed for a maximum of 7 days and with instruction for minimal applications. Long-term use can lead to thinning of the skin as well as ulceration and permanent damage to the delicate tissues of the perianal area. Excessive or continuous use increases the risk of adrenal suppression and systemic corticosteroid effects (Joint Formulary Committee, 2020).

The postnatal period

Haemorrhoids and anal fissures are very common in the postnatal period and may be a continuation of issues encountered in the pregnancy. In addition to the risk factors discussed for haemorrhoids and anal fissures, they are also thought to be exacerbated postnatally by prolonged active pushing in the second stage of labour and a baby with a birthweight of greater than 3800 g (Poskus et al., 2014). Topical haemorrhoid treatments are safe to use in the postnatal period, with only small amounts found in breast milk, but these should be prescribed by a clinician as perineal trauma may mean topical agents are contraindicated.

Third- and fourth-degree tears

Prevention of constipation is vital for the successful healing of severe perineal trauma (Table 15.3). The Royal College of Obstetricians and Gynaecologists asserts that there is considerable variation in the use of antibiotics, laxatives and physiotherapy and local guidelines will take into consideration local facilities and services. Laxatives are recommended during the postoperative period following obstetric anal sphincter injury (OASI) as passage of a hard stool may disrupt the repair. Use of stool softeners such as lactulose is recommended for around 10 days after repair. The dose of lactulose should be titrated to keep the stool soft but not loose. The use of a combination of lactulose with ispaghula husk is not recommended as it carries an increased risk of incontinence (RCOG, 2015).

Table 15.3   Perineal trauma classification.

Classification	Structures involved
First-degree tear	Injury to perineal skin and/or vaginal mucosa
Second-degree tear	Injury to perineum involving perineal muscles but not the anal sphincter
Third-degree tear	Injury to perineum involving the anal sphincter complex (consisting of internal anal sphincter [IAS], external anal sphincter [EAS] and puborectalis muscle)
3A	Less than 50% of EAS thickness torn
3B	More than 50% of EAS thickness torn
3C	Both EAS and IAS torn
Fourth-degree tear	Injury to perineum involving the anal sphincter complex (EAS and IAS) and anorectal mucosa

Source: Based on RCOG (2015).

Episode of care

Rehana gave birth to her first baby, a boy, 3 days ago. He was born in the operating theatre, by forceps delivery after a prolonged second stage in which Rehana was actively pushing for 90 minutes. The obstetrician carried out an episiotomy during the procedure which extended to a third-degree tear, classified as 3B. Rehana had suffered from constipation before and during her pregnancy, for which she took Fybogel. She is an inpatient on the postnatal ward and has not opened her bowels since her baby was born. She wants to go home but is very anxious about going to the toilet as she is experiencing pain from her perineum and perianal area. The midwife has examined the perineum today and there are no signs of infection and the swelling has reduced since yesterday. There are obvious, large external haemorrhoids visible, and all vital signs are within normal parameters.

Rehana has been prescribed antibiotics for prevention of infection, paracetamol and ibuprofen for pain relief, ferrous sulfate to increase her iron levels and lactulose, a laxative, which she has been taking regularly since her baby was born. The midwife has given Rehana the following advice about how to care for her perineum and prevent constipation, which could cause damage to her sutured wound.

Aim to drink 2 litres of fluid per day.

- Increase dietary fibre by eating plenty of fruits and vegetables.
- Eat protein-rich foods, which will aid the healing process.
- Take ferrous sulfate with orange juice, for vitamin C to aid with the absorption of iron.
- Continue laxative for at least 10 days.
- Continue regular analgesia.
- Take gentle exercise and regular pelvic floor exercises.

Conclusion

The use of medications for gastrointestinal disorders in pregnancy should be the subject of a more detailed assessment of the risks, benefits and recommendations, due to the large number of women accessing treatments and the lack of clinical trial data involving pregnant women (Meyer et al., 2021).

This chapter has provided an overview of some common gastrointestinal disorders in the perinatal period as well as the medication that may be used in their treatment. Each disorder has been discussed with a description of the normal physiology of pregnancy and its impact on the gastro-intestinal system. Non-pharmacological interventions as well as medications commonly prescribed to treat gastrointestinal disorders have been considered in view of national guidance and evidence that supports their use.

Find out more

The following is a list of conditions associated with the gastrointestinal tract. Take some time and write notes about each of the conditions. Think about the medications that may be used in order to treat these conditions and be specific about the pharmacokinetics and pharmacodynamics. Remember to include aspects of patient care. If you are making notes about women you have offered care and support to, you must ensure that you have adhered to the rules of confidentiality.

The condition	Your notes
Haemolysis, elevated liver enzymes & low platelets (HELLP syndrome)	
Intrahepatic cholestasis of pregnancy (ICP)	
Crohn's cisease	
Ulcerative colitis	
Weight loss surgery Gastric band Sleeve gastrectomy Gastric bypass	

Glossary

Acute   Sudden onset of symptoms

Antispasmodics   Drugs that inhibit smooth muscle contraction in the gastrointestinal tract

Chronic   Symptoms occurring over a long period of time

Colon   The large intestine

Constipation   Reduced stool frequency, hard stools, difficulty passing stools or painful bowel movements

D2 antagonists   A class of medicines that block dopamine receptors

Dehydration   An excessive loss of fluids from the body

Disorder   A disturbance in regular or normal function. An abnormal condition

Gastric   Related to the stomach

H1 antagonists   A class of medicines that block the action of histamine

H2 blockers   A class of medicines that reduce the amount of acid the stomach produces

Laxatives   A class of medicines used to treat constipation

Motility   Movement of content within the gastrointestinal tract

Perineum   The area of the body between the anus and the vulva

Proton pump inhibitors (PPI)   The strongest class of drugs for inhibiting acid secretion in the stomach

Quality of life   Perception of ability to meet daily needs, physical activities, well-being

Sphincter   Ring of muscle that opens and closes and acts as a valve at various points of the GI tract

Test yourself

Now review your learning by completing the learning activities for this chapter at www.wiley.com/go/pharmacologyformidwives.

References

About IBS (2014) Pregnancy and irritable bowel syndrome. https://aboutibs.org/living-with-ibs/pregnancy-and-ibs/ (accessed February 2022).

Bharj, K., Daniels, L. (2017) Confirming pregnancy and care of the pregnant woman. In: McDonald, S., Johnson, G. (eds) *Mayes' Midwifery*, 15th edn, pp.503–536. Elsevier: Edinburgh.

Bhakta, A., Goel, R. (2017) Causes and treatment of nausea and vomiting. *Prescriber*, **28**: 17–23.

Coad, J., Dunstall, M. (2011) *Anatomy & Physiology for Midwives*, 3rd edn. Churchill Livingstone: London.

Dean, C., Bannigan, K., Marsden, J. (2018) Reviewing the effect of hyperemesis gravidarum on women's lives and mental health. *British Journal of Midwifery*, **26**(2) 10.12968/bjom.2018.26.2.109 (accessed February 2022).

Delgado, C., Ring, L., Mushambi, M. (2020) General anaesthesia in obstetrics. *BJA Education*, **20**(6): 201–207.

Electronic Medicines Compendium (2018) Cyclizine 50mg tablets. www.medicines.org.uk/emc/medicine/27036#gref (accessed February 2022).

Electronic Medicines Compendium (2021) Gaviscon Advance Peppermint Flavour Oral Suspension. www.medicines.org.uk/emc/product/6715/smpc#gref (accessed February 2022).

Ferdinande, K., Dorreman, Y., Roelens, K., Ceelen, W., De Looze, D. (2018) Anorectal symptoms during pregnancy and postpartum: a prospective cohort study. *Colorectal Disease*, **20**(12):1109–1116.

Gyte, G.M.L., Richens, Y. (2006) Routine prophylactic drugs in normal labour for reducing gastric aspiration and its effects. *Cochrane Database of Systematic Reviews*, **3**: CD005298.

Herman, T., Santos, C. (2020) *The First Pass Effect*. www.ncbi.nlm.nih.gov/books/NBK551679/ (accessed February 2022).

Jarvis, S., Nelson-Piercy, C. (2011) Management of nausea & vomiting in pregnancy. *British Medical Journal*, *342*: d3606.

Johnson, R., Taylor, W. (2016) *Skills for Midwifery Practice*, 4th edn. Elsevier: London.

Joint Formulary Committee (2020) *British National Formulary*, 80th edn. BMJ Group and Pharmaceutical Press: London.

Koren, G., Madjunkova, S., Maltepe, C. (2014) The protective effects of nausea and vomiting of pregnancy against adverse fetal outcome – a systematic review. *Reproductive Toxicology*, **47**: 77–80.

Meteerattanapipat, P., Phupong, V. (2017) Efficacy of alginate-based reflux suppressant and magnesium aluminium antacid gel for treatment of heartburn in pregnancy: a randomized double-blind controlled trial. *Scientific Reports*, **7**: 44830.

Meyer, A., Fermaut, M., Drouin, J., Carbonnel, F., Weill, A. (2021) Drug use for gastrointestinal symptoms during pregnancy: a French nationwide study 2010–2018. *PLoS One*, **16**(1): e0245854.

Moosavi, S., Pimentel, M., Wong, M., Rezaie, A. (2021) Irritable bowel syndrome in pregnancy. *American Journal of Gastroenterology*, **116**(3): 480–490.

Moriarty, K., Irving, M. (1992) ABC of colorectal diseases. *Constipation. British Medical Journal*, **304**: 1237–1240.

National Institute for Health and Care Excellence (2014) Indigestion, heartburn and reflux in adults. www.nice.org.uk/guidance/cg184/resources/indigestion-heartburn-and-reflux-in-adults-pdf-250345039813 (accessed February 2022).

National Institute for Health and Care Excellence (2016) Topical haemorrhoidal preparations. https://cks.nice.org.uk/topics/haemorrhoids/prescribing-information/topical-haemorrhoidal-preparations/ (accessed February 2022).

National Institute for Health and Care Excellence (2017) Dyspepsia – pregnancy associated. https://cks.nice.org.uk/topics/dyspepsia-pregnancy-associated/prescribing-information/antacids-alginates/ (accessed February 2022).

National Institute for Health and Care Excellence (2019) Gastro-oesophageal reflux disease and dyspepsia in adults: investigation and management. www.nice.org.uk/guidance/cg184 (accessed February 2022).

National Institute for Health and Care Excellence (2020) Irritable bowel syndrome. https://cks.nice.org.uk/topics/irritable-bowel-syndrome/ (accessed February 2022).

Peate, I., Evans, S. (2020) *Fundamentals of Anatomy and Physiology for Nursing and Healthcare Students*, 4th edn. John Wiley & Sons.

Poskus, T., Buzinskienė, D., Drasutiene, G. et al. (2014) Haemorrhoids and anal fissures during pregnancy and after childbirth: a prospective cohort study. *British Journal of Obstetrics and Gynaecology*, **121**(13): 1666–1171.

Royal College of Obstetricians and Gynaecologists (2015) The management of third- and fourth-degree perineal tears. www.rcog.org.uk/globalassets/documents/guidelines/gtg-29.pdf (accessed February 2022).

Royal College of Obstetricians and Gynaecologists (2016) The management of nausea and vomiting of pregnancy and hyperemesis gravidarum. www.rcog.org.uk/globalassets/documents/guidelines/green-top-guidelines /gtg69-hyperemesis.pdf (accessed February 2022).

Rungsiprakarn, P., Laopaiboon, M., Sangkomkamhang, U., Lumbiganon, P. & Pratt, J. (2015) Interventions for treating constipation in pregnancy. *Cochrane Database of Systematic Reviews*, **9**: CD011448.

Verghese, T., Futaba, K., Latthe, P. (2015) *Constipation in pregnancy. Obstetrician & Gynaecologist*, **17**: 111–115.

Further reading

If you would like to explore specific areas of gastrointestinal care and medications used in more depth, you may want to consult some of the following resources and organisations.

National Institute for Health and Care Excellence: www.nice.org.uk
Royal College of Obstetricians and Gynaecologists: www.rcog.org.uk
British Society of Gastroenterology: www.bsg.org.uk
British Pharmacological Society: www.bps.ac.uk

Chapter 16

Medications and nutritional supplementation

Cathy Ashwin

University of Nottingham, Nottingham, UK

Aim

The aim of this chapter is to explore the medications and nutritional supplementation that may be required during pregnancy.

Learning outcomes

After reading this chapter the reader will be able to:
- Demonstrate the importance of well-being in association with nutritional supplementation before and during pregnancy
- Recognise the signs and symptoms of underlying nutritional deficiencies and the implications for the woman and fetus
- Gain an understanding of women who may require greater support to maintain good health during pregnancy
- Acknowledge and respect women's choices.

Test your existing knowledge

- Describe the main nutritional deficiencies that may present before and during pregnancy.
- Recall situations from practice that included giving nutritional information to women; what prompted these discussions?
- Which women may be at greater risk during pregnancy due to diminished nutritional health?
- Discuss potential risks if women wish to self-medicate with non-licensed medication.
- What information would you give a woman who has been prescribed iron tablets for anaemia in pregnancy to aid efficacy?

Fundamentals of Pharmacology for Midwives, First Edition. Edited by Ian Peate and Cathy Hamilton.
© 2022 John Wiley & Sons Ltd. Published 2022 by John Wiley & Sons Ltd.
Companion website: www.wiley.com/go/pharmacologyformidwives

Introduction

Most pregnant women are healthy and require little if any medication during pregnancy, labour or birth. However, the complexities of women's health during pregnancy are increasing as more women are entering the childbirth continuum with additional needs, both physically and psychologically. Consequently, not all women begin pregnancy in an optimum state of health. A further consideration is a widening disparity in the nutritional well-being of women of low-income and other disadvantaged families (National Institute for Health and Care Excellence (NICE), 2008). Maintaining a state of optimal health before and during pregnancy has far-reaching effects on the health of the baby which continues throughout life (Ho et al., 2016).

The nutritional requirements for a healthy pregnancy include macronutrients, such as carbohydrate and fibre, protein, fats and essential fatty acids, and micronutrients including vitamins, minerals and trace elements. These needs can be met by eating a healthy diet and having a healthy lifestyle. However, this may not be possible for all women without additional medication and nutritional supplementation that will be discussed further within this chapter.

To be competent in promoting health, providing women with evidence-based information on nutrition, midwives and allied health professionals must have the appropriate knowledge and skills. Furthermore, NICE (2008) states that these competencies should be the responsibility of the professional bodies. The International Federation of Gynecology and Obstetrics (FIGO) states that healthcare promotion is key in achieving good nutritional health (Hanson et al., 2015). This chapter will focus on the most used medications and nutritional supplements required for some women around pregnancy, birth and the postnatal period.

257

Assessing the needs of the woman

Health promotion should be at the forefront of our minds during each encounter with a woman of child-bearing age and her needs must be considered. It is therefore important to listen to the woman and take a detailed history of her medical and social background. This will aid understanding of her physical health before making any decisions about her care. Midwives and other healthcare professionals will encounter women from all parts of society who have emigrated from other countries prior to the COVID-19 pandemic. We belong to an increasingly diverse population and with that comes many illnesses and deficiencies we may not be so familiar with. Even within a presumed health-conscious nation, nutritional deficiency is not uncommon. For example, women may present with a history of anorexia and other eating disorders, dieting, drug use or with known underlying illnesses such as sickle cell disease and digestive disorders. Full blood screening will help to diagnose essential nutrients missing from the woman's diet. Women with little or no income may not be consuming enough nutritious food to maintain healthy levels of micronutrients to support themselves and the developing fetus. The woman's health may already be compromised before the pregnancy and as such cannot keep up with the body's demands at this crucial time in their lives.

At the other end of the spectrum, a woman may be so focused on maintaining a healthy pregnancy that she may take extra supplements without consultation with a health professional. It is important to assess any over-the-counter supplements the woman may be already taking as there is a danger of overdose which could potentially be harmful for the woman and her developing fetus.

This chapter will focus initially on the two main supplementations that may be required in pregnancy: folic acid and iron. Other nutritional supplements will be discussed, including those that should be avoided as they may be detrimental if taken in excessive amounts.

Folic acid

Ideally, healthy lifestyle should be discussed with a health professional before embarking on a pregnancy. During this discussion, the benefits of taking folic acid preconceptually will be covered (Table 16.1).

Folic acid (folate) is a B vitamin which is particularly important before conception and up to 12 weeks gestation. It is currently the only recommended supplement in the UK. Although folic acid is recommended in other countries, the uptake of this supplementation is not always observed in

Table 16.1 Folic acid medication and associated pharmacokinetics, pharmacodynamics and common side-effects.

Indications	Prevention of neural tube defects
Dose and frequency	400 micrograms daily taken before conception and until week 12 of pregnancy. Women at high risk should take 5 mg daily before conception and until week 12 of pregnancy
Interactions (examples relevant in pregnancy)	Risk of toxicity increased when given with capecitabine or fluorouracil. Predicted to decrease concentration of phenytoin, fosphenytoin and phenobarbital. Sulfasalazine predicted to decrease absorption of folic acid
Side-effects	Abdominal distension, decreased appetite, flatulence, nausea, vitamin B12 deficiency exacerbated
Absorption (A)	Folic acid is absorbed predominantly from the proximal part of the small intestine
Distribution (D)	Folic acid very quickly appears in the blood, where it is bound to plasma proteins. The liver is the principal storage site of folate; it is also actively concentrated in the CSF
Metabolism (M)	The amounts of folic acid absorbed from normal diets are rapidly distributed in body tissues and about 4–5 micrograms is excreted in the urine daily
Excretion (E)	Larger amounts of folate are rapidly excreted in the urine. Folic acid is removed by haemodialysis. Folate is distributed into breast milk

Source: BNF (2020).

women from ethnic minority populations or those with a low level of education (Kinnunen et al., 2017). Folic acid supplementation helps prevent neural tube defects (NTD), primarily major defects of the brain (anecephaly) and the spine (spina bifida). The production of thymidine, a component of DNA, is reliant on folic acid (Jordan and McOwatt, 2010). Furthermore, Jordan and McOwatt (2010) state that a deficiency of folic acid impairs cell division and thus impacts upon the developing embryo and blood cells. Folic acid is found naturally in food and the body requires 600 micrograms per day. The current guidelines and recommendations are to supplement the diet with 400 micrograms of folic acid daily in the form of a tablet prior to embarking on a pregnancy. This recommendation is for all pregnant women regardless of current health status (NICE, 2008; ACOG, 2021; NHS, 2020; Public Health England, 2018).

In addition, NICE (2008) recommends that a higher dose of 5 mg of folic acid should be prescribed preconception and in early pregnancy if the woman, her partner or previous baby have had a neural tube defect. This dosage should also be prescribed if the woman is diabetic or if there is a family history of neural tube defects. Other reasons for the higher dosage of 5 mg include:

- those with malabsorption syndrome
- sickle cell anaemia
- taking antiepileptic medication (BNF, 2020).

Potential concerns and adverse effects

Folic acid is generally tolerated by most women without serious adverse concerns apart from discoloration of the urine. It can be beneficial in decreasing the risk of anaemia due to increased serum ferritin and haemoglobin levels. However, care must be taken when prescribing to women with a history of epilepsy as the risk of convulsions is increased. The cause of the increased risk of convulsions is the drug interaction between the antiepileptic drugs and folic acid (Baxter, 2006; Ali and Asadi-Pooya, 2015). Furthermore, Aronson (2015) argues that folic acid supplementation may also impact upon the effects of an unknown Vitamin B12 deficiency.

Clinical consideration

Folic acid should ideally be commenced at least 3 months pre-pregnancy as it may not be as effective in preventing neural tube defects after conception. The risks and benefits should be carefully considered before recommending folic acid to women with epilepsy.

Iron

Iron deficiency is a frequent phenomenon in pregnant women, affecting over 2 billion people worldwide (Pavord et al., 2012). Low levels of iron can lead to anaemia which does not immediately show clinical signs (Table 16.2). Women may initially complain of tiredness but may dismiss this as 'normal in pregnancy'. However, left untreated, the clinical signs and symptoms may become apparent and treatment is required (Box 16.1).

Pregnant women are initially tested for iron deficiency anaemia when a full blood test is taken at their first antenatal appointment and at intervals during the pregnancy.

The World Health Organization (WHO, 2001) definition of anaemia in pregnancy is Hb <11 g/L and postpartum Hb <10.0 g/L. Serum ferritin levels less than 15 micrograms/L indicate iron deficiency and treatment in pregnancy should commence with levels below 30 micrograms/L.

Risk to mother and fetus

259

The effects of iron deficiency anaemia cover a broad spectrum from tiredness and lack of concentration through to risk of infection, haemorrhage and maternal death. The effects on the fetus are less clear as it is relatively protected in utero. However, iron deficiency may be seen in the first 3 months of life and behavioural problems in later life.

Table 16.2   Iron medication (ferrous fumarate) and the associated pharmacokinetics, pharmacodynamics and common side-effects.

Indications	Iron deficiency anaemia
Dose and frequency	210 mg tablets taken 1–3 times/day
Interactions (examples relevant in pregnancy)	Oral antacids decrease the absorption of oral iron. Methyldopa decreases the effect of oral iron. Oral iron is predicted to decrease absorption of oral penicillamine and tetracycline. Oral zinc is predicted to decrease the efficacy of oral iron and vice versa
Side-effects	Common: constipation, diarrhoea, gastrointestinal discomfort Uncommon: vomiting Frequency unknown: decreased appetite, faeces discoloured
Monitoring requirements	Haemoglobin concentration should rise by about 100–200 g/100 mL per day. Treatment should be continued for 3 months after reaching normal levels
Absorption (A)	Iron absorption occurs mainly in the duodenum and upper jejunum
Distribution (D)	Transported through gastrointestinal mucosal cells directly into the blood, where it is immediately bound to a carrier protein, transferrin, and transported to the bone marrow for incorporation into haemoglobin. Iron is highly protein bound
Metabolism (M)	Liberated by the destruction of haemoglobin but is conserved and reused by the body
Excretion (E)	Healthy people lose very minute amounts of iron each day. This loss usually through nails, hair, faeces and urine. Other sources of loss are in bile and sweat

Source: BNF (2020); Global Library of Women (n.d.).

Box 16.1   Clinical signs and symptoms of iron deficiency anaemia

- Fatigue
- Pallor
- Weakness
- Headaches
- Palpitations
- Dizziness
- Dyspnoea
- Irritability
- Feeling colder than usual

Source: Robson et al. (2014).

Episode of care

Definition of anaemia

Hb <110 g/L in first trimester

Hb <105 g/L in second and third trimesters

Hb <100 g/L postpartum

Underlying causes of anaemia

Anaemia is a deficiency of iron in the body that can arise from several causes and may be solely the result of lack of iron in the diet. However, it may also be caused by several other problems and pre-existing conditions.

- Previous menorrhagia (heavy periods)
- Sickle cell disease
- Thalassaemia
- Inflammatory disorders affecting the absorption of iron in the gut, i.e. inflammatory bowel disease, coeliac disease or previous surgery
- Multiple pregnancy, i.e. twins, triplets
- Teenage pregnancy
- Short interval between pregnancies
- History of anaemia in previous pregnancies
- Pre or postpartum haemorrhage

Some of the causes may be easily managed with oral supplementation, but others may require more intense treatment.

Management of iron deficiency

Initially, pregnant women should be given dietary advice alongside any medications or iron supplementation required. The amount of iron needed increases as the pregnancy progresses and encouraging a healthy diet rich in iron will support these needs. For women in difficult circumstances or those experiencing nausea and vomiting, eating a healthy well-balanced diet rich in sources of iron will be problematic.

Oral iron preparations are the first choice in managing anaemia, such as ferrous fumarate, ferrous sulfate and ferrous gluconate. The dosage of these preparations, usually in tablet form, is 100–200 mg per day, preferably with orange juice but before eating. Orange juice provides a source of vitamin C which aids absorption of the iron. The absorption of iron is increased by approximately 30% if taken with 200 mg of vitamin C. However, Jordan and McOwatt (2010) suggest that large doses of vitamin C (over 1 g per day) can potentially cause diarrhoea and renal calculi (kidney stones). For women with sickle cell disease, an excessive intake of vitamin C could trigger a crisis.

Non-compliance in taking oral preparations of iron is reported by some women due to the discomfort of the side-effects experienced (Box 16.2). However, for the majority of women iron supplementation is tolerated well. Women should be advised to take the medication at bedtime as it may be more tolerable and if more than one dose per day is required then the doses should be at least 6–8 hours apart. Dosages should be reduced if severe side-effects such as abdominal cramps and vomiting are experienced as this would indicate iron toxicity (Jordan and McOwatt, 2010).

Women taking iron supplementation should be advised to avoid coffee and tea as they both reduce the absorption of iron. Multivitamin and mineral supplements may also reduce the absorption of iron, such as calcium, zinc, folic acid and vitamin E. Therefore, it is important to take a detailed history from the woman before prescribing iron to ensure optimum absorption and effect on the body.

If iron levels are low and the woman is unable to tolerate oral iron supplements then liquid preparations are available or parenteral iron can be considered for women with conditions such as ulcerative colitis who are unable to absorb iron orally.

Box 16.2   Side-effects of oral iron supplementation

- Nausea
- Vomiting
- Stomach cramps
- Heartburn
- Constipation
- Diarrhoea

Episode of care

Beata Luttik aged 29 attended the midwife clinic for the first time in this pregnancy, having moved to the UK recently. The midwife spent time taking a detailed history from Beata, including her medical and social situation. Beata was late booking with the midwife as she said she had not had time to attend, with three other children and her partner working away. On examination, Beata appeared to be around 19 weeks pregnant. During the conversation, Beata commented she felt very tired, had headaches and felt nauseous in the evening, saying it was because she had no time to rest. The midwife was not alerted to any serious previous medical history to account for the symptoms apart from heavy periods prior to becoming pregnant. No treatment or investigations were undertaken for the heavy periods. The midwife took a blood sample to check for any abnormalities that may be the cause of the tiredness. Beata had not been taking any medication as she could not afford to buy over-the-counter supplements and ate little healthy food as she felt her children should eat first. Her blood results indicated that Beata was anaemic and would require iron supplementation to increase her haemoglobin levels. Ferrous sulfate tablets 200 mg three times a day were prescribed, but not folic acid as the neural tube would now be developed in the fetus. The midwife also gave Beata dietary advice on the best foods to support healthy iron levels and signposted her to other agencies to advise on her financial situation. Beata took the advice and continued to see the midwife regularly through pregnancy and her iron levels were at a normal level at birth.

Women should be advised that the colour of their urine and stools will alter during iron therapy, with stools taking on a black colouring. This is normal but other causes of this colouring should be considered if the woman is experiencing other symptoms. This may be an indicator of gastrointestinal bleeding.

When prescribing iron, the health professional must advise on the safe storage of this supplement as an accidental overdose is dangerous and could be fatal for small children. If an overdose is taken then desferrioxamine can be administered within an intensive care setting, so prompt referral is essential and potentially life saving.

Vitamin D and calcium

Vitamin D is an essential vitamin required to maintain normal blood levels of calcium and phosphate. This is particularly important not only for bone health but for all cells in the body (WHO, 2004). Calcium is also important for building and maintaining bones and vitamin D aids the effective absorption of calcium and regulation of phosphate in the body. Exposure to sunlight is the most effective way of getting vitamin D into the body. It is fat soluble and can also be obtained from a diet rich in fish liver oils, fatty fish, mushrooms, red meat, liver and egg yolks (Palacios et al., 2019; NHS, 2020). However, some of these food sources are not recommended for pregnant women; for example, liver is also rich in vitamin A.

The WHO (2020) does not currently recommend routine supplementation to all pregnant women, only to those with a known deficiency. Lack of vitamin D is becoming a more recognised issue in contemporary society as an increasing number of the population are not exposed to enough sunlight. This is particularly evident in those with an indoor occupation and women from Middle Eastern and Asian countries who for cultural reasons may be more concealed by their clothing. Women who have a darker skin pigment such as African, African-Caribbean or south Asian are less able to synthesise vitamin D than women with a lighter skin colour (WHO, 2020; NHS, 2020). Women with a BMI over 30 are also at greater risk of vitamin D deficiency (Royal College of Obstetricians and Gynaecologists (RCOG), 2014).

In addition to general requirements for vitamin D in the body, a deficit may also have further implications for pregnancy in the development of pre-eclampsia, gestational diabetes mellitus (GDM), prematurity and low birthweight.

If a woman presents with a known vitamin D deficiency or limited exposure, then it is advisable to supplement the diet with 200 iu (5 micrograms) per day. The WHO (2020) also recommends calcium supplements for women with a poor diet lacking in calcium-rich foods. Low calcium levels in pregnancy weaken the bones and teeth of the woman and, as with vitamin D deficiencies, may predispose to pre-eclampsia. The recommended dose of calcium supplement is 1.5–2.0 g daily taken orally and divided into three separate doses (WHO, 2020).

Taking vitamin D over a long period of time or taking when not deficient may result in too much calcium in the body which in turn will weaken rather than strengthen bones, and also possibly cause damage to the heart and kidneys (NHS, 2020).

Clinical consideration

If prescribing both calcium and iron, the woman should be advised to take these supplements several hours apart as they may interact with each other.

Vitamin B12

As discussed within this chapter, all the essential vitamins and minerals play a vital role in the development and normal growth of the fetus. Vitamin B12 (cobalamin) contributes to the formation of red blood cells, neural tube and brain development (Gluckman et al., 2014; Perry and Lowndes, 2020). The causes of vitamin B12 deficiency include pernicious anaemia, which is dysfunction of the intestinal tract where there is inadequate absorption. A vegan or vegetarian diet may also contribute to a deficiency of this vitamin. Only newly absorbed vitamin B12 is concentrated in the placenta so it is important that the pregnant woman consumes a nutritious diet containing adequate amounts of the vitamin (Gluckman et al., 2014). Although pregnancy will demand a greater amount of vitamin B12, the RCOG does not recommend routine supplementation. In most cases of vitamin B12 deficiency in pregnancy, treatment is not considered essential (Perry and Lowndes, 2020).

Currently, there are no UK guidelines for the administration of vitamin B12 but if the woman's consultant considers it necessary for the well-being of mother and fetus then vitamin B12 would be recommended. The administration of vitamin B12 would comprise intramuscular hydroxocobalamin which is not currently recommended for use in pregnancy (ADVANZ Pharma, 2018); however, clinical evidence supports its use during pregnancy (UK Teratology Information Service (UKTIS), 2017).

Dosage for vitamin B12

The dosage for vitamin B12 deficiency is the same for pregnant women as it is for the general population, but consideration should be given to women with additional obstetric concerns. In the UK the recommendations are to administer intramuscular hydroxocobalamin 1 mg three times a week for 2 weeks initially, then 1 mg every 2–3 months thereafter. If there is neurological involvement then administer intramuscular hydroxocobalamin 1 mg daily on alternate days until improvement ceases, then a maintenance dose of 1 mg every 2 months (Innes, 2020; BNF, 2020).

To date, no adverse effects of the treatment have been recorded and no additional fetal monitoring has been recommended (Innes, 2020).

Vitamin A

There is some debate around the requirements of vitamin A during pregnancy and whether intake should be increased during this period. Vitamin A is necessary for healthy development of the fetus and fetal stores. It also supports maternal tissue growth (Williamson, 2006). The requirements increase during pregnancy, peaking in the third trimester. Suggestions that low levels of vitamin A in pregnancy can be responsible for maternal death, stillbirth, perinatal death, premature birth and low birthweight have been put forward. However, McCauley et al. (2015) undertook an extensive review of 19 studies and concluded that taking vitamin A supplements does not reduce the incidence of these adverse effects.

Healthy pregnant women should maintain adequate levels of vitamin A during pregnancy through diet alone. Vitamin A is found in eggs, dairy products, some fruit and leafy vegetables including carrots. Beta-carotene is found naturally in green and yellow vegetables which also produce vitamin A. Dairy products, liver and fish liver oils contain retinol and excessive consumption should be avoided in pregnancy as retinol may be toxic to the developing fetus. Vitamin A supplements should not be taken during pregnancy as excess can cause birth defects in the developing embryo (Expert Group on Vitamins and Minerals (EVM), 2003).

- A typical 100 g portion of animal liver may contain 13 000–40 000 micrograms of vitamin A, which is over 18 times the reference nutrient intake (RNI) for pregnant women.
- Foods to avoid: liver, liver products such as paté, liver sausage, cod liver oil, supplements containing high-dose vitamins.

However, although vitamin A supplementation is not recommended for healthy pregnant women, for others who do not have access to nutritious foodstuffs it should be considered. The WHO (2011) recommends vitamin A supplementation for women in countries where the deficiency is a major health concern, for example in some African and Asian populations. For this group of women, a deficiency in vitamin A is a cause of night blindness.

The WHO recommendation on vitamin A deficiency causing a severe public health problem is 'if ≥25% over of women in a population have a history of night blindness in their most recent pregnancy in the previous 3–5 years that ended in a live birth, or if ≥20% of pregnant women have a serum retinol level of <0.70 µmol/L' (WHO, 2011).

The recommended intake of vitamin A is 100 micrograms per day rising to 700 micrograms in the third trimester, thus allowing adequate maternal storage available to the fetus.

Vitamin B6

Vitamin B6 (pyrodxine) is a water-soluble vitamin responsible for the development and functioning of the nervous system. Salam et al. (2015) suggest it has also been accredited with higher Apgar scores and birthweights. In addition, some evidence has been presented that claims a reduction in pre-eclampsia and congenital malformations. However, the authors of the Cochrane review (Salam et al., 2015) concluded there was insufficient evidence to support the supplementation of vitamin B6 during pregnancy.

Foods containing vitamin B6 include fish, meat, poultry, starchy vegetables and non-citrus fruit. A deficiency in vitamin B6 is uncommon unless there is a deficiency of other B vitamins at the same time (WHO, 2019).

Vitamin B6 has been used to alleviate the symptoms of nausea in pregnancy with varying results. Studies by Wibowo et al. (2012) found that women experiencing nausea and vomiting in pregnancy had lower levels of vitamin B6. However, after treating with vitamin B6 supplementation there was little difference in the severity of the nausea and vomiting. Moreover, Hu et al. (2020), comparing the use of herbal remedies such as ginger, found little difference in outcomes for alleviating the distressing effects of nausea and vomiting in pregnancy. If vitamin B supplementation is given to reduce the symptoms of nausea in pregnancy, the recommended dosage would be 30–75 mg daily in divided doses (Matthews et al., 2015). Moreover, Hisaro et al. (2010) support the use of vitamin B as a supplement for women who do not respond well to iron therapy when anaemic.

Episode of care

Josie Simmons, aged 23, was seen at home by the midwife after a call from her anxious partner. He reported that Josie was acting 'strangely' and appeared confused over the last few hours. The couple had assumed Josie had a stomach bug as she had been feeling nauseous over the past few days and vomiting frequently. The pregnancy had just been confirmed and on checking dates, Josie was about 7 weeks pregnant and this was her second pregnancy after miscarrying earlier in the year. After talking to the couple, the midwife confirmed that Josie was suffering from hyperemesis gravidarum (severe pregnancy sickness) and had become very dehydrated, contributing to her confusion. The sickness had started quite suddenly and so the couple were shocked at how quickly her condition had deteriorated. The midwife arranged for Josie to be admitted to hospital for rehydration and assessment of her condition. As Josie had first thought she had a stomach bug, she did not consider trying any known remedies or supplements for the sickness. In hospital, Josie required intravenous therapy to rehydrate her body. Blood tests revealed that she was also deficient in iron, vitamins and minerals so was advised to take vitamin supplements to allow her body to provide essential nutrients to the developing fetus. Josie continued to suffer from hyperemesis gravidarum for most of the pregnancy but with support from her partner and the midwife, coped well with her situation and gave birth to a healthy baby.

Vitamin E

Women eating a healthy diet during pregnancy should have sufficient vitamin E and not require supplementation. Vegetable oils, cereals, nuts and some leafy green vegetables are the main sources of gaining vitamin E through diet. As previously discussed, women who have difficulty in consuming healthy foods may suffer from a deficiency. As a result, a woman may be at risk of developing pre-eclampsia and the baby may be born small for gestational age. If diet is not an immediate cause for the vitamin E deficiency, then other causes should be considered such as too much iron. Therefore, it is important to ascertain whether the woman is self-medicating on iron supplementation which may affect her vitamin E levels.

Rumbold et al. (2015) reviewed the evidence for vitamin E supplementation in pregnancy and concluded that this should not be recommended as outcomes for mother and baby were not improved. Furthermore, it also does not help prevent stillbirth or baby deaths but may increase the risk of abdominal pain and term prelabour rupture of membranes. One positive outcome to emerge from the review was that vitamin E supplementation in pregnancy reduced the risk of placental abruption (Rumbold et al., 2015). However, further research is required as it was not determined whether vitamin E alone was the reason for this reduction or if other supplementation such as vitamin C contributed to it.

Vitamin K

Vitamin K (phytomenadione) is required for blood clotting in the body and a deficiency may precipitate haemorrhage. It is a fat-soluble vitamin stored in the liver. The clotting factors vitamin K forms are II, VII, IX and X; in the liver it forms anticlotting factors protein C and protein S. It helps maintain healthy bones in adults and is essential for the fetus as it aids bone formation (Jordan and McOwatt, 2010). It is found mainly in green leafy vegetables, cereals and to a lesser extent in meat and dairy products. Bacterial flora in the intestine contributes to vitamin K in the body and provides a significant amount to the daily requirement (Food Standards Agency (FSA), 2003). However, if absorption is impaired then the risk of vitamin K deficiency is increased. A deficiency in vitamin K puts the pregnant woman at risk of haemorrhage as the prothrombin levels drop and as such, blood takes longer to clot.

Although vitamin K supplementation is not usually required during pregnancy, there are exceptions, including women with coeliac disease or cystic fibrosis where absorption of the vitamin is compromised or with blood disorders such as factor VII (Shahrook et al., 2018; FSA, 2003). Consideration should also be given to women who have undergone bariatric surgery who may have vitamin K and other deficiencies, including anaemia. The dose of vitamin K will vary according to the disease and as such should be assessed by a health professional prior to supplementation.

Newborn babies require vitamin K at birth to reduce the risk of bleeding and intracranial haemorrhage particularly if the baby is preterm. It is also known that babies do have a deficiency of vitamin K at birth. Nonetheless, Shahrook et al. (2018) concluded that high levels of vitamin K in mothers did not increase levels in babies due to obstructed placental transfer at birth.

Shahrook et al. (2018) when undertaking a systematic review of the literature found that taking drugs such heparin or carbamazepine can adversely affect the woman's ability to metabolise vitamin K. Therefore, women taking antiepileptic drugs should be assessed and if required, prescribed vitamin K from 36 weeks of pregnancy either orally or intramuscular.

Vitamin K is an essential vitamin to aid blood clotting and levels must be assessed in pregnant women with additional complex needs such as:
- coeliac disease
- cystic fibrosis
- blood clotting disorders
- epilepsy
- previous bariatric surgery.

Vitamin K is found in two forms: water soluble and fat soluble. Only the fat-soluble preparation is recommended for use in neonates, infants and late pregnancy as the water-soluble preparation is contraindicated (BNF, 2020).

Zinc

Zinc is a mineral with several qualities for maintaining healthy bodies, including protein synthesis, cellular division, antioxidant defences, wound healing and visual health (Mousa et al., 2019). It is mainly found in milk, meat, seafood and nuts; however, high-fibre diets and some cereals may impede the absorption of zinc in the body. The recommended daily intake of zinc for pregnant women is 15 mg/day but up to 82% of women consume far less than this (Black et al., 2008).

Zinc deficiency can be attributed to a poor diet and the effects are seen more widely in low-income countries. Of approximately half a million maternal and child deaths worldwide, zinc deficiency is thought to be a contributory factor for this high figure and in addition can be associated with impaired immunity, prolonged labour, preterm and post-term births, low birthweight and pregnancy-induced hypertension. Both Ota et al. (2015) and Chaffee and King (2012) observed that supplementing the diet with zinc reduced preterm birth by 14% but did not make a difference to neonatal death or maternal hypertension. Mousa et al. (2019) argue that poor nutrition and maternal infection generally in low-income countries were more likely to be the cause of prematurity rather than lack of adequate zinc supplementation in pregnancy.

Magnesium

Magnesium can be used to treat pre-eclampsia and can reduce the risk of preterm birth by inhibiting uterine contractions. During pregnancy, magnesium supplementation may also alleviate the problem of leg cramps. A deficiency of magnesium may contribute to high blood pressure in pregnancy (Brown and Wright, 2020).

Makrides et al. (2014) agree that magnesium supplementation may improve outcomes for mother and baby by reducing pre-eclampsia and fetal growth restriction and increasing birthweight. However, their review concluded that there was insufficient evidence to support the benefit of supplementation during pregnancy. Conversely, Brown and Wright (2020) argue that many women worldwide do have a deficiency of magnesium and do not consume the recommended average intake of 300 mg per day.

Healthy women consuming a varied diet including dairy products, bread, cereals, nuts and legumes are less affected than more disadvantaged women in society. Therefore, further research is recommended to assess whether magnesium supplementation would be beneficial to all women during pregnancy or just for those with additional dietary needs. If magnesium supplementation is recommended during pregnancy, the dose should not exceed 350 mg per day and should be taken in divided doses to minimise the possible side-effect of diarrhoea. Excessive amounts may result in hypotension or weakness of the muscles (Brown and Wright, 2020).

Herbal and integrative supplementation and therapies

There is a paucity of evidence to confirm the safe or unsafe use of herbal supplementation in pregnancy or of the effects when taken with other supplements. It is important to understand that 'natural' does not always mean 'safe'. However, Tiran (2012) argues that the information available is often conflicting and does not always represent sound evidence. Furthermore, Tiran (2012) explains that any substances not commercially prepared as drugs are termed 'natural remedies', including nutritional supplements and herbal teas. Two examples of these are raspberry leaf tea and tablets and ginger. Raspberry leaf supplements are often used during the third trimester to help tone the muscles of the uterus and prevent haemorrhage. The leaves contain iron and vitamins A, C, B, E and calcium, manganese and magnesium. Raspberry leaf preparations are believed to strengthen uterine muscle and aid uncomplicated births (Ferguson, 2009). The recommended dosage is one cup of tea a day or one 300–400 mg tablet at 32 weeks of pregnancy, increasing to 3–4 cups or 3–4 tablets/day at regular intervals. The use of raspberry leaf is not considered safe in certain situations (Box 16.3) and women would be advised against the supplementation.

Box 16.3   Contraindications against the use of raspberry leaf supplementation

- Planned caesarean section or previous caesarean section in last 2 years
- Previous premature labour
- Previous rapid labour
- Placenta praevia, low-lying placenta or vaginal bleeding
- Multiple/breech birth
- High blood pressure
- Contraindicated if taking metformin or antidepressants
- Medical conditions: epilepsy, heart conditions, blood-clotting disorders, breast or ovarian cancer, endometriosis, fibroids

Source: Tiran, 2014; Mills et al. (2006).

Tannins found in raspberry leaf reduce the absorption of atropine, codeine, ephedrine, pseudoephedrine and aminophylline and these should not be used together (Ferguson, 2009).

Ginger as a supplement to alleviate the symptoms of nausea and sickness is often used by women rather than conventional medication. However, women should be informed of other possible effects ginger may produce such as lowering blood pressure, dizziness and anticoagulant effects (particularly for women taking non-steroidal anti-inflammatory drugs –NSAIDs) (Shawahna and Taha, 2017). On balance, ginger would appear safe to use in pregnancy if dosage were no more than 2 g per day (Lamia et al., 2017).

Ginger supplements should be discontinued if there is a history of blood-clotting problems, threatened miscarriage and 2 weeks prior to a planned caesarean section (Tiran, 2012). Box 16.4 also lists considerations that may preclude the safe use of ginger during pregnancy.

Facchinetti et al. (2012) examined the use of herbal supplements by pregnant women in Italy and found that they were frequently used, the most common being almond oil, chamomile and fennel. Some women experienced side-effects such as skin rashes when using almond oil for stretch marks. In addition, the women using almond oil had a higher incidence of preterm birth. The reasons for this theory are manifold, including stimulating the uterus by massage or due to the active constituents in almond oil – vitamins C and E. Both these vitamins have been associated with adverse outcomes including perinatal mortality, premature birth and premature rupture of membranes (Facchinetti et al., 2012). Almond oil could also be responsible for both stimulating or delaying uterine contractions as it contains high levels of oleic and linoleic acids (precursors of prostaglandins).

Use of non-commercially produced supplements should be discussed fully with the woman so an informed decision can be made if taken in pregnancy.

Box 16.4   Precautions in supplementing with ginger

Avoid if taking:

- blood-thinning drugs
- aspirin
- high blood pressure medication
- similar herbal supplements.

Factors affecting adequate vitamin and mineral intake during pregnancy

Nutritional deficiencies preconceptually and during pregnancy can have far-reaching and costly outcomes for society and cause personal distress for parents. Therefore, it is vital that women are in the best of health during the childbirth continuum. The health professional caring for the woman is well placed to provide information and signpost to other agencies where there is a need. Although many women are well informed and seek out health information, others are not so fortunate or are misguided by current trends and health fads.

When considering the nutritional status of a pregnant women during a consultation, consider the following points that may lead you to suspect a nutritional deficiency

- Nausea /hyperemesis
- Eating disorders: anorexia, bulimia, obesity
- Coeliac/Crohn's disease
- Cystic fibrosis
- Blood disorders
- Smoking
- Alcohol
- Substance misuse
- Diets (vegan, vegetarian, slimming diets)
- Self-supplementing (recognised supplements, alternative/herbal preparations)
- Poverty

Factors affecting adequate dietary intake fall mainly into two groups: complex medical and social needs, with some cross-over for some women. The Red Flag box below highlights the points to consider when taking the medical and social history of a pregnant woman and how this may affect her nutritional status and that of the fetus.

Conclusion

Medications and nutritional supplementation in pregnancy can be a complex area with both positive and negative outcomes for mother and child. This chapter has explored supplementation and given a brief overview of some of these. The issues around safety and efficacy have been explored along with the importance of understanding the woman's medical and social background to ensure optimum nutritional status can be gained during pregnancy for the safety and well-being of both mother and child. It is paramount for all health professionals to give holistic care with shared decision making and be respectful of the woman's beliefs regarding her health.

Find out more

The following is a list of conditions associated with medication and nutritional supplements in pregnancy. Take some time and write notes about each of the conditions. Think about the medications that may be used in order to treat or reduce the risk of these conditions and be specific about the pharmacokinetics and pharmacodynamics. Remember to include aspects of patient care. If you are making notes about people you have offered care and support to, you must ensure that you have adhered to the rules of confidentiality.

The condition	Your notes
Neural tube defect	
Anaemia	
Night blindness	
Low prothrombin levels	
Gastric banding	

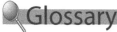

Glossary

Anorexia   Lack or loss of appetite for food

Bariatric surgery   Weight loss surgery such as a gastric bypass

Bulimia   Eating disorder characterised by eating and then purging

Coeliac disease   An immune condition in which eating gluten causes damage to the gut

Cystic fibrosis   Hereditary disease affecting lungs and digestive system

Endometriosis   A condition where tissue similar to the lining of the uterus grows in other places in the body

Factor VII   Protein produced in the liver, important for blood clotting

Gestational diabetes mellitus   High blood sugar that develops during pregnancy and usually resolves after birth

Hypotension   Low blood pressure

Iron deficiency anaemia   Low levels of iron in the blood so not enough red blood cells are produced

Malabsorption syndrome   Disorder in which the small intestine is unable to absorb adequate amounts of nutrients

Neural tube defect   A birth defect of the brain, spine or spinal cord which occurs in early pregnancy

Neonatal death   Death of a baby in the first 28 days of life

Placental abruption   Separation of the placenta from the uterus during pregnancy

Postpartum   Period after birth, not less than 10 days

Postterm birth   Birth after 42 weeks gestation

Pre-eclampsia   Condition affecting some pregnant women; symptoms include high blood pressure and proteinuria. This can progress to eclampsia, a serious and potentially life-threatening condition for mother and fetus

Prelabour rupture of membranes   The amniotic sac ruptures before labour commences

Preterm birth   A birth before 37completed weeks of gestation

Prothrombin   A protein made by the liver that aids clotting

Sickle cell anaemia   An inherited blood disorder causing lack of healthy red blood cells. The red blood cells are 'sickle shaped'

Thalassaemia   An inherited blood disorder in which the red blood cells are abnormally formed and are destroyed, causing severe anaemia

Trimester   One of three periods of pregnancy comprising week 1 to end of 12th week, week 13 to end of week 26 and week 27 to the end of pregnancy (usually 40 weeks)

Test yourself

Now review your learning by completing the learning activities for this chapter at www.wiley.com/go/pharmacologyformidwives.

References

ADVANZ Pharma (2018) Summary of Product Characteristics. Hydroxocobalamin 1mg/1ml solution for injection. www.medicines.org.uk/emc/product/6620/smpc#gref(accessed February 2022).

Ali, A., Asadi-Pooya, A. (2015) High dose folic acid supplementation in women with epilepsy: are we sure it is safe? *Seizure*, **27**: 51–53.

American College of Obstetrics and Gynecology (2021) Nutrition during pregnancy. www.acog.org/womens-health/faqs/nutrition-during-pregnancy?utm_source=redirect&utm_medium=web (accessed February 2022).

Aronson, J.K. (ed.) (2015) *Meyler's Side Effects of Drugs: The International Encyclopedia of Adverse Drug Reactions and Interactions*. Elsevier: New York.

Baxter, K. (2006) *Stockley's Drug Interactions*, 7th edn. Blackwell Science: Oxford.

Black, R.E., Allen, L.H., Bhutta, Z.A. et al.(2008). Maternal and child undernutrition: global and regional exposures and health consequences. *Lancet*, **371**: 243–260.

BNF (2020) *British National Formulary*. https://bnf.nice.org.uk/ (accessed February 2022).

Brown, B., Wright, C. (2020) Safety and efficacy of supplements in pregnancy. *Nutrition Reviews*, **78**: 813–826.

Chaffee, B.W., King, J.C. (2012) Effect of zinc supplementation on pregnancy and infant outcomes: a systematic review. *Paediatric and Perinatal Epidemiology*, **26**(suppl. 1): 118–137.

Expert Group on Vitamins and Minerals (2003) Safe Upper Levels for Vitamins and Minerals. cot.food.gov.uk/sites/default/files/vitmin2003.pdf (accessed February 2022).

Facchinetto, F., Pedrielli, G., Benoni, G. et al. (2012) Herbal supplements in pregnancy: unexpected results from a multicentre study. *Human Reproduction*, **27**(11): 3161–3167.

Ferguson, P. (2009) Raspberry leaves: turning over a new leaf for pregnancy. www.rcm.org.uk/news-views/rcm-opinion/raspberry-leaves-turning-over-a-new-leaf-for-pregnancy/#:~:text=The%20outcome%20indicated%20that%20raspberry,incidence%20of%20delivery%20by%20forceps (accessed February 2022).

Food Standards Agency (2003) Expert Group on Vitamins and Minerals. Part 2 Fat Soluble Vitamins. Webarchive. nationalarchives.gov.uk/201205180.154-161

Global Library of Women (n.d.) Ferrous sulfate. https://glowm.com/resources/glowm/cd/pages/drugs/f011.html (accessed February 2022).

Gluckman, P., Hanson, M., Seng, C.Y. et al. (eds) (2014) *Vitamin B$_{12}$ (cobalamin) in pregnancy and breastfeeding. In: Nutrition and Lifestyle for Pregnancy and Breastfeeding*. Oxford University Press: Oxford.

Hanson, M.A., Bardsley, A., De-Regil, L.M. et al. (2015) The International Federation of Gynecology and Obstetrics (FIGO) Recommendations on Adolescent, Preconception, and Maternal Nutrition: "Think Nutrition First." *International Journal of Gynecology and Obstetrics*, **131**(suppl. 4): S213–254.

Hisano, M., Suzuki, R., Sago, H. et al. (2010. Vitamin B6 deficiency and anemia in pregnancy. *European Journal of Clinical Nutrition*, **64**: 221–223.

Ho, A., Flynn, A.C., Pasupathy, D. (2016) Nutrition in pregnancy. *Obstetrics Gynaecology & Reproductive Medicine*, **26**(9). doi:10.1016/J.ORGM.2016.06.005.

Hu, Y., Amoah, A., Zhang, H. et al. (2020) Effect of ginger in the treatment of nausea and vomiting compared with vitamin B6 and placebo during pregnancy: a meta-analysis. *Journal of Maternal-Fetal & Neonatal Medicine*, **35**: 187–196.

Innes, A. (2020) How should vitamin B$_{12}$ deficiency in pregnancy be treated? www.sps.nhs.uk (accessed February 2022).

Jordan, S., McOwatt, R. (2010). Nutritional supplements in pregnancy: iron and folic acid. In: Jordan, S. (ed.) (2010) *Pharmacology for Midwives*, 2nd edn. Palgrave Macmillan: London.

Kinnunen, T.I., Sletner, L., Sommer, C., Post, M.C., Jeneum, A.K. (2017) Ethnic differences in folic acid supplement use in a population-based cohort of pregnant women in Norway. *BMC Pregnancy and Childbirth*, **17**: 143.

Lamia, A., Alfalasi, M., Abdelrahim, M., Al Kaabi, R. (2017) The efficacy of ginger for pregnancy-induced nausea and vomiting: a systematic review. *Journal of Natural Remedies*, **17**(2): 48–56.

Makrides, M., Crosby, D.D., Bain, E., Crowther, C. (2014) Magnesium supplementation in pregnancy. *Cochrane Database of Systematic Reviews*, **4**: CD000937.

Matthews, A., Haas, D.M., O'Mathuna, D.P. et al. (2015) Interventions for nausea and vomiting in early pregnancy. *Cochrane Database of Systematic Reviews*, **9**: CD007575.

McCauley, M.E., van den Broek, N., Dou, L., Othman, M. (2015) Vitamin A supplementation during pregnancy for maternal and newborn health outcomes. www.cochrane.org/CD008666/PREG_vitamin-supplementation-during-pregnancy-maternal-and-newborn-health-outcomes (accessed February 2022).

Mills, E., Duguoa, J-J., Perri, D., Koren, G. (2006) *Herbal Medicines in Pregnancy and Lactation: An Evidence-Based Approach*. Taylor and Francis: Oxford.

Mousa, A., Naqash, A., Lim, S. (2019) Macronutrient and micronutrient intake during pregnancy: an overview of recent evidence. *Nutrients*, **11**(2): 443.

NHS (2020)Vitamins, minerals and supplements in pregnancy. www.nhs.uk (accessed February 2022).

National Institute for Health and Care Excellence (2008) *Maternal and Child Nutrition*. NICE: London

Ota, E., Mori, R., Middleton, P. et al. (2015) Zinc supplementation for improving pregnancy and infant outcome. *Cochrane Database of Systematic Reviews*, **2**: CD000320.[

Palacios, C., Kostiuk, L.K., Peña-Rosas, J.P. (2019) Vitamin D supplementation for women during pregnancy. *Cochrane Database of Systematic Reviews*, **7**:CD008873.

Pavord, S., Myers, B., Robinson, S., Allard, S., Strong, J., Oppenheimer, C. (2012) UK guidelines on the management of iron deficiency in pregnancy. *British Journal of Haematology*, **156**: 588–600.

Perry, D.J., Lowndes, K. (2020) Blood disorders in pregnancy. In: Firth, J., Conlon, C., Cox, T. (eds) *Oxford Textbook of Medicine*, 6th edn. Oxford University Press: Oxford.

Public Health England (2018) Health matters: reproductive health and pregnancy planning. www.gov.uk/ government/publications/health-matters-reproductive-health-and-pregnancy-planning/health-matters-reproductive-health-and-pregnancy-planning (accessed February 2022).

Robson, E., Marshall, J.E., Doughty, R., McLean, M. (2014) Medical conditions of significance to midwifery practice. In: Marshall, J., Raynor, M. (eds) *Myles Textbook for Midwives*, 16th edn, pp.273–274. Churchill-Livingstone Elsevier: Edinburgh.

Royal College of Obstetricians and Gynaecologists (2014) Healthy eating and vitamin supplements in pregnancy. www.rcog.org.uk/ (accessed February 2022).

Rumbold, A., Ota, E., Hori, H., Miyazaki, C., Crowther, C.A. (2015) Vitamin E supplementation in pregnancy. *Cochrane Library Database of Systematic Reviews*, **9**: CD004069.

Salam, R.A., Zuberi, N.F., Bhutta, Z.A. (2015) Pyridoxine (vitamin B6) supplementation during pregnancy or labour for maternal and neonatal outcomes. *Cochrane Database of Systematic Reviews*, **6**: CD000179.

Shahrook, S., Ota, E., Hanada, N., Sawada, K., Mori, R. (2018) Vitamin K supplementation during pregnancy for improving outcomes: a systematic review and meta-analysis. *Scientific Reports*, **8**: 11459.

Shawahna, R., Taha, A. (2017) Which potential harms and benefits of using ginger in the management of nausea and vomiting of pregnancy should be addressed? A consensual study among pregnant women and gynecologists. *BMC Complementary and Alternative Medicine*, **17**: 204.

Tiran, D. (2012) Ginger to reduce nausea and vomiting during pregnancy. *Complementary Therapies in Clinical Practice*, **18**: 22–25.

Tiran, D. (2014) Raspberry leaf tea in pregnancy. www.expectancy.co.uk/Content/Media/PDFs/LEAFLET_ RASPBERRY_LEAF.pdf (accessed February 2022).

UK Teratology Information Service (2017) Vitamin B12 in Pregnancy. www.toxbase.org (accessed February 2022).

Wibowo, N., Purwosunu, Y., Sekizawa, A., Farina, A., Tambunan, V., Bardosono, S. (2012) Vitamin B6 supplementation in pregnant women with nausea and vomiting. *International Journal of Gynecology & Obstetrics*, **116**(3): 206–210.

Williamson, C.S. (2006) *Nutrition in Pregnancy. Briefing paper*. British Nutrition Foundation: London.

World Health Organization (2001) *Iron Deficiency Anaemia: Assessment, Prevention and Control*. World Health Organizatin: Geneva.

World Health Organization (2004) *Vitamin and Mineral Requirements in Human Nutrition*, 2nd edn. World Health Organization: Geneva.

World Health Organization (2011) *WHO Recommendations on Antenatal Care for a Positive Pregnancy Experience. Vitamin A Supplementation*. World Health Organization: Geneva.

World Health Organization (2019) Vitamin B supplementation during pregnancy. www.who.int (accessed February 2022).

World Health Organization (2020) *Antenatal Care Recommendations for a Positive Pregnancy Experience. Nutritional Interventions Update: Vitamin D Supplements During Pregnancy*. World Health Organization: Geneva.

Further reading

Allied and Complementary Medicine Database, Tetrology Information Service, Health Care Information Service of the British Library: www.bl.uk

Complementary and Natural Healthcare Council: http://cnhc.org.uk

NHS Start4life: www.nhs.uk/start4life

271

Chapter 17

Medications and the nervous system

Cathy Hamilton

University of Hertfordshire, Hatfield, UK

Aim

The aim of this chapter is to introduce the reader to medicines that may be required during pregnancy, childbirth and the postnatal period to treat women with common neurological conditions.

Learning outcomes

After reading this chapter the reader will:
- Recognise the role of the midwife in supporting women with common neurological conditions (namely headache, migraine and epilepsy) to make the most appropriate decisions about taking medication during pregnancy and the postnatal period
- Gain an understanding of the issues associated with taking antiepileptic drugs (AEDs) during pregnancy, including the types of drugs most commonly prescribed and the associated teratogenic risk
- Be aware of recommendations from the Mothers and Babies Reducing Risk through Audits and Confidential Enquiries across the UK Report (MBRRACE-UK) in relation to the management of care for women with epilepsy during pregnancy and the postnatal period
- Acknowledge and respect women's choice when deciding on the most appropriate medication options.

Test your existing knowledge

- How should a midwife support a woman suffering from recurring headaches during pregnancy?
- Why is it important that women with epilepsy continue to take their prescribed medication throughout pregnancy?
- Which AEDs are considered safe to take during pregnancy?
- A pregnant woman who experiences migraine headaches informs the midwife that she has visual disturbances. What plan of care should the midwife instigate?
- Why may a woman with epilepsy be at increased risk of having seizures when she becomes pregnant?

Fundamentals of Pharmacology for Midwives, First Edition. Edited by Ian Peate and Cathy Hamilton.
© 2022 John Wiley & Sons Ltd. Published 2022 by John Wiley & Sons Ltd.
Companion website: www.wiley.com/go/pharmacologyformidwives

Introduction

The nervous system is the body's main communicating and control system. It works in collaboration with the endocrine (hormonal) system to control bodily functions. The endocrine system normally responds in a slower, more sustained way with the nervous system producing a quicker but shorter-lived response (McErlean and Migliozzi, 2016). The two bodily systems work in tandem to achieve homeostasis. The nervous system consists of two parts: the central nervous system (CNS), comprising the brain and spinal cord, and the peripheral nervous system which carries sensory (afferent) nerve impulses to the CNS and motor (efferent) nerve impulses out of the CNS (McErlean and Migliozzi, 2016). Neurology is the medical science that studies the nervous system and disorders affecting it, including diagnosis and treatment.

Prescribing medication and managing specific treatment for pregnant women with a neurological condition such as epilepsy are beyond the scope of practice of the midwife. However, some neurological conditions are common within the general population and it is inevitable that midwives will be involved in the care of women with a neurological disorder who have been prescribed medication by a specialist medical practitioner. As stated in the Standards of Proficiency for Midwives (Nursing and Midwifery Council (NMC), 2019), at the point of registration midwives are required to demonstrate a knowledge and understanding of pharmacology, including being able to recognise the positive and adverse effects of medication across the continuum of care. This should include knowledge of side-effects as well as contraindications to pregnant women taking certain medicines and the teratogenic effect they may have on the developing fetus.

This chapter aims to introduce the reader to medication associated with the most commonly encountered neurological conditions, namely headache, migraine and epilepsy. It is acknowledged that there are numerous other neurological conditions which midwives may encounter during their career. However, it is beyond the scope of this chapter to include detailed information about more than these three conditions. Similarly, only the most common medications associated with the conditions have been included here. The reader is referred to the British National Formulary (BNF) (Joint Formulary Committee, 2021) for information about other relevant drugs, and a medical neurology textbook and/or midwifery textbook with a focus on medical disorders for more detailed information on the diagnosis, management and treatment of other neurological disorders such as multiple sclerosis, myasthenia gravis, Bell's palsy and cerebrovascular accident.

273

Episode of care

Selma is 30 weeks pregnant with her first baby and at her antenatal appointment, she informs her midwife that she is suffering from a severe, frontal headache. She states that prior to her pregnancy she was prone to recurring headaches, often during times of stress. She also says that she has not been sleeping well recently and thinks that her tiredness is making the pain worse. She asks her midwife if she can take any medication to relieve the pain as she is worried that anything she takes will adversely affect her baby.

How should the midwife manage care for Selma and what advice can be given?

Headache and migraine

Headache is a common neurological disorder, 'tension' headache being the type most frequently reported, affecting approximately 4% of the general population (Manzoni and Stovner, 2010). Tension headaches occur when the muscles in the scalp contract, leading to a feeling of pressure in the head and sometimes behind the eyes (McAuliffe et al., 2013). About one in three women will experience headaches during their pregnancy (Martin and Foley, 2005). Headaches may be related to stress and anxiety as well as fatigue, dehydration, excessive noise, lack of sleep, depression and staring at a computer or television screen for long periods (McAuliffe et al., 2013). Diagnosis is based on a careful history taking to exclude potentially serious secondary conditions such as subarachnoid haemorrhage, cerebral venous thrombosis, meningitis, intracranial lesions and, for pregnant women, pre-eclampsia (Jarvis et al., 2018). During pregnancy, secondary causes of headaches usually manifest after 12 weeks gestation and require urgent assessment (Robbins et al., 2015). Around two-thirds of headaches in pregnancy have no underlying pathology (Robbins et al., 2015).

Migraine is a chronic neurological condition that may be linked to genetics as it is known to occur in families. It is characterised by a moderate to severe throbbing headache sometimes accompanied by nausea and heightened sensitivity to light and/or sound (McAuliffe et al., 2013). Migraine headaches are caused by activation of trigeminal ganglia in the brain leading to the nerves supplying the meningeal blood vessels becoming inflamed, which causes the blood vessels to open and dilate (Duong et al., 2010).

During pregnancy, 50–75% of women with migraine will notice an improvement, particularly during the third trimester (Macgregor, 2012). Despite an improvement during pregnancy, migraines often return during the postpartum period and may even present for the first time in around 5% of women. For some women, the symptoms of migraine can become debilitating, causing dehydration, inadequate nutrition and stress, all of which have the potential to adversely affect the fetus. This leads women to seek medication to help relieve the distressing symptoms associated with the condition.

Treatment of headaches and migraine during pregnancy

Non-pharmacological strategies are initially recommended for pregnant women to see if symptoms can be relieved without resorting to medication (Jarvis et al., 2018). These include ensuring adequate hydration (unless contraindicated, at least 2 litres of water per day), reducing caffeine intake (bearing in mind that a sudden reduction in caffeine intake can lead to a so-called 'caffeine withdrawal' headache), not going for long periods without food, ensuring adequate sleep including the avoidance of mobile phone/screen use just before going to bed (Jarvis et al., 2018). Massage and meditation can help with relaxation and the use of ice packs may relieve the headache.

The first choice of medicine for both headaches and migraines during pregnancy is paracetamol (Bhatia et al., 2020; UKTIS, 2016). Paracetamol is classified as a General Sales List medicine and as such is readily available to the general public, allowing women to self-medicate without requiring a prescription. It is important therefore that midwives remind women to follow the guidance in relation to taking paracetamol and to ensure that no more than six 500 mg tablets are taken in any 24-hour period. If pregnant women feel they need to take paracetamol regularly for recurring headache then this suggests the possibility of a potentially serious underlying cause and the woman should be encouraged to consult a doctor as further investigation may be required to ascertain the cause of the pain.

Opiates (such as codeine) should not normally be prescribed to treat pain associated with headache or migraine during pregnancy because they can increase nausea, decrease gastric motility and cause constipation. Prolonged use of opiates can also lead to what is known as 'overuse headache' (Jarvis et al., 2018). Non-steroidal anti-inflammatory drugs (NSAIDs) such as ibuprofen can be used during pregnancy although safety data is not so prevalent as it is for paracetamol. Ibuprofen use should be avoided in the third trimester because studies have shown that it can increase the risk of premature closure of the ductus arteriosus in the fetus (Flint et al., 2016; Bhatia et al., 2020).

If migraine is accompanied by nausea and vomiting, antiemetics such as prochlorperazine, ondansetron and metoclopramide are safe to use during pregnancy (Koren, 2017). Metoclopramide, however, should not be used on a long-term basis due to the risk of developing mobility disorders such as involuntary tremors and muscle contractions. These are referred to as extrapyramidal side-effects (Koren, 2017).

Serotonin receptor agonists (known as triptans) are effective in the treatment of migraine although they do not prevent migraine attacks (Spielmann et al., 2018). Triptans relieve a migraine headache by binding to the serotonin 5-HT receptors, leading to constriction of the blood vessels and prevention of nerve inflammation (Duong et al., 2010). Well-established triptan medicines, for example sumatriptan, are safe to take even during the first trimester as no teratogenic effect has been identified (UKTIS, 2016).

For recurrent migraine, beta-blockers such as propranolol 10–40 mg three times a day can be considered as a preventive measure (Macgregor, 2012). Early research suggested that use of beta-blockers during pregnancy led to an increased risk of intrauterine growth restriction (Sibai et al.,

1987) but more recent studies highlight that this finding may have been associated with high-dosage beta-blockers and does not appear to be a significant issue if lower doses are prescribed. The risk of congenital abnormalities has not been found to be increased in women taking beta-blockers during pregnancy (Bergman et al., 2017).

Jarvis et al. (2018) suggest that low-dose aspirin (75 mg once daily) can be used to prevent migraines and highlight a randomised controlled trial which demonstrated that it can be used safely until 36 weeks gestation (Rolinik et al., 2017). Despite this, the National Institute for Health and Care Excellence (NICE, 2015) does not recommend taking aspirin to prevent migraine in pregnant or breast-feeding women.

A group of medicines known as ergot alkaloids (for example, ergotamine) may be used to treat the throbbing headache associated with migraine in the non-pregnant patient. These drugs work by narrowing the blood vessels in the brain and altering the way that blood flows through the brain. They have, however, been shown to have a teratogenic effect during pregnancy (Wells et al., 2016; Goadsby et al., 2008).

Feverfew is a herbal remedy used by some people to reduce the frequency of migraines although its value is questioned (NICE, 2015). However, as it also contains ergot alkaloids it is contraindicated during pregnancy and women should be advised to avoid using it (Migraine Trust, 2021; NICE, 2015).

Antiepileptic drugs (AEDs) can be used to treat migraine but as they have a known teratogenic effect, they should not be used during pregnancy when other safer medication is available (Wells et al., 2016). The teratogenic effects associated with AEDs will be discussed later in the chapter.

Epilepsy

Epilepsy is a common neurological condition characterised by at least two or more recurrent sei-zures (colloquially called 'fits') (McAuliffe et al., 2013). The seizures are caused by a sudden but temporary burst of electrical activity in the brain leading to disruption of the normal communication pathways between brain cells. There are many possible causes for epilepsy ranging from brain injury to hereditary factors but often no specific cause can be found. It affects about 1 in 100 people (Epilepsy Society, 2019a) and this includes between 0.5–1% of pregnant women (Kapoor and Wallace, 2014). Epilepsy is the most common neurological condition seen in pregnant women (Morley, 2018).

The type of seizure evoked is dependent on the site and extent of the excessive electrical activity within the brain. Seizures can be classified into two specific categories: focal (previously called partial), affecting one specific area of the brain, and generalised, affecting the whole brain (Epilepsy Action, 2019).

Sudden unexpected death in epilepsy (SUDEP) affects 500 people a year and is an unexplained phenomenon whereby a person with epilepsy dies suddenly for no obvious physiological reason. The biggest risk factor in this condition is epilepsy associated with uncontrolled generalised tonic clonic seizures. This is why it is so important that women with epilepsy receive the required treat-ment to prevent seizures.

Epilepsy and maternal mortality

The most recent report into maternal deaths during pregnancy produced by Mothers and Babies: Reducing Risk through Audits and Confidential Enquiries across the United Kingdom (MBRRACE-UK) (Knight et al., 2020) demonstrated a significant increase in the number of women who died from conditions relating to epilepsy during and up to a year after the end of pregnancy in the UK and Ireland from 2016 to 2018. During this period, 22 women died from epilepsy-related causes com-pared with 13 deaths in the previous report (2013–2015). The latest report highlighted concern that 18 women died from SUDEP compared to eight women previously. A further two women died following status epilepticus and two drowned. Of the 19 women for whom information was avail-able, four were not taking medication to control their epilepsy and eight out of 15 were taking lamotrigine, an AED which is known to be less effective during pregnancy when serum levels fall following the physiological haemodilution of pregnancy (Knight et al., 2020). A small number of the women who died had preconceptual counselling relating to their epilepsy; most had uncontrolled epilepsy and less than half received a specialist review from a neurologist (Knight et al., 2020).

Recommendations have been made about the care of women with epilepsy before, during and following pregnancy and this includes the importance of appropriate specialist input into their care and ensuring that medication is taken appropriately to control seizures and prevent SUDEP (Knight et al., 2020) (Figure 17.1).

Whilst it is acknowledged that responsibility for the medical care of women with epilepsy lies with the neurologist working in collaboration with the obstetrician, the midwife plays an important role in ensuring that women get the information and specialist care they need to make informed choices about their epilepsy treatment during pregnancy and beyond. This relies on midwives having up-to-date knowledge of medication options (Hugill and Meredith, 2017).

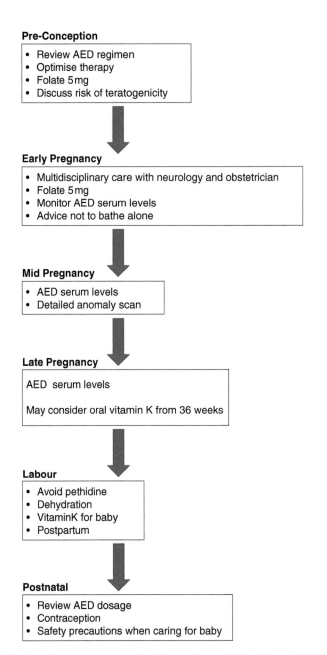

Pre-Conception
- Review AED regimen
- Optimise therapy
- Folate 5 mg
- Discuss risk of teratogenicity

Early Pregnancy
- Multidisciplinary care with neurology and obstetrician
- Folate 5 mg
- Monitor AED serum levels
- Advice not to bathe alone

Mid Pregnancy
- AED serum levels
- Detailed anomaly scan

Late Pregnancy

AED serum levels

May consider oral vitamin K from 36 weeks

Labour
- Avoid pethidine
- Dehydration
- VitaminK for baby
- Postpartum

Postnatal
- Review AED dosage
- Contraception
- Safety precautions when caring for baby

Figure 17.1 Algorithm for the management of epilepsy. *Source*: McAuliffe et al. (2013)/with permission of John Wiley & Sons.

Episode of care

A woman had increased seizures following the birth of her first baby. She was advised at the neurology clinic to increase her dose of the antiepileptic drug lamotrigine. She became pregnant again very soon after the birth and returned to her GP in early pregnancy reporting a further increase in seizures. Her GP advised her to contact the neurology clinic and book antenatal care with the midwife. She died from SUDEP 2 weeks later. It is not known if she ever contacted either her midwife or the neurology clinic (based on Knight et al., 2020).

Antiepileptic drugs

The treatment of epilepsy involves the careful selection of AEDs to control the severity of the seizures experienced. The aim of AED therapy is to use the lowest effective dose, balancing control of seizures against the severity of any side-effects from the medication (Hugill and Meredith, 2017).

The pharmacology of individual and combined AEDs is not always predictable because branded and generic versions of the same AED can have different effects on different individuals (Hugill and Meredith, 2017; Joint Formulary Committee, 2021). In AED therapy, the general rule is to begin with a single drug (monotherapy) and if this proves to be ineffective in controlling seizures, an alternative drug is tried. If seizures remain uncontrolled then a cocktail of different drugs is used (polytherapy). The AED regimen will require regular review through various life changes including puberty, pregnancy, menopause and the ageing process (Hugill and Meredith, 2017).

Some AEDs are enzyme inducing, which means that they may increase the levels of enzymes in the body that then break down hormones. This may influence contraceptive choices for women taking enzyme-inducing AEDs as they will affect the hormones contained in contraceptives, leading them to break down more rapidly and so potentially reducing the effectiveness of the contraceptive in preventing pregnancy. Zhao et al. (2014) state that prescribing AEDs for women requires greater consideration than it does for men as their menstrual cycles and contraceptive choices have the potential to affect both the efficacy of the AED and some hormonal contraceptive methods.

Antiepileptic drugs and how they work

Antiepileptic drugs cannot cure epilepsy or treat the reason for the condition. They are prescribed to prevent seizures. Except for emergency medication used to control status epilepticus, most AEDS do not stop a seizure once it has started (Epilepsy Society, 2019b).

Antiepileptic drugs make the brain less likely to have seizures by reducing the level of electrical activity within the neurones. There are various types of AED and they have differing effects on brain cells. It is still not completely understood how they all work. We do know that AEDs prevent seizures by targeting specific areas in the brain. For example, they may affect neurotransmitters responsible for transmitting messages within the brain or they may attach themselves to the surface of neurones, so altering how ions move in and out of the neurones (Alarcón and Valentín, 2012).

Some AEDs (for example, phenytoin, lamotrigine and carbamazepine) work on the sodium channels of neurones. They bind to the sodium ion channels and this stops the channel from becoming activated. This prevents neurones from firing repetitive electrical discharges via sodium ions moving through the sodium channels (Alarcón and Valentín, 2012; Epilepsy Society, 2020).

Other AEDs (for example, zonisamide and topiramate) work by blocking calcium ion channels. Calcium channels are involved specifically in sending a message from one neurone to another by influencing the release of neurotransmitters across the gap or synapse where neurones meet. Calcium channels also influence the movement of calcium ions into the receiving neurone. By blocking calcium channels, the AED prevents messages being sent across the synaptic gap from one neurone to another by either preventing the release of neurotransmitters or preventing calcium from entering the next neurone (Alarcón and Valentín, 2012; Epilepsy Society, 2020).

Gamma-amino butyric acid (GABA) is an inhibitory neurotransmitter in the brain which prevents electrical messages from being transmitted around the brain. It works by assisting chloride ions to move into neurones which then affects the resting membrane potential of the cell, making it difficult for the neurone to transmit messages (Epilepsy Society, 2020; Doyle et al., 2016). Certain AEDs (for example, gabapentin) work on the GABA system by increasing the movement of chloride into cells,

277

so increasing the 'switch off' of messages within the brain. They are known as 'agonists' as they assist another substance to work more effectively. Gabapentin works by increasing the amount of GABA in the brain while other AEDS such as sodium valproate and vigabatrin work by reducing the breakdown of GABA (Doyle et al., 2016).

Benzodiazepines (for example, clonazepam and clobazam) work by increasing how frequently GABA receptors open while barbiturates (such as phenobarbitone) increase the amount of time that the receptors are open for. Whether the AED increases the production of GABA, reduces its breakdown or increases its movement through the neurones, the cumulative effect is that the level of GABA in the brain is increased. Higher GABA levels inhibit the transmission of electrical messages through the brain, leading to a reduction in the electrical activity that is known to cause seizures (Doyle et al., 2016).

Glutamate, an amino acid, is an excitatory neurotransmitter in the brain. The movement of sodium and calcium ions into cells and potassium out of cells is assisted by glutamate as it binds to neuroreceptors situated in the cell membrane. AEDs such as perampanel works on glutamate receptors while others, such as topiramate, work on glutamate receptors and other targets (Epilepsy Society, 2020).

The National Institute for Health and Care Excellence (2020) recommends dividing AED choices into seizure types to assist prescribers in their decision making regarding the most appropriate treatment for an individual depending on how their condition manifests. There are about 25 AEDs currently licensed for use in the UK (Epilepsy Society, 2019).

Antiepileptic drugs which may be commonly prescribed in women of child-bearing age and in pregnancy include the following.

- Levetiracetam (Keppra®)
- Clobazam (Frisium®)
- Lamotrigine (Lamictal®)

Antiepileptic drugs commonly avoided in pregnancy include the following.

- Sodium valproate (Epilim®)
- Carbamazepine (Tegretol®).
- Phenytoin (Epanutin®)

It is beyond the scope of this chapter to provide a detailed description of all the AEDs currently in use. However, four of the most commonly used will be described. Two of these are not usually prescribed during pregnancy due to their high teratogenic risk. However, the midwife needs to be aware of these drugs so that questions can be asked and further specialist guidance sought if a pregnant woman has been prescribed them.

Carbamazepine

Carbamazepine (marketed as Tegretol®) is one of the older AEDs and is used to treat tonic clonic seizures. It exerts its therapeutic action by blocking sodium channels in the neurones, leading to the conducting nerve remaining inactive. Usually given orally, it is absorbed in the gastrointestinal tract and metabolised in the liver. Side-effects may include drowsiness, skin rashes, dizziness, dry mouth, fatigue and gastrointestinal disturbance (BNF, 2021a). Studies by Peterson et al. (2017) and Bromley et al. (2017) give a major congenital malformation (MCM) risk associated with carbamazepine use during pregnancy of 3.3–3.7%. This means that other AEDs carrying a lower MCM risk are likely to be the first choice for use during pregnancy. Carbamazepine is excreted in breast milk, but the amount is negligible and too small to cause harm to the baby (Joint Formulary Committee, 2021).

Sodium valproate

Sodium valproate is an older AED particularly effective in preventing tonic clonic, absence and myoclonic seizures (Crouch and Chapelhow, 2008). Valproate medications (marketed as Epilim®, Depakote® and Valpal®) are also licensed for use in treatment of bipolar disorder and prescribed, albeit off licence, for the prevention of migraines.

Sodium valproate is contraindicated in women of child-bearing age (NICE, 2020; MHRA, 2018). This is due to the high risk of MCM (10.9%) (Bromley et al., 2017) in addition to a 30–40% risk of neurodevelopmental disorders in the child (Bromley, 2016). Some women of child-bearing age may continue to be prescribed sodium valproate if it is effective in managing their epilepsy provided conditions of the Pregnancy Prevention Programme are met (Morley, 2018; MHRA, 2018).

Clinical consideration

Valproate Pregnancy Prevention Programme Checklist
All female patients taking valproate medicines:

- understand the risks associated with valproate use during pregnancy ☑
- have signed a risk acknowledgement form ☑
- are taking effective contraception if required ☑
- will see their neurology specialist once a year ☑

Source: Based on MHRA (2018).

Clinical consideration

If a woman is taking valproate and thinks she might be pregnant, she is advised to contact her doctor. She should not stop taking the medicine without medical guidance. If women have questions or concerns about taking valproate during pregnancy, midwives should advise them to discuss these with their doctor, pharmacist, obstetrician or neurology specialist. They can also contact a patient support network such as Epilepsy Action (www.epilepsy.org.uk/), the Epilepsy Society (https://epilepsysociety.org.uk/) or Mind (www.mind.org.uk/).

If a child has been affected by valproate medicines, families can also contact a support network such as the Organisation for Anti-Convulsant Syndrome (OACS) (www.oacscharity.org/), the Independent Fetal Anti-Convulsant Trust (IN-FACT) (https://infactuk.com/about-in-fact/) and the Fetal Anti-Convulsant Syndrome Association (FACSA) (https://facsassociation.org/).

Source: MHRA (2018).

Lamotrigine
Lamotrigine is one of the newer AEDs and works by blocking the release of two neurotransmitters, glutamate and aspartate, in the neurones of the brain. It is known to be effective in the treatment of focal and tonic clonic seizures (Joint Formulary Committee, 2021). Studies have shown that the risk of MCM is low, at 2.3% (Bromley et al., 2017) (Table 17.1).

Levetiracetam
Levetiracetam is another new AED and is used for the treatment of focal seizures (Joint Formulary Committee, 2021). It is believed to work by interfering with neurotransmitter release at the synaptic gap although the exact mode of action remains unclear (Lewis, 2014). Side-effects include skin rashes, dizziness, nausea, headache and loss of appetite although again it is usually well tolerated. It has also been found to exacerbate depression in women who are prone to this (Table 17.2).

Preconceptual issues for women taking AEDs
It is recommended that all women prescribed AEDs receive preconceptual counselling at least 1–2 years before becoming pregnancy (Fiest et al., 2017; Knight et al., 2020). This may come in the form of verbal and written information on the risks of stopping AEDs without seeking medical advice and the effects of seizures and AEDs on the developing fetus, the pregnancy, breast feeding and

Table 17.1 Lamotrigine and associated pharmacokinetics, pharmacodynamics and common side-effects.

Indications	Monotherapy of focal seizures Monotherapy of primary and secondary generalised tonic clonic seizures
Dose and frequency	Initially 25 mg once daily for 14 days, increasing to 50 mg for 14 days and then increased in steps of up to q100 mg daily every 7–14 days. Maintenance dose 100–200 mg daily in 1–2 divided doses, increased up to 500 mg daily
Side-effects	*Common or very common:* aggression, agitation, joint pain, diarrhoea, dizziness, drowsiness, dry mouth, fatigue, headache, irritability, pain, rash, sleep disorders, tremor, vomiting *Uncommon:* alopecia, movement disorders, vision disorders *Rare or very rare:* confusion, conjunctivitis, face oedema, fever, hallucination, meningitis, disseminated intravascular coagulation, multiorgan failure, tic
Monitoring requirements	Plasma-drug concentration should be monitored before, during and after pregnancy, and doses adjusted according to response
Absorption (A)	Readily absorbed from the gastrointestinal tract and peak serum levels are obtained within 1–3 hours
Distribution (D)	The mean volume of distribution (Vd/F) following oral administration ranges from 0.9 to 1.3 L/kg. Accumulated in the kidney of the male rat and is thought to do the same in humans
Metabolism (M)	Lamotrigine is inactivated by glucuronidation in the liver. It is metabolised mainly by glucuronic acid conjugation. The main metabolite is an inactive 2-N-glucuronide conjugate
Excretion (E)	Most excreted via urine with minimal amounts via faeces

Source: BNF (2021b).

contraception. It is important that seizures are controlled with appropriate medication before a pregnancy begins, as highlighted in the latest MBRRACE-UK report (Knight et al., 2020).

Preconceptual care should include a review of current medication with a neurologist. If a woman has not experienced seizures for at least 2 years, then consideration may be given to stopping the AED at least until the end of the first trimester when development of fetal organs (organogenesis) is complete. Implications of a possible recurrence of seizures and the impact this may have on the woman's life, including her ability to drive, balanced against the risk of congenital abnormality of the fetus, must be discussed so that she is empowered to make an informed choice (Morley, 2018).

It is known that AEDs have a teratogenic effect on the fetus (discussed later) and increase the risk of folate deficiency, neural tube defects such as spina bifida and other MCMs. Studies have found that treatment with a single AED reduces the risk of MCM when compared with polytherapy (Crawford, 2005; Bromley et al., 2017; Peterson et al., 2017). As a result of an increased risk of folate deficiency in women taking AEDs, folic acid supplementation of 5 mg daily should be commenced from 12 weeks before pregnancy until the end of the first trimester (Royal College of Obstetricians and Gynaecologists (RCOG), 2016). Asadi-Pooya (2015) found that there can be significant interactions with some AEDs and high doses of folate and recommended that women taking AEDS should be provided with specific guidance about the required folate dose by their neurologist.

Teratogenic effect of AEDs

The most common MCMs associated with AED exposure during pregnancy are congenital heart disease, cleft lip and palate, neural tube defects and urogenital abnormalities (Bromley et al., 2017). As Hugill and Meredith (2017) highlight, a teratogenic effect is unsurprising considering the intended neurological impact of these drugs coupled with the enhanced sensitivity of the developing fetal brain.

Table 17.2 Levetiracetam and associated pharmacokinetics, pharmacodynamics and common side-effects.

Indications	Monotherapy of focal seizures with or without secondary generalisation
Dose and frequency	Initially 250 mg once a day for 1–2 weeks, increasing to 250 mg twice daily, increasing in steps of 250 mg twice daily (maximum dose 1.5 g twice daily) adjusted according to response. Dose to be increased every 2 weeks if needed
Side-effects	*Common or very common*: anxiety, loss of appetite, lack of energy, cough, depression, diarrhoea, dizziness, drowsiness, headache, insomnia, nausea, skin reactions, vertigo, vomiting *Uncommon*: alopecia, poor concentration, confusion, hallucination, muscle weakness, muscle pain, paraesthesia, psychotic disorder, suicidal behaviour, vision disorders, change in weight *Rare or very rare*: kidney and liver disorders, pancreatitis, personality disorder, hyponatraemia
Monitoring requirements	Clinical response should be monitored during pregnancy – plasma concentrations decrease (by up to 60% in the third trimester)
Absorption (A)	Almost completely absorbed from the small intestine. Food does not interact with absorption; however, for best therapeutic outcomes it should be taken consistently either with food or on an empty stomach
Distribution (D)	The volume of distribution (Vd/F) following oral administration ranges from 0.5 to 0.7 L/kg. The drug and its metabolites pass through the body mainly unbound to plasma proteins (less than 10%)
Metabolism (M)	Minimally metabolised within the body. The main metabolic pathway is the enzymatic hydrolysis of its acetamide group producing an inactive carboxylic acid metabolite, L057. This amounts to 24% of the total dose. The enzyme(s) leading to this reaction are unknown but are independent of hepatic cytochrome P450 (CVP) enzymes and thought to be driven by type B esterases in the blood and other tissues
Excretion (E)	Most of the drug is excreted in the urine as unchanged drug; a small amount of the total dose is excreted via faeces

Source: BNF (2021c).

Research studies (Patel and Pennell, 2016; Baker et al., 2015; Bromley et al., 2017) confirm that fetal and neonatal teratogenic effects are directly related to specific drug dosage and exposure to AEDs while the fetus is in utero. Bromley et al. (2017) demonstrated that sodium valproate is most harmful, particularly when administered at a high dose or as part of poly-therapy. This study demonstrated a MCM rate of 10.9% in 2565 pregnancies compared to a 2.3% malformation rate in 4195 women taking lamotrigine. Peterson et al. (2017) demonstrated similar results (Table 17.3).

Evidence about the teratogenic effects of newer AEDs (for example, lamotrigine and leveti-racetam) is limited but does appear to indicate a lower risk of MCM (Dolk et al., 2016; Bromley et al., 2017; Peterson et al., 2017). This research has inevitably led to concern amongst women with epilepsy and explains why some decide to stop taking AEDs prior to embarking on a pregnancy, sometimes without seeking medical guidance, thereby putting themselves at risk of SUDEP.

Morley (2018) highlights the importance of midwives encouraging women to register their pregnancy anonymously with the UK Epilepsy and Pregnancy Register. It should be emphasised that data collected via this register will add to the body of knowledge regarding the teratogenic effects of various AED regimens and will assist future decision making as women and clinicians weigh up the various risks and benefits associated with the use of AEDs during pregnancy (Morley, 2018; RCOG, 2016).

Table 17.3 Antiepileptic drug use and MCMs.

Study	AED	Number of pregnancies	MCM %
Peterson et al. (2017)	Sodium valproate	229	6.6
	Lamotrigine	357	2.7
	Carbamazepine	334	
	No AEDS	239 151	2.2
Bromley et al. (2017)	Valproate	2565	10.9
	Lamotrigine	4195	2.3
	Carbamazepine	224	3.7
	Levetiracetam	817	1.8
	No AEDs	2154	2.5

Source: Morley (2018).

Episode of care

Bhavna has been taking lamotrigine for 8 years (100 mg twice a day). It has controlled her focal impaired awareness epilepsy and she has been seizure free for 5 years. Bhavna is now planning a pregnancy with her partner. She informs her neurologist and says that she would like to stop taking the AED as she is aware that there is a risk of congenital abnormality in the baby. The neurologist informs her that lamotrigine carries a smaller risk of abnormality than many other AEDs but not taking it at all will remove that negligible risk. However, there is a risk that her seizures will return, and this may affect her quality of life, including her ability to drive as individuals must be at least a year without seizures before they are permitted to drive. Bhavna and her partner discuss the benefits of taking lamotrigine during pregnancy balanced against the risk of congenital abnormality in their baby. Bhavana has an office-based job and does not need to drive to get to work. She has only experienced focal impaired seizures involving her losing awareness for a few seconds.

Bhavna decides that she wants to stop lamotrigine prior to conception with a view to recommencing it after 12 weeks gestation. The neurologist supports Bhavna in her decision and lamotrigine is gradually reduced and eventually stopped.

When Bhavna becomes pregnant, she continues to see her neurologist regularly. She also informs her midwife about her epilepsy and her midwife asks her about the frequency of seizures at every appointment. Bhavna also keeps a diary monitoring seizures so that she can recognise any potential triggers and avoid these. Bhavna notices that her seizures do return, and they occur once or twice a week. She takes steps to protect herself from harm including not bathing when she is home alone and not doing activities alone that might put her at risk if she has a seizure. She also informs the Driving and Vehicle Licensing Agency (DVLA) and her driving licence is revoked. At 4 months gestation, her neurologist prescribes lamotrigine and Bhavna takes it for the remainder of her pregnancy.

Bhavna is pleased with the care she receives during her pregnancy and felt well informed in order to make a decision that was right for her.

AED use during pregnancy

The woman's AED regimen will require close monitoring throughout her pregnancy, to ensure that she is taking the lowest effective dose of medication. For example, serum lamotrigine levels have been found to decrease throughout pregnancy, meaning that an increase in dosage is required for most women in order to ensure that seizures are controlled (Doyle et al., 2016). Serum levels drop because the metabolism of lamotrigine is increased during pregnancy due to higher levels of oestradiol, which in turn affects liver function and increases renal excretion (Doyle et al., 2016).

Any AED regimen should be managed by neurologists at a combined neurology/obstetric clinic and the midwife must ensure that a plan of care is put in place and that the woman is informed of the importance of attending appointments with both consultants (Morley, 2018).

Enzyme-inducing AEDs such as carbamazepine, phenytoin and phenobarbital produce enzymes that reduce the fetal uptake of vitamin K, thus increasing the risk of haemorrhagic disease of the newborn (RCOG, 2016; Shahrook et al., 2018). Despite this, the RCOG guidelines (RCOG, 2016) state that there is a lack of evidence supporting the routine practice of prescribing oral vitamin K in late pregnancy for women taking enzyme-inducing AEDs (Yamasmit et al., 2006). It is recommended that routine administration of 1 mg of vitamin K by injection is provided to all babies born to mothers prescribed enzyme-inducing AEDs (NICE, 2020; RCOG, 2016).

Midwives should ask the woman at every antenatal appointment if she is continuing to take her AEDs as prescribed. Any woman who discontinues AEDs on her own initiative should be referred to a neurology specialist (Morley, 2018). Whilst it is important to respect women's autonomy and their right to make decisions, the risks of self-discontinuation of AEDs should be made clear and midwives must feel able to challenge potentially unsafe decisions as this could save a woman's life. Skilful and sensitive communication is needed, especially where epilepsy co-exists with adverse psychological or social conditions (RCOG, 2016; Knight et al., 2020).

Medication during labour for women with epilepsy

Seizures occur in about 1–2% of women with epilepsy during labour, with a further 1–2% occurring within 24 hours after birth (RCOG, 2016; NICE, 2020). Holistic care including adequate analgesia should be provided by the midwife to avoid trigger factors for a seizure such as fatigue, insomnia, stress and dehydration (Morley, 2018). Options for analgesia include transcutaneous electrical nerve stimulation (TENS), nitrous oxide and oxygen (Entonox®) and regional anaesthesia.

Morley (2018) highlights that excessive vomiting during labour can lead to reduced AED absorption and the midwife should assess the need for an antiemetic, rehydration and further AED treatment. Pethidine should be used with caution during labour as it may be metabolised to norpethidine and this may trigger a seizure (RCOG, 2016; McAuliffe et al., 2013). Diamorphine is the preferred alternative to pethidine.

Women should continue to take their prescribed AEDS during labour. If these cannot be tolerated via the oral route, they should be administered parenterally (RCOG, 2016; McAuliffe et al., 2013).

Postnatal care and AEDS

Prior to discharge from the maternity services, women with epilepsy should be offered contraceptive advice to avoid future unplanned pregnancies (RCOG, 2016). The midwife should approach this subject sensitively to avoid any implication of judgement, particularly if the previous pregnancy had been unplanned. The risks of women with epilepsy embarking on another pregnancy when their condition is unstable have already been discussed. This makes it an important and potentially life-saving topic for the midwife to broach during the postpartum period.

The risk of potential contraceptive failure should also be discussed with the woman since certain forms of hormonal contraception may be compromised by the effects of some AEDs. For example, enzyme-inducing AEDS such as carbamazepine, phenytoin and topiramate may cause progesterone-only contraception (including intrauterine devices containing progesterone) to be excreted more rapidly from the body, thus reducing their efficacy (Hugill and Meredith, 2017). In addition, oestrogen-based contraceptives when used with lamotrigine can lower the concentration of the drug in plasma, thus weakening its therapeutic effect (NICE, 2020). It should be noted that although lamotrigine is not an enzyme-inducing AED, it still influences the reliability of hormonal contraception (Table 17.4).

For these reasons, wherever possible, tailored advice should be given by a person with specialist contraceptive knowledge such as a family planning nurse or sexual health practitioner.

Regardless of proposed contraception methods, during the postpartum period haemodynamic changes occur in the woman's body which eventually reverse the effects of those which occurred during pregnancy. This may result in changing serum levels of AEDs, so to ensure that women

Table 17.4   Enzyme-inducing and non-enzyme-inducing antiepileptic drugs.

Enzyme-inducing AEDs	Non-enzyme-inducing AEDs
Phenobarbital	Clobazam
Primidone	Clonazepam
Carbamazepine	Gabapentin
Phenytoin	Sodium valproate
Topiramate	Levetiracetam
Rufinamide	Lamotrigine[a]
	Zonisamide
	Ethosuximide
	Tiagabine

[a] Lamotrigine, although non-enzyme inducing, does interact with the therapeutic action of oestrogen-containing hormonal contraception to reduce its efficacy in preventing pregnancy
Source: McAuliffe et al. (2013)/with permission of John Wiley & Sons.

continue to receive medication at the lowest dose to prevent seizures, their drug regimen will need to be reviewed and monitored by the neurological team. Morley (2018) suggests that having a plan of care in place during the antenatal period is good practice in order to facilitate this process.

Antiepileptic drugs are secreted in breast milk. However, research shows that breast-fed babies exposed to AEDs demonstrated higher IQ scores and better speech development at ages 3 and 6 compared to AED-exposed babies who were not breast fed (Meador et al., 2014). This research is reassuring for mothers as it demonstrates that there is no increase in poor cognitive outcomes when babies are exposed to breast milk containing AEDs. It also means that midwives can confidently support women taking AEDs to breast feed in order to facilitate the many health benefits associated with breast milk for both mother and baby (Meador et al., 2014; RCOG, 2016; Hugill and Meredith, 2017).

Conclusion

This chapter has focused on the midwife's role in supporting pregnant women with their choice of medication when treating the most common neurological conditions. It has demonstrated that medicines taken during pregnancy (particularly during the first trimester) can have an adverse effect on the developing fetus, suggesting that trying other non- pharmaceutical methods (such as rest, ice packs, massage, relaxation techniques) for treating headache and/or migraine is preferable as first-line treatment. However, if the condition remains unresolved, the midwife's role is to ensure that pregnant women are aware of how to take medicines safely. The fact that headache or migraine could be caused by a potentially serious condition secondary to pregnancy is also acknowledged and midwives need to be alert to this and prepared to refer a woman to a medical practitioner.

Antiepileptic drug treatment regimens are highly individualised, meaning that sensitive holistic care on the part of the midwife is required to ensure that women with epilepsy are empowered to make appropriate decisions about their medication. The increase in deaths from SUDEP in the latest MBRRACE-UK report (Knight et al., 2020) is highlighted alongside the fact that AEDs are teratogenic, some leading to a particularly high risk of MCM in the fetus.

Sharing care of a woman with epilepsy between the multidisciplinary team and involving women in decision making is the best way to ensure that optimum care is provided throughout the childbirth continuum.

Find out more

The following is a list of conditions associated with the nervous system. Take some time and write notes about each of the conditions. Think about the medications that may be used to treat these conditions and be specific about the pharmacokinetics and pharmacodynamics. Remember to include aspects of women's care. If you are making notes about women you have offered care and support to, you must ensure that you have adhered to the rules of confidentiality.

The condition	Your notes
Bell's palsy	
Multiple sclerosis	
Carpal tunnel syndrome	
Cerebrovascular disease and stroke	
Status epilepticus	

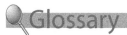

Glossary

Enzyme   A substance that acts as a catalyst in living organisms

Epilepsy   A central nervous system disorder in which brain activity becomes abnormal, causing seizures or periods of unusual behaviour, sensations and sometimes loss of awareness

Focal seizure   Seizure affecting one specific area of the brain, usually the temporal lobe; previously called partial seizure

Generalized seizure   When focal seizures spread to involve the whole brain

Migraine   A headache characterised by severe throbbing pain or a pulsing sensation, usually on one side of the head. Often accompanied by nausea, vomiting and sensitivity to light and sound.

Seizure   A burst of uncontrolled electrical activity in brain cells causing temporary abnormalities in muscle tone or movement, behaviours, sensations or states of awareness

Teratogen   A substance that may cause birth defects via a toxic (teratogenic) effect on an embryo or fetus

Tonic clonic seizure   The whole body contracts, leading to the individual falling to the ground. This is followed by generalised twitching of the limbs. This may last a few minutes and is frequently accompanied by incontinence

Test yourself

Now review your learning by completing the learning activities for this chapter at www.wiley.com/go/pharmacologyformidwives.

References

Alarcón, G., Valentín, A. (2012) *Introduction to Epilepsy*. Cambridge University Press: Cambridge.

Asadi-Pooya, A. (2015) High dose folic acid supplementation in women with epilepsy: are we sure it is safe? *Seizure*, **27**: 51–53.

Baker, G.A., Bromley, R.L., Briggs, M. et al. on behalf of the Liverpool and Manchester Neurodevelopment Group (2015) IQ at 6 years after in utero exposure to antiepileptic drugs: a controlled cohort study. *Neurology*, **84**(4): 382–390.

Bergman, J.E.H., Lutke, L.R., Gans, R.O.B. et al. (2017) Beta-blocker use in pregnancy and risk of specific congenital anomalies: a European case-malformed control study. *Drug Safety*, **41**: 415–427.

Bhatia, M., Mahtani, K.R., Rochman, R., Collins, S.L. (2020a) Primary care assessment and management of common physical symptoms in pregnancy. *British Medical Journal (Clinical research edition)*, **370**: m2248.

British National Formulary (2021a) Carbamazepine. https://bnf.nice.org.uk/drug/carbamazepine.html# indicationsAndDoses (accessed February 2022).

British National Formulary (2021b) Lamotrigine. https://bnf.nice.org.uk/drug/carbamazepine.html#Search? q=Lamotrigine%20 (accessed February 2022).

British National Formulary (2021c) Levetiracetam. https://bnf.nice.org.uk/drug/levetiracetam.html (accessed February 2022).

Bromley, R. (2016) The treatment of epilepsy in pregnancy: the neurodevelopmental risks associated with exposure to antiepileptic drugs. *Reproductive Toxicology*, **64**(64): 203–210.

Bromley, R., Weston, J., Marson, A. (2017) Maternal use of antiepileptic agents during pregnancy and major congenital malformations in children. *Journal of the American Medical Association*, **318**(17): 1700–1701.

Crawford, P. (2005) Best practice guidelines for the management of women with epilepsy. *Epilepsia*, **46**(suppl 9): 117–124.

Crouch, S., Chapelhow, C. (2008). *Medicines Management: A Nursing Perspective*. Routledge Taylor and Francis: London.

Dolk, H., Wang, H., Loane, M. et al. (2016) Lamotrigine use in pregnancy and risk of orofacial cleft and other congenital anomalies. *Neurology*, **86**(18): 1716–1725.

Doyle, L., Geraghty, S., Folan, M. (2016) Epilepsy in pregnancy: pharmacodynamics and pharmacokinetics. *British Journal of Midwifery*, **24**(12): 830–835.

Duong, S., Bozzo, P., Nordeng, H. (2010) Safety of triptans for migraine headaches during pregnancy and breastfeeding. *Canadian Family Physician*, **56**(6): 537–539.

Epilepsy Action (2019) Epileptic seizures explained. www.epilepsy.org.uk/info/seizures-explained (accessed February 2022).

Epilepsy Society (2019a) What is Epilepsy? https://epilepsysociety.org.uk/sites/default/files/2020-04/What-is-epilepsy-January-2019.pdf (accessed February 2022).

Epilepsy Society (2019b) *Epilepsy treatment*. www.epilepsysociety.org.uk/treatment (accessed February 2022).

Epilepsy Society (2020) How anti-epileptic drugs work. https://epilepsysociety.org.uk/anti-epileptic-drugs/how-anti-epileptic-drugs-work (accessed February 2022).

Fiest, K.M., Sauro, K.M., Wiebe, S. et al. (2017) Prevalence and incidence of epilepsy. A systematic review and meta-analysis of international studies. *Neurology*, **88**(3): 296303.

Flint, J., Panchal, S., Hurrell, A. et al. (2016) British Society for Rheumatology (BSR) and British Health Professionals in Rheumatology (BHPR) Standards, Guidelines and Audit Working Group. BSR and BHPR guideline on prescribing drugs in pregnancy and breastfeeding-Part II: analgesics and other drugs used in rheumatology practice. *Rheumatology*, **55**: 1698–1702.

Goadsby, P.J., Goldberg, J., Silberstein, S.D. (2008) Migraine in pregnancy. *British Medical Journal*, **336**(7659): 1502–1504.

Hugill, K., Meredith, D. (2017) Caring for pregnant women with long term conditions: maternal and neonatal effects of epilepsy. *British Journal of Midwifery*, **25**(5): 301–307.

Jarvis, S., Dassan, P., Nelson-Piercy, C. (2018) Managing migraine in pregnancy. *British Medical Journal*, **360**: k80.

Joint Formulary Committee (2021) *BNF British National Formulary*. bnf.nice.org.uk (accessed February 2022).

Kapoor, D., Wallace, S. (2014) Trends in maternal deaths from epilepsy in the United Kingdom: a 30-year retrospective review. *Obstetric Medicine*, **7**(4): 160–164.

Koren, G. (2017) Safety considerations surrounding use of treatment options for nausea and vomiting in pregnancy. *Expert Opinion on Drug Safety*, **16**: 1227–1234.

Knight, M., Bunch, K., Tuffnell, D. et al. (eds) (2020) Saving lives, improving mothers' care: lessons learned to inform maternity care from the UK and Ireland Confidential Enquiries into Maternal Deaths and Morbidity 2015–18. www.npeu.ox.ac.uk/mbrrace-uk/reports (accessed February 2022).

Lewis, S.A. (2014) Newer drug treatments for focal-onset epilepsy. *British Journal of Neurosciences Nursing*, **10**(1): 9–12.

Macgregor, E.A. (2012) Headache in pregnancy. *Neurologic Clinics*, **30**: 835–866.

Manzoni, G.C., Stovner, L.J. (2010) Epidemiology of headache. *Handbook of Clinical Neurology*, **97**: 3–22.

Martin, S.R., Foley, M.R. (2005) Approach to the pregnant patient with headache. *Clinical Obstetrics and Gynaecology*, **48**(1): 2–11.

McAuliffe, F., Burns-Kent, D., Frost, E., Howarth, E. (2013) Neurological disorders. In: Robson, S.E., Waugh, J. (eds) *Medical Disorders in Pregnancy: A Manual for Midwives*. John Wiley and Sons: Chichester.

McErlean, L., Migliozzi, J. (2016) The nervous system. In: Peate, I., Nair, M. (eds) *Fundamentals of Anatomy and Physiology for Nursing and Healthcare Students*, 2nd edn, pp. 447–482. Wiley-Blackwell: Chichester.

Meador, K.J., Baker, G.A., Browning, N. et al. for the Neurodevelopmental Effects of Antiepileptic Drugs (NEAD) Study Group (2014) Breastfeeding in children of women taking antiepileptic drugs: cognitive outcomes at age 6 years. *JAMA Paediatrics*, **168**(8): 729–736.

Medicines and Healthcare products Regulatory Agency (2018) Valproate use by women and girls. www.gov.uk/guidance/valproate-use-by-women-and-girls (accessed February 2022).

Migraine Trust (2021) Treatments: Feverfew. www.migrainetrust.org/living-with-migraine/treatments/feverfew/ (accessed February 2022).

Morley, K. (2018) Epilepsy in pregnancy: the role of the midwife in risk management. *British Journal of Midwifery*, **26**(9): 564–573.

National Institute for Health and Care Excellence (2015) Headaches in over 12s; diagnosis and management. CG150. www.nice.org/guidance/CG150 (accessed February 2022).

National Institute for Health and Care Excellence (2020) Epilepsies: diagnosis and management. CG137. www.nice.org.uk/guidance/cg137/chapter/Introduction (accessed February 2022).

Nursing and Midwifery Council (2019) Standards of Proficiency for Midwives. www.nmc.org.uk/globalassets/sitedocuments/standards/standards-of-proficiency-for-midwives.pdf (accessed February 2022).

Patel, S.I., Pennell, P.B. (2016) Management of epilepsy during pregnancy: an update. *Therapeutic Advances in Neurological Disorders*, **9**(2): 118–129.

Petersen, I., Collings, S.L., McCrea, R.L. et al. (2017) Antiepileptic drugs prescribed in pregnancy and prevalence of major congenital malformations: comparative prevalence studies. *Clinical Epidemiology*, **9**(9): 95–103.

Robbins, M.S., Farmakidis, C., Dayal, A.K., Lipton, R.B. (2015) Acute headache diagnosis in pregnant women: a hospital-based study. *Neurology*, **85**(12): 1024–1030.

Rolnik, D.L., Wright, D., Poon, L.C. et al. (2017) Aspirin versus placebo in pregnancies at high risk for preterm preeclampsia. *New England Journal of Medicine*, **377**(7): 613–622.

Royal College of Obstetricians and Gynaecologists (2016) *Epilepsy in pregnancy. Green-top Guideline 68*. RCOG: London.

Shahrook, S., Ota, E., Hanada, N., Sawada, K., Mori, R. (2018) Vitamin K supplememtation during pregnancy for improving outcomes: a systematic review and meta-analysis. *Scientific Reports*, **8**: 11459.

Sibai, B.M., Gonzalez, A.R., Mabie, W.C., Moretti, M. (1987) A comparison of labetalol plus hospitalization versus hospitalization alone in the management of preeclampsia remote from term. *Obstetrics and Gynaecology*, **70**(3): 323–327.

Spielmann, K., Kayser, A., Beck, E., Meister, R., Schaefer, C. (2018) Pregnancy outcome after anti-migraine triptan use: a prospective observational cohort study. *Cephalalgia*, **38**(6): 1081–1092.

United Kingdom Teratology Information Service (2016) Treatment of migraine in pregnancy. www.medicinesinpregnancy.org/bumps/monographs/TREATMENT-OF-MIGRAINE-IN-PREGNANCY (accessed February 2022).

Wells, R.E., Turner, D.P., Lee, M., Bishop, L., Strauss, L. (2016) Managing migraine during pregnancy and lactation. *Current Neurology and Neuroscience Reports*, **16**(4): 40.

Yamasmit, W., Chaithongwongwatthana, S., Tolosa, J.E. (2006) Prenatal vitamin K1 administration in epileptic women to prevent neonatal haemorrhage: is it effective? *Journal of Reproductive Medicine*, **51**(6): 463–466.

Zhao, Y., Hebert, M.F., Venkataramanan, R. (2014) Basic obstetric pharmacology. *Seminars in Perinatology*, **38**(8): 475–486.

Chapter 18

Medications and mental health

Emmanuel Ndisang

University of Hertfordshire, Hatfield, UK

Aim

The aim of this chapter is to provide the reader with a broad overview of the medicines used in mental health with a focus on psychotropic medications in the perinatal period.

Learning outcomes

After reading this chapter, the reader will:
- Be able to demonstrate an awareness of general mental health presentations
- Understand some psychotropic medications and their use in pregnancy and lactation
- Be able to list psychotropic medications that are linked to teratogenicity
- Have some understanding of the risk–benefit analysis in relation to mental health medications during the perinatal period.

Test your existing knowledge

- What are psychotropic medications? Give two examples and when they are used.
- Discuss the precautions you would take when administering psychotropic medication to someone considering pregnancy or who is pregnant.
- Describe some of the developmental abnormalities associated with psychotropic medications.
- Discuss some of the risk–benefit considerations of psychotropic medications used in pregnancy.

Introduction

More than ever before, our mental and physical health are being inextricably linked, and sometimes have common origins even when they manifest differently. Psychosomatic presentations are becoming more common with ongoing research on some physical illnesses of apparently psychological or unexplained origins. In some instances, unexplained body pains such as backache or headache

Fundamentals of Pharmacology for Midwives, First Edition. Edited by Ian Peate and Cathy Hamilton.
© 2022 John Wiley & Sons Ltd. Published 2022 by John Wiley & Sons Ltd.
Companion website: www.wiley.com/go/pharmacologyformidwives

are manifestations of prodromal or even moderate to severe depression (De Ridder et al., 2021; McTeague et al., 2020; Serafini et al., 2019). From depression to bipolar disorders and psychosis, mental and physical health conditions share a close connection with biological and psychosocial influences. This means treatment interventions in mental health should straddle medication together with other psychosocial and environmental approaches. This chapter will focus on psycho-tropic medications during the perinatal period, their efficacy and effectiveness, acknowledging that these will be influenced by various aspects of the individual's environment and psychosocial factors.

Severe anxiety, depression, bipolar disorder and psychosis are a few of the common mental health manifestations which need to be carefully managed before, during and after pregnancy, with cautious use of psychotropic medication where indicated. The use of these medicines during the perinatal period is particularly challenging because of the risk of a potential relapse to the mother if untreated, and the possible behavioural, developmental, cognitive and teratogenic risk to the fetus and child. It is therefore relevant for women with a history or an existing mental health condi-tion to seek specialist advice from their mental health services if they plan to become pregnant, as this would require good understanding and close monitoring for any complications that could affect the mother or her baby.

For some psychotropic medications, there is data for tens of thousands of pregnancy exposures, with varying safety profiles, while for others there are relatively limited studies or just a few case reports. It is important not to interpret the absence of evidence of harm as a general licence for use or evidence of safety.

Medications and mental health presentations

Depression is a cluster of symptoms that include feeling low with loss of motivation, concentration, interests or pleasure in activities most days of the week, over a sustained duration of at least 2 weeks. Severity is determined by the number and intensity of symptoms and the degree of functional impairment. Pregnancy can be a challenging period, during which many biological, physical, psy-chosocial and lifestyle changes can lead to re-emergence or exacerbation of some of these symptoms.

Many hormonal and neurotransmitter activities help to maintain normal euthymic functioning. Some of the biological markers of mood changes and depression include dysregulation or defi-ciency in neurotransmitters such as serotonin, noradrenaline and dopamine in specific brain regions. Almost all current antidepressants work by boosting one or a combination of these neurotransmit-ters. Hormones also play a significant role in how we feel and are particularly implicated in preg-nancy. Hormones such as cortisol and corticosteroids play a crucial part in regulating stress responses. Studies now show a link between increased stress activation and depression (LeMoult et al., 2020; Gustavo et al., 2015) and stress is implicated in almost all mental health presentations and particularly relevant during the perinatal period. For most women, a fine balance between progesterone and oestrogen levels helps maintain euthymia (normal mood) and disruption of this homeostatic balance at certain times of the reproductive cycle has been linked to low mood and symptoms of depression (Albert and Paul, 2019; Soares and Zitek, 2008). Pregnancy and the post-partum period come with significant changes in the progesterone–oestrogen ratio which, together with physical changes, emotional, social and environment stressors, leave some women particularly vulnerable to mood swings and depression.

Antidepressants are mainly indicated for moderate to severe depression. They may also be indi-cated for persistent subthreshold depression that has not responded to other remedies, including psychological and psychosocial interventions. There are different classes of antidepressants with different properties and mode of action. The selective serotonin reuptake inhibitors (SSRIs) are cur-rently relatively more widely used in pregnancy. Table 18.1 shows the main classes of antidepres-sants, their safety categorisation and indication for use in pregnancy. The categorisation is based on the A, B, C, D, X and N Food and Drug Administration (FDA) system (FDA, 2021) (Box 18.1).

It is worth noting that such categorisations of pregnancy medication safety can be too simplistic, and they should therefore be interpreted with caution, as every woman has a unique profile, history and response to medication.

Table 18.1 Different classes of antidepressant and their use in pregnancy.

Antidepressants	Examples	Safety category	Use in pregnancy
SSRI	Sertraline, citalopram, escitalopram, fluoxetine, paroxetine[a]	Mainly C Paroxetine[a] D	Use with caution where benefits outweigh potential risk
SNRI	Venlafaxine, desvenlafaxine, duloxetine	C	
NaSSA	Mirtazapine	C	
Tricyclic antidepressants	Amitriptyline, clomipramine, lofepramine, desipramine, dosulepin, imipramine, doxepin, nortriptyline[b]	Mainly C Nortriptyline D	Not currently widely used. However, if stable on the treatment, use with caution where benefits outweigh potential risk
MAOI	Phenelzine, tranylcypromine	C	Not widely used. Use with caution
Others	Trazodone, nefazodone, bupropion	C	

Source: Zhong et al. (2020); Berard et al. (2016).

[a] Paroxetine: cautious use in pregnancy as studies show increase in congenital cardiac defects when taken in the first trimester, maladaptive syndrome and persistent pulmonary hypertension in the newborn when taken in the third trimester.
[b] No controlled studies in humans. Variable indications for its use in pregnancy and breast feeding. Relatively small amounts secreted in breast milk compared to the other tricyclic antidepressants.
Note that none of the antidepressants has a category A or B rating.
MAOI, monoamine oxidase inhibitor; NaSSA, noradrenergic and specific serotonergic antidepressant; SNRI, selective serotonin and noradrenaline reuptake inhibitor; SSRI, selective serotonin reuptake inhibitor; TCA, tricyclic antidepressant.

Box 18.1   Safety categorisation

- Category A drugs are the safest, with no fetal risk associated with the medication in controlled human studies
- Category B indicates no known risk to humans although some found in studies with animals
- Category C suggests risks in humans cannot be ruled out but the drug could be used where benefits outweigh the potential risk
- Category D drugs are those with positive evidence of risk to the fetus but could be used with caution where benefits outweigh potential risk
- X drugs are contraindicated and should not be used in pregnancy
- N drugs are those yet to be categorised

Source: Based on FDA (2021).

Psychosis is characterised by distortions of reality and perceptual dysfunction which include various forms of hallucinations or irrational thoughts or delusions. Like depression, psychosis is linked to biological, psychosocial and environment exposure. Increased neurotransmitter activity in certain brain regions has led to both the dopamine and glutamate hypotheses of schizophrenia, a particular type of psychosis. During the perinatal period, exposure to various changes could increase sensitivity or even susceptibility to hormonal or neurotransmitter fluctuations. Recent studies have suggested more susceptibility to psychosis during low oestrogen periods (Reilly et al., 2020), although these findings are still premature with a need for replicable large-scale studies. Nevertheless, psychosis in pregnancy could pose a significant risk to the mother, the fetus and baby if not carefully managed (Kucukgoncu et al., 2020).

Antipsychotic medications are widely used to manage psychosis, and effectively too in many cases. They work by reducing dopamine activity in the mesolimbic pathway of the brain. Some of the side-effects could lead to weight gain and movement disorders. Nevertheless, antipsychotic medications play a crucial role in managing psychosis (Wang et al., 2021; Vigod, 2015) and, in combination with psychosocial interventions, lead to better management and treatment outcomes during the perinatal period (Galbally et al., 2014) (Box 18.2).

Box 18.2   Recommendations for starting, using and stopping antidepressant treatment

When choosing a TCA, SSRI or SNRI, take into account:

- the woman's previous response to these drugs
- the stage of pregnancy (for example, there is a small increased risk of postpartum haemorrhage with SSRI and SNRI antidepressant medicines when used in the month before delivery)
- what is known about the reproductive safety of these drugs (for example, the risk of fetal cardiac abnormalities and persistent pulmonary hypertension in the newborn baby)
- the uncertainty about whether any increased risk to the fetus and other problems for the woman or baby can be attributed directly to these drugs or may be caused by other factors
- the risk of discontinuation symptoms in the woman and neonatal adaptation syndrome in the baby with most TCAs, SSRIs and SNRIs, in particular paroxetine and venlafaxine.

When assessing the risks and benefits of TCAs, SSRIs or SNRIs for a woman who is considering breast feeding, the following should be taken into account:

- the benefits of breast feeding for the woman and baby
- the uncertainty about the safety of these drugs for the breast-feeding baby
- the risks associated with switching from or stopping a previously effective medication.

Professional advice should be sought from a specialist (preferably a specialist perinatal mental health service) if there is uncertainty about specific drugs. See also the United Kingdom Drugs in Lactation Advisory Service (2021) for information on the use of specific drugs.

Source: Modified from NICE (2020a).

Clinical consideration

When psychotropic medication is started in pregnancy and the postnatal period:

- consider seeking advice, preferably from a specialist in perinatal mental health
- choose the drug with the lowest risk profile for the woman, fetus and baby, taking into account the woman's previous response to medication
- use the lowest effective dose (this is important when the risks of adverse effects to the woman, fetus and baby may be dose related), but note that subtherapeutic doses may also expose the fetus to risks and may not treat the mental health problem effectively
- use a single drug, if possible, rather than two or more drugs
- consider that dosages may need to be adjusted in pregnancy.

Source: Modified from NICE (2020a).

291

Psychotropic medication in the perinatal period

Perinatal mental health

Maintaining stable maternal mental health is fundamental to ensuring the overall well-being of both the mother and the infant. So, unless a psychotropic medication is contraindicated during this period, it is preferable to continue its treatment during pregnancy and after birth. This is more so because untreated mental ill health could lead to apathy, demotivation, poor nutrition, overweight, smoking, poor physical health, drug and alcohol use and self-harm. These all have potentially detrimental consequences to the mother and the fetus. In severe cases, the pregnancy itself may not be sustained, with placental abnormalities, pre-eclampsia, low birthweight and prematurity, neonatal hypoglycaemia, stillbirth, fetal discomfort or distress and congenital defects, as well as the potential for adverse neurodevelopmental outcomes independent of any risk associated with exposure to psychotropic medication (Galbally et al., 2014; Abel et al., 2014). As such, for many women, maintaining medication treatment during this period is essential for the woman, the pregnancy and the infant.

Antenatal and postnatal medication

Placebo randomised controlled trials on psychotropic medications are not permissible for women during pregnancy, due to often complex ethical considerations, not least depriving pregnant women of their treatment (Teodorescu et al., 2017). This means most of the information about the effects of medication during this period has been gleaned from naturalistic case–control studies. The longer and more widely used a medication has been, the better is our understanding of its safety profile during pregnancy. Typically, the older generation psychotropic medications, for which there has been more exposure, have more data on their safety during pregnancy.

Due to physiological changes during pregnancy, the increased body mass, blood flow, liver, kidney and metabolic output mean that some drugs may need to be prescribed at a higher dose to maintain euthymia or prevent relapse. However, this must be considered alongside a possible increased risk to the fetus which means the lowest possible effective dose is preferable during this period as the fetus has lower liver function, lower plasma protein binding, relatively increased cardiac throughput and greater blood–brain barrier permeability (Stowe and Nemeroff, 1998). These physiological, metabolic, pharmacokinetic and pharmacodynamic changes point to the importance of cautious prescribing during pregnancy, the need for monotherapy and lowest possible therapeutic doses of psychotropic medications, and close monitoring and follow-up for possible side-effects, to protect both the mother and fetus (Lassiter and Manns-James, 2017; Kohen, 2004).

Depot formulation of antipsychotic medications should normally be avoided during pregnancy due to their pharmacokinetics and pharmacodynamic in the body with prolonged duration, effects and half-life.

The trimesters of pregnancy come with different physiological changes, which means that some psychotropic medications are best avoided at certain times of pregnancy, and particularly during the first trimester when most of the neural and vital organs are being formed. However, some psychotropic drugs (SSRIs, for example), when given during the third trimester, increase the possibility of embryotoxicity or maladaptive neonatal syndrome of the newborn (Kalra et al., 2005; Yonkers et al., 2014). Table 18.2 shows some psychotropic medications and their effects at different times of pregnancy.

Serotonergic antidepressants such as SSRIs are newer drugs compared to MAOIs and TCAs but are more widely prescribed. As a class, they are relatively well tolerated but with specific cautionary exceptions as noted in Table 18.2.

Infants exposed to SSRIs during pregnancy have a one in three chance of developing poor neonatal adaptive syndrome (PNAS), characterised by irritability, difficulty feeding, jitteriness, restlessness, increased muscle tone and rapid breathing. These tend to self-limit after a couple of weeks or within days for some infants. However, there have been isolated reports of poorer fine motor

Table 18.2   Psychotropic medications in the perinatal period.

Antidepressant	Use in pregnancy	Passage into breast milk	Effect on fetus or breast milk
SSRI	Use if benefits outweigh any potential harm	Varying degree of passage in breast milk	Small increase in congenital heart defect if taken in the first trimester and neonatal maladaptive syndrome and persistent pulmonary hypertension in the newborn if taken in the third trimester
Citalopram		Present but too small to have a harmful effect. Use with caution	
Escitalopram		Present. Preferable to avoid if breast feeding	
Fluoxetine		Present; long half-life. Avoid	As above plus sedation and colic
Paroxetine[a]	Caution	Present: low. Caution	Increased risk of the above
Sertraline	Use if benefits outweigh any potential harm	Present but too small to have a harmful effect	As above for SSRIs
Fluvoxamine	As above	Present. Preferable to avoid if breast feeding	
Vortioxetine[b]	Limited data. Avoid unless benefits outweigh risk	Present in animal studies. Avoid if breast feeding	
SNRI			
Venlafaxine[c]	Caution	Present. Preferable to avoid if breast feeding	Withdrawal symptoms in the newborn
Duloxetine	Use if potential benefits outweigh risk. Avoid in stress incontinence		Neonatal withdrawal symptoms if used the third trimester
Bupropion	Limited information available		Limited information available
TCA			
Amitriptyline	Use if benefits outweigh risk	Too small to be harmful	Caution. Limited data
Clomipramine	Use if benefits outweigh risk		Neonatal withdrawal symptoms if used in the third trimester
Dosulepin	Use if benefits outweigh risk	Only use if benefits outweigh risk	Caution. Limited information available.

293

(Continued)

Table 18.2 (Continued)

Antidepressant	Use in pregnancy	Passage into breast milk	Effect on fetus or breast milk
Doxepin[d]	Limited information available. Avoid	Low. However, potential of accumulation of metabolites	Metabolites may cause sedation and respiratory depression in newborns. Avoid
Lofepramine	Use if benefits outweigh risk	Too small to be harmful	Neonatal withdrawal symptoms if used in the third trimester
Nortriptyline[e]	Use only if potential benefit outweighs risk	Too small to be harmful	Limited data

Paroxetine[a], Venlafaxine[c], Doxepin[d] and Nortriptyline[e] – avoid in pregnancy or only use where the benefits outweight the risks.
Vortioxetine[b], limited data on vortioxetine as it is relatively new.

development even at 6 months post partum (Galbally et al., 2017; Kieviet et al., 2016). Symptoms tend to lessen in breast-fed babies. Nevertheless, infants exposed to SSRIs or SNRIs in the third tri-mester and through breast feeding should be closely monitored for sedation and neonatal adaptive syndrome, and possibly serum levels of the drugs should be measured to rule out neonatal toxicity where there is a concern.

Sertraline is generally considered safer during pregnancy with few known adverse effects to the mother or fetus (Kolding et al., 2021). Paroxetine, however, has been linked with congenital heart defects if taken in the first trimester and neonatal maladaptive syndrome and persistent pulmonary hypertension in the newborn if taken in the third trimester (British National Formulary (BNF), 2021a). Fluoxetine has a long half-life and is associated with sedation and colic for some babies and therefore is not the first choice of antidepressant to commence post partum (BNF, 2021b). Vortioxetine is a relatively new antidepressant with not much data on its safety profile in pregnancy (BNF, 2021c).

Other classes of antidepressants, although not contraindicated during the perinatal period, are not widely used because their side-effects tend to be higher or not well studied. For example, doxepin is a TCA with cases of hypotonia and poor suckling. MAOIs such as phenelzine and tranyl-cypromine are now rarely used, owing to the development of newer antidepressants such as SSRIs and SNRIs. There are few reliable reports on safety of MAOIs in pregnancy. It is therefore not advis-able for pregnant women to be prescribed these drugs and if a woman is already on the medication, it is preferable to discuss switching to newer options with a mental health specialist prior to preg-nancy where possible.

Antipsychotic medications are relatively safe during pregnancy. However, more research is needed in this area, with specific caution with some medications. Current evidence suggests there is no significant increased risk of miscarriage or stillbirth and studies with over 10 000 women during pregnancy did not show a significant increase in risk of birth defects (McAllister et al., 2017; Huybrechts et al., 2016). However, there is a small increased risk of birth defects with risperidone affecting from 3 in every 100 babies to 4 in every 100 babies (Huybrechts et al., 2016) although this has not been shown in other studies.

Box 18.3 shows the main classes of antipsychotic medications. The first-generation antipsychotic medications (FGAs) (also known as conventionals or typicals) have been in use much longer than the second generation (SGAs) (atypicals), with better data on their tolerability in pregnancy. Because of their high dopamine affinity in the tuberoinfundibular pathway, FGAs tend to increase prolactin levels, which for some women make it harder to become pregnant. Prolactin levels should normally be checked at least yearly for patients on these medications and if becoming pregnant becomes difficult, it is advisable to discuss this with the psychiatrist or perinatal mental health service for consideration of alternative medications, more likely one of the atypical antipsychotics.

Box 18.3   The two main classes of antipsychotic medications

Second generation	First generation
Risperidone	Haloperidol
Quetiapine	Chlorpromazine
Olanzapine	Fluphenazine
Paliperidone	Perphenazine
Ziprasidone	Thioridazine
Luraridone	
Aripiprazole	
Clozapine	

First-generation antipsychotics such as haloperidol do not appear to show increased risk of teratogenicity, although chlorpromazine may show a small but not statistically significant increased risk of non-specific teratogenic effects with first trimester exposure (BNF, 2021d). Transient complications have been documented in the infant, including withdrawal symptoms, extrapyramidal signs (tremors, motor restlessness, feeding difficulties, abnormalities of tone and underdeveloped reflexes), neonatal jaundice and intestinal obstruction (BNF, 2021d; Yonkers et al., 2004). There have been reports of these symptoms lasting up to 10 months, although most resolve within days (Galbally et al., 2014; Slone et al., 1977).

Second-generation antipsychotics can lead to cardiovascular problems such as weight gain, metabolic syndrome and diabetes. Some antipsychotic medication like olanzapine and clozapine could double the risk of gestational diabetes from 2 in every 100 to 4 in every 100 pregnant women (Park et al., 2018; Petersenet al., 2016). Box 18.4 gives some recommendations about the use of antipsychotic medication during and after pregnancy.

Box 18.4   Recommendations for using antipsychotic medication in pregnancy

- When assessing the risks and benefits of antipsychotic medication for a pregnant woman, consider risk factors for gestational diabetes and excessive weight gain.
- When choosing an antipsychotic, bear in mind that there are limited data on the safety of these drugs in pregnancy and the postnatal period.
- Measure prolactin levels in women who are taking prolactin-raising antipsychotic medication and planning a pregnancy, because raised prolactin levels reduce the chances of conception. If prolactin levels are raised, consider a prolactin-sparing antipsychotic.
- If a pregnant woman is stable on an antipsychotic and likely to relapse without medication, advise her to continue the antipsychotic.
- Advise pregnant women taking antipsychotic medication about diet and monitor for excessive weight gain, in line with the NICE (2020a) guideline on weight management before, during and after pregnancy.
- Monitor for gestational diabetes in pregnant women taking antipsychotic medication in line with the NICE (2020b) guideline on diabetes in pregnancy and offer an oral glucose tolerance test.
- Do not offer depot antipsychotics to a woman who is planning a pregnancy, pregnant or considering breast feeding, unless she is responding well to a depot and has a previous history of non-adherence with oral medication.

Sources: NICE (2020a, 2020b, 2020c).

Although many women with a bipolar disorder will go through pregnancy with no complications, the condition will require careful management during pregnancy due to an increased susceptibility to relapse from various stressors, including environmental, physical, psychosocial, and biological changes. Relapse can lead to major depressive episodes, hypomania or mania with sleep disturbances, substance use and various cognitive, behavioural and lifestyle changes which could pose significant risks during pregnancy.

Medication used for bipolar disorders include antipsychotics and mood stabilisers. Many of the mood stabilisers, including sodium valproate, are also indicated for epilepsy and seizures and have been addressed in other chapters (see Chapter 17). Sodium valproate and its derivatives should not be used during pregnancy or in women of child-bearing potential because of their increased teratogenicity and developmental risks. Lithium, carbamazepine and lamotrigine are some of the other mood stabilisers that could be used in pregnancy with caution and close monitoring. Table 18.3 shows some of the possible effects of these medications on the fetus and baby.

It is not recommended to offer lithium to women who are planning a pregnancy or are pregnant, unless an antipsychotic medication alternative has not been effective (Poels et al., 2018; NICE, 2020a). Lithium levels vary through pregnancy, with a reduced level during the first trimester and higher levels in the third trimester. This means close monitoring of these levels (and more frequently if abnormal)

Table 18.3 Mood stabilisers and their use in pregnancy.

Mood stabiliser	Effects on mother	Effects on fetus	Risk in pregnancy	Risk in lactation
Lithium	Used for bipolar depression, hypomania and mania. Monitor lithium levels, thyroid and renal function	Increased risk of congenital (Munk-Olsen et al., 2018) or cardiac (Patorno et al., 2017) malformations after first-trimester lithium exposure A small increased risk of heart defects – Ebstein's anomaly	D	Avoid in breast feeding
Lamotrigine	More effective in bipolar depression. Generally, well tolerated	Relatively safer in pregnancy. No significant risk of preterm delivery, birth weight or maladaptive syndrome of the newborn	C	Moderately safe in breast feeding
Carbamazepine	More effective for hypomania and mania	Teratogenic: neural tube defect, craniofacial defects, cardiac and urinary defects. Low birthweight	D	Avoid in breast feeding (MHRA, 2021)
Oxycarbazepine	Mixed but better as an antimanic agent	Limited data	Limited data	
Sodium valproate	Used for bipolar depression, hypomania and mania. Not recommended for women of child-bearing age. Many side-effects	Teratogenic: neural tube defects around 5 in 100, spina bifida around 12 in 100. Developmental delays and neurocognitive difficulties. Increased risk of autism	Not recommended in pregnancy	Not recommended in breast feeding

Box 18.5   Recommendations for lithium management in pregnancy

- Do not offer lithium to women who are planning a pregnancy or are pregnant, unless antipsychotic medication has not been effective.
- If antipsychotic medication has not been effective and lithium is offered to a woman who is planning a pregnancy or pregnant, ensure that:
  - the woman knows that there is a risk of fetal heart malformations when lithium is taken in the first trimester, but the size of the risk is uncertain
  - the woman knows that lithium levels may be high in breast milk with a risk of toxicity for the baby
  - lithium levels are monitored more frequently throughout pregnancy and the postnatal period.

If a woman taking lithium becomes pregnant, consider stopping the drug gradually over 4 weeks if she is well. Explain to her that:
- stopping medication may not remove the risk of fetal heart malformations
- there is a risk of relapse, particularly in the postnatal period, if she has bipolar disorder.

If a woman taking lithium becomes pregnant and is not well or is at high risk of relapse, consider:
- switching gradually to an antipsychotic or
- stopping lithium and restarting it in the second trimester (if the woman is not planning to breast feed and her symptoms have responded better to lithium than to other drugs in the past) or
- continuing with lithium if she is at high risk of relapse and an antipsychotic is unlikely to be effective.

If a woman continues taking lithium during pregnancy:
- check plasma lithium levels every 4 weeks, then weekly from the 36th week
- adjust the dose to keep plasma lithium levels in the woman's therapeutic range
- ensure the woman maintains an adequate fluid balance
- ensure the woman gives birth in hospital
- ensure monitoring by the obstetric team when labour starts, including checking plasma lithium levels and fluid balance because of the risk of dehydration and lithium toxicity
- stop lithium during labour and check plasma lithium levels 12 hours after her last dose.

Source: NICE (2020).

297

throughout the course of pregnancy with necessary dose adjustments to avoid toxicity, with lowest effective doses during late pregnancy. Two- to three-weekly lithium checks are recommended until week 36 and then weekly thereafter (Poels et al., 2018; McAllister-Williams et al., 2017). Thyroid and renal functions also need to be concurrently monitored as these are directly affected by lithium (Poels et al., 2018). Box 18.5 shows some recommendations for lithium management in pregnancy.

Lamotrigine is more effective in treating bipolar depression and generally better tolerated in pregnancy. Because of increased renal clearance, dose adjustments may be necessary for more effective outcomes. There is relatively no significant risk of miscarriage, preterm delivery, low birth-weight, maladaptive syndrome of the newborn or neurocognitive developmental effects associated with lamotrigine.

Psychotropic medications and lactation

It is beyond the scope of this chapter to provide detailed information on the safety of women taking psychotropic drugs whilst breast feeding and the reader is referred to Chapter 20 of this text. If a breast-feeding woman requires ongoing treatment, caution is needed as close monitoring of the infant for signs of drug-related toxicity and adverse effects, mainly extrapyramidal symptoms, sedation and weight monitoring will be needed. In view of this, referral to a mental health specialist is recommended.

Episode of care

Joan was a 26-year-old woman diagnosed with schizophrenia for the past 8 years. She attended hospital once for her mental health issues during that period. Joan had been mentally stable for 2 years prior to her pregnancy. She had a good response in the past to risperidone, lurasidone and aripiprazole.

Joan took risperidone during her pregnancy and remained asymptomatic. Her baby was born at 40 weeks gestation with no problems. The baby was bottle fed in hospital because of concerns about Joan's medications. However, she wanted to breast feed her baby and asked if she could do so prior to her discharge from the postnatal ward. She was concerned about weight gain so aripiprazole and lurasidone were good options as they have less effect on weight. However, aripiprazole may have an adverse effect on milk production. As risperidone had kept her well for several years and has no effect on milk supply, the advice from her mental health specialist was to continue taking risperidone and if excessive weight gain became a problem, to consider weight management regimes including exercise and nutrition advice or referral to the dietician. If any weight gain was still not managed, then aripiprazole could be considered as an alternative once milk production was fully established.

Source: Adapted from Osborne (2021).

Clinical consideration

When a woman with a severe mental illness decides to stop psychotropic medication in pregnancy and the postnatal period, it is recommended that her mental health specialist discusses with her:

- her reasons for doing so
- the possibility of:
  - restarting the medication
  - switching to another medication
  - having a psychological intervention
  - increasing the level of monitoring and support.

Ensure she knows about any risks to herself, the fetus or baby when stopping medication.

Source: NICE (2020a).

Conclusion

As shown in this chapter, it is recommended that mental health specialists discuss medications, their safety profiles and treatment options with a woman prior to during and after pregnancy and child birth wherever possible in order to decide the preferred course of treatment. Women should be fully informed and involved in all decisions about their medications during the perinatal period. There are alternatives to psychotropic medications for women who may prefer these, where indicated. They include psychological and psychosocial interventions. In many instances, talking therapies or seeing a psychologist can be helpful during pregnancy. However, for most women, a concomitant antipsychotic medication treatment will still be necessary to stay well, especially for those with a current, recent or past history of mental ill-health. On balance with the exception of those contraindicated, the medication that has normally kept the woman well would usually rank higher during these considerations.

Glossary

Antidepressant   Medication used to treat depression and some anxiety disorders. These medications work by increasing the activity and levels of certain chemicals in the brain, helping to lift an individual's mood

Antipsychotic medication   Medication used primarily to treat psychosis and now, bipolar disorders. The main symptoms of psychosis are hallucinations and delusions

Bipolar disorder   A mental health problem in which a person has periods of hypomania or mania and periods of depression

Depression   A common mental health problem; the main symptoms include losing pleasure in things that were once enjoyable and losing interest in everyday activities and other people

Mania   Feelings of elation, extreme happiness or feeling 'high' or irritability, or both. Those with mania can also feel overconfident, sleep less than usual, can have 'speeded-up thoughts' and may take unnecessary risks

Post-traumatic stress disorder   A type of anxiety disorder that can sometimes follow a threatening or traumatic event

Psychosis and schizophrenia   Mental health problems, the main symptoms of which are hallucinations and delusions

Test yourself

Now review your learning by completing the learning activities for this chapter at www.wiley.com/go/pharmacologyformidwives.

299

References

Abel, K.M., Au, K., Howard, L.M. (2014) Schizophrenia, psychopharmacology, and pregnancy. In: Galbally, M., Snellen, M., Lewis, A. (eds) *Psychopharmacology and Pregnancy*, pp.119–138. Springer: Berlin.

Albert, K.M., Paul, P.A. (2019) Estrogen, stress, and depression: cognitive and biological interactions. *Annual Review of Clinical Psychology*, **15**: 399–423.

Bérard, A., Iessa, N., Chaabane, S., Muanda, F.T., Boukhris, T., Zhao, J.P. (2016) The risk of major cardiac malformations associated with paroxetine use during the first trimester of pregnancy: a systematic review and meta-analysis. *British Journal of Clinical Pharmacology*, **81**(4): 589–604.

British National Formulary (2021a). Paroxetine. https://bnf.nice.org.uk/drug/paroxetine.html#pregnancy (accessed February 2022).

British National Formulary (2021b) Fluoxetine. https://bnf.nice.org.uk/drug/fluoxetine.html#pregnancy (accessed February 2022).

British National Formulary (2021c) Vortioxetine. https://bnf.nice.org.uk/drug/vortioxetine.html#pregnancy (accessed February 2022).

British National Formulary (2021d) Chlorpromazine hydrochloride. https://bnf.nice.org.uk/drug/chlorpromazine-hydrochloride.html#pregnancy (accessed February 2022).

De Ridder, D., Adhia, D., Vanneste, S. (2021) The anatomy of pain and suffering in the brain and its clinical implications. *Neuroscience and Biobehavioral Reviews*, **130**: 125–146.

Food and Drug Administration (2021) FDA Pregnancy Risk Information: An Update. www.drugs.com/pregnancy-categories.html (accessed February 2022).

Galbally, M., Snellen, M., Power, J. (2014) Antipsychotic drugs in pregnancy: a review of their maternal and fetal effects. *Therapeutic Advances in Drug Safety*, **5**(2): 100–109.

Galbally, M., Spigset, O., Johnson, A.R., Kohan, R., Lappas, M., Lewis, A.J. (2017) Neonatal adaptation following intrauterine antidepressant exposure: assessment, drug assay levels, and infant development outcomes. *Pediatric Research*, **82**: 806–813.

Gustavo, E., Tafet, M.D., Nemeroff, C.B. (2015) The links between stress and depression: psychoneuroendocrinological, genetic, and environmental interactions. *Journal of Neuropsychiatry and Clinical Neuroscience*, **28**: 77–88.

Huybrechts, K.F., Hernández-Díaz, S., Patorno, E. et al. (2016) Antipsychotic use in pregnancy and the risk for congenital malformations. *JAMA Psychiatry*, **73**(9): 938–946.

Kalra, S., Einarson, A., Koren, G., Motherisk Team (2005) Taking antidepressants during late pregnancy. How should we advise women? *Canadian Family Physician*, **51**(8): 1077–1078.

Kieviet, N., Van Keulen, V., Van de Ven, P., Dolman, K., Deckers, M., Honig, A. (2016) Serotonin and poor neonatal adaptation after antidepressant exposure in utero. *Acta Neuropsychiatrica*, **29**(1): 43–53.

Kohen, D. (2004) Psychotropic medication in pregnancy. *Advances in Psychiatric Treatment*, **10**: 59–66.

Kolding, L., Pedersen, L.H., Petersen, O.B., Uldbjerg, N., Sandager, P. (2021) Sertraline use during pregnancy and effect on fetal cardiac function. *Journal of Maternal-Fetal & Neonatal Medicine*, **34**(22): 3631–3638.

Kucukgoncu, S., Guloksuz, S., Celik, K. et al. (2020) Antipsychotic exposure in pregnancy and the risk of gestational diabetes: a systematic review and meta-analysis. *Schizophrenia Bulletin*, **46**(2): 311–318.

Lassiter, N.T., Manns-James, L.E. (2017) Pregnancy.In: Brucker, M.C., King, T.L. (eds) *Pharmacology for Women's Health*, 2nd edn, pp.1025–1059. Jones and Bartlett Learning: Burlington.

LeMoult, J., Humphreys, K.L., Tracy, A., Hoffmeister, J.A., Ip, E., Gotlib, I.H. (2020) Meta-analysis: exposure to early life stress and risk for depression in childhood and adolescence. *Journal of the American Academy of Child & Adolescent Psychiatry*, **59**: 842–855.

McAllister-Williams, R.H., Baldwin, D.S., Cantwell, R. et al. (2017) British Association for Psychopharmacology consensus guidance on the use of psychotropic medication preconception, in pregnancy and postpartum. *Journal of Psychopharmacology*, **31**: 519–552.

McTeague, L.M., Rosenberg, B.M., Lopez, J.W. et al. (2020) Identification of common neural circuit disruptions in emotional processing across psychiatric disorders. *American Journal of Psychiatry*, **177**: 411–421.

Medicines and Healthcare products Regulatory Agency (2021) Antiepileptic drugs: review of safety of use during pregnancy. www.gov.uk/government/publications/public-assesment-report-of-antiepileptic-drugs-review-of-safety-of-use-during-pregnancy/antiepileptic-drugs-review-of-safety-of-use-during-pregnancy (accessed February 2022).

Munk-Olsen, T., Liu, X., Viktorin, A. et al. (2018) Maternal and infant outcomes associated with lithium use in pregnancy: an international collaborative meta-analysis of six cohort studies. *Lancet Psychiatry*, **5**(8): 644–652.

National Institute for Health and Care Excellence (2020a) Mental health in pregnancy and the year after giving birth. www.nice.org.uk/guidance/cg192/resources/mental-health-in-pregnancy-and-the-year-after-giving-birth-pdf-250640652229 (accessed February 2022).

National Institute for Health and Care Excellence (2020b) Weight management before, during and after pregnancy. www.nice.org.uk/guidance/ph27 (accessed February 2022).

National Institute for Health and Care Excellence (2020c) Diabetes in pregnancy: management from preconception to the postnatal period. www.nice.org.uk/guidance/ng3 (accessed February 2022).

Osborne, M.L. (2021) Antipsychotics during breastfeeding. Psychopharmacology Institute. https://psychopharmacologyinstitute.com/section/antipsychotics-during-breastfeeding-2615-5075?utm_medium=email (accessed February 2022).

Park, Y., Hernandez-Diaz, S., Bateman, B.T. et al. (2018) Continuation of atypical antipsychotic medication during early pregnancy and the risk of gestational diabetes. *American Journal of Psychiatry*, **175**(6): 564–574.

Patorno, E., Huybrechts, K.F., Bateman, B.T. et al. (2017) Lithium use in pregnancy and the risk of cardiac malformations. *New England Journal of Medicine*, **376**(23): 2245–2254.

Petersen, I., McCrea, R.L., Sammon, C.J. et al. (2016) Risks and benefits of psychotropic medication in pregnancy: cohort studies based on UK electronic primary care health records. *Health Technology Assessment*, **20**: 1–176.

Poels, E.M.P., Bijma, H.H., Galbally, M. et al. (2018) Lithium during pregnancy and after delivery: a review. *International Journal of Bipolar Disorders*, **6**: 26.

Reilly, T.J., Sagnay de la Bastida, V.C., Joyce, D.W., Cullen, A.E., McGuire, P. (2020) Exacerbation of psychosis during the perimenstrual phase of the menstrual cycle: systematic review and meta-analysis. *Schizophrenia Bulletin*, **46**(1): 78–90.

Serafini, R.A., Pryce, K.D., Zachariou, V. (2019) The mesolimbic dopamine system in chronic pain and associated affective comorbidities. *Biological Psychiatry*, **87**(1): 64–73.

Slone, D., Siskind, V., Heinonen, O.P., Monson, R.R., Kaufman, D.W., Shapiro, S. (1977) Antenatal exposure to the phenothiazines in relation to congenital malformations, perinatal mortality rate, birth weight, and intelligence quotient score. *American Journal of Obstetrics and Gynecology*, **128**: 486–488.

Soares, C.N., Zitek, B. (2008) Reproductive hormone sensitivity and risk for depression across the female life cycle: a continuum of vulnerability? *Journal of Psychiatry and Neuroscience*, **33**(4): 331–343

Stowe, Z.N., Nemeroff, C. B. (1998) Psychopharmacology during pregnancy and lactation. In: Schatzberg, A.F., Nemeroff, C.B. (eds) *Textbook of Psychopharmacology*, pp.823–837. American Psychiatric Press: Washington, DC.

Teodorescu, A., Ifteni, P., Moga, M.A. et al. (2017) Dilemma of treating schizophrenia during pregnancy: a case series and a review of literature. *BMC Psychiatry*, **17**: 311.

United Kingdom Drugs in Lactation Advisory Service (2021) www.sps.nhs.uk/articles/ukdilas/ (accessed February 2022).

Vigod, S.N., Tara Gomes, T., Wilton, A.S., Taylor, V.H., Ray, J.G. (2015) Antipsychotic drug use in pregnancy: high dimensional, propensity matched, population based cohort study. *British Medical Journal*, **350**: h2298.

Wang, Z., Brauer, R., Man, K.K.C. et al. (2021) Prenatal exposure to antipsychotic agents and the risk of congenital malformations in children: a systematic review and meta-analysis. *British Journal of Clinical Pharmacology*, **87**: 4101–4123.

Yonkers, K.A., Wisner, K.L., Stowe, Z. et al. (2004) Management of bipolar disorder during pregnancy and the postpartum period. *American Journal of Psychiatry*, **161**:608–620.

Yonkers, K.A., Blackwell, K.A., Glover, J., Forray, A. (2014) Antidepressant use in pregnant and postpartum women. *Annual Review of Clinical Psychology*, **10**: 369–392.

Zhong, X., Harris, G., Smirnova, L. et al. (2020) Antidepressant paroxetine exerts developmental neurotoxicity in an iPSC-derived 3D human brain model. *Frontiers in Cellular Neuroscience*, **14**: 25.

Further reading

Action on Postpartum Psychosis: the national charity for women and families affected by postpartum psychosis, a severe mental illness which begins suddenly following childbirth. www.app-network.org

MIND: information on postnatal depression and perinatal mental health. www.mind.org.uk/information-support/types-of-mental-health-problems/postnatal-depression-and-perinatal-mental-health/about-maternal-mental-health-problems/

Royal College of Psychiatrists: information on mental health in pregnancy. www.rcpsych.ac.uk/mental-health/treatments-and-wellbeing/mental-health-in-pregnancy

Tommy's: mental health before, during and after pregnancy. www.tommys.org/pregnancy-information/im-pregnant/mental-wellbeing/mental-health-during-and-after-pregnancy

Chapter 19

Medications and the immune system

Janet G. Migliozzi and Cathy Hamilton

University of Hertfordshire, Hatfield, UK

Aim

The aim of this chapter is to introduce the reader to issues relating to the immune system during pregnancy, birth and the postnatal period.

Learning outcomes

After reading this chapter the reader will be able to:
- Explain the difference between various types of immunity and the basic immune response to a vaccine
- Identify the different types of vaccines currently used in the UK
- Explain the midwife's role in relation to vaccination
- Discuss specific issues relating to vaccines currently offered to child-bearing women in the UK.

Test Your existing knowledge

- What are the differences between innate and acquired immunity?
- What are RNA vaccines?
- At what stage of pregnancy should the influenza vaccine be offered?
- When is the optimal time for the pregnant woman to receive the pertussis vaccine?
- Why did screening for rubella immunity during pregnancy cease?

Introduction

The midwife has a key role to play in providing women with information in order to make fully informed decisions about whether to accept vaccination during pregnancy (Regan et al., 2016). Most pregnant women are anxious about taking medication that might have an adverse effect on their unborn baby and they need to know the benefits of accepting the vaccine weighed against

Fundamentals of Pharmacology for Midwives, First Edition. Edited by Ian Peate and Cathy Hamilton.
© 2022 John Wiley & Sons Ltd. Published 2022 by John Wiley & Sons Ltd.
Companion website: www.wiley.com/go/pharmacologyformidwives

the risk of contracting a disease if they choose not to be vaccinated. The use of vaccinations during pregnancy will be discussed in this chapter, including a summary of how vaccination might be managed in the postnatal period in order to protect a future pregnancy from infection.

Immunity

The environment contains many substances and organisms that are harmful to health and will cause disease if they enter the body. Organisms gain entry to the body by both active and passive means, e.g. through inhalation, ingestion or an open wound. However, whatever an organism's point of entry, the body has various defence mechanisms to either physically prevent pathogens from entering the body or destroy them if they do.

Immunity is the means by which the body recognises and resists infection, resulting from antigens on the surface of micro-organisms or other toxins, chemicals, drugs or foreign objects that may be harmful. An antigen is any substance that stimulates the body's immune system to produce antibodies against it. Penetration of the body's external barriers by micro-organisms leads to activation of the body's immune system which recognises the invading infectious agent as not belonging to the host and then seeks to eliminate it.

There are two main types of immunity: innate and acquired (Figure 19.1).

Innate immunity

Innate immunity does not require contact with a disease-causing organism or pathogen for responses to occur as this type of immunity is inherent. The response and defence provided by the innate immune system are quick, non-specific and short-acting. The first line of defence provided by these components of the immune system is the body's physical and mechanical barriers, chemical barriers, phagocytic cells and the complement system. It is important to note that innate immunity has no memory.

303

Acquired immunity

Acquired or adaptive immunity is the body's second line of defence. The immune system learns to recognise specific disease-causing pathogens and if they are encountered again, is able to challenge and ward them off. This is because acquired immunity has the capacity to develop an immunological memory.

Acquired immunity can be natural or artificial and acquired through active and passive means.

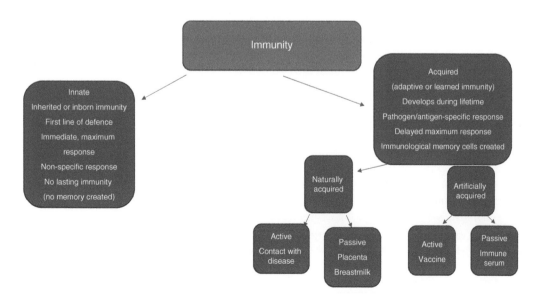

Figure 19.1 Types of immunity.

Naturally acquired immunity

Active means of gaining natural immunity are when antigens enter the body naturally, i.e. from being exposed to a disease-causing organism/infection, and the body produces antibodies and specialised lymphocytes in response to this.

Passive means of naturally acquired immunity involve antibodies from the mother passing to the fetus via the placenta or to the baby from breast milk.

Artificially acquired immunity

Active means of gaining artificial immunity are introducing antigens via vaccination which will lead to the body producing antibodies and specialised lymphocytes in response to this.

Passive means of artificially acquired immunity include the injecting of preformed antibodies in the form of an immune serum taken from purified blood products of humans or animals who are immune to the disease to individuals who are not.

Immunity in pregnancy

The establishment, maintenance and completion of a healthy pregnancy are dependent on the critical role played by the maternal immune system. During a normal pregnancy, the immune system undergoes predictable and precisely timed changes in order that the pregnant woman's body does not reject the fetus. As the developing fetus contains genetic information from both parents, the pregnant woman's immune system must be regulated as it will perceive the presence of the father's cells as foreign material and there is a risk that the woman's immune system will seek to destroy them.

The alterations in immune function that occur during pregnancy aim not only to protect the developing fetus from immunological attack but also to maintain protection against infection (Aghaeepour et al., 2017).

Vaccines

Vaccination takes advantage of the immune system's ability to develop an *immunological memory*, so that it can effectively mobilise a cellular response to fight infection in a timely manner. The goal of all vaccines is to ensure that when an individual is again exposed to a micro-organism, an immune response will occur and the individual has protection from the disease.

There are two main types of pathogen that can be vaccinated against, bacteria and viruses, and vaccines contain the same antigens found in the pathogens that cause the associated disease; however, exposure to the antigen in the vaccine is controlled. This is achieved by 'priming' the immune system through artificial induction of immunity to protect against infectious disease. Vaccinations involve the administration of one or more antigens that can produce immunity to a disease-causing organism or toxin (poison). When an individual is later exposed to environmental disease-causing organisms, the immune system can destroy them before they can cause disease.

Types of vaccines

Attenuated live vaccines

These vaccines use live micro-organisms that have been 'weakened' or attenuated to make them less pathogenic. Attenuated live vaccines are usually not offered to individuals with weakened immune systems as, due to the absence of a normal immune response, there is the risk that the live micro-organisms contained within the vaccine can replicate quickly and cause serious infection. Box 19.1 outlines attenuated live vaccines used in the UK.

Inactivated (whole-pathogen) vaccines

These vaccines contain whole pathogens that have been killed so that they are unable to infect or replicate and cause disease. Because inactivated vaccines cannot replicate, they can only elicit a weak and short-lived immune response (unlike attenuated live vaccines). Consequently, repeated doses of the vaccine are required to achieve an adequate immune response and maintenance of immunity requires booster vaccinations. Because inactivated live vaccines contain no viable pathogenic organisms, they are safe to give to individuals with compromised immune systems.

Box 19.1 Attenuated live vaccines used in the UK

MMR (measles, mumps and rubella)
Nasal flu
Shingles
Chickenpox
Rotavirus

Subunit vaccines

Subunit vaccines contain components of natural antigens found within bacterial cell walls and viral envelopes that would normally trigger antibody production during infection. Therefore, unlike inactivated vaccines, they contain no intact bacterial or viral particles and are particularly useful for highly pathogenic micro-organisms as the lack of any pathogenic material within the vaccine means that they are very safe to use even in the immunocompromised patient as infection is impossible (Liu, 2019). Many of the vaccines developed for use against the coronavirus pandemic are subunit vaccines; for example, the AstraZeneca vaccine uses a spike from the SARS-Cov-2 virus inserted into a harmless chimpanzee virus which when injected, infects target cells to produce SARS-Cov-2 spike protein and triggers antibody production. If the vaccinated individual then comes into contact with SARS-Cov-2, they are able to target the virus and prevent infection (Mahase, 2020). Figure 19.2 provides an overview of how subunit vaccines work.

DNA and RNA vaccines

Recent advances in molecular biology that allow the manipulation of DNA have led to the design and production of a new generation of vaccines. These vaccines, known as DNA and RNA vaccines, use the body's own cells to make antigenic components of bacteria and viruses to trigger an immune response (Liu, 2019). For example, inserting the sequence of a viral protein into a plasmid (a small piece of DNA) and then injecting this into a muscle allows the muscle cells to use the information contained within the plasmid to make the viral protein, which then stimulates the production of antibodies.

One of the first SARS-Cov-2 vaccines to undergo clinical trials in America was an RNA-based vaccine. Similar RNA vaccines developed by Pfizer and BioNtech became the first SARS-Cov-2 vaccines to receive regulatory approval in the UK (Mahase, 2020). Figure 19.3 outlines how RNA-based vaccines work.

305

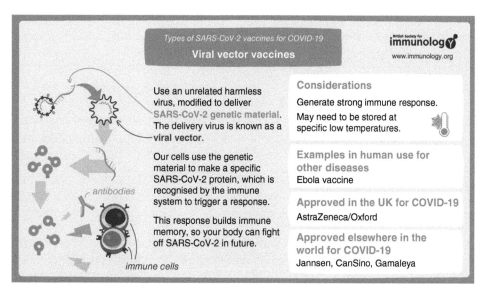

Figure 19.2   Subunit vaccines.
Source: British Society for Immunology (2021).

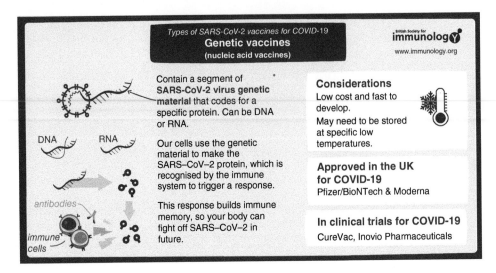

Figure 19.3   RNA-based vaccines.
Source: British Society for Immunology (2021).

Clinical consideration

Immunisation procedures

Preparation of vaccines
In order to avoid errors and maintain vaccine efficacy, each vaccine should be reconstituted and drawn up when required rather than being drawn up in advance of an immunisation session.

Before use, the colour and composition of the vaccine must be examined to ensure that it conforms to its given description and vaccines should not be used after their expiry date.

Different vaccines should not be mixed in the same syringe unless recommended for such use and the right product, right route and correct dose must be checked prior to administration.

Vaccine administration
Any individual giving vaccinations must have received training in the management of anaphylaxis and have immediate access to appropriate equipment.

Prior to administration, the individual giving the vaccination should ensure that:

- consent has been obtained
- there are no contraindications to the vaccine being given
- the person receiving the vaccine is fully informed about the vaccine to be given, understands the vaccination procedure and is aware of possible adverse reactions and how to treat them.

Route of vaccination
Most vaccines should be given by an intramuscular (IM) injection which deposits medication into deep muscle tissue under the subcutaneous tissue and is a common technique for vaccine administration. Administration of vaccines by this route also minimises local reactions. Vaccines should not be given intravenously.

Vaccines not given by the IM route include the BCG vaccine, which is given by intradermal injection, varicella vaccines, which are given by deep subcutaneous (SC) injection, and cholera vaccine which is given by mouth.

The angle for administration of an IM injection is 90° and a needle length from 25 mm to 38 mm will be required, depending on the patient's BMI. Suitable sites for vaccination include the anterolateral aspect of the thigh or the deltoid area of the upper arm. Due to the risk of sciatic nerve damage, immunisations should not be given into the buttock. During administration of an IM injection, the skin should be stretched, not bunched, and it is not necessary to aspirate the syringe after insertion into the muscle.

Source: Based on The Green Book. https://assets.publishing.service.gov.uk/government/uploads/system/uploads/attachment_data/file/147915/Green-Book-Chapter-4.pdf

Safety in vaccination programmes

Before the development of vaccines, mortality and morbidity from infectious diseases that are now preventable were very high. However, as more and more vaccines have been developed, the risk of adverse events arising from their use is increasing. Where rapid vaccine development has been needed (as in the case of the COVID-19 pandemic) and the evidence supporting a new vaccine's development has been conducted via a rolling review, it is even more important that any adverse reactions that are suspected to be vaccine related are reported via the Medicines and Healthcare products Regulatory Agency (MHRA) Yellow Card scheme (https://yellowcard.mhra.gov.uk/the-yellow-card-scheme/).

Clinical consideration

Suspected reactions following vaccination

Any suspected reaction following a vaccination should be reported to the MHRA via the Yellow Card scheme. A Yellow Card should be submitted when a causal association is suspected between the vaccine administered and the condition experienced by the patient. Newly licensed vaccine products are subject to enhanced surveillance and are given 'black triangle' status (indicated by an inverted triangle) on the product information. For such products, all serious and non-serious suspected ADRs should be reported. For vaccines that have been marketed for 2 years or more, any serious suspected ADRs should be reported.

307

Cold chain storage of vaccines

Vaccines are biological products that are temperature sensitive and must be stored and transported at the recommended temperature. The system of transporting and storing vaccines is called the 'cold chain' and vaccine storage recommendations are set by the manufacturer and are part of the licensing conditions. This is a necessary requirement as when a vaccine is stored at too hot or cold a temperature, it becomes less effective or possibly inactive. Most vaccines require storage at 2–8 °C in specialised medical refrigerators. However, some vaccines require temperatures as cold as -20 °C and in the case of the newer vaccines, for example the Pfizer-BioNTech COVID-19 vaccine, ultra-low temperatures of -70 °C are required.

UK routine immunisation schedule

In the UK, routine immunisations are provided to protect against the vaccine-preventable infections shown in Box 19.2.

A summary of the national immunisation programme currently offered in the UK can be found at www.gov.uk/government/publications/immunisation-schedule-the-green-book-chapter-11.

Vaccination during pregnancy

Live vaccines are not usually advocated for use during pregnancy unless the risk of infection is greater than the risk of the vaccination to the pregnant woman as there is the possibility that the fetus can become infected. Live vaccines that should be avoided include:

- BCG (vaccination against tuberculosis)
- MMR (measles, mumps and rubella)

Box 19.2   UK routine immunisation schedule

Diphtheria
Haemophilus influenzae type b (Hib)
Hepatitis B
Human papillomavirus
Influenza
Measles
Meningococcal disease
Mumps
Pertussis (whooping cough)
Polio
Pneumococcal disease
Polio
Rotavirus
Rubella
Shingles
Tetanus

Source: Public Health England (PHE, 2019).

- oral polio (which forms part of the 5-in-1 vaccine given to infants)
- oral typhoid
- yellow fever.

The following vaccines are inactive and are therefore considered safe to administer during pregnancy.

- Influenza vaccine
- Whooping cough vaccine
- COVID-19 vaccine

The role of the midwife in vaccination of pregnant women

Midwives can help to dispel myths and inaccurate information associated with certain vaccines, bearing in mind that women will have different levels of understanding. For example, women may have additional learning needs or may speak English as a second language. Healthcare information that is confusing or contradictory may lead people to mistrust the system and seek their own information from alternative, possibly unreliable sources (Berger et al., 2020). This is supported by research undertaken by the Royal Society for Public Health (RSPH, 2021) which demonstrated a lack of trust within black, Asian and minority ethnic (BAME) communities in relation to the COVID-19 vaccine. Many respondents stated that they might accept the vaccine if they received appropriate information from a healthcare professional. However, although midwives may recommend a course of action to women based on current medical evidence, the individual woman has the right to make the final decision. The midwife as the woman's advocate must support her in whatever decision she reaches (NMC, 2018).

When midwives administer vaccines, they do so on the basis of a prescription written by medical practitioner or a Patient Group Direction. It is important that midwives are fully versed in the mode of action of vaccines, contradictions to their use and any potential side-effects. They also need to be prepared to instigate emergency measures in the unlikely event that a woman has an anaphylactic reaction to the vaccine. This includes knowing how to summon emergency assistance, particularly when working in a community setting.

Many vaccines cause systematic effects in some people a day or two after administration. Side-effects may include a sore arm at the site of injection, muscular aches and pains, nausea, headache and a general feeling of malaise. These symptoms are bound to raise anxiety in a pregnant woman who will be concerned that her being unwell will have an effect on her baby. The midwife should alert women to potential side-effects so that they know what is normal and when they should seek medical help in case symptoms are due to a cause unrelated to the vaccine.

National influenza vaccination programme

Vaccinating pregnant women against influenza is an important public health strategy to prevent serious illness in women and their babies during the first 6 months of life (Regan et al., 2018). Pregnant women are known to be at high risk of developing serious complications following infection with influenza, especially if they contract it during the second and third trimesters (Duncan, 2020). This is due to their altered immunity instigated by the physiological adaptations of pregnancy (Jamieson et al., 2006; Dodds et al., 2007). The increased risk to pregnant women if they get influenza was seen during the 2009–2010 H1N1 (swine flu) pandemic when 12 women died in the UK from August 2009 to January 2010 as a result of the virus (Modder, 2010). In addition to protecting women from contracting the infection, antenatal vaccination directly protects newborn babies through transplacental transfer of maternal antibodies.

Prevention through immunisation is a vital aspect in the Department of Health and Social Care's management of influenza strategy (NHS England, 2020). The national flu immunisation programme is geared to protect those individuals who are at high risk of flu- related morbidity and mortality (NHS England, 2020), including pregnant women.

Since 2010, routine influenza immunisation in the UK has been extended to include all pregnant women. Inactivated influenza vaccine is offered to women at any stage of their pregnancy, preferably between October and January to incorporate the winter season when influenza cases are most prevalent (NHS, 2020). Clinical judgement should be used to decide whether vaccination is warranted outside these months. The level and severity of the influenza strain circulating in any year along with the presence of other risk factors in the woman and the availability of inactivated influenza vaccine are factors that need to be considered (NHS England, 2020).

Vaccination in the UK is available free on the NHS and women are encouraged to discuss their options for receiving the vaccine with their midwife during early pregnancy. In some areas it is administered at hospital antenatal clinics whilst in others it is offered at the GP surgery (Vaccine Knowledge Project, 2019).

However, despite pregnant women being identified as a priority group for influenza vaccination, studies indicate that uptake remains low and may be below 50% (Regan et al., 2016; Dabrera et al., 2014). The national influenza vaccine uptake for pregnant women in the winter of 2019–20 demonstrated a reduction, to 43% of all pregnant women compared to 45.2% in the winter of 2018–19 (PHE, 2020).

Further studies have shown that concern amongst women about the safety of having a vaccine whilst pregnant and the potential adverse effect it may have on their developing baby is the main reason behind this reluctance to be vaccinated (Yuen and Tarrant, 2014). This concern is reflected amongst healthcare providers who find that product information provided by vaccine manufacturers stating that official recommendations for vaccination during pregnancy are merely 'considered' contradicts the message to have the vaccine promoted by national public health programmes (Proveaux et al., 2016).

Despite these concerns, there are a plethora of studies demonstrating the safety of the influenza vaccine during pregnancy when administered in its inactivated form. A systematic review by Giles et al. (2019), based on studies involving over 100 000 women, confirmed the safety of the influenza vaccine during pregnancy and highlighted its protective effect against preterm birth and low birthweight. There was no associated increase in preterm birth, low birthweight, small for gestational age, congenital malformations, miscarriage or stillbirth.

Other studies investigating reasons behind the low uptake of the flu vaccine have consistently identified advice given by healthcare providers as being the strongest factor in deciding whether a pregnant woman will accept or refuse the vaccine (Mak et al., 2015; Regan et al., 2016). Midwives have an important role to play in promotion of the influenza vaccine during pregnancy given the regular contact they have with women. Regan et al. (2018) argue that professional development for midwives is needed to enable them to recommend and administer vaccines to pregnant women with confidence. This position is supported by the Royal College of Midwives which also recommends that all frontline workers involved in direct patient care receive the seasonable influenza vaccine (RCM, 2020) (Box 19.3).

Episode of care

Penny is a 35-year-old woman with moderate learning difficulties. She is pregnant with her first baby. She visits her midwife at the local doctor's surgery in the early stages of pregnancy with her partner, Tony, who also has moderate learning needs. They live together independently with minimal input from the social services. The midwife talks to Penny about having the flu vaccination. Penny and Tony have both heard of the 'flu jab' but Penny informs the midwife that she is frightened of needles and does not want to have it. The midwife explains to the couple that although the injection might hurt momentarily, it will protect both Penny and her baby from flu and is well worth having as women can get very unwell if they get the flu while they are pregnant. She reassures Penny that it is safe to take during pregnancy and won't hurt the baby but will protect it from getting infected with flu. She explains that the practice nurse will give Penny the injection and talks her through what will happen. Penny has met the practice nurse before and feels reassured by this. The midwife finds some leaflets produced by MENCAP explaining the 'flu jab' in clear language with pictures showing what will happen during the vaccination appointment. Penny and Tony take these away to look at together.

A few days later, Penny makes an informed decision that she will have the flu vaccination despite her fear of needles. She returns the following week for an appointment with the practice nurse and although she is very nervous, she is surprised at how little the 'jab' hurts. She leaves the surgery feeling pleased that she is protecting both herself and her baby and the vaccination won't hurt the baby but will protect it from getting infected with flu.

Pertussis (whooping cough) maternal vaccination programme

Pertussis, commonly known as whooping cough, is a highly infectious disease. There is an initial catarrhal stage following by a cough that increases in severity to become paroxysmal usually within 1–2 weeks. The paroxysms are followed by the very characteristic 'whoop' that gives this disease its name (PHE, 2016). If contracted by babies, pertussis is a significant cause of serious illness and death. Most hospitalisations occur in babies less than 6 months old and many of them require care in paediatric intensive care units due to the severity of the illness (Crowcroft et al., 2003). Infants are at risk of contracting the disease from older children and adults which highlights the importance of an ongoing national vaccination programme.

In January 2016, the Joint Committee on Vaccination and Immunisation (JCVI) advised that maternal pertussis vaccination should be administered from 16 weeks gestation (Eberhardt et al.,

Box 19.3   Quadrivalent influenza vaccine

Indications	Immunity against influenza for eligible pregnant women
Dose and frequency	0.5 mL × 1 dose
Contraindications	Known history of confirmed anaphylactic reaction to a preceding dose of the vaccine or any component of the influenza vaccine
Side-effects	Common side-effects include local reaction at the injection site, fatigue, headache, joint and muscle aches and chills

2016: JCVI, 2016). A study showed that early second trimester maternal vaccination significantly increased the number of neonatal antibodies produced (Eberhardt et al., 2016). This meant that widening the immunisation window from the second trimester would further improve seroprotection. It would also offer extra protection to infants born prematurely who are likely to be vulnerable to complications associated with pertussis and would benefit from extra antibodies. The JCVI (2016) also recommended that the maternal programme, although initially introduced as a temporary measure, should continue to be offered indefinitely.

The introduction of the maternal pertussis vaccination programme has been very effective in reducing the numbers of infants with pertussis. From 2012 to 2013, maternal vaccine effectiveness in England was estimated to be 91% with average vaccine coverage across the country being 64% (Amirthalingam et al., 2014). Another study in England and Wales using a case–control approach demonstrated an adjusted vaccine effectiveness of 93% (Dabrera et al., 2014).

During 2012 there were 14 infant deaths from pertussis reported in England and Wales, all born before the start of the maternal vaccination programme in October 2012. From the beginning of the programme to the end of October 2014, 10 infant deaths from pertussis were reported, nine of these were to unvaccinated mothers, all 10 babies being too young to have received the first dose of the pertussis-containing vaccine (PHE, 2014).

Research has raised no concerns about the safety of pertussis-containing inactivated vaccine being administered at any stage of pregnancy. Inactivated vaccines do not contain any live organisms and therefore cannot replicate to cause infection in either the woman or fetus. A large observational cohort study based on 18 000 vaccinated women (Donegan et al., 2014) showed no evidence of increased stillbirth risk or any other adverse effects following vaccination, with similar rates of normal healthy births in vaccinated as in unvaccinated women.

Pertussis-containing vaccines are also safe for breast-feeding women and there is evidence to demonstrate that pertussis antibodies in breast milk are increased after vaccination during pregnancy. It should be highlighted, however, that this extra protection is still not enough to replace the need for the breast-fed baby to complete the recommended neonatal immunisation programme (PHE, 2016).

Recommended pertussis vaccine during pregnancy

Single pertussis vaccines are not currently available so pregnant women are offered low-dose diphtheria, tetanus, pertussis and inactivated poliomyelitis vaccine (dTA P/IPV). Since July 2014 the recommended vaccine has been Boostrix®-IPV which is licensed as a booster vaccine from 4 years of age containing low-dose diphtheria vaccine suitable for adults.

dTAP/IPV is supplied as a single 0.5 mL dose in a prefilled syringe and is usually administered as an intramuscular injection into the upper outer quadrant of the deltoid muscle in the arm. Any healthcare professional who plans to be involved in a vaccination programme should ensure that they read the Patient Group Direction and Summary of Product Characteristics so they are familiar with the product and how it should be used prior to administration. Very few women are unable to receive pertussis-containing vaccines although it is contraindicated for any individuals who have suffered a confirmed anaphylactic reaction to a previous pertussis-containing vaccine or to any component of the vaccine, including polymyxin and neomycin. As dTAP/IPV is an inactivated vaccine, it can be used safely at the same time as anti-D treatment or the flu vaccine.

If dTA/IPV is inadvertently given prior to 16 weeks gestation, it should be given again once the woman reaches 16 weeks or around the time of her fetal anomaly scan. Repeating the dose in this way means that the fetus benefits from the optimal transfer of maternal antibodies. However, to reduce the risk of a local reaction, it is advised that there are at least 4 weeks between each dose.

COVID-19

COVID-19 was first recognised as a severe respiratory infection in Wuhan, China, in late 2019 (WHO, 2020). A SARS-CoV-2 pandemic was declared by the WHO in March 2020.

Studies indicate that the risk to pregnant women and babies following COVID-19 infection is relatively low compared to other groups. Over 50% of pregnant women who test positive for COVID-19 show no symptoms and there is no increase in stillbirth or neonatal death when babies are exposed to the infection in utero (Allotey et al., 2020). It remains unclear whether the infection can be transmitted vertically from mother to unborn baby and only 2% of babies born to women known to be infected with COVID-19 test positive themselves. However, risks to the pregnant woman and her baby do increase if the woman shows symptoms. In this case, there is a 2–3-fold increase in preterm birth, usually as a result of medical intervention to deliver the baby so as to improve the woman's oxygen levels (Vousden et al., 2021).

The largest worldwide review of COVID-19 to date indicates that pregnant women are more likely to be admitted to the intensive care unit with COVID-19 than their non-pregnant counterparts (Mullins et al., 2021). Risk factors for pregnant women having the more severe form of infection include them being overweight, from a BAME background, being over the age of 35 and with other diseases such as diabetes, asthma and hypertension (Vousden et al., 2021; Allotey et al., 2020).

As inactivated vaccines are unable to replicate, they do not cause infection in either the woman or her fetus (Kroger et al., 2013). Although the AstraZeneca COVID-19 vaccine does contain a live adenovirus vector, this is not replicating so will not cause the infection in the recipient (PHE, 2021).

Testing of the COVID-19 vaccines (Pfizer-BioNTech, Moderna and AstraZeneca) has taken place in animals and at the time of writing no concerns have been raised regarding their use in pregnant women (PHE, 2021). Indeed, similar vaccines have been used widely already to vaccinate pregnant women against the Ebola virus with no adverse effect on either the woman or her baby (PHE, 2021).

It is acknowledged that as these new vaccines were developed rapidly in response to the onset of the COVID-19 pandemic, extensive testing on pregnant women is still to take place. However, the JCVI advises that pregnant women should be offered the vaccine at the same time as non-pregnant women, the decision being based on their age and clinical risk category (JCVI, 2021). Midwives should advise pregnant women on the benefits and risks of accepting the vaccine whilst acknowledging that to date there is limited evidence on the safety of the vaccine in pregnancy.

In March 2021, a rare condition involving excessive blood clotting (thrombosis) accompanied by a low platelet count (thrombocytopenia) was reported in a small number of cases following vaccination with the AstraZeneca product (Greinacher et al., 2021). At the time of writing, the reported rate of this condition in the UK is just over 10 cases per million vaccinations administered so it remains rare.

Consequently, the WHO, JCVI and MHRA continue to support using the vaccine, highlighting that the benefits of the vaccine outweigh the small risk, particularly for individuals in vulnerable clinical groups and those over 40. In other words, individuals in these priority groups are more at risk of the adverse effects of contracting COVID-19 than they are from this rare adverse reaction to the vaccine itself. However, for individuals under 40 who are not so much at risk of serious illness if they are infected, it is recommended that one of the other vaccines should be used wherever possible. Pregnant women and women who have recently given birth or are receiving treatment for infertility may all be at increased thrombotic risk due to hormonal influences on blood viscosity. However, the latest Royal College of Obstetricians and Gynaecologists guidance suggests that there is currently no clear link between this adverse effect and the higher thrombotic risk associated with childbirth (RCOG, 2021).

The Pfizer-BioNTech (Box 19.4) and Moderna vaccines have the most detailed safety data available currently and are therefore the preferred options for pregnant women. However, if a pregnant woman received AstraZeneca as her first dose then she should receive the same product for her second dose. If a woman discovers she is pregnant shortly after being vaccinated, then she should

Box 19.4   Pfizer COVID-19 vaccine

Indications	Immunity against COVID-19 infection for eligible pregnant women
Dose and frequency	0.5 mL ×2 doses, a minimum of 28 days apart
Contraindications	Known history of severe allergic reaction to any component of the Pfizer-BioNTech COVID-19 vaccine
Side-effects	Common side-effects include local reaction at the injection site, fatigue, headache, joint and muscle aches and chills

Clinical consideration

Information for pregnant women about vaccines

Influenza vaccine

During pregnancy, your immune system (the body's natural defence) is weakened to protect the pregnancy. This can mean you're less able to fight off infections. As the baby grows, you may be unable to breathe as deeply, increasing the risk of infections such as pneumonia.

These changes can raise the risk from flu – pregnant women are more likely to get flu complications than women who are not pregnant and are more likely to be admitted to hospital.

Whooping cough vaccine

Whooping cough is a very serious infection, and young babies are most at risk. Most babies with whooping cough will be admitted to hospital.

When you have the whooping cough vaccination in pregnancy, your body produces antibodies to protect against whooping cough. These antibodies pass to your baby, giving them some protection until they're able to have their whooping cough vaccination at 8 weeks old.

Travel vaccinations during pregnancy

It may not always be possible to avoid areas that require vaccinations when you're pregnant. If this is the case, talk to a midwife or GP, who can tell you about the risks and benefits of any vaccinations you might need.

If there's a high risk of infection in the area you are travelling to, it's often safer to have a vaccine rather than travel unprotected as most diseases will be more harmful to your baby than a vaccine.

continue to complete the course with the same product. There is no need for the vaccinator to question women about potential pregnancy or a menstrual history prior to administration of the vaccine.

As these are inactive vaccines, they can be administered to breast-feeding women although again full safety data is not yet available for use of the vaccine during breast feeding. Midwives need to alert women to this risk (albeit small) of receiving a vaccine which has currently not been extensively tested. However, currently the benefits of receiving it do outweigh the risks and although the decision is up to the individual woman, midwives can confidently support the recommendation that pregnant and breast-feeding women can have the vaccine.

Rubella

Rubella (more commonly known as 'German measles' after its German name of *Rotln*) was once an epidemic in the UK (Green and Webb, 2016). If pregnant women contract this infection in the first 8–10 weeks of pregnancy, 90% of their infants will be born with congenital rubella syndrome (CRS). This condition is characterised by mild to significant hearing loss, microcephaly, cataracts, inflammation of the brain, lungs and bone marrow, amongst other things (PHE, 2013). Some infants, although appearing healthy at birth, may have deafness detected later (Plotkin and Ornenstein, 2004). The particularly high infection rate is because a fetus is unable to mount an effective immune response to fight the infection at this early stage of development (Banatvala and Peckham, 2007).

In 2003 and 2012, the UK National Screening Committee (NSC) reviewed the evidence relating to the prevalence of rubella in the country and uptake of the vaccine. Following a period of stakeholder consultation, it made the decision to stop routine rubella screening in pregnancy from April 2016 (UK NSC, 2012). The committee based its decision on the fact that rubella infection levels in the UK were low, mainly due to the effectiveness of the national immunisation programme. Consequently, rubella infection in pregnancy was rare with less than 1 case of CRS per 100 000 live births. It was highlighted that being fully vaccinated with the MMR vaccine prior to becoming pregnant is the most effective way of protecting the woman against becoming infected whilst pregnant (UK NSC, 2012). Indeed, screening for rubella immunity during pregnancy has no protective effect on the fetus. Women found to lack immunity following screening were advised to stay away from any potential cases of rubella if they became aware of them and to get vaccinated as soon as possible during the postnatal period to protect future pregnancies. The serum screening test can also provide inaccurate results, causing undue stress and anxiety for pregnant women (PHE, 2016).

All women who lack evidence of two documented doses of the MMR vaccine should be offered the vaccine postnatally. The MMR vaccine can be given safely to breast-feeding women although they should be advised to avoid conceiving for at least 1 month following administration of the vaccine, so a reliable form of contraception is needed.

Episode of care

Tania attends her first antenatal appointment with the midwife at her local doctor's surgery. She is 6 weeks pregnant. When discussing her past medical history, Tania informs her midwife that she only had one of the recommended two doses of MMR vaccine when she was a toddler. Her mother had told her that she worried about taking her for her second dose because of concerns about a link between the MMR vaccine and childhood autism.

Tania's midwife ordered a blood test to ascertain if she was immune to rubella. The results demonstrated that Tania was not immune. The midwife reassured her that rubella rates in the community are very low and as most children are now fully vaccinated, she was unlikely to become infected. However, while she is pregnant, she should avoid people who are complaining of a rash in case they are infected.

It is unsafe to give a live vaccine during pregnancy, so Tania was offered the MMR vaccine when she was in hospital following the birth of her son. Tania was advised to avoid getting pregnant again for at least a month after receiving the vaccine.

Conclusion

This chapter has provided information about immunisation during pregnancy and highlighted the vital role of midwives in supporting women to make their own individual decision. Midwives need to keep themselves fully updated on current evidence in relation to this topic in order to provide the most effective woman-centred care.

Find out more

The following is a list of conditions that are associated with the immune system. Take some time and write notes about each of the conditions. Think about the medications that may be used in order to treat these conditions and be specific about the pharmacokinetics and pharmacodynamics. Remember to include aspects of patient care. If you are making notes about people you have offered care and support to, you must ensure that you have adhered to the rules of confidentiality.

The condition	Your notes
Neutropenia	
Systemic lupus erythematosus	
Anaphylaxis	
Leukaemia	
Myasthenia gravis	

Glossary

Active immunity   Immunity developed inside the body as a result of encountering infectious agents

Anaphylaxis   A severe allergic (hypersensitivity) response to a chemical introduced into the body

Antibody   An immunoglobulin protein secreted by B lymphocytes. Antibody synthesis is induced by specific antigens

Antigen   Any substance that induces the immune system to produce *antibodies* against it

Attenuation   The process of weakening a pathogen so that it is able to stimulate an immune response without causing the disease

Bacteria   Microscopic single-celled organisms, some of which are capable of causing disease

Booster   A vaccine dose given to stimulate the immune system's memory response

DNA vaccine   A vaccine made from sections of a pathogen's DNA

Fetus   An unborn offspring of a mammal, particularly an unborn human more than 8 weeks after conception

Herd immunity   Indirect protection against disease that results from a sufficient number of individuals in a community having immunity to that disease

Immune system   The collection of organs and cells that make up the body's response to a disease or foreign substance threat

Immunisation   The process of either transferring antibodies to someone or inducing an immune reaction safely

Immunity   The body's response to infection, damage or other diseases

Inactivated vaccine   A type of vaccine in which the vaccine pathogen is killed or altered so that it cannot cause infection but can still stimulate an immune response

Influenza   An infectious disease caused by influenza viruses. Symptoms range from mild to severe and often include fever, runny nose, sore throat, muscle pain, headache, coughing and fatigue

Innate immunity   The immunity with which we are born

Inoculation   The introduction of material into a person in order to provoke immunity to a disease

Passive immunisation   A form of temporary immunity, created by giving disease-specific antibodies

Pathogen   An agent that causes disease, e.g. virus, bacterium, fungus

Pertussis   Commonly known as whooping cough, this is a highly contagious respiratory disease caused by the bacterium *Bordetella pertussis*. It is known for uncontrollable, violent coughing which may make it difficult to breathe

Rubella   Commonly known as German measles, rubella is a contagious viral infection that occurs most often in children and young adults. Most individuals have a mild illness, with a low-grade fever, sore throat and a rash that starts on the face and then spreads to the body

Seroprotection   An antibody response capable of preventing infection

Serum   The liquid obtained after allowing blood to clot and removing the solid matter

Toxin   Poisonous substance capable of causing disease

Vaccination   Introduction into the body of material designed to provoke an immune response that will provide protection from a related disease

Vaccine   A suspension of inactivated (or dead) micro-organisms that stimulates the body to develop immunity to a particular disease

Test yourself

Now review your learning by completing the learning activities for this chapter at www.wiley.com/go/pharmacologyformidwives**.**

References

Aghaeepour, N., Ganio, E.A., Mcilwain, D. et al. (2017) An immune clock of human pregnancy. *Science Immunology*, **2**(15): eaan2946.

Allotey, J., Stallings, E., Bonet, M. et al. for PregCOV-19 Living Systematic Review Consortium (2020) Clinical manifestations, risk factors, and maternal and perinatal outcomes of coronavirus disease 2019 in pregnancy: living systematic review and meta-analysis. *BMJ (Clinical Research Edition)*, **370**: m3320.

Amirthalingam, G., Andrews, N., Campbell, H. et al. (2014) Effectiveness of maternal pertussis vaccination in England: an observational study. *Lancet*, **384**(9953): 1521–1528.

Banatvala, J., Peckham, C. (eds) (2007) Rubella viruses. In: *Perspectives in Medical Virology*, vol. **15**. Elsevier: Oxford.

Berger, Z.D., Evans, N.G., Phelan, A.L., Silverman, R.D. (2020) Covid-19: control measures must be equitable and inclusive. *British Medical Journal*, **368**: m1141.

British Society for Immunology (2021) Coronavirus. www.immunology.org/coronavirus (accessed February 2022).

Crowcroft, N.S., Booy, R., Harrison, T. et al. (2003) Severe and unrecognised: pertussis in UK infants. *Archives of Disease in Childhood*, **88** (9): 802–806.

Dabrera, G., Zhao, H., Andrews, N. et al. (2014) Effectiveness of seasonal influenza vaccination during pregnancy in preventing influenza infection in infants, England, 2013/14. *Euro Surveillance*, **19**(45): 20959.

Dodds, L., McNeil, S.A., Fell, D.B. et al. (2007) Impact of influenza exposure on rates of hospital admissions and physician visits because of respiratory illness among pregnant women. *Canadian Medical Association Journal*, **176**(4): 463–468.

Donegan, K., King, B., Bryan, P. (2014) Safety of pertussis vaccination in pregnant women in UK: observational study. *British Medical Journal*, **349**: g4219.

Duncan, D. (2020) Influenza and pregnancy. *British Journal of Midwifery*, **28**(2): 78–82.

Eberhardt, C.S., Blanchard-Rohner, G., Lemaître, B. et al. (2016) Maternal immunization earlier in pregnancy maximizes antibody transfer and expected infant seropositivity against pertussis. *Clinical Infectious Diseases*, **62**(7): 829–836.

Giles, M.L., Krishnaswamy, S., Macartney, K., Cheng, A. (2019) The safety of inactivated influenza vaccines in pregnancy for birth outcomes: a systematic review. *Human Vaccines & Immunotherapeutics*, **15**(3): 687–699.

Green, D., Webb, S. (2016) Cessation of rubella susceptibility screening in pregnancy and its implications for practice nursing. *British Journal of Midwifery*, **27**(12): 571–574.

Greinacher, A., Thiele, T., Warkentin, T.E., Weisser, K., Kyrle, P.A., Eichinger, S. (2021) Thrombotic thrombocytopenia after ChAdOx1 nCov-19 vaccination. *New England Journal of Medicine*, **384**: 2092–2101.

Jamieson, D.J., Theiler, R.N., Rasmussen, S.A. (2006) Emerging infections and pregnancy. *Emerging Infectious Diseases*, **12**(11): 1638–1643.

Joint Committee on Vaccination and Immunisation (2016) Minute of the meeting held on 3 February 2016. www.nitag-resource.org/media-center/document/2164-minute-of-the-meeting-on-3-february-2016 (accessed February 2022).

Joint Committee on Vaccination and Immunisation (2021) JCVI issues new advice on COVID-19 vaccination for pregnant women. www.gov.uk/government/news/jcvi-issues-new-advice-on-covid-19-vaccination-for-pregnant-women (accessed February 2022).

Kroger, A.T., Bahta, L., Hunter, P. (2021) General best practice guidelines for immunization. www.cdc.gov/vaccines/hcp/acip-recs/general-recs/index.html (accessed February 2022).

Liu, M.A. (2019) A comparison of plasmid DNA and mRNA as vaccine technologies. *Vaccines*, **7**: 37.

Mahase, E. (2020) Covid-109: UK approves Pfizer and BioNTech vaccine with rollout due to start next week. *British Medical Journal*, **369**: m2612.

Mak, D.B., Regan, A.K., Joyce, S., Gibbs, R., Effler, P.V. (2015) Antenatal care provider's advice is the key determinant of influenza vaccination uptake in pregnant women. *Australian & New Zealand Journal of Obstetrics & Gynaecology*, **55**(2): 131–137.

Modder, J. (2010) Review of maternal deaths in the UK related to A H1N1 2009 influenza (Centre for Maternal and Child Enquiries). www.hqip.org.uk/resource/cmace-and-cemach-reports/#.YJfrMLVKi70 (accessed February 2022).

Mullins, E., Hudak, M.L., Banerjee, J. et al. (2021) Pregnancy and neonatal outcomes of COVID-19: coreporting of common outcomes from PAN-COVID and AAP-SONPM registries. *Ultrasound in Obstetrics & Gynecology*, **57**(4): 573–581.

NHS England (2020a) Annual flu immunisation programme 2020–2021. www.gov.uk/government/collections/annual-flu-programme (accessed February 2022).

Nursing and Midwifery Council (2018) *The Code: Professional standards of practice and behaviour for nurses, midwives and nursing associates*. Nursing and Midwifery Council: London.

Plotkin, S.A., Orenstein, W. (eds) (2004) *Vaccines*, 4th edn. WB Saunders: Philadelphia.

Proveaux, T., Lambach, P., Ortiz, J.R., Hombach, J., Halsey, N.A. (2016) Review of prescribing information for influenza vaccines for pregnant and lactating women. *Vaccine*, **34**(45): 5406–5409.

Public Health England (2013) Rubella. In: *The Green Book of Immunisation*. https://assets.publishing.service.gov.uk/government/uploads/system/uploads/attachment_data/file/148498/Green-Book-Chapter-28-v2_0.pdf (accessed February 2022).

Public Health England (2014) Laboratory confirmed pertussis in England: data to end October 2014. https://assets.publishing.service.gov.uk/government/uploads/system/uploads/attachment_data/file/388854/hpr4714_prtsss.pdf (accessed February 2022).

Public Health England (2016) Pertussis. https://assets.publishing.service.gov.uk/government/uploads/system/uploads/attachment_data/file/514363/Pertussis_Green_Book_Chapter_24_Ap2016.pdf (accessed February 2022).

Public Health England (2019) The United Kingdom immunisation schedule. In: The Green Book of Immunisation. https://assets.publishing.service.gov.uk/government/uploads/system/uploads/attachment_data/file/855727/Greenbook_chapter_11_UK_Immunisation_schedule.pdf (accessed February 2022).

Public Health England (2020b) Seasonal influenza vaccine uptake in GP patients: winter season 2019 to 2020. Final data for 1 September 2019 to 29 February 2020. https://assets.publishing.service.gov.uk/government/uploads/system/uploads/attachment_data/file/912099/Annual-Report_SeasonalFlu-Vaccine_GPs_2019-20_FINAL_amended.pdf (accessed February 2022).

Public Health England (2021) COVID-19- SARS-CoV-2. https://assets.publishing.service.gov.uk/government/uploads/system/uploads/attachment_data/file/984310/Greenbook_chapter_14a_7May2021.pdf (accessed February 2022).

Regan, A.K., Mak, D.B., Hauck, Y.L., Gibbs, R., Tracey, L., Effler, P.V. (2016) Trends in seasonal influenza vaccine uptake during pregnancy in Western Australia: implications for midwives. *Women and Birth*, **29**(5): 423–429.

Regan, A.K., Hauck, Y., Nicolaou, L. et al. (2018) Midwives' knowledge, attitudes and learning needs regarding antenatal vaccination. *Midwifery*, **62**: 199–204.

Royal College of Midwives (2020) Position Statement: Flu vaccination. www.rcm.org.uk/media/4354/flu-vaccination_4.pdf (accessed February 2022).

Royal College of Obstetricians and Gynaecologists (2021) RCOG statement in response to change in guidance around the Oxford AstraZeneca vaccine. www.rcog.org.uk/en/news/rcog-statement-in-response-to-change-in-guidance-around-the-oxford-astra-zeneca-vaccine/ (accessed February 2022).

Royal Society for Public Health (2021) Public attitudes to a COVID-19 vaccine. www.rsph.org.uk/our-work/policy/vaccinations/public-attitudes-to-a-covid-19-vaccine.html (accessed February 2022).

UK National Screening Committee (2012) Rubella Susceptibility. https://view-health-screening-recommendations.service.gov.uk/rubella-susceptibility/ (accessed February 2022).

Vaccine Knowledge Project (2019) Flu vaccine in pregnancy. https://vk.ovg.ox.ac.uk/vk/flu-vaccine-pregnancy (accessed February 2022).

Vousden, N., Bunch, K., Morris, E. et al. (2021) The incidence, characteristics and outcomes of pregnant women hospitalized with symptomatic and asymptomatic SARS-CoV-2 infection in the UK from March to September 2020: a national cohort study using the UK Obstetric Surveillance System (UKOSS). *PLoS One*, **16**(5): e0251123.

World Health Organization (2020) Novel coronavirus – China. www.who.int/csr/don/12-january-2020-novel-coronavirus-china/en/ (accessed February 2022).

Yuen, C.Y., Tarrant, M. (2014) Determinants of uptake of influenza vaccination among pregnant women – a systematic review. *Vaccine*, **32**(36): 4602–4613.

Chapter 20

Medications and breast feeding

Deborah Sharp and Zoi Vardavaki

University of Hertfordshire, Hatfield, UK

Aim

The aim of this chapter is to provide the reader with an understanding of the impact of the administration of medication to breast-feeding women and the key points related to this.

Learning outcomes

After reading this chapter, the reader will:
- Understand the transfer of medication into breast milk
- Gain knowledge about medications provided to women during the intrapartum and postnatal period and how this may affect breast feeding
- Gain knowledge about medications that are safe to use while breast feeding
- Understand professional duties when caring for breast-feeding women requiring administration of medication
- Understand where to signpost women to sources of information about medications whilst breast feeding.

Test your existing knowledge

- During the colostrum period, the transfer of medication into the breast milk is lower or higher? What do you think and why?
- Is labetalol a recommended antihypertensive medication during the lactating period?
- On a postnatal ward, you are called to provide breast-feeding support to a woman who had fentanyl during labour as pain relief. What assessment would you carry out? What feeding advice would you give her based on the risk factors?
- Where would you access accurate information about medications and their effect on breast feeding?
- What management plan of care are you able to develop for a woman with mastitis?

Fundamentals of Pharmacology for Midwives, First Edition. Edited by Ian Peate and Cathy Hamilton.
© 2022 John Wiley & Sons Ltd. Published 2022 by John Wiley & Sons Ltd.
Companion website: www.wiley.com/go/pharmacologyformidwives

Introduction

The management and administration of medication is an essential skill for midwives. Equally, promoting breast feeding and supporting women's infant feeding choices are essential skills for midwives. It is important that midwives and student midwives have knowledge around the use of medication during the lactating period in order to provide safe and effective care for breast-feeding women. This chapter will focus on the role of the midwife and student midwife in administration of medication to breast-feeding women and the key points related to this. As part of this process, it is necessary that midwives and student midwives understand the transfer of medication into breast milk and use the most up-to-date knowledge about medicines management and breast feeding. This is essential in order to provide accurate and evidence-based information to women, enabling them to make an informed choice (Nursing and Midwifery Council (NMC), 2018).

This chapter will also explore some safe medication that can be used during the lactation period and common challenges arising while women breast feed and how these can be managed with and without the use of medicine.

Transfer of medication in breast milk

Before prescribing a medication for a breast-feeding woman, it is necessary to decide on the safety of the medication for the mother–infant dyad. The midwife as the individual administering a medication has to consider if the specific medication is appropriate to be used while the woman is breast feeding, due to the potential effect on the infant and the production of milk. It is important to know the route of administration, the volume, potential side-effects, how it will be absorbed, half-times/pick time of the medication and the ability of the lactating mother to absorb, metabolise and excrete the given medication. Hamilton (2014) highlighted that a midwife should refer to another healthcare professional for specialised knowledge on potential side-effects of a medication should there be any doubt. Similarly, it is necessary to have an awareness of the ability of the infant to absorb, metabolise, detoxify and excrete the medication passed through the breast milk (Mattison and Halbert, 2013). Another important issue is the age of the infant and how regularly they are fed in order to make a decision on what medication should be prescribed (Hamilton, 2014; Jones, 2018).

It is therefore necessary to be able to assess the transfer of a medication in breast milk. This assessment can be complex and may be difficult to undertake. Adverse effects on infants of medications passed from their lactating mother are rare and so serious events are not frequent (Anderson et al., 2003). However, precautions need to be taken when prescribing a medication to the breast-feeding mother in order to avoid the discontinuation of breast feeding.

Clinical consideration

Is oxytocin the medication of choice for painful engorgement?

Oxytocin stimulates the milk ejection reflex (also known as the 'let-down reflex'). Therefore, it is a medication of choice for painful engorgement. It also encourages uterine involution in the postnatal period (Schaefer et al., 2007).

Passage of medication during the intrapartum period

It is known that the breast-feeding infant's previous exposure to medication during the antenatal and intrapartum period can have an enhanced adverse effect during breast feeding (Mattinson, 2013). Midwives and student midwives looking after women during pregnancy, labour and birth and the postnatal period need to provide support and guidance on medication. Medication is administered routinely to women, especially during the intrapartum period, which means that the infant may be born having been exposed to maternal medication and this may have an impact on breast feeding. In the UK, breast-feeding rates are lower than in other European countries (Rollins et al., 2016) and failure to breast feed increases mortality and morbidity in mothers and their infants

(Victora et al., 2016). Therefore, unnecessary administration of medication during the intrapartum period should be avoided to minimise the impact on breast feeding.

Evidence shows that uterotonics used for management of the third stage of labour and prostaglandins used for induction of labour are associated with reduced breast-feeding rates (Jordan et al., 2009; Cadwell and Brimdyr, 2017; Erickson and Emeis, 2017). Brown and Jordan (2014) highlighted that prophylactic administration of uterotonics for the management of the third stage of labour does not affect the initiation of breast feeding but it may reduce the duration of it and women may need additional breast-feeding support. The National Institute for Health and Care Excellence (NICE, 2017) recommends that women should be informed about their choices on the management of the third stage of labour during the antenatal period and when in labour. Midwives and healthcare professionals should discuss with women their preference on this and the potential impact on breast feeding, especially when they plan to breast feed their infant.

The use of pain relief in labour has an impact on infant feeding behaviours. Wildstrom et al. (2019) found that high levels of intrapartum epidural fentanyl were associated with physiological compromise in newborns shortly after birth compared to mothers who had no exposure. Such compromised behaviours included less efficient crawling when newborns are skin to skin after birth, self-attachment to the breast and suckling, all of which will have an impact on initiation of breast feeding (Wildstrom et al., 2019).

Other studies have found an association between the use of intrapartum epidurals and suckling issues in the first few hours of life, exclusive breast-feeding rates following discharge and at 6 weeks postnatally while other studies failed to find a link between epidural use and breast feeding (Brimdyr et al., 2015; Wiklund et al., 2009). Jordan et al. (2005) highlighted that use of epidural in labour is linked to shorter duration of breast feeding. The use of intramuscular pethidine for pain management during labour is also associated with more admissions to neonatal units and less skin-to-skin contact which may have an impact on breast feeding (Fleet et al., 2017). In any case, women with interventions or complications during labour and birth tend to have higher rates of pain, be less mobile after birth, may be separated from their newborn infant and are less likely to have skin-to-skin contact. All these will contribute to fewer breast feeds and therefore less milk production.

The midwife's role is crucial to ensure accurate information is shared with women on the use of analgesia during labour in order for women to make an informed decision, especially if they aim to breast feed (NICE, 2017; NMC, 2018). Furthermore, the use of opioids should be taken into consideration when providing education to women who intend to breast feed (Fleet et al., 2017). To aid such discussions, the Royal College of Association of Anaesthetists has produced a guidance document (Mitchell et al., 2020). See also Chapter 8 of this text for a detailed discussion of the pharmacology and analgesia used in pregnancy.

Passage of medication in the immediate postnatal period

The transfer of medication into breast milk occurs via several factors such as the oral bioavailability of the drug, its half-life and plasma protein binding, the milk–plasma ratio, the extent to which the drug undergoes first-pass metabolism and the relative infant dose (Jones, 2018; Mattison and Halbert, 2013). Medications are transferred from the maternal plasma, through the capillary walls and the alveolar epithelium and enter into the milk. There are four diffusion mechanisms of drug transfer, the transcellular route via the alveolar cell being the most common (Mattison and Halbert, 2013). The intercellular diffusion route allows transfer of the medication into breast milk due to the intercellular gaps that are wide open at delivery and gradually tighten over the following 4 days, allowing more medication to pass into breast milk on day 1 compared to day 3 after delivery (Jones, 2018). In the following days (days 4–6 postnatally), the alveolar cells enlarge and these gaps are tightened, resulting in a reduced amount of medication entering the breast milk (Hale and Rowe, 2017). The solubility of the medication is also very important for transfer into breast milk. The more lipid soluble a medication is, the greater its ability to penetrate the alveolar cells and pass into the breast milk (Hale and Rowe, 2017). Some medications cannot pass through the closed gaps but have to dissolve through the cellular membranes of the alveolar cells to enter the breast milk, while other medications are actively transported through the alveolar cells into the breast milk (Figure 20.1).

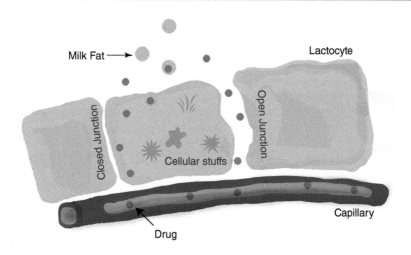

Figure 20.1   Transfer of medication in the immediate postnatal period.

The transfer of medication into breast milk depends on a variety of factors, discussed below.

Oral bioavailability of a medication

This refers to the percentage of the medication being absorbed into the system having passed through the gut or the liver for first-pass metabolism (Jones, 2018). Medication given by injection only (i.e. low molecular weight heparinoids or insulin) have poor oral bioavailability because they are not absorbed from the gut. So, medication with low oral bioavailability is safer for a breast-feeding mother to take.

Half-life of the medication

This is the time that a medication takes to clear from the mother's body and milk. Five half-lives have to elapse to ensure that a safe and steady state is reached (Jones, 2018; Mattison and Halbert, 2013). For the lactating mother, when a medication is prescribed it is important to remember that the longer the half-life, the greater the risk of accumulation in the infant's body and the higher the possibility of adverse effects. That is why naproxen is not a preferred non-steroidal anti-inflammatory drug (NSAID) during the postnatal period (first 6 weeks after birth); instead, ibuprofen is recommended as its half-life is 1.8–2 hours (Bushra and Aslam, 2010).

Plasma protein binding

This is the extent to which a medication becomes bound to the plasma protein in the maternal bloodstream and the amount that remains free (Jones, 2018; Mattison and Halbert, 2013). The free medication can be passed to the infant through the milk. Therefore, high protein-binding medications are preferred for the lactating mother. During the early postnatal period, some medications compete for binding sites that would normally be occupied by bilirubin, with the risk of bilirubin displacement. Such displacement of the unconjugated bilirubin can cause kernicterus and brain damage to the infant (Jones, 2018) and therefore it is important to avoid prescribing such medication for lactating mothers.

Episode of care

Mary, a primigravida, gave birth to her infant 4 days ago and was been discharged. In the last 38 hours, Mary developed some pain in the lower abdomen and burning when passing urine, which seemed to be a common issue as she had recurrent urinary tract infections (UTIs) during her pregnancy. She spoke to the GP on the phone and was diagnosed with a UTI. Mary was advised to collect the prescribed medication from the nearest pharmacy. Ellie, the community midwife, visited Mary for a routine postnatal visit. During the visit, Ellie discussed with Mary her infant feeding choices and noted that Mary was breast feeding effectively. Mary also mentioned that because of her UTI symptoms, she was prescribed co-trimoxazole that she had collected from the pharmacy earlier in the day – but she had not taken any yet. Ellie contacted the GP to discuss the prescribed medication as there is a risk of kernicterus and it is not recommended for a lactating mother. The GP had not seen Mary before, and he was not aware of her infant feeding choice. Following the discussion with Ellie, the GP decided to change the medication and cephalexin was prescribed instead as it is a commonly used first-generation cephalosporin antibiotic to be used while breast feeding.

Further activity

- Describe are the signs and symptoms of UTI.
- Considering the physiology of lactation, what are the priorities for managing this and enabling Mary and her child to successfully continue breast feeding?
- Where can Mary get additional help about breast feeding from?

Milk/plasma (m/p) ratio

This refers to the concentration of the protein-free fractions in milk and plasma (Jones, 2018). It is advisable for lactating mothers to avoid medication with a milk/plasma ratio over 1. For instance, iodine has a m/p ratio up to 26 (Jones, 2018) and therefore should be avoided during the lactating period as it can cause an increased level of iodine in breast milk which can result in transient hypo-thyroidism in breast-fed infants.

Extent to which the drug undergoes first-pass metabolism

This relates to the phenomenon of medication metabolism whereby the concentration of a medication when absorbed from the gut is greatly reduced before it reaches the systemic circulation and is carried to the liver. In the liver, it may be converted to active or inactive metabolites. Inactive metabolites will be excreted without any effect. Active metabolites may pass through the liver unchanged or they will have a therapeutic effect (Jones, 2018). Medications with an inactive first-pass metabolism are safer for use during lactation as they will be excreted without any effect on mother and the infant.

Relative infant dose (RID)

The relative infant dose is one of the most important parameters to determine the safety of a medication entering the breast milk. The simplest way to calculate the RID is the dose in the infant in milligrams per kilogram per day divided by the dose in the mother in the same way (Hale and Rowe, 2017). Therefore, to calculate the RID the equation below is used.

$$RID = \frac{infant\ dose\ mg\ /\ kg\ /\ day}{mother\ dose\ mg\ /\ kg\ /\ day}$$

Hale (2017) and Jones (2018) state that a safe option for percentage of RID is less than 10% for full-term infants. However, when deciding about medication prescription and thinking about the RID, every case should be evaluated based on the individual medication and its toxicity. The age of the infant is therefore important when considering the RID in a preterm infant as the dose should be decreased appropriately in order to ensure the safest option is provided and the potential increased medication is not passed through the breast milk to the infant.

Maturity and age of the infant

When considering the risk of medication being transferred into the breast milk, it is important to know the maturity and age of the infant (Jones, 2018). Premature infants have immature hepatic and renal function and a lower percentage of body fat and therefore cannot metabolise and excrete medication effectively. In contrast, a 10-week-old infant will be able to better detoxify and excrete medication than a premature infant or a newborn. The age of the infant matters as this is linked to the volume of milk the infant will consume and therefore the potential risk of transferring medication into the breast milk (Jones, 2018). For instance, a newborn infant who exclusively breast feeds will have more feeds during 24 hours which results in consumption of a higher volume of milk and therefore the level of medication transferred to the newborn infant is higher. The risk of drug exposure via the breast milk is decreased after 2 months of life in exclusively breast-fed infants and even more when breast milk is no longer the only food for the infant or toddler (Anderson et al., 2003; Soussan et al., 2014).

It is important to note that if the medication passed through the breast milk to the infant has a therapeutic range, then an effect on the infant might be noted, but in most of cases the amount of medication passed to the infant is below the therapeutic level and therefore no side-effects are noted (Jones, 2018). If the amount of medication passing through breast milk is above the therapeutic level, then the infant will have side-effects from this medication (Jones, 2018).

During the immediate postnatal period, breast-feeding women are commonly prescribed more medication (e.g. pain relief, anti-inflammatory medication, medication for haemorrhoids, laxatives and low molecular weight heparinoids). The midwife's role is not only to ensure necessary and safe treatment is provided to the breast-feeding mother but also to consider the impact on breast feeding and the infant, especially if the latter is premature. Information on the transfer of medication into breast milk is not readily available to healthcare practitioners and therefore it is important to ensure that available specialised resources are used. In addition, involving parents in decision making is necessary and therefore sufficient information about the relative risks of all the options should be provided to women to allow them to make an informed decision. Midwives should ensure they practise in accordance with the NMC Code in terms of administration of medication and its use to preserve the safety of the woman (NMC, 2018), bearing in mind the severity of her situation and the maturity and age of her child (Hamilton, 2014).

Maternal diseases and medication in the breast-feeding mother

With advances in medical treatment and medication, there has been a significant increase in the number of women with pre-existing medical conditions and increasing complexity becoming pregnant and having a baby (Knight et al., 2020). Increased awareness of the potential teratogenic effects of medication on the fetus has resulted in caution when prescribing for pregnant women. When medication is required for chronic conditions, this requires careful monitoring and/or a review of medication by a medical specialist, to minimise the harmful effects when known contraindications exist (Robson and Waugh, 2008; NICE, 2021a).

The midwife's role is to identify any medical and mental health conditions and medications taken and refer to the appropriate team as early as possible (NICE, 2021a). This practice of referral, review and caution is now standardised practice within maternity care (NICE, 2021a). However, it is suggested that some healthcare practitioners' lack of knowledge about the known effects of medications on breast feeding results in women being given incorrect or conflicting advice that they cannot breast feed or must stop. It should, however, be recognised that medication is a barrier to breast feeding for some women, which needs to be addressed within the healthcare system (Jones, 2018).

The advantages of breast feeding should never be underestimated nor should the wishes of a mother to continue to breast feed and the right of the infant to continue to receive it (Jones, 2018). It is important to remember that most medications for acute and chronic maternal disorders are safe to use during lactation. It has been reported that serious acute adverse reactions from drugs in breast milk are uncommon and cautionary warnings about not using a drug in lactation may sometimes be based on one reported incident (Anderson et al., 2015; Jones, 2018).

This is complicated by the advice provided in standard reference sources of information on medications such as the British National Formulary (BNF), which often present minimal information on certain drugs and applies an 'avoid if breast feeding' advisory line (Jones, 2018). Upon receipt of this advice, women have described feeling that they have no alternative other than to formula feed (Jones, 2018). This inaccurate information may be a contributory factor affecting the 1% exclusive breast-feeding rates in the UK at 6 months (McAndrew et al., 2012). Whilst it is acknowledged that the decision to breast feed and to continue to breast feed is multifactorial and complex, it is argued that a lack of correct accessible information may contribute to three out of five women stopping breast feeding before they want to (Brown et al., 2015; McAndrew et al., 2012). Additional sources such as the Breastfeeding Network Drugs in Breastmilk information service (www.breastfeedingnet-work.org.uk/detailed-information/drugs-in-breastmilk/) provide more detailed evidence to inform decision making, often providing safer alternatives for mothers who are breast feeding which enable them to continue breast feeding as opposed to stopping.

Two examples of a common medical condition and a breast-feeding challenge that the student midwife is likely to encounter on a regular basis, postnatal depression and mastitis, are presented below. An overview of the considerations needed when caring for the breast-feeding woman who needs medication is presented. Pharmacological and non-pharmacological approaches will be discussed. A full exploration of the pharmacological management of all medical conditions and the effects of medications on breast feeding is beyond the remit of this chapter and this book. For more detailed information about specific conditions, drugs and the effect on breast feeding, other sources need to be accessed.

Postnatal depression

Having a baby is an extremely emotional event resulting in physical, social and psychological adaptations. Establishment of a close loving relationship between a mother and baby is vital for maternal and neonatal physical, mental health and well-being, in both the short and long term (Gerhardt, 2015; NICE, 2021a, 2021b; UNICEF, 2017). The importance of promoting secure mother–infant attachment for neurological development is now widely recognised (NICE, 2021a, 2021b; UNICEF, 2017). It is estimated that 10–20% of mothers experience some form of depression, from mild depression and anxiety-related symptoms to the rarer severe pschiatric disorders, during pregnancy and the first year of the baby's life (NICE 2014, 2021). This can significantly affect the development of this precious mother–baby relationship (Brown et al., 2015; Gerhardt, 2015; Jones, 2018; UNICEF, 2017). A full discussion of postnatal depression is beyond the remit of this chapter and as such the focus will be on issues related to medication and the midwife's role in recognition and referral. See Chapter 18 for more information.

The relationship between breast feeding and the development and continuation of depression is complex, with some studies suggesting that when breast-feeding challenges are encountered, these can contribute to the development of depression (Brown et al., 2015). However, it is also argued that a positive breast-feeding experience can prevent postnatal depression (Kendall-Tackett et al., 2011; Ystrom, 2012). There is evidence to suggest that many women with pre-existing depression or who develop depression stop taking antidepressants or are reluctant to take them postnatally if breast feeding because of perceived concerns about the effect on the baby through transference in breast milk (Mohrbacher, 2010; NICE, 2014).

Despite this concern, many modern antidepressants, particularly selective serotonin uptake inhibitors (SSRIs), are considered compatible with breast feeding as studies have demonstrated that accumulation in the breast-fed baby is minimal, particularly in babies whose mothers have been medicated with sertraline (see below for more detail) (Jones, 2018). It is suggested that in most cases, depression in the breast-feeding mother can be successfully managed. Therefore, the need to medicate a mother with antidepressants should not be a reason to suggest discontinuation of breast feeding. Furthermore, if medication is suddenly stopped because of these perceived concerns or depression is not appropriately recognised and treated, this could have dire consequences as described above (Knight et al., 2020; NICE, 2014, 2021b).

Antidepressants commonly used

Most manufacturers have not conducted clinical trials on the use of antidepressants in lactation and in the Summary of Product Characteristics recommend that they are not used by breast-feeding mothers. However, evidence from studies that have examined levels in neonates should be considered when having conversations with women to inform their decisions (Jones, 2018). To assist these discussions, women could be directed to the Breastfeeding Network antidepressant factsheet (www.breastfeedingnetwork.org.uk/antidepressants/).

Prior to the mother being prescribed medication by a medical practitioner, other strategies should be explored such as talking therapies.

324

The treatment for depression usually involves SSRIs such as sertraline (Lustral®), citalopram (Cipramil®), paroxetine (Seroxat®) and fluoxetine (Prozac®) which act by inhibiting reuptake of serotonin into neurones in the central nervous system (Jones, 2018). Studies have reported varying effects on the neonate, depending on which drug is given. Jones (2018) suggests that due to the shorter half-life of sertraline, accumulation in the baby is unlikely and therefore this SSRI is normally the choice for a breast-feeding woman if she has not had a previous antidepressant which was effective for her (Breastfeeding Network, 2021).

Episode of care

Depression

Khajal had an uncomplicated pregnancy and delivery, and gave birth to a boy called William who is now 2 weeks old. Khajal is breast feeding William who is gaining weight and breast feeding 8–12 times in 24 hours with yellow stools and at least six wet nappies in a 24-hour period. The midwife visiting Khajal knows her well as the trust where Khajal delivered is implementing a continuity of care model.

When the midwife arrives, Khajal is in bed saying that she is just so tired, with no energy. The midwife undertakes a full assessment of both mother and baby and has no concerns about their physical well-being. During this visit, Khajal starts crying and shares with the midwife that she is crying a lot for no reason, isn't really bothered with anything, just wants to sleep all the time and is finding it hard to even think about going out or seeing friends or family. Following this conversation, Khajal recognises that she was trying to do too much and is going to spend more time with William in skin-to-skin contact as she finds this calming. Khajal feels better after this discussion; the midwife provides helpline numbers and has a further discussion with the couple about signs of postnatal depression.

When the midwife visits next, Khajal states that she has done the things that were suggested but is still crying a lot and does not really feel any different to when the midwife came before. She is aware of the possibility of developing depression but feels that she can't see her GP as she is worried what she will think of her. She loves William and desperately wants to breast feed as she feels this is the only thing that she is doing well. She is asthmatic and has eczema and knows that breast feeding can protect William against this and doesn't want to have to formula feed. The midwife recognises that Khajal is showing signs of depression and has a conversation with her about this and tries to encourage her to see her GP. It is revealed that Kahajl has heard that if she is prescribed medication then she will have to stop breast feeding. The midwife discusses this with her and encourages her to look at the Breastfeeding Network drug factsheet.

Khajal does this and is seen by the GP who is supportive and confirms that she is depressed and in discussion with Khajal prescribes sertraline 25 mg increasing to 50 mg after 1 week and also encourages Khajal to access the local mother and baby group. The midwife visits Khajal following this and is pleased to see that she is feeling more positive about having been to the doctor and is able to continue to breast feed William.

Discussion points

- What factors contributed to the disclosure about how Khajal was feeling?
- What professional considerations must the midwife remember?
- During postnatal care and discharge from midwifery care, who in the multidisciplinary team could the midwife liaise with to support Khajal further?

Mastitis

The management of mastitis is controversial as it does not always need antibiotic treatment. This is normally only recommended if an infection is present. It can be difficult to determine if the mastitis is caused by an inflammation or infection but with prompt recognition and non-pharmacological management, antibiotics can often be avoided. Whilst many antibiotics are considered safe for use in breast feeding, it is also documented that breast-fed babies often develop colic, abdominal pain and diarrhoea. This together with the overuse of antibiotics are valid reasons to avoid taking them unless necessary. Conservative non-pharmacological management should occur with careful

325

observation and the mother being advised of what signs to look for regarding deterioration. However, if the condition worsens oral antibiotic treatment may be necessary.

Episode of care

Mandi is breast feeding her baby Carlie which was going well. However, when the midwife visits her on day 5 the midwife identifies as part of the physical assessment that Mandi's left breast is displaying early signs of a potential mastitis that is becoming painful. Carlie is also feeding constantly and not settling between feeds. At this stage the midwife feels that antibiotics are not needed. However, as Mandi has pain and the mastitis at this stage is suggestive of an inflammatory response, the midwife suggests she takes paracetamol and ibuprofen regularly which are considered safe whilst breast feeding.

Two days later Mandi's symptoms have developed further, and she is now feeling unwell. Mandi visits her GP who prescribes an antibiotic, amoxicillin, that is considered safe whilst breast feeding. The GP is aware of the importance of checking that medications are compatible with breast feeding and has accessed the Breastfeeding Network antibiotic and mastitis factsheet and has assured Mandi that she should continue to breast feed during the treatment with frequent milk removal as well as regular analgesia.

Note: The use of antibiotics does not necessitate suspension or cessation of breast feeding (Jones, 2018).

Further activity

- Describe the signs and symptoms of mastitis.
- What are the likely causes of the mastitis? What else needs to be determined to answer this question and to rectify this for Mandi?
- Considering the physiology of lactation, what are the priorities for managing this and enabling Mandi and Carlie to successfully continue breast feeding?
- Where can Mandi get additional help about breast feeding?
- Describe the non-pharmacological management plan that the midwife can suggest both before starting the antibiotics and during treatment?
- What considerations are needed before the mother takes ibuprofen?
- What is the maximum dose of paracetamol that the mother can take in a 24-hour period?

Over-the-counter medicines

There are many medications available without prescription, including simple analgesics, antihistamines, cough and cold preparations, decongestants, gastrointestinal preparations, herbal remedies and alternative therapies. Caution needs to be exercised whilst breast feeding as transference to the breast milk and baby can occur. If the breast-feeding mother asks the student midwife about the suitability of taking such medications, she should be advised that she should always discuss this with a pharmacist, advising them of the fact that she is breast feeding. She should also be directed to one of the additional sources of information as described below. The Breastfeeding Network, for example, has extensive factsheets on over-the-counter medications.

Midwife's role

The decision to treat depression or any other medical condition in a woman who is breast feeding is one for the medical practitioner in conjunction with the woman and not the midwife. However, the student midwife/midwife's role is to advise the mother and family about the possibility and signs of illness, in this case depression and mastitis, as well as recognising deviation from the normal in the postnatal mother. Upon recognition, it is appropriate to refer to a medical practitioner and consider referring to a specialist service as well as accessing information about breast feeding and the condition (NICE, 2014, 2021b).

If treatment or advice is required about specific conditions and/or drugs for the breast-feeding mother that is beyond the remit and knowledge of the student midwife/midwife, a timely referral to an appropriate practitioner should always be made (NMC, 2018). The skills of advocacy could be used to support the mother's discussion with such practitioners, to facilitate an informed decision-making process about the most appropriate medication and management (NMC, 2019). It is suggested that the midwife/student midwife could signpost both the mother and the professional to reliable, effective information (see Further reading). A breast-feeding mother should be advised to always share the fact that she is breast feeding with a pharmacist or any healthcare practitioner prescribing medications as well as practitioners providing any alternative therapies before taking or applying any medications.

Breast feeding and medications information

Sources of information about medication whilst breast feeding include the Breastfeeding Network (BfN) which is a registered charity and an independent source of support and extensive information for breast-feeding women and healthcare professionals. This charity operates a Drugs in Breast milk service for parents and professionals which is run by volunteer qualified pharmacists and produces factsheets on a range of topics related to medications and breast feeding. Additionally, there are online lactation-specific databases such as the UK Drugs in Lactation Advisory Service (UKDILAS) and the Drug and Lactation database (LactMed). It is recommended that student midwives familiarise themselves with these resources in order to effectively signpost the mother to them for more information.

Conclusion

Taking any medications whilst breast feeding should always be undertaken with caution. Many women who have medical conditions can breast feed. Most drugs pass into breast milk but at low levels and it is suggested that very few are totally contraindicated during breast feeding (Jones, 2018). Whilst most medications can be taken as the amount transferred in the breast milk is minimal, there is always a possibility of the baby having a reaction. New medications are being developed all the time and it is not possible to clearly define which are suitable for breast feeding, but it is the responsibility of the practitioner to search for studies that determine the safety and effect in the neonate.

There should be a careful decision-making process to ensure that the advantages of taking the medication for the mother's health outweigh the small risks to the baby. These decisions should be aided by healthcare professionals to enable the mother to make an informed decision, thus ensuring that breast feeding is protected and women are supported to breast feed for as long as they wish. Requiring medication should not be a reason for a woman to stop breast feeding and safe alternatives should always be sought.

Find out more

The following is a list of conditions. Take some time and write notes about each of them . Be specific about the pharmacokinetics and pharmacodynamics and how these may affect breast feeding. Remember to include aspects of patient care. It may be helpful to think of actual examples you have seen, but ensure that you have adhered to the rules of confidentiality.

Condition	Your notes
Oral thrush in the baby.thrush in the mother's breast	
Cold/flu	
Urinary tract infection	
Hayfever	

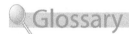

Glossary

Bioavailability A measure of absorption or the fractional extent to which the drug dose reaches its site of action

Half-life Defined as the time taken for the concentration of a medication in blood or plasma to fall to half its maximum value

Kernicterus High plasma concentration of bilirubin in the newborn which can lead to neurological damage

Mastitis An inflammation of the breast tissue that may or may not be accompanied by infection. It is often caused by poor attachment of the baby to the breast and ineffective removal of breast milk. If untreated, it can result in painful breast feeding

Over-the-counter medication A medication sold directly to the public without a prescription

Therapeutic range The desirable range for concentration of the medication in plasma and tissues to achieve the desired therapeutic effect. Above the therapeutic range, toxic effects will appear and below the therapeutic range, the medication is less likely to have the desired effect

Test yourself

Now review your learning by completing the learning activities for this chapter at www.wiley.com/go/pharmacologyformidwives.

References

Anderson, P.O., Pochop, S.L., Manoguerra, A.S. (2003) Adverse drug reactions in breastfed infants: less than imagined. *Clinical Pediatrics*, **42**(4) : 325–340.

Anderson, P., Manoguerra, A., Valdez, V. (2015) A review of adverse reactions in infants from medications in breast milk. *Clinical Pediatrics*, **5**(3): 236–244.

Breastfeeding Network (2021) Antidepressants and breastfeeding. www.breastfeedingnetwork.org.uk/antidepressants/ (accessed February 2022).

Brimdyr, K., Cadwell, K., Widström, A.-M. et al. (2015) The association between common labor drugs and suckling when skin-to-skin during the first hour after birth. *Birth*, **42**: 319–328.

Brown, A., Jordan, S. (2014) Active management of the third stage of labor may reduce breast feeding duration due to pain and physical complications. *Breastfeeding Medicine*, **9**(10): 494–502.

Brown, A., Rance, J., Bennett, P. (2015) Understanding the relationship between breast feeding and postnatal depression: the role of pain and physical difficulties. *Journal of Advanced Nursing*, **72**: 273–282.

Bushra, R., Aslam, N. (2010) An overview of clinical pharmacology of ibuprofen. *Oman Medical Journal*, **25**(3): 155–1661.

Cadwell, K., Brimdyr, K. (2017) Intrapartum administration of synthetic oxytocin and downstream effects on breast feeding: elucidating physiologic pathways. *Annals of Nursing Research and Practice*, **2**(3): 1024.

Erickson, E.N., Emeis, C.L. (2017) Breast feeding outcomes after oxytocin use during childbirth: an integrative review. *Journal of Midwifery & Women's Health*, **62**(4): 397–417.

Fleet, A.J., Jones, M., Belan, I. (2017) The influence of intrapartum opioid use on breast feeding experience at 6 weeks post partum: a secondary analysis. *Midwifery*, **50**: 106–109.

Gerhardt, S. (2015) *Why Love Matters*. Routledge: London.

Hale, T., Rowe, H. (2017) *Medications and Mother's Milk*. Springer: New York.

Hamilton, C. (2014) Medication and the midwife. In: Peate, I., Hamilton, C. (eds) *The Student's Guide to Becoming a Midwife*. Wiley-Blackwell: Oxford.

Jones, W. (2018) *Breast feeding and Medications*. Routledge: London.

Jordan, S., Emery, S., Bradshaw, C., Watkins, A., Friswell, W. (2005) The impact of intrapartum analgesia on infant feeding. *British Journal of Obstetrics & Gynaecology*, **112**: 927–934.

Jordan, S., Emery, S., Watkins, A., Evans, J.D., Storey, M., Morgan, G. (2009) Associations of drugs routinely given in labour with breast feeding at 48 hours: analysis of the Cardiff Births Survey. *British Journal of Obstetrics & Gynaecology*, **116**(12): 1622–1629.

Kendall-Tackett, K., Cong, Z., Hale, T.W. (2011) The effect of feeding method on sleep duration, maternal well-being and postpartum depression. *Clinical Lactation*, **2**(2): 22– 26.

Knight, M., Bunch, K., Tuffnell, D. et al. (2020) Saving Lives, Improving Mothers' Care: Lessons learned to inform maternity care from the UK and Ireland Confidential Enquiries into Maternal Deaths and Morbidity 2016–18. www.npeu.ox.ac.uk/mbrrace-uk/reports (accessed February 2022).

Mattison, D., Halbert, L. (eds) (2013) *Clinical Pharmacology During Pregnancy*. Elsevier: St Louis.

McAndrew, F., Thompson, J.. Fellows, L., Large, A., Speed, M., Renfrew, M. (2012) Infant Feeding Survey 2010. https://sp.ukdataservice.ac.uk/doc/7281/mrdoc/pdf/7281_ifs-uk-2010_report.pdf (accessed February 2022).

Mitchell, J., Jones, W., Winkley, E., Kinsella, S.M. (2020) Guideline on anaesthesia and sedation in breast feeding women 2020. *Anaesthesia*, **75**: 1482–1493.

Mohrbacher, N. (2010) *Breastfeeding Answers Made Simple*. Hale: London.

National Institute for Health and Care Excellence (2014) Antenatal and postnatal mental health: clinical management and service guidance (CG 192). www.nice.org.uk/guidance/cg192 (accessed February 2022).

National Institute for Health and Care Excellence (2017) Intrapartum care for healthy women and babies (CG190). www.nice.org.uk/guidance/cg190 (accessed February 2022).

National Institute for Health and Care Excellence (2021a) Antenatal care (NG201). www.nice.org.uk/guidance/ng201 (accessed February 2022).

National Institute for Health and Care Excellence (2021b) Postnatal care (NG194). www.nice.org.uk/guidance/ng194 (accessed February 2022).

Nursing and Midwifery Council (2018) The Code: Professional standards of practice and behaviour for nurses, midwives and nursing associates. www.nmc.org.uk/standards/code/ (accessed February 2022).

Nursing and Midwifery Council (2019) Standards of proficiency for midwives. www.nmc.org.uk/standards/standards-for-midwives/standards-of-proficiency-for-midwives/ (accessed February 2022).

Robson, E., Waugh, J. (2008) *Medical Disorders in Pregnancy*. Blackwell: Oxford.

Rollins, N.C., Bhandari, N., Hajeebhoy, N. et al. (2016).Why invest, and what it will take to improve breast feeding practices? *Lancet Breastfeeding Series*, **387**: 491–504.

Schaefer, C., Peters, P.W.J., Miller, R.K., Miller, R.K. (eds) (2007) *Drugs During Pregnancy and Lactation: Treatment Options and Risk Assessment*. Elsevier: St Louis.

Soussan, C., Gouraud, A., Portolan, G. et al. (2014) Drug-induced adverse reactions via breast feeding: a descriptive study in the French Pharmacovigilance Database. *European Journal of Clinical Pharmacology*, **70**: 1361–1366.

UNICEF (2017) Guide to the Baby Friendly Initiative Standards. www.unicef.org.uk/babyfriendly/baby-friendly-resources/implementing-standards-resources/guide-to-the-standards/ (accessed February 2022).

Victora, C.G., Bahi, R., Barros, A.J.D. et al. (2016) Breast feeding in the 21st century: epidemiology, mechanisms and lifelong effect. *Lancet Breastfeeding Series*, **387**: 475–490.

Widström, A.M., Brimdyr, K., Svensson, K., Cadwell, K., Nissen, E. (2019) Skin-to-skin contact the first hour after birth, underlying implications and clinical practice. *Acta Paediatrica*, **108**: 1192–1204.

Wiklund, I., Norman, M., Uvnas-Moberg, K., Ransjo-Arvidson, A.-B., Andolf, E. (2009) Epidural analgesia: breast-feeding success and related factors. *Midwifery*, **25**: e31–e38.

Ystrom, E. (2012) Breast feeding cessation and symptoms of anxiety and depression: a longitudinal cohort study. *BMC Pregnancy and Childbirth*, **12**(1): 36.

Further reading

Breastfeeding Network (2019) Drugs In Breast milk – Is It Safe? www.breast feedingnetwork.org.uk/drugs-in-breast milk/

Breastfeeding Network drugs factsheets: www.breast feedingnetwork.org.uk/drugs-factsheets/

UK Drugs in Lactation Advisory Service (UKDILAS): www.sps.nhs.uk/articles/ukdilas/

Drug and Lactation database (LactMed): www.ncbi.nlm.nih.gov/books/NBK501922/

Chapter 21

Medications and sexually transmitted infections

Celia Wildeman

University of Hertfordshire, Hatfield, UK

Aim

This chapter provides an introduction to the pharmacology associated with sexually transmitted infections (STIs) in pregnancy.

Learning outcomes

After reading this chapter the reader will be able to:

- Define sexually transmitted infections
- Discuss medications and associated pharmacology that may be required for the treatment of women with sexually transmitted infections
- Discuss the role and responsibilities of the midwife and healthcare practitioner from the perspectives of quality, respect, equality of care and the safety of clients
- Apply practice-based experience of sexually transmitted infections to the care and support of women and their infants
- Evaluate current medicines management, including the significance of stewardship in the context of medicines management.

Test your existing knowledge

- What common sexually transmitted infections can be acquired in pregnancy?
- How is the midwife involved in the medicines management of women with sexually transmitted infections?
- Why is it so important for the midwife to have knowledge and practical experience of caring for women with sexually transmitted infections?
- What are the common medicines currently prescribed and administered to women who are affected by an infection acquired sexually?
- A pregnant woman diagnosed with a sexually transmitted infection informs you that she is concerned that her partner will know that she has developed a sexually transmitted infection. How might this situation be managed?

Fundamentals of Pharmacology for Midwives, First Edition. Edited by Ian Peate and Cathy Hamilton.
© 2022 John Wiley & Sons Ltd. Published 2022 by John Wiley & Sons Ltd.
Companion website: www.wiley.com/go/pharmacologyformidwives

Introduction

Sexually transmitted infections (STIs) are amongst the most emotive and contentious topics that may affect society. The dynamic changes in diagnosis, treatment and medicines management over decades have ensured that the subject remains critical in an ever-changing world. Rogstad et al. (2015) state how important it is to consider the history of previous efforts that have addressed different aspects of STIs. Indeed, the epidemiology of STIs during the twentieth and twenty-first centuries has shown remarkable changes. These infections are primarily acquired by someone who has had sexual activity with a person who has the infection. Cultural attitudes towards sex and sexuality have always affected responses to STIs. These responses are also intertwined with the social and political aspects of a culture. It seems that from a historical perspective, medical interventions have failed to address the Complexity of these social illnesses.

This chapter will focus on the most common STIs: *Chlamydia trachomatis* (chlamydia), gonorrhoea, syphilis (bacterial infections), human immunodeficiency virus (HIV), human papillomavirus (HPV), hepatitis B virus (HBV) and parasites (Trichomonas vaginalis). How these are implicated in pregnancy and child bearing and the related pharmacology will also be addressed.

Infectious organisms are implicated in at least half of all human disease (Janson-Cohen, 2020). The body is constantly exposed to pathogenic invasion and certain conditions determine whether an infection will occur, for example lowering of the body's resistance as occurs in the pregnant woman. STIs are common, diverse and dangerous to health, extending from bacterial diseases that may be readily treatable once diagnosed to viral infections such as HIV that could be life threatening and currently have no cure. STIs can lead to low self-esteem, stigma and sexual dysfunction. Moreover, some STIs are transmitted from mother to child, such as syphilis, and thereby lead to poor pregnancy, neonatal and child health outcomes, for example stillbirth and blindness (Low et al., 2017) or are transmitted through breast milk (Wood and Gudka, 2018).

Currently, there are more than 30 micro-organisms, including bacteria, viruses and parasites, that are transmissible through vaginal, anal and oral sex or genital skin-to-skin contact. A brief overview of the three main micro-organisms that are implicated in the transmission of STIs will be given to explain how and why medicines employed to treat these infections influence their management and the course of the disease.

331

Bacteria

Microbiological studies identify bacteria as single-cell organisms (prokaryotic) that grow in a wide variety of environments and are invisible to the naked eye. They exist inside and outside organisms and can live independently from a host. They are part of a large group of organisms which have cell walls but lack organelles and an organised nucleus, including some that can cause disease. They are a few micrometres in length. Bacteria can carry out all seven life processes (movement, reproduction, sensitivity, nutrition, excretion, respiration and growth) (Janson-Cohen, 2020). They contain DNA and use their enzymes and ribosomes to manufacture proteins that allow their growth and reproduction to occur. Each bacterial type has a different shape: bacilli are rod shaped, cocci are round and spirochaetes are spiral/corkscrew shaped.

Bacteria can be harmless, pathogenic or beneficial to humans. Beneficial bacteria inhabit the intestine and help to extract nutrients from food and fight off pathogens that could cause disease. Bacteria comprise the largest group of pathogens. These pathogenic bacteria are most at home within the human body. Suitable living conditions enable bacteria to reproduce by simple cell division. However, the body has a number of natural defences to protect against harmful organisms including the skin, mucous membranes and the immune system. Bacteria that succeed in overwhelming the immune system can cause damage in two ways: by producing poisons (toxins) or by entering body tissues and growing within them.

Antibacterial medications: mode of action

Antibacterial medications have six modes of action which are interference with cell wall synthesis, inhibition of protein synthesis, interference with nucleic acid synthesis, inhibition of a metabolic pathway, inhibition of membrane function and inhibition of ATP synthase. Therefore, according to their mechanism of action, the targets of antibacterial drugs include the cell membrane, cell wall, protein synthesis, nucleic acid synthesis and biological metabolic compound synthesis (Kirmusaoglu et al., 2019). See also Chapter 9 of this text.

Viruses

Viruses are extremely small infectious agents that can multiply only within living cells. Viruses are not cellular and have no enzyme system. They consist of a nucleic acid core, either DNA or RNA, surrounded by a coat of protein. Viruses are classified according to the type of nucleic acid and are single stranded or double stranded. They contain genetic material and can reproduce; for example, with chlamydia, they can grow only within living cells as they are obligate intracellular parasites (Janson-Cohen, 2020). Viruses are not susceptible to antibacterial agents and must be treated with antiviral drugs.

Antiviral medications: mode of action

Antiviral medications can increase the cell's resistance to a virus (interferons), suppress the virus absorption in the cell or its diffusion into the cell and its deproteinisation process in the cell (amantadine) along with antimetabolites that cause the inhibition of nucleic acid synthesis (Kauser et al., 2021).

Parasites

Although more than 30 identified pathogens are known to be transmitted sexually, eight of these have been clearly linked to the greatest amount of morbidity (Gottlieb et al., 2014). Three are bacterial STIs.

* *Chlamydia trachomatis* (chlamydia)
* *Neisseria gonorrhoeae* (gonorrhoea)
* *Treponema pallidum* (syphilis)

One parasitic STI (Trichomonas vaginalis, causing trichomoniasis) is currently curable. Four viral STIs – HPV, HIV, herpes simplex virus (HSV) and HBV – can be chronic. Medication, which will be discussed later in this chapter, can modify symptoms and influence the course of the disease.

Antiparasitic medications: mode of action

Antiparasitics are indicated for the treatment of parasitic diseases such as protozoa, among others. They target the parasite agents of the infection, including cell membrane and ionic channel, energy metabolism enzymes, cytoplasmic microtubules, DNA synthesis, ribosomal protein synthesis and free radical damage (Miguel, 2018).

Episode of care

Anne-Marie is a 20-year-old woman. This is her first pregnancy and she has recently moved away from her home in the north of England. She knows only her partner's family. Anne-Marie is having her first antenatal appointment and is 12 weeks pregnant. During the antenatal discussion, she informs you that she is concerned about a vaginal discharge that she has noticed. After questioning her further about the nature of the discharge (that is: colour, quantity, consistency, whether itchy, causing discomfort or pain and whether there is any offensive odour), you reassure her and explain that it is a normal vaginal discharge that occurs in pregnancy. You document your discussion in her antenatal case notes. This complies with the Nursing and Midwifery Council's (NMC, 2018) guidance that states 'Good record-keeping is an integral part of nursing and midwifery practice and is essential to the provision of safe and effective care'.

Clinical consideration

Leucorrhoea, a vaginal discharge that occurs in the early stages of pregnancy, is caused by the surge in oestrogen levels. This causes more blood flow towards the vagina. The discharge is usually white in colour, thin and odourless. Vaginal discharge is a common presenting symptom in pregnancy. It is usually physiological and is subject to hormonal variations in consistency and quantity.

Physiological changes occur in pregnancy to nurture the developing fetus and prepare the mother for birth. Some of these changes influence normal biochemical values while others may mimic symptoms of medical disease (Arthy et al., 2016). It is therefore important to differentiate between normal physiological changes and disease pathology. Rice et al. (2016) noted that vaginal discharge is a clinical feature, not a diagnosis, and that history and examination of the patient should be the first line in deciding whether investigations and treatment are required, as observed in the episode of care discussed above.

The classification of STIs is shown in Table 21.1.

Table 21.1   Classification of STIs with responsible organism.

Organism	Infection	Signs and symptoms	In pregnancy
Bacterium	Chlamydia	- In 70% no symptoms - Pain when urinating - Unusual vaginal discharge - Abdominal pain - Pelvic pain - Pain during sexual intercourse - Bleeding after sex - Vaginal itching - Rectal pain	- Premature rupture of membranes - Preterm birth - Baby may develop conjunctivitis or pneumonia
Bacterium	Gonorrhoea	- Symptoms show after a week - Some people are asymptomatic - Fever - Vaginal discharge - Pain or burning on urination - Urinating frequently - Pain during sexual intercourse - Sharp pain in lower abdomen - Sore throat	Newborn baby may pick up the infection during birth, leading to ophthalmia neonatorum (sticky eye)
Bacterium	Syphilis	Symptoms vary as condition progresses **Primary stage:** - enlarged lymph nodes near groin - Small painless sores on the skin - Sores inside the rectum and vagina **Secondary stage:** - small reddish brown sores on the skin, mouth, vagina and anus - Fever and swollen lymph glands - Weight loss - Hair loss - Headaches - Muscle loss - Extreme fatigue	May cross the placenta, causing developmental problems in the baby

333

(Continued)

Table 21.1   (Continued)

Organism	Infection	Signs and symptoms	In pregnancy
		Latent stage: • no symptoms for many years but person is still extremely contagious **Tertiary stage:** • permanent organ damage • Death	
Virus	Human papillomavirus	May be asymptomatic Genital warts: flat, small cauliflower-like or small stem-like protrusions on the vulva, cervix or anus Common warts: hard, grainy growth of skin generally found on the heel or balls of the feet	Unlikely to affect pregnancy, although genital warts may grow more rapidly
Virus	Hepatitis B virus	• Symptoms occur 3 months after exposure • Fatigue • Nausea and vomiting • Pain in joints • Headache • Fever • Dark-coloured urine • Pale clay-coloured faeces • Jaundice	Greater than 90% chance that baby will also develop hepatitis B without treatment at birth • Preterm birth • Placenta abruption • Fetal growth restriction
Virus	Human immunodeficiency virus (HIV)	• Flu-like illness • Infection • Raised temperature • Body rash • Tiredness • Joint pain • Muscle pain • Swollen glands Later, immune system gets severely damaged, leading to • weight loss • Chronic diarrhoea • Night sweats • Skin problems • Recurrent infection • Serious life-threatening illness	Breast feeding by HIV-positive mothers may cause HIV in the baby and should be avoided
Protozoan parasite	Trichomonas vaginalis	• Abnormal vaginal discharge • Itching in vagina • Dysuria • Strawberry cervix • Urethral infection	• Two- to three-fold increase in preterm delivery • Low birthweight

Chlamydia trachomatis (chlamydia)

The World Health Organization (WHO, 2017) found that globally every year, about 131 million infections are diagnosed in individuals with a new sexual partner. Chlamydia is one of the two most commonly reported infections. Females have a higher incidence rate over males, 4.2.% over 2.7% positivity rates (Garcia, 2010). The risk is highest for those who are sexually active between the ages of 15 and 29 years, individuals with two or more partners in the preceding year, individuals with a new sexual partner and men who have sex with men (MSM).

Control of chlamydia is extremely challenging because 70–90% of infected women and over 50% of infected men are asymptomatic and this can remain for years. In cases where the infection remains undetected and untreated, chlamydia-positive individuals will spread the infection to subsequent sexual partners, even in the absence of symptoms. Treatment is also necessary because, left untreated, persistent chlamydia leads to serious and potentially permanent complications such as pelvic inflammatory disease (PID) and tubal factor infertility in women (Land et al., 2019). Screening is therefore essential to detect chlamydia in asymptomatic individuals to prevent the spread of infection and minimise the potential for complications arising from untreated cases.

Barlow (2011) asserts that chlamydial infection is greatly on the increase. Reported cases rose from 59 461 in 1999 to 89 431 in 2003 and 126 882 in 2008 (Barlow, 2011). STIs bear a high burden of disease and subsequent high health costs globally. STIs continue to be the most frequently notified conditions in the notifiable surveillance system.

Diagnosis

Sexually transmitted infection screening is a critical initiative that aims to reduce the increasing global prevalence of many common STIs, such as chlamydia. The often asymptomatic nature of the infection means that another different infection may be implicated. Screening is the only way to identify and treat them (Wood and Gudka, 2018). In this way, the transmission of STIs can be reduced and the health implications of an untreated STI reduced.

Screening for chlamydia involves testing a specimen using nucleic acid amplification testing (NAAT) (Lim et al., 2012). NAAT detects part of the bacterium rather than the whole organism. The test tends to be highly sensitive but at the expense of specificity, which results in some false positives (Barlow, 2011). NAAT is the preferred test recommended by the WHO as it is highly sensitive and specific. It can also be used for a wide range of samples (WHO, 2017), including self-collected samples. Gender and risk factors influence the type of specimen collected (Wood and Gudka, 2018).

Traditionally, to access chlamydia screening, the person needed to make and attend an appointment with the GP or present to a genitourinary medicine (GUM) clinic or a family planning clinic. The health provider or person collects the relevant specimen for screening and waits for the pathology results. Antibiotic treatment will be commenced if the result is positive.

Once diagnosed, chlamydia is easily treated with readily available antibiotics. Management guidelines recommend azithromycin 1 gram orally single dose or erythromycin 500 mg twice daily for 14 days as first-line treatment for uncomplicated chlamydial infection.

There are a number of well-documented barriers to existing screening pathways, including embarrassment, inconvenience, fear of invasive sample collection and low motivation to self- refer for screening (Hughes and Field, 2015). Therefore, screening rates in general practice remain low so alternative sources of chlamydia screening are necessary. One such alternative is the purchase of chlamydia screening kits which can be bought over the counter from some pharmacies. Another is for the person to self-collect a urine or vaginal sample for which a prepaid postal bag is made available for return of the sample to be analysed. Diagnosis is then possible and results are given to the person usually by telephone, text messaging, email or a website with a secure log-in. The person will be directed to an appropriate service for necessary treatment. It is important to be vigilant about test results, particularly the possibility of false negatives and false positives (Barlow, 2011).

Complications

Chlamydia is the most common cause of pelvic infection although infertility does not automatically follow (Barlow, 2011). PID can result in ectopic pregnancy and chronic pelvic pain. Confined to the cervix, chlamydia does no harm although it can infect a male partner (discussed later in the chapter). Problems arise when the infection spreads internally to the uterus, fallopian tubes and other pelvic contents. Acute salpingitis is a serious condition characterised by fever and severe lower abdominal pain. Chronic salpingitis results in a more constant pain without fever and may or may not be associated with active infection. However, antibiotics are given to be on the safe side. The pain of acute and chronic salpingitis is exacerbated by sexual intercourse with deep dyspareunia. Successful antibiotic treatment that removes all traces of infection may still result in sticky inflammation from the fluid and pus. This can leave the contents of the pelvis with adhesions.

The chlamydia that causes non-specific urethritis (NSU) can also infect the eyes. Conjunctivitis is uncommon but can occur when genital secretions contaminate the eyes. The eyelids are red and inflamed when pulled back. Eye infection can spread to the middle ear (otitis media) with temporary hearing loss. Chlamydial conjunctivitis needs to be treated with antibiotics orally.

Infection in babies

Ophthalmia neonatorum is seen babies soon after birth. It is a significant cause of neonatal morbidity and chlamydia is the most common infectious cause of ophthalmia neonatorum in high-income countries (Zar, 2005). It has an equal incidence with gonorrhoea acquired eye infection. It may take a week or longer to appea,r by which time both mother and baby are likely to have been discharged home. Systemic antibiotic treatment is required by mouth because, like adults, the infection may spread to the ears and lungs. Erythromycin 12.5 mg every 6 hours is administered orally. Additional topical therapy is unnecessary. In approximately 20–30% of infants, initial therapy will not eradicate the organism and the infant may require a repeat oral course of antibiotics.

Parents and carers should be advised to seek medical attention if vomiting or irritability with feeding occurs in infants during treatment. There is a risk of infantile hypertrophic pyloric stenosis after exposure to erythromycin during infancy (MHRA CHM, 2020).

Side-effects of treatment with erythromycin include decreased appetite, diarrhoea, skin rashes and vomiting.

Treatment

Azithromycin

This is the drug of choice for the treatment of chlamydia and is cost-effective. It is an antibiotic that fights bacteria, including those implicated in STIs. It should not be taken if the woman is allergic to it or to a similar drug. The woman should be advised to inform the doctor if she is pregnant or intending to become pregnant though azithromycin is not known to be harmful in pregnancy (BNF, 2022). It can be taken with or without food. It is advisable to take this medicine for the full prescribed length of time as symptoms may improve before the infection is completely cleared. Skipping doses may also increase the risk of further infection that is resistant to antibiotics. It should be stored at room temperature away from moisture and heat.

Avoid taking antacids that contain aluminium or magnesium within 2 hours before or after taking azithromycin. This includes Gaviscon® and milk of magnesia. These antacids can make azithromycin less effective when taken at the same time.

Azithromycin can result in increased photosensitivity. Exposure to sunlight and tanning beds can cause sunburn more easily therefore protective clothing and sunscreen (SPF 30 or higher) should be applied when out of doors.

Common side-effects
- Diarrhoea
- Nausea and vomiting
- Stomach pain
- Headache

Drug interactions
- Blood thinners (for example, warfarin)
- Vitamins and herbal products

Pregnancy
- No control data in human pregnancy (Drugs.com, 2021).
- AUTGA pregnancy category B1: Drugs that have been taken by only a limited number of pregnant women and women of child-bearing age, without an increase in the frequency of malformation

or other direct/indirect harmful effects on the human fetus having been observed. Studies in animals have not shown evidence of an increased occurrence of fetal damage.

- Use is not recommended unless clearly needed.

Breast feeding

Azithromycin is excreted in breast milk (Goldstein et al., 2009). Breast-fed infants should be monitored for gastrointestinal side-effects, for example diarrhoea, and fungal infections and sensitisation. Some experts recommend discontinuing breast feeding during treatment and discarding milk during and up to 2 days after discontinuation of azithromycin. Other experts recommend use if alternative agents are not available, such as erythromycin or clarithromycin. The levels of azithromycin in breast milk are so low that it would not be expected to cause adverse effects.

Erythromycin

Erythromycin can be used in the treatment of chlamydia. The dose varies from 500 mg to 1000 mg orally for 14 days.

Interactions

Erythromycin can interact with corticosteroids, for example, methylprednisolone which may be taken by the woman as treatment for asthma. In this case it is important to monitor and adjust the dose.

Side-effects

Vomiting, nausea, diarrhoea.

Pregnancy

Use only if adequate alternatives are not available.

Breast feeding

Erythromycin is present in breast milk. It should only be used if no other suitably alternative exists (BNF, 2017–2018).

Episode of care

Baby Olivia is now 7 days old. You are carrying out her daily postnatal care at her home as delegated by the community midwife. You notice that there is a purulent discharge from both of the baby's eyes. Her mother Jasmine has been diagnosed with chlamydia and has had a course of antibiotics. She is formula feeding Olivia. Jasmine is concerned that she may have passed the infection to Olivia and is very distressed. You have reported your findings to the community midwife. Apart from the discharging eyes, Olivia appears to be thriving.

Clinical consideration

It is important to reassure Jasmine that pathology tests will be carried out to confirm whether Olivia is infected with chlamydia and that if it is confirmed, treatment will be successful. The midwife should be informed of your findings and swabs should be taken from both eyes (a separate swab from each eye), ensuring local policy and procedure are adhered to, and sent to the laboratory for microscopy, culture and sensitivity to antibiotics. The GP should be informed and antibiotic treatment will be commenced. All findings and midwifery management of care should be documented in the baby's care notes.

The midwife as a skilled practitioner is ideally placed to recognise any changes that may lead to complications (NMC, 2019) and indeed, to provide additional care for women and newborn infants with complications. The midwife also has a role in 'effective health protection through understanding and applying the principles of infection prevention and control, communicable disease surveillance and antimicrobial resistance and stewardship' (NMC, 2019).

Gonorrhoea

The WHO (2017) estimates that there are 78 million new cases of *Neisseria gonorrhoeae* every year worldwide. The greatest incidence is seen in the western Pacific, South-East Asia and African regions. Global prevalence is 0.6% in men and 0.82% in women. Cases in England are at the highest level since records began more than 100 years ago. A total of 70 936 cases were reported in 2019 (BBC statistics, 2020), up by more than a quarter on 2018 (Table 21.2).

Gonorrhoea is almost exclusively acquired sexually by penetrative vaginal or rectal sexual intercourse and oral sex. It is unknown how infectious the disease is. However, a man with gonorrhoea might have a 95% chance of passing it on from one episode of vaginal sex. On the other hand, if a woman has gonorrhoea, the risk to the man will be less. It is unknown how rapidly the recipient becomes infectious but there have been anecdotes of transmission within an hour or two of being exposed to gonorrhoea (Barlow, 2011).

Gonorrhoea is implicated in the list of common infections in pregnancy. Indeed, its significance for the midwife was demonstrated when it was found that pregnant women were more significantly likely to be undertreated when positive for infection compared to non-pregnant women (Bergquist et al., 2020) and significantly less likely to be overtreated when negative for infection. One prevalence study identified that up to 80% of pregnant women with STIs can be undertreated and lost to follow-up (Krivochenitser et al., 2013). STIs including gonorrhoea can have serious consequences for women, the fetus and neonate and the potential asymptomatic nature of the disease can prevent effective management. For example, screening for many STIs is not explicit in the UK antenatal guidelines and as a consequence these infections may be overlooked. It is therefore essential to consider a woman's risk of STIs regularly throughout pregnancy and to know how and when to undertake an appropriate sexual history and relevant testing.

The key principles to successfully managing STIs in pregnancy are early diagnosis and effective treatment together with minimising the risk of reinfection and vertical transmission.

Management in pregnancy may differ depending on gestation age, stage of infection and contraindications to drugs. Test of cure (TOC) is often advised (Thwaites et al., 2016) to confirm successful treatment. Mode of birth is not commonly influenced by the presence of an STI, with the exception of herpes.

Non-sexual modes of transmission include:

- newborn babies via vertical transmission
- prepubertal girls
- passed from objects like towels or flannels.

Gonorrhoea in pregnancy and breast feeding

Neisseria gonorrhoeae is associated with a number of adverse pregnancy and newborn outcomes. Information about these associations is necessary as this can improve understanding of the evidence of causality and help to determine the potential impact of preventive interventions (Vallely et al., 2021). Chorioamnionitis leads to premature rupture of the membranes, preterm birth, if diagnosed in the first trimester of pregnancy, lowbirth weight and postpartum infection. The infection is transmitted to the neonate in 30–50% of cases (Thwaites et al., 2016). This occurs during birth and less commonly before birth when there was prolonged rupture of the membranes. It is more common for ophthalmia neonatorum of the newborn with profuse purulent conjunctival discharge to occur (Thwaites et al., 2016). This invariably causes blindness if untreated and so the neonate should receive prophylactic erythromycin ophthalmic ointment at birth irrespective of mode of birth.

Table 21.2   Annual number of cases of gonorrhoea in England 2012–2019 per 100 000 population.

Year	Number of cases
2012	50.3
2013	57.9
2014	68.4
2015	75.5
2016	66.2
2017	80.5
2018	100;5
2019	126

In 2017, 422 females were newly diagnosed in Wales, the highest number of cases.
In 2019, 951 cases were diagnosed in Northern Ireland.
Source: Greenfield, M. (2021) Sexual Health in the United Kingdom. Hearst magazine, London.

Diagnosis

The three criteria for diagnosis are:

- Gram negative (GN)
- intracellular (I)
- diplococci (D).

Public Health England confirmed that although detection of gonorrhoea by NAAT is more sensitive than culture, it is culture that allows confirmatory identification and antimicrobial susceptibility testing (PHE, 2013). A culture should be taken in all cases diagnosed by NAAT. Microscopy of Gram-stained genital specimens allows direct visualisation of *Neisseria* as monomorphic Gram-negative diplococci within polymorphonuclear leucocytes. Local GUM clinics should inform laboratories about samples specifically requiring culture. Public health figures also show that while infection is still relatively uncommon in the general UK population, it is significant among those with other risk factors such as co-infection and is more prevalent in the under 25s. Additionally, Thwaites et al. (2016) believe that early diagnosis and treatment, partner notification and multidisciplinary management with genitourinary physicians, microbiologists and paediatricians are key to securing good outcomes for mother and child.

National Institute for Health and Care Excellence (NICE) guidelines on STIs (2019) advised health professionals to be proactive and ask people about their sexual history at key points of contact. This form of questioning of those at risk of contracting an STI should include a discussion about prevention and testing. A comprehensive sexual history that identifies the risk of STIs is important. This history should include the gender of the sexual partner, the type of sexual contact and sites of exposure (oral, anal, vaginal), condom use/barrier use and, importantly, whether properly used, relationship with the partner, for example live-in, regular or casual, duration of the relationship and whether the partner can be contacted, including the time interval since the last contact (NICE, 2019).

The midwife has a professional responsibility to take an adequate sexual history during the antenatal period and to ensure that this is carried out at regular intervals as necessary. This aspect of the midwife's role is clearly identified by the NMC, which states that the midwife has a role in assessment, screening and care planning (NMC, 2019). Supporting people who have been diagnosed with an STI to notify their partner can help to prevent reinfection and reduce the transmission of STIs. It can also ensure that their partners are tested and, if necessary, treated as soon as possible to prevent health complications. To facilitate these requirements, screening is routinely offered and recommended to all pregnant women in England.

Complications

- Local infection of glands around the vulva leading to bartholinitis, painful swelling of the labia, or skenitis a similar condition next to the urethra.
- Endometriosis followed by involvement of the fallopian tubes, salpingitis and into the pelvis to cause pelvic peritonitis which can lead to ectopic pregnancy.
- Lower abdominal pain with pelvic inflammation and can be combined with deep dyspareunia (discomfort felt on intercourse).
- Fitz-Hugh–Curtis syndrome. The lining outside the liver can become inflamed, a perihepatitis. This is hard to diagnose as pain under the right rib is difficult to reconcile with an infection originally contracted through sex.
- Rarely gonorrhoea spreads via the bloodstream to elsewhere in the body, including the skin and joints.

Treatment

Gonorrhoea is an issue of global health concern. It is asymptomatic in most affected individuals and antibiotic-resistant strains of *Neisseria gonorrhoeae* have been emerging in recent years. Resistant strains are reducing the effectiveness of some antibiotic treatments (Wood and Gudka, 2018). The WHO guidelines for gonorrhoeal treatment recommend that local resistance data should guide treatment choice. If the antibiotic susceptibility is unknown, treatment requires a combination of two antibacterial medications of differing mechanisms of action. This strategy improves treatment effectiveness and can slow the occurrence of antibiotic resistance in *Neisseria gonorrhoeae*.

Ceftriaxone

Prescribed for bacterial infections, e.g. uncomplicated gonorrhoea.

Pregnancy

The manufacturer advises use only if the benefit outweighs the risk; limited data available but not known to be harmful in animal studies. No evidence of embryotoxicity, fetotoxicity or teratogenicity, Specialist sources indicate that it is suitable for use in pregnancy.

- Compatible with breast feeding; present in milk in low concentration but limited effects on breast-fed infants.
- Occasionally disruption of the infant's gastrointestinal flora, resulting in diarrhoea or thrush, has been reported with cephalosporins but these effects have not been adequately evaluated. Acceptable in breast-feeding mothers.

Spectinomycin

Considered safe for use in pregnancy and can be used during lactation. Spectinomycin is in FDA pregnancy category B, which means that it is not expected to be harmful to an unborn baby. It is not known if spectinomycin passes into breast milk. There are no restrictions on food, beverages or activities during treatment.

Side-effects

Difficulty breathing, swelling of the throat, lips, tongue or face, and hives. The woman is advised to stop taking the spectinomycin and seek emergency medical attention if these effects occur. Less serious effects include nausea, dizziness and fever.

Interactions

Can interact with vitamins, minerals and herbal products.

Erythromycin ophthalmic ointment

Applied up to six times a day for eye infections. Applied one time in the hospital soon after birth to prevent eye infection in newborn babies. Can be used in breast-feeding infants.

Wash hands before using eye medication. Side-effects are unlikely with topical application.

Syphilis

Syphilis has been described as the most common congenital infection worldwide (Howe et al., 2018). The WHO estimates that globally, 1.5 million pregnancies are affected each year and up to 50% of those untreated will result in adverse outcomes. Syphilis is relatively uncommon in the UK but incidence of the disease has risen at an alarming rate since 2013.

The bacteria enter the body and usually leave behind at least one small painless lesion, a chancre that heals on its own within a week. This is known as primary syphilis. This is followed a few weeks later by secondary syphilis. Typically a rash can be seen and this can cover the whole body. This rash can be accompanied by wart-like oral or genital lesions and flu-like symptoms. This stage can last from a few weeks to a year, during which the infection becomes latent with no obvious signs or symptoms. At this stage the infection becomes tertiary syphilis.

The NICE (2019) guidelines specify that professionals should ensure that people with suspected infection but who decline testing, or those with confirmed syphilis who decline treatment but knowingly transmit the infection via sexual contact or non-sexual contact with extragenital lesions, are made aware that these acts could result in prosecution. This professional responsibility emphasises the legislative role of the midwife in the demonstration of 'effective health protection through understanding and applying the principles of infection prevention and control, communicable disease surveillance and antimicrobial resistance and stewardship' (NMC, 2019).

Diagnosis

The National Institute for Health and Care Excellence clearly stated that screening for syphilis should be offered to all pregnant women at an early stage in antenatal care because treatment of syphilis is beneficial to mother and baby (NICE, 2019). PHE is supportive of this view; it confirmed that all women must receive information about antenatal screening tests early in pregnancy before they are asked to make screening decisions (PHE, 2018).

Serological tests, such as enzyme immunoassays and *T. pallidum* particle agglutination assays, detect antibodies to treponemal proteins or non-treponemal antigens, such as damaged host cells or lipoidal antigens. Treponemal serological tests must be confirmed by further serology, for example, a non-treponemal serological test, because there is a genuine risk of false reactivity, especially with other infections or inflammatory conditions such as systemic lupus erythematosus. These tests will be reported as reactive or non-reactive and although they may suggest infection, they do not give any information about the stage of infection or whether it has been treated (Henao-Martinez and Johnson, 2014).

Treatment

In cases of early, primary, secondary and latent syphilis in pregnancy, treatment with a single-dose intramuscular injection of benzathine penicillin G 2.4 MU is recommended if administered in the first or second trimester of pregnancy or two doses if administered later (Townsend et al., 2017). Currently British guidelines also advise retreatment if there is uncertainty over the efficacy of past treatment. For latent treatment in pregnancy, three doses of benzathine penicillin are recommended (Townsend et al., 2017).

Other possible medications are amoxicillin 500 mg and probenecid 500 mg , both orally, four times per day.

A second dose is recommended when treating early infection in the third trimester because there are lower serum levels of the drug and a risk of treatment failure. For women who report possible sensitivity to penicillin and who can tolerate cephalosporins, the alternative is ceftriaxone 500 mg intramuscularly, daily for 10 days (Howe et al., 2018).

For a woman who is not allergic to penicillin but who is unable to tolerate an intramuscular regimen, the alternative is amoxicillin 500 mg and probenecid 500 mg, both orally, four times per day for 14 days.

Table 21.3 lists the antibiotics used in each stage of pregnancy. It should be remembered that each woman is individually assessed, and care tailored to meet her needs.

Clinical consideration

It is important to be aware of the Jarisch–Herxheimer reaction during the treatment of syphilis. This can complicate up to 45% of syphilis treatments in pregnancy. This is thought to be associated with large numbers of *T. pallidum* being destroyed which in turn release excessive cytokines, initiating an acute inflammatory reaction. Symptoms typically occur within the first 24 hours of treatment and include fever, rigors and skin rash. In pregnancy, there are also case reports of uterine contractions induced by the Jarisch–Herxheimer reaction. The reaction is particularly common during the management of early disease, occurring in 50% of cases of primary syphilis and as many as 90% of cases of secondary syphilis and in the latent phase, 25% (Henao-Martinez et al., 2014).

Table 21.3   Antibiotics used to treat syphilis in each stage of pregnancy, by stage of disease.

Early disease: primary/ secondary or latent <2 years	Late disease: latent/unknown duration
Benzathine penicillin 2.4 MU (IM) single dose	Benzathine penicillin 2.4 MU (IM) weekly for 3 weeks

IM, intramuscular.
Source: WHO (2016).

Hepatitis B virus

Hepatitis B infection is one of the major public health burdens worldwide (Pan et al., 2020). The WHO (2019) estimated that 296 million people had chronic hepatitis in 2019, with 1.5 million new infections each year.

Perinatal transmission, vertical transmission and mother-to-child transmission (MTCT) of HBV are the primary pathways of infection. The active-passive immune prophylaxis strategy has reduced perinatal transmission rates to 10–15%. Maternal hepatitis B e antigen (HBeAg) positivity and high HBV-DNA levels are associated with increased transmission despite universal immune prophylaxis programmes (Chen et al., 2017). The risk of becoming chronically infected is inversely proportional to the age at exposure, with 90% of perinatal transmissions leading to chronic HBV infection (Bergin et al., 2018). Clearly, then, the two greatest risk factors for MTCT are high maternal viral load and HBeAg positivity.

Diagnosis

Hepatitis B virus can only be differentiated from other types of viral hepatitis by laboratory confirmation (Lallemand et al., 2016). A blood sample is tested for the presence of HBV surface antigens (HbsAG), using enzyme immunoassay techniques. Screening is recommended (Lallemand et al., 2016; Land et al., 2019) in pregnant women, adults at increased risk of transmission and people who are hepatitis C (HCV) positive or HIV positive due to the increased risk of co-infection.

Treatment

There is no cure for HBV. Treatment in acute infections is aimed at relieving symptoms and replacing fluid loss caused through vomiting and diarrhoea. Medication can be used to manage chronic infection, but treatment is complex and case specific. The deciding factors relevant to treatment include the duration of the infection, presence of symptoms and complications arising from chronic infection. Life-long antiviral medication such as tenofovir (TDF) can be used to slow down the ability of the virus to multiply in chronic HBV infection.

Despite the safety record of TDF in pregnancy, some guidelines recommend against its use during breast feeding. Authors have compared the dose levels of TDF-exposed fetuses, breast-fed infants and children receiving TDF treatment. They found that breast-fed infants were exposed to only

0.5–16% of the TDF dose that fetuses experienced via placental transfer. Based on the safety data from fetuses and children exposed to TFD, and the comparatively negligible exposure dosage from breast feeding, it was concluded that mothers should be encouraged to breast feed (Hu et al., 2019). The WHO agreed that chronic HBV infection of the mother should not be a reason to avoid breast feeding (Pan et al., 2020).

Telbivudine

Telbivudine used to treat high viraemic women during late pregnancy has been shown to decrease perinatal transmission of HBV (Chen et al., 2017). However, there is limited data concerning telbivudine therapy initiated from the second trimester and transmission rates for HBV pregnant patients with low viral loads. Overall, Chen et al. (2017) suggest that more research is necessary before antepartum antiviral therapy is routinely recommended in women with detectable viral loads.

Tenofovir disoprovil

Tenofovir for the treatment of chronic HBV works by blocking the enzyme reverse transcriptase which is responsible for Hep B replication (NICE, 2009). The adult dose is 245 mg once daily.

Indications

Chronic HBV infection with compensated liver disease (with evidence of viral replication and histologically documented active liver inflammation or fibrosis) and chronic HBV infection with decompensated liver disease.

Side-effects

When treating chronic HBV with tenofovir, monitor liver function tests every 3 months and viral markers for HBV every 3–6 months (continue to monitor for at least 1 year after discontinuation of treatment). Test renal function and serum phosphate before treatment then every 4 weeks (more frequently if at increased risk of renal impairment).

Rare side-effects include nephrogenic diabetes insipidus, proximal renal tubulopathy and renal failure.

343

Pregnancy

Mitochondrial dysfunction has been reported in infants exposed to nucleoside reverse transcriptase inhibitors in utero. The main effects include haematological, metabolic and neurological disorders. All infants whose mothers receive nucleoside reverse transcriptase inhibitors during pregnancy should be monitored for relevant signs and symptoms (BNF, 2017–18).

Interactions

If taken with ibuprofen, can increase the risk of nephrotoxicity.

Human papillomavirus

Human papillomavirus is a normal consequence of having sexual intercourse and is common regardless of sexual orientation. Evidence suggests that about 80% of all women who have had sexual intercourse have a lifetime risk of becoming infected with one or more of the STI HPV types (WHO, 2017). It is a common STI and part of the HPV family of viruses, of which there are more than 200 types. Some cause benign skin warts or papillomas. Approximately 40 types affect the genital area. They can be subdivided into those that are low risk for cervical cancer (HPV 6 and 11), which are also responsible for some genital warts, and those which are high risk for cervical cancer (HPV 16 and 18). These are responsible for approximately 70% of cervical cancer cases (WHO, 2014). In a minority of women, the virus can become persistent and this may result in changes to the cells of the cervix or cervical abnormalities known as cervical intraepithelial neoplasia (CIN). This is the abnormal growth of precancer cells in the cervix.

Although high-risk HPV is the cause of 99.7% of all cervical cancers, certain factors have been shown to increase the risk of developing the disease, including persistent and chronic infection with one or more of the high-risk oncogenic types of HPV (RCN, 2020).

Treatment and prevention

Condoms and dental dams offer a degree of protection against the initial transmission of HPV infections as HPV is spread by skin-to-skin and genital tract contact; however, condoms will not provide complete protection. There is no treatment for HPV but as most infections are cleared rapidly by the immune system, it is considered unnecessary to treat a virus which may not cause ill health (RCN, 2020).

HPV vaccination

This was introduced in the UK in September 2008 for girls and boys 12–13 years old and in school year 8 or from the age of 11 in Scotland. The vaccination helps to protect against the two most high-risk types of HPV (16 and 18) which are responsible for more than 70% of cervical cancers. Girls and boys missed the vaccination in school can request it through the NHS up to the age of 25 (Jo's Cervical Cancer Trust, 2019).

Human immunodeficiency virus (HIV)

The latest WHO estimates indicate that 37 million people are infected with HIV globally and of these, nearly half are unaware of their HIV status (WHO, 2017). HIV infection causes a chronic immune deficiency that usually first presents as a flu-like illness 2 weeks after exposure. It is currently incurable but if detected early, lifelong combination antiretroviral therapy (ART) tailored to the individual will lower the viral load, prevent HIV transmission and prevent progression from HIV to acquired immune deficiency syndrome (AIDS).

Diagnosis

Pregnant women in the UK are cared for in accordance with the British HIV Association (BHIVA) guidelines. Improvements are advocated (Raffe et al .,2017) to ensure timely referral and ART initiation that will ensure the best outcome for mother and child. Antenatal screening was introduced in 2000 and the take-up rate has remained consistently high at >90% in all UK regions. Currently, about 1300 HIV-positive women have given birth in the UK (Raffe et al., 2017).

Neonatal testing

The mother who is exclusively non-breast feeding her infant should be HIV tested with an HIV, DNA or RNA PCR test. The test should be performed at the following times:

- 2 weeks after birth
- when the baby is 6 weeks old
- when the baby is 12 weeks old (Peters et al., 2018).

HIV antibody testing should be performed at 18–24 months of age to rule out rare cases of HIV seroconversion in the infant without detectable virus on PCR. A breast-feeding woman's infant should have additional tests performed.

Complications – mother-to-child transmission

The potential for HIV transmission from a pregnant woman to her unborn child has been recognised since 1982 (Raffe et al., 2017). Planning for an appropriate mode of birth is an important factor in the prevention of MTCT, and recommendations are dependent on the maternal viral load at or after 36 weeks gestation. However, prevention of MTCT is complex. Interventions are aimed at reducing risks throughout pregnancy, birth and the postnatal period. Facilitating this aim requires a specialist multidisciplinary team including HIV clinicians, midwives, obstetricians and paediatricians.

Transmission can occur antenatally, perinatally or postnatally (through breast feeding). Previously, advice for mode of birth was for caesarean section to reduce the risk of perinatal transmission (Hamlyn and Barber, 2018). More recently, evidence has shown that there is no difference in transmission rates in those women who birth vaginally compared to caesarean section as long as the woman is taking ART and has achieved viral suppression (defined as <50 copies/mL at 36 weeks) prior to birth (Peters et al., 2018).

Identified reasons for MTCT

- Undiagnosed breast feeding is a factor in postnatal transmission (one-fifth of infants born to diagnosed women).
- Declined HIV testing in pregnancy accounting for nearly half of undiagnosed women.
- Seroconversion (around 25%), late antenatal booking, breast feeding, preterm birth.
- Seroconversion in pregnancy or postnatally after an earlier negative antenatal HIV test occurred in around 25% of women (PHE, 2015).

Infant feeding

While ART can significantly reduce the risk of postnatal HIV transmission, it does not abolish it completely. The current guidance is that all HIV-positive women should be advised to exclusively formula feed their baby. These women can opt for breast feeding as long as they are virally suppressed (this should not be considered a child protection issue and the woman should be offered intensive support) (Peters et al., 2018).

Treatment

The BHIVA recommend that all women beginning ART during pregnancy should start treatment by the beginning of week 24 and those with a viral load >30 000 copies/mL should start treatment by 16 weeks gestation.

Zidovudine (AZT)

All infants born to HIV-positive women are offered postexposure prophylaxis (PEP) in all cases where the mother is virally suppressed prior to birth.

Trichomonas vaginalis (TV)

This is a very common STI, caused by infection with a protozoan parasite. The parasite passes from an infected person during sexual intercourse. In women, the most commonly infected part of the body is the lower genital tract (vulva, vagina, cervix and urethra). It is uncommon for the parasite to spread to other parts of the body such as the hand, mouth or anus. About 30% of people have symptoms though it is possible for infection to be passed on without symptoms.

Signs and symptoms

Mild irritation to severe inflammation develop 5–28 days after being infected. Women notice:

- abnormal vaginal discharge (thin or increased in volume) that can be clear, white, yellowish or green
- pruritus
- dysuria
- itching, burning, redness or soreness of the genitals
- painful sex.

The characteristic feature of the infection is the strawberry cervix. This appears as a friable erythematous cervix with punctate areas of exudate (Rice et al., 2016).
Urethral infection is present in 90% of cases.

Diagnosis

Reliability depends on laboratory testing. Increased local polymorph leucocytes are the main host response to the infection. Sites for sampling are by high vaginal swabs from the posterior fornix, self-taken vaginal swab or urine samples.
Methods for detection of TV include the following.

- *NAAT*: a highly sensitive method for detection of TV. It can detect 3–5 times more than wet preparations using direct microscopy. It is now considered the gold standard for detection of TV. Specimens are usually retrieved from the vagina, endocervix or urine. This method detects the protozoal RNA with a high sensitivity of 95.3–100% (Rice et al., 2016).

- *Direct microscopy*: this is the method of choice for screening. A wet preparation has a low sensitivity of 50–70%. Vaginal discharge mixed with a drop of saline on a glass slide can be used to detect TV motility. TV lose their motility quickly, therefore the wet preparation should be read within 10 minutes of collection.
- *Cervical smear*: the PAP test can incidentally detect TV but the false-positive and false-negative rates make it unreliable as a diagnostic tool.

Treatment

The only effective treatment against TV are nitroimidazoles such as metronidazole and tinidazole. The cure rate for metronidazole is 84–98% while that for tinidazole, a more expensive drug, is 92–100%.

Indications for treatment

- Testing positive for TV regardless of symptoms.
- Treatment of sexual partner is recommended.
- A single dose of 2 g metronidazole orally or a single dose of 2 g tinidazole orally.

Alternative regimen

Twice daily 500mg Metronidazole orally for 7 days.

Pregnancy

Trichomonas vaginalis is a risk factor for the vertical transmission of HIV, therefore screening and treatment of TV are recommended for HIV-positive pregnant women. These individuals should have a repeat test 3 months after treatment. Infection in pregnancy is associated with a two-fold increase in preterm delivery and low birthweight. Treatment may prevent genital or respiratory infection in the newborn. (Rice et al., 2016). Metronidazole can be prescribed at any gestation, if indicated, although it crosses the placenta. There is no evidence of teratogenicity.

Metronidazole is secreted in breast milk but only low plasma levels are found in breast-fed babies of women using this medication (Rice et al., 2016). However, some obstetricians recommend deferring breast feeding for at least 24–48 hours after completion of treatment.

Due to limited data regarding the safety of tinidazole in pregnancy, it is best avoided. Breast feeding should be deferred for at least 72 hours following a 2 g tinidazole dose (Rice et al., 2016).

Women with HIV should be given a 7-day course of metronidazole to ensure treatment of the infection.

Retesting after 3 months may be necessary in some cases.

Conclusion

Medications employed in the management of STIs have advanced in the twenty-first century and the knowledge and expertise discussed in this chapter would suggest that medicines will continue to play a significant role in the treatment of these diseases. Midwives have a significant part to play by demonstrating knowledge and understanding of pharmacology and to ensure they can recognise the positive and adverse effects of medicines. These include allergies, drug sensitivities, side-effects, contraindications, incompatibilities, adverse reactions, prescribing errors and the impact of polypharmacy and over-the-counter medication usage (NMC, 2019).

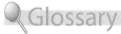 ## Glossary

Bacteria   Single-cell micro-organisms

Dyspareunia   Difficult or painful sexual intercourse

Infantile hypertrophic pyloric stenosis   A condition in neonates characterised by an acquired narrowing of the pylorus

Lesion   A region in an organ or tissue which has suffered damage through injury or disease

Leucorrhoea   A whitish or yellowish discharge of mucus from the vagina

Ophthalmia neonatorum   An acute inflammation of the eyes of a newborn from infection acquired during passage through the vaginal canal

Parasite An organism that lives in or on an organism of another species (its host) and benefits by deriving nutrients at the other's expense

Pelvic inflammatory disease Inflammation of the female genital tract, accompanied by fever and lower abdominal pain

Photosensitivity An extreme sensitivity to ultraviolet rays from the sun and other light sources

Salpingitis Inflammation of the fallopian tubes

Virus Very small infectious agent that can multiply only within living cells

Test yourself

Now review your learning by completing the learning activities for this chapter at www.wiley.com/go/pharmacologyformidwives.

References

Arthy, A., Nelson-Piercy, C., Heli, T. et al. (2016) Physiological changes in pregnancy. *International Journal of Reproduction, Contraception, Obstetrics and Gynaecology*, **10**(4): 89–94.

Barlow, D. (2011) *Sexually Transmitted Infections: The Facts*, 3rd edn. Oxford University Press: Oxford.

BBC Statistics (2020) www.bbc.co.UK/newsbeat-54011133 (accessed February 2020).

Bergin, H., Wood, G., Walker, S. P., Hui, L. (2018) Perinatal management of hepatitis B virus: clinical implementation of updated Australasian management guidelines. *Obstetric Medicine*, **11**(1): 23–27.

Bergquist, E., Trolard, A., Kuhlmann, A. (2020) Undertreatment of chlamydia and gonorrhoea amongst pregnant women in emergency department. *International Journal of Sexually Transmitted Disease and AIDS*, **31**(2): 166–173.

British National Formulary (2017–2018) https://bnf.nice.org.uk/ (accessed February 2022).

British National Formulary (2022) Azithromycin. https://bnf.nice.org.uk/drug/azithromycin.html (accessed February 2022).

Chen, Z., Gu, G., Bian, Z. et al. (2017) Clinical course and perinatal transmission of chronic HB during pregnancy: a real world prospective cohort study. *Journal of Infection*, **75**(2): 146–154.

Drugs.com (2021) Prescription Drugs Information – interactions. www.drugs.com (accessed February 2022).

Garcia, P.J. (2010) Historical perspective of sexually transmitted infections. *International Journal of STD and AIDS*, **21**(4): 242–245.

Goldstein, L.H., Berlin, M., Tsuy, L. et al. (2009) The safety of macrolides during lactation. *Breastfeeding Medicine*, **4**: 197–200.

Gottlieb, S., Low, N., Newman, L. et al. (2014) Towards global prevention of sexually transmitted infections: the need for STI vaccines. *Vaccine*, **32**(14): 1527–1535.

Hamlyn, E., Barber, T.J. (2018) Management of HIV in pregnancy. *Obstetrics, Gynaecology and Reproductive Medicine*, **28**(7): 203–207.

Henao-Martinez, A.F., Johnson, S.E. (2014) Diagnostic tests for syphilis: new tests and new algorithms. *Neurology Clinical Practice*, **4**: 114–122.

Howe, B., Foster, K., Waldram, A. (2018) Challenges in the management of syphilis in pregnancy: completing a multi-centre audit cycle with mixed outcomes. *International Journal of STDs and AIDS*, **29**(4): 418–420.

Hu, X., Wang, L., Xu, F. (2019) Guides concerning tenofovir exposure via breastfeeding: a comparison of drug dosages by developmental stage. *International Journal of Infectious Diseases*, **87**: 8–12.

Hughes, G., Field, N. (2018) The epidemiology of sexually transmitted infections in the UK: impact of behavior, services and interventions. *Future Microbiology*, **10**(1): 35–51.

Janson-Cohen, B. (ed.) (2020) *The Human Body in Health and Disease*, 11th edn. Lippincott Williams & Wilkins: London.

Jo's Cervical Cancer Trust (2019) Having the HPV vaccine in school. www.jostrust.org.uk/information/hpv-vaccine/school (accessed February 2022).

Kausar, S., Said, K., Ishaq, M. et al. (2021) A review: mechanisms of action in antiviral drugs. *Interational Journal of Immunopathology and Pharmacology*, **35**: 20587384211002621.

Kirmusaoglu, S., Gareayaghi, N., Kocazeybek, B. (2019) The action mechanisms of antibiotics and antibiotic resistance. In: *Antimicrobials, Antibiotic Resistance, Antibiofilm Strategies and Activity Methods*. InTechOpen: London.

347

Krivochenitser, R., Jones, J.S. ,Whalen, D. et al. (2013) Underrecognition of Neisseria, gonorrhoea and chlamydia infections in pregnant patients. *Emergency Medicine*, **31**: 661–663.

Lallemand, A., Bremer, V., Jansen, K. et al. (2016) Prevalence of Chlamydia trachomatis infection in women, heterosexual men and MSM visiting HIV counselling institutions. *BMC Infectious Diseases*, **16**(1): 610.

Land, J., VanBergen, J., Posma, M., Morve, S. (2019) Epidemiology of Chlamydia trachomatis infection in women and the cost-effectiveness of screening. *Human Reproductive Update*, **16**(2): 198–204.

Lim, M.S., Collier, J.L., Guy, R. (2012) Correlates of Chlamydia trachomatis infections in a primary care sentinel surveillance network. *Sexual Health*, **9**(3): 247–253.

Low, N., Broutet, N., Turner, R. (2017) A collection on the prevention, diagnosis and treatment of STIs. *PLoS Medicine*, **14**(6): e1002333.

Medicines and Healthcare products Regulatory Commission on Human Medicines (2020) *Erythromycin: update on known risk of infantile hypertrophic pyloric stenosis*. Department of Health: London.

Miguel, F. (2018) *Protozoan Parasitism*. Cambridge University Press: Cambridge

National Institute for Health and Care Excellence (2009) *Guidelines on the Management of Uncomplicated Genital Chlamydia*. NICE: London.

National Institute for Health and Care Excellence (2019) *Guidelines on Sexual Health*. QS178. NICE: London.

Nursing and Midwifery Council (2018) *Standards of Proficiency for Registered Nurses*. NMC: London.

Nursing and Midwifery Council (2019) *Standards of Proficiency for Midwives*. NMC: London.

Pan, Y., Jia, Z., Wang, Y. et al. (2020) The role of caesarean section and non-breastfeeding in preventing mother to child transmission of Hep B. *Journal of Viral Hepatitis*, **27**(10): 1032–1043.

Peters, H., Thorne, C., Tookey, P.A. (2018) National audit of perinatal HIV infections in the UK, 2006–2013: what lessons can be learnt? *HIV Medicine*, **19**(4): 280–289.

Public Health England (2013) *Public Health Outcomes Framework for England*. Department of Health: London.

Public Health England (2015) Antenatal screening for infectious diseases in England: summary report for 2014. https://assets.publishing.service.gov.uk/government/uploads/system/uploads/attachment_data/file/482642/hpr4315_ntntlscrng.pdf (accessed February 2022).

Public Health England (2018) *Antenatal Screening Standards*. Department of Health: London.

Raffe, S., Curtis, H., Tookey, P. (2017) UK National Clinical Audit: management of pregnancies in women with HIV. *BMC Infectious Diseases*, **17**(1): 1–6.

Rice, A., Elwerdany, M., Hadoura, E. et al. (2016) Vaginal discharge. *Obstetric Gynaecology and Reproductive Medicine*, **26**(11): 317–323.

Rogstad, K., Ashby, J., Forsyth, S. et al. (2015) Sexually transmitted infections. *Sexual Health*, **15**(5): 447–451.

Royal College of Nursing (2020) *Human Papilloma Virus, Cancer Screening and Cervical Cancer*. RCN: London.

Thwaites, A., Iveson, H., Datta, S. et al. (2016) Non-HIV sexually transmitted infections in pregnancy. *Obstetrics, Gynaecology and Reproductive Medicine*, **26**(9): 253–258.

Townsend, C.L., Francis, K., Peckham, C.S., Tookey, P.A. (2017) Syphilis screening in pregnancy in the United Kingdom, 2010–2011: a national surveillance study. *British Journal of Obstetrics and Gynaecology*, **124**(1): 79–86.

Vallely, L., Egli-Gany, D., Wand, H. et al. (2021) Adverse pregnancy and neonatal outcomes associated with N gonorrhoeae: systematic review and meta-analysis. *Sexually Transmitted Infections*, **97**(2): 104–111.

Wood, H., Gudka, S. (2018) Pharmacist-led screening in sexually transmitted infections: current perspectives. *Integrated Pharmacy Research & Practice*, **7**: 67–82.

World Health Organization (2014) *Vaccines. WHO position paper*. www.who.int/wer/2014/wer8943pdf?ua=1 (accessed February 2022).

World Health Organisation (2016). *Guidelines for the treatment of Treponema Palladium Syphilis*. Geneva: WHO.

World Health Organization (2017) Sexual and reproductive health. http://who.int/reproductivehealth/topics/rtis/en/ (accessed February 2022).

World Health Organization (2019) Hepatitis B key facts. www.who.int/news-room/fact-sheets/detail/hepatitis-b (accessed February 2022).

Zar, H. (2005) Neonatal chlamydial infections: prevention and treatment. *Paediatric Drugs*, **7**(2): 103–110.

Further reading

Faculty of Reproductive and Sexual Health (FRSH): www.fsrh.org/home/

NHS Inform (2021) Sex and sexual health in pregnancy. www.nhsinform.scot/ready-steady-baby/pregnancy/relationships-and-wellbeing-in-pregnancy/sex-and-sexual-health-in-pregnancy

Royal College of Midwives (2017) Stepping Up to Public Health: A New Maternity Model for Women and Families, Midwives and Maternity Support Workers.www.rcm.org.uk/media/3165/stepping-up-to-public-health.pdf

Royal College of Paediatrics and Child health (n.d.) Sexual Health.www.what0-18.nhs.uk/pregnant-women/staying-healthy-pregnancy/sexual-health

Chapter 22

Medications and recreational drug use

Laura Abbott and Karen Mills

University of Hertfordshire, Hatfield, UK

Aim

The aim of this chapter is to engage the reader in knowledge, practice, analysis and understanding of recreational drug use and the child-bearing woman.

Learning outcomes

By the end of this chapter, the reader will:
- Have a good understanding of illegal substances commonly accessed, their effects and psychosocial impact
- Have a good understanding of risks associated with recreational drug use in pregnancy
- Understand the role of the midwife when supporting women who engage in recreational drug use
- Begin to examine the role which recreational drugs play in life and the impact using them can have on the dynamics of care.

Test your existing knowledge

- Why might a woman who is addicted to illegal drugs book late for midwifery care?
- What are the characteristics of stimulant drugs?
- What are the potential impacts upon a baby whose mother is addicted to cocaine?
- What are the symptoms of fetal alcohol syndrome?
- Can a woman who is taking methadone breast feed?

Introduction

Midwives support women through the watershed moments of pregnancy and childbirth. For women who use drugs or alcohol, this can be a time which reinforces stigma or which incentivises positive change. Starting by exploring the nature of drugs and drug use generally and in the lives

Fundamentals of Pharmacology for Midwives, First Edition. Edited by Ian Peate and Cathy Hamilton.
© 2022 John Wiley & Sons Ltd. Published 2022 by John Wiley & Sons Ltd.
Companion website: www.wiley.com/go/pharmacologyformidwives

of women, this chapter looks at the risks which these drugs present to women, their unborn children and the impact after birth.

The chapter explores risk in a wider context of complex personal and structural issues and the pharmacodynamic impact drug use can have. It challenges the reader to reflect on the place which drugs have in their own lives in order to provide holistic, woman-centred care for pregnant women who use drugs.

Role of midwives working with women who use drugs

It was estimated that 43 000 babies under 1 year of age in England are living with a parent who has used an illegal drug in the past year (NSPCC, 2013). Nevertheless, these figures do not reflect the true number as frequently substance misuse will not be revealed to health professionals. The Centre for Behavioural Health Statistics and Quality (2019) stated that 15.4% of women aged 18 years or older consumed illegal drugs in the past year. In pregnancy, polysubstance (individual use of at least three different forms of substances) (Connor et al., 2014; Biggar et al., 2017) use is common (Forray, 2016; Jarlenski et al., 2020). It is understood that women who misuse multiple substances may also experience psychiatric conditions alongside complex social issues and many are survivors of childhood trauma. All of these can have health consequences for both the mother and unborn baby.

The recent confidential enquiry into maternal deaths in the UK (MBRRACE-UK, 2017) found that two-thirds of the women who died had 'pre-existing physical or mental health problems'. This underlines the evidence that drug use is seldom the only issue in a woman's life and that the triangulation of drug risks with other factors (most often domestic violence and mental ill health) should not be discounted (Sidebotham et al., 2016).

The role of the midwife is to prioritise the woman's care and safety whilst distinguishing her individual needs (Nursing and Midwifery Council (NMC), 2018). Women who use drugs report that they experience increased anxiety due to the potential stigma of being addicted to illicit drugs and/or alcohol (Steele et al., 2020). Midwives must be mindful of this experience of shame and its impact. It is essential for midwives to behave in a non-judgemental manner in order to elicit a trusting relationship, especially as women are more likely to book late with maternity services and may be less likely to attend antenatal appointments if they are substance misusers (National Institute for Health and Care Excellence (NICE), 2010). In response to this complexity, the importance of multiagency working and integrated care from an educated, respectful and compassionate multiprofessional team has been endorsed to ensure optimal outcomes for mother and baby (Geraghty et al., 2019; Steele et al., 2020).

Drugs of misuse

Introduction

Under the Misuse of Drugs Act 1971 (MDA), illegal drugs in the UK are classified into three rankings – A, B and C. At first glance, drugs classified as Class A might be thought to cause the most harm. Possession, manufacture and dealing of drugs in this group are subject to the most stringent sanctions; often they are the substances which receive most negative press attention and users of these drugs suffer significant social stigma. However, it is important to explore this more fully. Drug classification is based in historical, social and political constructs, influenced by moral panics or popular discourse. Alcohol and tobacco, for example, are legal and socially acceptable, having been a part of the nation's culture for hundreds of years (House of Commons Health Committee, 2009). They remain a significant part of people's recreational life, with over 29 million people drinking each week and 6.9 million smoking (Office for National Statistics (ONS), 2017, 2020a) despite associated harms (7000+ alcohol-specific deaths and 77 600 associated with smoking) (ONS, 2019, 2020a).

In comparison, in 2019, 2160 drug poisoning deaths involved opiates. While this is an all-time high, the figure remains substantially lower than those for either alcohol or tobacco (Mahase, 2020;

ONS, 2020b). Illicit drug users may choose substances that are rapidly absorbed into the central nervous system with a short half-life (e.g. cocaine). Nutt et al. (2007) made an attempt to evaluate this scale of harms based on three conceptualisations: physical harm (physical damage or death), psychological harm (dependence, injury or psychological impairment) and social harm (whether personal, for example relationship breakdown, or societal, including economic harms and crime). Scaling drugs using these criteria delivered a scale of harm which looked somewhat different to the current legal classification. For example, while heroin remined high in the scale, it was superseded by alcohol which causes significant problems in all areas, despite being legal in the UK.

In addition, there are drugs which are not classified under the MDA. The early part of this century saw a proliferation of new psychoactive substances (NPS) (European Monitoring Centre for Drugs and Drug Addiction (EMCDDA), 2021b). Initially marketed as legal alternatives to cannabis, ecstasy or cocaine, these 'legal highs' proliferated and manufacturers changed compounds very frequently in order to evade law enforcement (Corazza and Roman-Urrestarazu, 2017). The government ultimately opted for a blanket ban, passing the Psychoactive Substances Act in 2016. This kind of prohibition can be seen as just as problematic as the staged approach of the MDA (Reuter and Pardo, 2017); it is not connected to the harms caused and a definition of what is actually 'psychoactive' is fractured terrain. It is fair to say, however, that no other government has found a better alternative to the issue.

These attempts remind us that in working with women, it is important to assess the impact and effect of drugs themselves and respond to individual circumstances rather than make global judgements based on flawed classification systems.

As a starting point, Table 22.1 outlines some of the main drugs classified under the MDA/Psychoactive Substances Act together with details of their effects.

New psychoactive substances controlled under the Psychoactive Substances Act (2016)

Drugs containing chemicals which produce similar effects to cannabis, cocaine or ecstasy. These drugs have widely different effects and strengths. Table 22.2 depicts legal drugs and NPS (Mind, 2021).

Impact of drugs on the body

An alternative way of categorising drug use, not related to harm or society's views, is by considering their impact on the body. This can be useful as it can help to develop an insight and can potentially generate a discussion which is freer from judgement, using as a starting point a consideration of the effect which a person is seeking, and why.

Stimulants

As the name suggests, stimulants speed up the metabolism. In doing so, they can make a person feel energised, physically active and quick-thinking. Along with this can come an experience of greater confidence, sometimes bordering on euphoria. A person taking stimulants may be talkative and outgoing. Examples are:

- amphetamines
- cocaine
- ecstasy
- mephedrone.

Sedatives/depressants

Depressant drugs serve to depress key parts of the central nervous system and can result in feelings of relaxation, happiness and freedom from anxiety and emotional or physical pain. Examples include:

- alcohol
- heroin/opiates/opioids
- benzodiazepines
- GHB/GBL.

Table 22.1   Main drugs classified under the MDA/Psychoactive Substances Act.[a]

Class	Drug and some common names	Appearance	Effects
Class A	Crack cocaine Cocaine Freebase (C, Coke, Charlie, White, Snow, Sniff, Stones, White Lady)	Cocaine is a white powder. Crack looks like small rocks. Freebase appears crystallised	Happy, excited, confident and powerful. Also raised heart rate, temperature; anxiety and paranoia
	Ecstasy (MDMA) (E, Beans, Dolphins, Pills)	Swallowed as a tablet – may be many different colours	High energy, happiness, followed by calmness. Jaw stiffness, anxiety, potential for overheating and excessive thirst
	Heroin (Smack, Junk, H, Brown, Gear, Skag) NB: Also synthetic opioids such as fentanyl/carfentanyl	Grey, white or brown powder Synthetic opioids as white powder, patches or pills	Drowsiness, amnesia, physical pain relief
	LSD (Acid, Blotter, Dots, Liquid Acid, Microdots, Tabs, Trips)	Small squares of paper are ingested, often with animation designs/ pictures on them. Also, a liquid or pellets	Hallucinations, increased awareness. May change the way someone hears or sees. Euphoria, excitement. A bad experience ('trip') can cause immense fear, suspicion or anxiety
	Magic mushrooms (Liberties, Mushies, Magics, Shrooms)	Small mushrooms, tan in colour. Fly agarics look like red and white spotted toadstools. Usually only available during the autumn months. They are ingested (cooked or raw) and can be smoked or made into a tea	Hallucinations. Giggly, excited or confused. Possibly anxious/paranoid, distorted sound/vision
	Methadone (Linctus, Mixture)	Green liquid. Occasionally tablets	Reduced pain. Relaxation and warmth
Class B	Amphetamines (Speed, Billy, Whizz, Phet)	Off-white or pinkish powder. Sometimes like crystals. Also, as a white/grey paste, damp and gritty	Feel energised and excited. It is an appetite suppressant, therefore may be used for weight loss
	Barbiturates (Barbs, Barbies, Blue Bullets, Blue Devils, Gorillas, Nembies, Pink Ladies, Red Devils, Sleepers)		

(Continued)

Table 22.1 (Continued)

Class	Drug and some common names	Appearance	Effects
	Cannabis (Marijuana, Dope, Weed, Skunk, Grass, Hash, Pot, Sensimilia, Ganga, Zoot, Spliff, Green) NB: See also synthetic cannabinoids below	Strong-smelling dry herb or hard, crumbly resin	Relaxation, chattiness, giggly. Also lethargy, paranoia and forgetfulness
	Codeine (Co-codamol, cough syrup, Nurofen Plus/Max)	Small white tablets; also a syrup	Relaxation, drowsiness. Also, confusion, nausea, itchiness, constipation
	Ketamine (Green, K, Special K, Super K)	White/brown powder. When used as a medicine, a clear liquid. Occasionally tablets	Altered perception, relaxation, euphoria, hallucinations. Can cause loss of consciousness and numbness, loss of the ability to move
	Mephedrone (Meow Meow, M-Cat, Drone, Bubbles, Bounce)	Fine white/off-white/yellow powder	Described as a cross between ecstasy, speed and cocaine. Euphoria, vigilance and feelings of affection. Can cause anxiety and paranoia
	Methamphetamine (Crystal Meth, Glass, Ice, Tina and Christine, Yaba)	Tablets, powder or crystals	Elated and wide awake and aroused. Also, paranoid, confused, belligerent
	Methylphenidate (Ritalin®)	White/off-white powder, crystals or tablets	Awake and excited, appetite suppressant. Also agitated and aggressive
Class C	Anabolic steroids	Tablets or liquid	Builds muscle mass, faster recovery when exercising. Also, paranoia, irritability, mood swings and violence
	Benzodiazepines (Benzos, Blues, Diazepam, Valium®, Vallies)	Tablets, capsules in a wide variety of colours. Also, as injections	Sleepy, relaxed and calm. Possibly confused and disorientated
	Gamma-hydroxybutyrate (GHB) Gamma-butyrolactone (GBL)	Colourless liquid. (Rarely) as capsules or powders	Euphoria, insomnia and reduced inhibitions. Dangerous when taken with alcohol
	Khat (Qat, Quat, Chat)	The leaves of the green plant are chewed and ingested	Appetite suppressant; energetic and talkative. Also, insomnia. Can cause high blood pressure
	Piperazines (BZP)	Pills in a variety of shapes and colours, sometimes with an impression (fly, crown, heart). Also as an off-white powder and a liquid	Euphoria, high energy, sleeplessness, loss of appetite. Similar to ecstasy but not as potent, dose for dose

353

[a] Drugs are constantly changing. The production of synthetics especially is in constant flux; new drugs emerge and street names evolve. This table is a guide, to be used in conjunction with contemporary detail.

Table 22.2   New psychoactive substances and legal drugs.

Class	Drug and some common names	Appearance	Effects
New psychoactive substances (NPS)	Synthetic cannabinoids (Amsterdam Gold, Black Mamba, Clockwork Orange Spice) NB: Some synthetic cannabinoids have been legal in the past. Some contain drugs which are illegal under the MDA. These are Class B. Black Mamba would be an example of a mixture of this type	Solids or oils added to plant matter to look somewhat like cannabis	Feelings of euphoria and relaxation, drowsiness. Hallucinations are more common than with natural cannabis. Can cause anxiety and paranoia
	Volatile substances (solvents)	Many are normal household products. Can include aerosols containing hairspray, deodorants, air fresheners, dry cleaning fluid, butane gas, nail varnish removers and/or glue	Dizziness, light-headed, feeling like being drunk. Can cause fainting, nausea and vomiting
Legal drugs	Alcohol (Bevvy, Booze)	Wide range of drinks with different tastes, colours and smells. Wide variety of strengths	Reduced anxiety/inhibition. Increased sociability, sex drive, risk taking and aggression. Slurred speech, lack of co-ordination, memory loss
	Poppers (Amyls, Liquid Gold, TNT) NB: Poppers are regulated under the Medicines Act 1968, legal to sell but not for human consumption	Liquid sold in small bottles. Strong solvent smell	Head rush, euphoria, increased sex drive. Also, sick or faint with headache or chest pain
	Tobacco (Baccy, Ciggies, Roll-Ups, Smokes)	Leaves dried and cut to a flaky mixture	Raised heart rate. Users report relaxation and reduced experience of stress

Source: Based on Mind (2021).

Hallucinogenic drugs

Hallucinogenic or psychedelic drugs alter perceptions and can induce feelings of detachment from daily life, sometimes a sense of being enlightened, with accompanying euphoria. They can cause hallucinations (seeing and/or hearing things that aren't there). Examples of hallucinogenic drugs are:

- ketamine
- LSD
- magic mushrooms.

It should be noted that not all drugs are easily compartmentalised. Cannabis, for example, has effects which cross over between these labels.

Absorption, distribution, metabolism and excretion (ADME) of drugs

The main way in which all drugs are metabolised is via the liver, although other organs (e.g. intestines, lung, kidney) also support the metabolisation of drugs (McLeod and He, 2020). The absorption of a drug occurs from the area where it was administered (e.g. injection, inhalation) and it is distributed throughout the body (e.g. circulation to major organs). Excretion (removal of drugs from the body through urine, sweat, bile, saliva, milk) occurs mainly via the kidney and liver (McLeod and He, 2020). These principles are applied to both legal and illegal substances.

Cocaine is usually snorted via the nose and is well absorbed via mucous membranes, intranasally. Peak concentrations occur within 60 minutes after intranasal administration and cocaine has a shorter half-life than amphetamines, with blood levels dropping rapidly, usually within an hour (Isenschmid, 2020). Alcohol ingested orally is metabolised by absorption, distribution and elimination through the liver and excreted through the breath, sweat and urine. When smoking tobacco, nicotine reaches its peak blood level concentration within 5 minutes and the majority of it will also be metabolised via the liver, together with the lung membranes, brain and kidneys. Alsherbiny and Li (2019) report that when smoking marijuana, metabolism occurs via the liver and the concentrations in blood plasma reduce quickly as the drug is distributed into the tissues. Rook et al. (2009) described the effect of heroin taken intravenously as being a sensation of a warm rush, with a sense of euphoria and numbness. The metabolism of heroin occurs in the central nervous system via the blood circulation and tissues (Huecker et al., 2017).

Understanding the role drugs play in the lives of women

Another key factor in working holistically with women who use drugs is a consideration of the role which drugs play in a person's life. Becker coined the idea of a drug-using 'career' as early as 1963 (Becker, 2008). In this model, people move through stages in their patterns of drug use, influenced by context, peers and ultimately the action of the drug physically and psychologically. A first introduction to alcohol or drugs (whether legal or illegal) might be described as 'experimental'. Most commonly associated with young people, experimental users are often introduced to drugs by peers or partners. People are drawn by curiosity, fashion or reputation. In this stage, drug use might be relatively short term, perhaps only a single episode of use. There is no pattern of use, and while this means that intervention models are of limited use, the risks are related to medical complications or infections.

For a variety of reasons, however, a large number of drug and alcohol users move to the next stage and become 'recreational' drug users. According to Rassool (2017), the most common recreational drugs are alcohol, caffeine, nicotine, cannabis, LSD and ecstasy. The inclusion of these first three, and the word 'recreation' itself, indicate how prevalent this type of use is and remind us that although drug use is stigmatised and drug users 'othered' in the popular imagination (Johnson et al., 2004), it is a feature in the lives of most people. Recreational use is social, pleasurable and relaxing. Recreational users come from all sections of society and users weigh the benefits of that pleasure against the health and legal risks of their drug use (Parker et al., 1998). Many such users are healthcare professionals working with and advising women (Watson et al., 2006) and this personal experience of drug and alcohol use seems to affect risk screening as well as the nature and style of advice provided to women (Olusanya and Barry, 2020).

Some drug users progress to a level of use which might be described as 'problematic'. The EMCDDA (2021a) defines problem drug use as 'injecting drug use or long duration or regular use of opioids, cocaine and/or amphetamines'. Nutt combines physical, social and dependence-related harms to recommend a re-examination of drug classification laws (Nutt et al., 2007), while the popular press associate harm with Class A drugs, often in association with crime (UKDPC, 2010). These definitions focus on macro responses and consider drugs as a socio-economic issue. As such, they are less helpful to midwives seeking to engage women. Problems might include issues of employment or relationships; drug use might have an impact on a woman's wider health or might lead to criminality or

Episode of care

In what way do your views affect the conversations you have with women? Consider the following scenario.

Sheila is a community midwife working in an area of high poverty and disadvantage. She runs a weekly clinic from a GP surgery. One woman has not attended for the last three booked appointments. This is 19-year-old Chanel, a primigravida who is 27 weeks pregnant. Chanel was placed into foster care from the age of 4 because of domestic violence and neglect in the home she shared with her biological mother and stepfather. Sheila is concerned about the well-being of Chanel and visits her at the home she shares with her boyfriend's family. Chanel tells Sheila that she does not like going to the GP surgery because she feels like 'everyone is looking' at her. Chanel confides in Sheila that she takes marijuana and ecstasy on occasions. Chanel is measuring small for gestational age and is worried about her unborn baby being removed from her care at birth.

- What approach should Sheila take when communicating with Chanel?
- What services should Sheila work with to support Chanel in the best way?
- What impact does marijuana have on the fetus?
- What impact does ecstasy have on the fetus?
- What do reports suggest about women who attend for antenatal care late in their pregnancy?
- Would you consider that Chanel needs a referral to the child protection team and/or social services?
- How do you feel when you consider a pregnant woman who takes illegal drugs?
- What impact do you think the sensation of shame and stigma has upon the likelihood of a woman engaging with the multidisciplinary team, especially if she is a survivor of childhood trauma?

Table 22.3   Selected drugs – effect on the fetus.

Drug	Impact
Alcohol	- Increased risk of miscarriage, fetal alcohol syndrome
Tobacco	- Risk of stillbirth - Placental abruption/placenta praevia - Premature labour - Low birthweight (Crume, 2019)
Cocaine	- Miscarriage/stillbirth - Premature labour due to increased blood pressure/tachycardia - Placental abruption - Withdrawal once born/seizures
Ecstasy (MDMA)	- Possible risk of premature birth
Opioids	- Miscarriage - Preterm labour - Reduced birthweight
Cannabinoids	- Possible low birthweight - Possible sudden infant death syndrome (SIDS) NB: Both of these may be due to cannabis use in conjunction with tobacco
Benzodiazepines	- Association with social issues, and consequently low birthweight and premature birth.

problems with the law. Delap (2021) suggests that there are some 'types of traumatic events, and some ways of experiencing them that can lead to a person's increased likelihood of suffering from ill health, being affected adversely by social factors and choosing harmful behaviours throughout their life'. Underpinning all of these might be issues due to adverse childhood experiences (ACES) of trauma, past or current, for which drug use is often a self-prescribed medication. ACES response to childhood trauma suggests that addiction is not the primary problem but rather an attempt to solve problems of deep emotional pain (Maté, 2018). Working in a woman-centred way, it might be more profitable to consider the problems which drug use causes in individuals' lives.

In pregnant women or those who are breast feeding, the demarcation between recreational and problematic use becomes blurred as the health risks to the fetus and infant potentially supersede the unfettered choices of women. Such risks are not inconsiderable and the impact on the fetus of a number of drugs can be seen in Table 22.3.

Drug use, pregnancy and risks

Drugs used in pregnancy can affect the health of the woman as well as causing complications in her pregnancy and affecting the fetus. In considering risk issues and so offering appropriate advice to women, the first step must be to have a secure knowledge base. Table 22.4 shows a number of the drugs discussed so far, with links to the impact they have on the fetus. These effects are most

Table 22.4   Drugs and their effects on the fetus.

Drug	Impact
Tobacco	• Low birthweight • Respiratory problems • Increased risk of SIDS (Andrade et al., 2020; Crume, 2019)
Alcohol	• Learning difficulties • Behavioural problems • Fetal alcohol syndrome (FAS) (McQuire et al., 2020) Symptoms include: • poor growth • distinct facial features • learning and behavioural problems
Cocaine	• Growth restriction • Risk of baby withdrawal once born/seizures • Microcephaly • Higher risk of necrotising enterocolitis, with rather late onset of disease – Cardiovascular anomalies
Ecstasy (MDMA)	• Possibly birth defects • Mental and motor development may be decreased in babies up to 12 months–2 years old (Singer et al., 2012; 2016; Smets, 2020)
Opioids	• Neonatal abstinence syndrome (NAS) • Increased risk of SIDS (Smets, 2020)
Cannabinoids	• Cognitive disorders in children from 3 years • Behavioural problems in children • Potential for future psychiatric conditions and depressive disorders • Some suggestions of potential for acute non-lymphoblastic leukaemia in child (Smet, 2020)
Benzodiazepines	• Withdrawal symptoms (e.g. seizures) • Unable to regulate temperature • Respiratory problems

likely where drug use is heavy and problematic. More moderate use during pregnancy may not lead to these problems and as can be seen, there are some drugs where complications are few or are associated with factors other than the illegal drug consumed. Indeed, suddenly stopping use of heroin or other opiate drugs during pregnancy can be dangerous to the fetus and it may be safer for the woman to delay withdrawal until after the birth.

Impact of drugs post birth

Low birthweight (babies of smokers are, on average, 200 g lighter than expected) is implicated in use of a number of drugs and the complications which result from this (difficulty in keeping warm or increased risk of infection) are complicated by the withdrawal syndrome which a baby might experience.

Use of some drugs is associated with a withdrawal syndrome in the baby after birth (opiates, benzodiazepines, nicotine and alcohol). Withdrawal from opiates or benzodiazepines may need pharmacological intervention and in the case of opiates, this may be by methadone treatment.

An initial dose of methadone for treatment of neonatal withdrawal is 0.1–0.2 mg/kg/day and a maximum dose is 1 mg/kg/day, indicating that a breast-fed infant of a mother receiving 90 mg/day of methadone is exposed to the medicine at a dose ranging from 15–45% of the low end of the typical starting dose of methadone (Table 22.5).

Breast feeding and drug use

According to recent evidence-based research, women who take methadone who wish to breast feed their baby should be supported to do so (Hicks et al., 2018; Tsai and Doan, 2016; Doerzbacher and Chang, 2019; Yonke et al., 2020). Evidence suggests that babies born to mothers who are dependent on methadone are at increased risk of neonatal abstinence syndrome (NAS) but if women breast feed, their babies are less likely to require treatment (Wu and Carre, 2018). It is suggested that the dose of methadone administered to breast-feeding women should be kept low and taken post breast feed (Clark, 2019). However, caution should be exercised if a woman wishes to cease breast feeding in case the baby experiences withdrawal symptoms (Lembeck et al., 2020).

Breast feeding while using some other drugs is not advised. Moderate alcohol use in breast-feeding women is relatively common (Greiner, 2019), along with the misconception that if a woman expresses her breast milk following alcohol consumption, alcoholic content in the bloodstream will be reduced (Pham et al., 2020). This is not the case and Pham et al. (2020) recommended that women refrain from drinking alcohol whilst breast feeding.

Table 22.5   Doses of methadone for treatment of opiate withdrawal.

Dose	Route	Mechanism of action	Side-effects
Initially 10–30 mg daily, increased in steps of 5–10 mg daily if required until no signs of withdrawal nor evidence of intoxication Dose to be increased in the first week, then increased every few days as necessary up to usual dose, maximum weekly dose increase of 30 mg; usual dose 60–120 mg daily	By mouth using oral solution	An opiate agonist interacting primarily with the mu receptor to suppress opiate withdrawal, cravings and the reinforcing effects of opioids	Suppression of cough reflex, respiratory depression, drowsiness, change in mood, euphoria, dysphoria, mental blurring, nausea and vomiting, excessive sweating, reduced creation of saliva, dry mouth, gum disease, tooth decay

Source: Based on Tran et al. (2017).

Many women cease smoking tobacco during pregnancy, only to relapse postpartum (Crume, 2019). However, the composition of breast milk in women who smoke would seem to be altered, being lower in calories, lipids and proteins (Macchi et al., 2021). Pham et al. (2020) found that milk volume was reduced for women who smoke, which may have implications for those substances that are inhaled due to reduction in prolactin. Bartu et al. (2009) found that amphetamines passed into breast milk following recreational use and suggested that breast feeding should be withheld for at least 48 hours after recreational amphetamine use.

Risks from drug use extend throughout pregnancy and childhood. As has been seen elsewhere in this chapter, however, all these risk associations are far stronger where there is a cluster of risk factors, including violence or poor mental health and/or structural factors such as poverty and housing. For example, poverty increases the risk of stillbirth or subsequent death in childhood and is associated with premature labour, low birthweight and SIDS. These are exacerbated by poor housing and this in turn causes stress. In this context, co-existing drug use might be viewed as both an aggravating risk factor and a response to that stress. Working through the COVID-19 pandemic, it is important to be aware of the amplification of these issues and Kar et al. (2021) point out the increased anxiety and depression which pregnant women face with alcohol and drug use as a coping mechanism.

Traditional, patriarchal perspectives on pregnancy and childbirth view women during pregnancy as the vehicle for the unborn child (O'Brien, 1981). Though a fetus is not recognised in law as a legal 'person' until birth (Birthrights, 2021), the state can and does intervene in the lives of women whose behaviour towards that fetus might be seen as reckless, and preparations for care proceedings are not infrequently undertaken by social workers (Lushey et al., 2018). Ettorre (2004) comments power-fully on this in relation to drug-using women, stating that unlike 'normal' women, their bodies are viewed *as* 'lethal foetal containers'. It is a phrase which underlines the stigma which drug-using women face in perinatal care.

Nixon (2010) considers whether legal change is required, to amend the status of the unborn child. Doing so might resolve issues legally but does not help midwives in the field as they try to engage women in a process of harm minimisation and personal change (Mills, 2021). When working with women, the issues are not solely pharmacological. Drug use in pregnancy can be such an emotive issue that it clouds other factors such as poverty and deprivation. But the stigma associated with drug use, and the primacy given to what may, in fact, be a presenting problem can act to drive the most vulnerable women away from services (Mills, 2021).

Anyone working in this field must balance risky behaviours with the rights of the woman and factor in the need to be gender sensitive, trauma informed, engaged and non-judgemental. The full complexity of a woman's situation, including structural factors, must be considered. Negotiating this leads to practical and ethical considerations which are best addressed in the context of the relationship between the woman and her midwife.

Hooks (2019) found that compassion from student midwives improved following education about substance misuse and Geraghty et al. (2019) suggest that education does influence the atti-tudes of midwives towards pregnant addicts. Pezaro et al. (2020) undertook a systematic review and found that midwives were likely to partake in harmful alcohol consumption often in relation to long working hours. Some student midwives were more likely to smoke tobacco or cannabis alongside drinking alcohol as a form of escapism. The impact of health professionals as substance misusers meant that there was potential for associated medical errors and stress leading to suicidal ideation and self-harm along with disinclination to pursue support for themselves. Even at a recreational level, using drugs can have an impact on the style and type of advice which women receive (Watson et al., 2006) as midwives' psychological response to their own drug use affects the dynamics of their professional relationships (Olusanya and Barry, 2020).

Conclusion

This chapter has explored issues in relation to illegal substances to engage the reader in knowledge, practice, analysis and understanding of drug use and the perinatal woman. The chapter has enhanced understanding of the illegal substances commonly accessed and their effects and considered how multiagency working can ensure the best outcomes for mother and baby. The role of the midwife has been considered when supporting women who engage in recreational drug use. The complexity of women's lives has been discussed as well as the dynamics of relationship building. Empathy has been highlighted in understanding the lives of women, and attention has been drawn to the importance of personal reflection: understanding the role which drugs play in the lives of midwives themselves.

Glossary

Addiction   Habitual physiological need for and use of a habit-forming substance (such as heroin or nicotine)

Adverse childhood experiences (ACES)   Traumatic experience in a person's life happening before the age of 18 (e.g. bereavement, childhood sexual abuse)

Drug classification   Illicit drugs are classified by the effects they have on the user. There are four major types: depressants, stimulants, hallucinogens and narcotics

Fetal alcohol syndrome   A condition in a child that results from alcohol exposure during the mother's pregnancy and may cause brain damage and growth problems

Illegal drugs   Drugs forbidden by law

Neonatal abstinence syndrome (NAS)   Physical and developmental conditions caused when a baby withdraws from certain drugs that they were exposed to in utero. NAS is most often caused when a woman takes opioids during pregnancy

Novel psychoactive substances (NPS)   Designer drugs that evade legal categorisation guidelines

Substance misuse   The use of alcohol, illegal drugs or over-the-counter or prescription medications in an excessive or inappropriate manner

Test yourself

Now review your learning by completing the learning activities for this chapter at www.wiley.com/go/pharmacologyformidwives.

Find out more

The following is a list of common drugs. Take some time and think about how women you have cared for have shared their experiences of drug use with you. Consider the reasons why women may use drugs. Where do you think the person was in their drug-using 'career' (Becker, 2008)? Remember to include aspects of woman-centred care. If you are making notes about people you have offered care and support to, you must ensure that you have adhered to the rules of confidentiality. Also, consider your own drug use and the place which drugs have in your life. How does your experience of the positive/negative impact it has had in your life affect how you might discuss that drug with women?

The drug	Experiences people have shared with you	Your notes on your own experience
Alcohol		
Tobacco		
Caffeine		
Benzodiazepines		

The drug	Experiences people have shared with you	Your notes on your own experience
Heroin		
Cocaine		
Crack cocaine		
Amphetamines		
LSD		
Marijuana		
NPS		
Ecstasy		

References

Alsherbiny, M.A., Li, C.G. (2019) Medicinal cannabis – potential drug interactions. *Medicines*, **6**(1): 3.

Andrade, E.D.Q., Sena, C.R.D.S., Collison, A. et al. (2020) Association between active tobacco use during pregnancy and infant respiratory health: a systematic review and meta-analysis. *BMJ Open*, **10**(9): e037819.

Bartu, A., Dusci, L.J., Ilett, K.F. (2009) Transfer of methylamphetamine and amphetamine into breast milk following recreational use of methylamphetamine. *British Journal of Clinical Pharmacology*, **67**(4): 455–459.

Becker, H.S. (2008) *Outsiders*. Simon and Schuster: New York.

Biggar Jr, R.W., Forsyth, C.J., Chen, J., Burstein, K. (2017) The poly-drug user: examining associations between drugs used by adolescents. *Deviant Behavior*, **38**(10): 1186–1196.

Birthrights (2021) Human rights in maternity care. www.birthrights.org.uk/factsheets/human-rights-in-maternity-care/ (accessed February 2022).

Clark, R.R. (2019) Breastfeeding in women on opioid maintenance therapy: a review of policy and practice. *Journal of Midwifery & Women's Health*, **64**(5): 545–558.

Centre for Behavioral Health Statistics and Quality.(2019) Results from the 2016 National Survey on Drug Use and Health: Detailed Tables. www.samhsa.gov/data/sites/default/files/NSDUH-DetTabs-2016/NSDUH-DetTabs-2016.pdf (accessed February 2022).

Connor, J.P., Gullo, M.J., White, A., Kelly, A.B. (2014) Polysubstance use: diagnostic challenges, patterns of use and health. *Current Opinion in Psychiatry*, **27**(4): 269–275.

Corazza, O., Roman-Urrestarazu, A. (2017) *Novel Psychoactive Substances: Policy, Economics and Drug Regulation*. Springer International Publishing: Cham.

Crume, T. (2019) Tobacco use during pregnancy. *Clinical Obstetrics and Gynaecology*, **62**(1): 128–141.

Delap, N. (2021) Trauma-informed care of perinatal women. In: Abbott, L. (ed.) *Complex Social Issues and the Perinatal Woman*. Springer: Cham.

Doerzbacher, M., Chang, Y.P. (2019) Supporting breastfeeding for women on opioid maintenance therapy: a systematic review. *Journal of Perinatology*, **39**(9):1159–1164.

Ettorre, E. (2004) Revisioning women and drug use: gender sensitivity, embodiment and reducing harm. *International Journal of Drug Policy*, **15**(5-6): 327–335.

European Monitoring Centre for Drugs and Drug Addiction (2021a) Methods and Definitions. www.emcdda.europa.eu/stats07/PDU/methods (accessed February 2022).

European Monitoring Centre for Drugs and Drug Addiction (2021b) Risk assessment report on a new psychoactive substance: methyl 2-{[1-(4-fluorobutyl)-1H-indole-3-carbonyl]amino}-3,3-dimethylbutanoate (4F-MDMB-BICA) in accordance with Article 5c of Regulation (EC) No 1920/2006 (as amended). www.emcdda.europa.eu/publications/risk-assessments/4f-mdmb-bica_en (accessed February 2022).

Forray, A. (2016) Substance use during pregnancy. www.ncbi.nlm.nih.gov/pmc/articles/PMC4870985/ (accessed February 2022).

Geraghty, S., Doleman, G., De Leo, A. (2019) Midwives' attitudes towards pregnant women using substances: informing a care pathway. *Women and Birth*, **32**(4): e477–e482.

Greiner, T. (2019) Alcohol and breastfeeding, a review of the issues. *World Nutrition*, **10**(1): 63–88.

Hicks, J., Morse, E., Wyant, D.K. (2018) Barriers and facilitators of breastfeeding reported by postpartum women in methadone maintenance therapy. *Breastfeeding Medicine*, **13**(4): 259–265.

Hooks, C. (2019) Attitudes toward substance misusing pregnant women following a specialist education programme: an exploratory case study. *Midwifery*, **76**: 45–53.

House of Commons Health Committee (2009). *First Report – Alcohol*. Stationery Office: London.

Huecker, M.R., Koutsothanasis, G.A., Abbasy, M.S.U., Marraffa, J. (2017) *Heroin*. StatPearls: Treasure Island.

Isenschmid, D.S. (2020) Cocaine. In: Levine, B., Kerrigan, S. (eds) *Principles of Forensic Toxicology*, pp.371–387. Springer: Cham.

Jarlenski, M.P., Paul, N.C., Krans, E.E. (2020) Polysubstance use among pregnant women with opioid use disorder in the United States, 2007–2016. *Obstetrics and Gynecology*, **136**(3): 556–564.

Johnson, J.L., Bottorff, J.L., Browne, A.J., Grewal, S., Hilton, B.A., Clarke, H. (2004) Othering and being othered in the context of health care services. *Health Communication*, **16**(2): 255–271.

Kar, P., Tomfohr-Madsen, L., Giesbrecht, G., Bagshawe, M., Lebel, C. (2021) Alcohol and substance use in pregnancy during the COVID-19 pandemic. *Drug and Alcohol Dependence*, **225**: 108760.

Lembeck, A.L., Tuttle, D., Locke, R. et al. (2020) Breastfeeding and formula selection in neonatal abstinence syndrome. *American Journal of Perinatology*, **38**: 1488–1493.

Lushey, C.J., Barlow, J., Rayns, G., Ward, H. (2018) Assessing parental capacity when there are concerns about an unborn child: pre-birth assessment guidance and practice in England. *Child Abuse Review*, **27**(2): 97–107.

Macchi, M., Bambini, L., Franceschini, S., Alexa, I.D., Agostoni, C. (2021) The effect of tobacco smoking during pregnancy and breastfeeding on human milk composition – a systematic review. *European Journal of Clinical Nutrition*, **75**(5): 736–747.

Mahase, E. (2020) Drug deaths: England and Wales see highest number since records began. *BMJ*, **371**: m3988.

Maté, G. (2018) *In the Realm of Hungry Ghosts*. Penguin Random House: London.

McLeod, H.L., He, Y. (2020) Pharmacokinetics for the prescriber. *Medicine*, **48**(7): 433–438.

McQuire, C., Daniel, R., Hurt, L., Kemp, A., Paranjothy, S. (2020) The causal web of foetal alcohol spectrum disorders: a review and causal diagram. *European Child & Adolescent Psychiatry*, **29**(5): 575–594.

Mills, K. (2021) Balancing risk and need: substance misuse and perinatal women. In: Abbott, L. (ed.) *Complex Social Issues and the Perinatal Woman*. Springer: Cham.

Mind (2021) Recreational drugs and alcohol. www.mind.org.uk/information-support/types-of-mental-health-problems/drugs-recreational-drugs-alcohol/types-of-recreational-drug/ (accessed February 2022).

Mothers and Babies: Reducing Risk Through Audits and Confidential Enquiries Across the UK (MBRRACE-UK) (2017) www.npeu.ox.ac.uk/mbrrace-uk (accessed February 2022).

National Institute for Health and Care Excellence (2010) *Pregnancy and Complex Social Factors: A Model for Service Provision for Pregnant Women with Complex Social Factors*. NICE: London.

Nixon, D. (2010) Should UK law reconsider the initial threshold of legal personality? A critical analysis. *Human Reproduction & Genetic Ethics*, **16**(2): 182–217.

NSPCC (2013) *All Babies Count: Spotlight on Drugs and Alcohol*. NSPCC: London.

Nursing and Midwifery Council (2018) *The Code: Professional Standards of Practice and Behaviour for Nurses and Midwives*. NMC: London.

Nutt, D., King, L.A., Saulsbury, W., Blakemore, C. (2007) Development of a rational scale to assess the harm of drugs of potential misuse. *Lancet*, **369**(9566): 1047–1053.

O'Brien, M. (1981) *The Politics of Reproduction*. Routledge & Kegan Paul: New York.

Office for National Statistics (2017) *Adult Drinking Habits in Great Britain: 2017*. ONS: London.

Office for National Statistics (2019) *Alcohol-specific Deaths in the UK: Registered in 2019*. ONS: London.

Office for National Statistics (2020a) *Adult Smoking Habits in the UK: 2019*. ONS: London.

Office for National Statistics (2020b) *Deaths Related to Drug Poisoning in England and Wales: 2019 Registrations*. ONS: London.

Olusanya, O.A., Barry, A.E. (2020) Dissemination of prenatal drinking guidelines: a preliminary study examining personal alcohol use among midwives in a southwestern US state. *Journal of Midwifery & Women's Health*, **65**(5): 634–642.

Parker, H.J., Parker, H., Aldridge, J., Measham, F. (1998) *Illegal Leisure: The Normalization of Adolescent Recreational Drug Use*. Psychology Press: London.

Pezaro, S., Patterson, J., Moncrieff, G., Ghai, I. (2020) A systematic integrative review of the literature on midwives and student midwives engaged in problematic substance use. *Midwifery*, **89**: 102785.

Pham, Q., Patel, P., Baban, B., Yu, J., Bhatia, J. (2020) Factors affecting the composition of expressed fresh human Milk. *Breastfeeding Medicine*, **15**(9): 551–558.

Rassool, G.H. (2017) *Alcohol and Drug Misuse: A Guide for Health and Social Care Professionals*, 2nd edn. Routledge: London.

Reuter, P., Pardo, B. (2017) Can new psychoactive substances be regulated effectively? An assessment of the British Psychoactive Substances Bill. *Addiction*, **112**(1): 25–31.

Rook, E.J., Huitema, A.D., Ree, J.M.V., Beijnen, J.H. (2006P Pharmacokinetics and pharmacokinetic variability of heroin and its metabolites: review of the literature. *Current Clinical Pharmacology*, **1**(1): 109–118.

Sidebotham, P., Brandon, M., Bailey, S. et al. (2016) *Pathways to Harm, Pathways to Protection: A Triennial Analysis of Serious Case Reviews 2011 to 2014*. Department for Education: London.

Singer, L.T., Moore, D.G., Min, M.O. et al. (2012) One-year outcomes of prenatal exposure to MDMA and other recreational drugs. *Pediatrics*, **130**(3): 407–413.

Singer, L.T., Moore, D.G., Min, M.O. et al. (2016) Motor delays in MDMA (ecstasy) exposed infants persist to 2 years. *Neurotoxicology and Teratology*, **54**: 22–28.

Smets, K. (2020) Long term consequences of illicit drug use during pregnancy. *International Archives of Pediatrics & Neonatology*, **2**.

Steele, S., Osorio, R., Page, L.M. (2020) Substance misuse in pregnancy. *Obstetrics, Gynaecology & Reproductive Medicine*, **30**: 347–355.

Tran, T.H., Griffin, B.L., Stone, R.H., Vest, K.M., Todd, T.J. (2017) Methadone, buprenorphine, and naltrexone for the treatment of opioid use disorder in pregnant women. *Pharmacotherapy*, **37**(7): 824–839.

Tsai, L.C., Doan, T.J. (2016) Breastfeeding among mothers on opioid maintenance treatment: a literature review. *Journal of Human Lactation*, **32**(3): 521–529.

UK Drug Policy Commission (2010) *Representations of Drug Use and Drug Users in the British Press. A Content Analysis of Newspaper Coverage*. Loughborough Communications Research Centre: Loughborough.

Watson, H., Whyte, R., Schartau, E., Jamieson, E. (2006) Survey of student nurses and midwives: smoking and alcohol use. *British Journal of Nursing*, **15**(22): 1212–1216.

Wu, D., Carre, C. (2018) The impact of breastfeeding on health outcomes for infants diagnosed with neonatal abstinence syndrome: a review. *Cureus*, **10**(7): e3061.

Yonke, N., Jimenez, E.Y., Leeman, L., Leyva, Y., Ortega, A., Bakhireva, L.N. (2020) Breastfeeding motivators and barriers in women receiving medications for opioid use disorder. *Breastfeeding Medicine*, **15**(1): 17–23.

Further reading

Breastfeeding Network's Drugs in Breastmilk Service:

druginformation@breastfeedingnetwork.org.uk
www.drugs.gov.uk
www.drugscope.org.uk/
www.talktofrank.com/

Chapter 23

Medications used in emergency midwifery situations

Jayne E. Marshall

University of Leicester, Leicester, UK

Aim

The aim of the chapter is to provide the reader with an understanding of specific medications and their actions in emergency midwifery situations.

Learning outcomes

After reading this chapter, the reader should be able to:
- Understand the midwife's professional responsibilities in administering medicines in emergency situations
- Recognise the most common drugs used in maternity emergencies
- Understand the basic pharmacokinetics of drugs commonly used in maternity emergencies
- Recognise the drugs used during cardiopulmonary resuscitation.

It is not the purpose of this chapter to provide in-depth detail of specific emergencies the midwife may experience as these are well documented elsewhere, but to focus on the medicines used in such situations and their impact in childbirth.

Test your existing knowledge

- How would you define a maternity emergency?
- What are the midwife's professional responsibilities in relation to medicines administration in a maternity emergency?
- List the reversible causes of maternal collapse using the acronym *THE*.
- At what stage in the ABCDE process would resuscitative drugs be administered in a maternity emergency?
- In what circumstances would a perimortem caesarean section be undertaken?

Fundamentals of Pharmacology for Midwives, First Edition. Edited by Ian Peate and Cathy Hamilton.
© 2022 John Wiley & Sons Ltd. Published 2022 by John Wiley & Sons Ltd.
Companion website: www.wiley.com/go/pharmacologyformidwives

Principles of managing maternity emergencies

Midwifery practice is based on the understanding that the childbirth continuum is a physiological process for healthy women. However, it is acknowledged that complications and emergencies can occur during pregnancy and childbirth. Many women now present in pregnancy with complex co-morbidities. Midwives must therefore be familiar with and proficient in identifying early those women at risk of developing morbidity due to pregnancy and childbirth as well as managing emergencies when they arise in order to protect the well-being of child-bearing women and their babies. This includes understanding the role that specific medicines play in the management of maternal emergencies to improve health and save lives.

Midwives should be able to manage emergencies in all settings where birth takes place: this could be in the home, in a birthing unit/centre or in a hospital. Knight et al. (2020) endorse that when a woman collapses out of hospital, good communication should ensure senior review at admission and multidisciplinary involvement (obstetric, anaesthetic, critical care and neonatal specialists) to determine a prompt diagnosis and enable rapid appropriate treatment. However, where there are limited details of the epidemiology and management of the less common emergencies, such as amniotic fluid embolism, the UK Obstetric Surveillance System (UKOSS), which is a database of voluntary notifications, has been established to collect information to inform earlier diagnosis with the aim of leading to better outcomes.

Although with careful history taking and vigilant observation and screening, it is possible to prevent or mitigate certain emergencies, there will still be some instances where they present with little or no warning (Knight et al., 2020). The midwife should remain calm and aim to keep the woman and her partner fully informed in order to obtain her consent and co-operation for procedures and administration of any medicines that may be required (Nursing and Midwifery Council (NMC), 2018a). Abnormalities in maternal vital signs often precede deterioration in maternal condition. The purpose of using an obstetric modified early warning score chart is to detect a window of deterioration which can be reversed by treatment interventions ahead of catastrophic collapse. In pregnant women, this window may be very small (Knight et al., 2020; Chu et al., 2020).

The national maternity review (NHS England, 2016) and the independent review of maternity services (Ockenden 2022) highlight the importance of multiprofessional education and training in emergency situations to enhance safety in maternity care. Emergency skills training for midwifery and medical staff should facilitate the opportunity to practise and maintain skills in the management of maternity emergencies and provide an update on the signs and symptoms of critical illness in respect of midwifery, obstetric and non-obstetric causes. Effective communication between the multiprofessional team is essential to ensure that when a child-bearing woman suddenly becomes ill, the outcome for her and her baby is the best it possibly can be in the circumstances (Knight et al., 2020; Ockenden 2022).

Communication

Poor communication is what health and maternity services are often criticised for when the outcome is unexpected. NHS Improvement (2018) endorses that effective communication involves the sharing of accurate and precise information among healthcare professionals, particularly in emergency situations. The SBAR communication tool consists of standardised prompt questions about the condition of an individual in four stages: *Situation, Background, Assessment and Recommendations* (Haig et al., 2006). These prompts can assist the midwife to assertively and effectively share concise and focused information about a woman's condition, reducing repetition. The SBAR tool can be used in *all* clinical conversations such as in escalation of a situation, transferring care from one setting to another and in shift handover, on a face-to face basis, by telephone or through collaborative multiprofessional team meetings. An example of how the SBAR tool can be used in practice is shown in the Episode of care.

As Pillay and Smith (2019) explain, it may take some effort on the part of the healthcare professional to adapt their communication and be assertive when making recommendations, particularly to senior colleagues, if they are an inexperienced midwife/student midwife. Making recommendations is a vital stage of the SBAR process as it conveys the action that the *sender* requires from the

Episode of care

SBAR communication tool

Step	Action	Example
Situation	Describe the current situation, identifying the woman by name and the reason for your report/referral, your concerns and provide details of their vital signs	*This is midwife Emily Mann in triage. I have Priti Panasar with me who is booked for midwife-led care. She has a 3-day history of vomiting and is complaining of left leg pain, mainly in the buttock and posterior thigh. On admission her pulse was 110 bpm, blood pressure 120/90 mmHg, respiration rate 18 breaths/minute. Her temperature was 37.4 °C*
Background	State the reason for the woman's admission, explain any significant medical history and provide the woman's background including: · Diagnosis on admission · Date of admission · Prior procedures · Current medications · Any allergies · Significant laboratory results · Other diagnostic results of relevance gathered from observational records	*Priti is 14 weeks pregnant and was referred today by her community midwife to come to hospital. She has been unable to tolerate any food although she has had no diarrhoea. Her previous three pregnancies have also been complicated by vomiting. However, this is the first time she has experienced constant left iliac fossa pain that appears to worsen on climbing stairs. She is currently taking folic acid and states she has no known allergies*
Assessment	Summarise the facts and provide an assessment by critically considering the underlying cause for the woman's condition, having reviewed your findings and consolidating them with other objective indicators, such as laboratory results	*I have undertaken an antenatal examination and the fundus is just about palpable abdominally compatible with the gestational age. There is no vaginal bleeding. However, her left leg is very swollen from the foot to the groin, feels warm to the touch and is tender over the calf and shin, but there are no varicosities or cellulitis evident. From my observations, I believe Priti is showing signs of a DVT*
Recommendation	Explain what you need/recommend, being specific about your request *and* time-frame, making suggestions about the course of action and subsequent care. REPEAT your request/recommendation to ensure clarity and accuracy	*She needs urgent review by the obstetric team. In the meantime I have commenced a fluid balance chart. Do you wish me to obtain IV access and organise leg Doppler studies before anticoagulant therapy is commenced? When are you likely to get here to review Priti as she requires urgent review?*

recipient. Having a supportive preceptor or practice supervisor/lecturer to assist the midwife or student midwife respectively in practising using the tool to allay anxiety and develop personal confidence is a valuable strategy to consider (NHS Improvement, 2018).

The closed loop communication tool (Hargestam et al., 2013) is a further means of communication which can be used in emergency situations to ensure that any instructions are clearly conveyed so they are fully understood among team members and action is promptly taken. This is a three-stage process that is shown with an example in the following Episode of care.

Closed loop communication (Hargestam et al., 2013) also provides the opportunity for further clarification, particularly in respect of specific drug, dosage and route of administration, as shown in the example. As a consequence, it is an effective framework that midwives can use during clinical conversations that require *immediate* focus and action, including drug administration. Accuracy and quality of documentation as a communication tool to inform decisions, and to facilitate continuity of care, are professional requirements, being the mark of a skilled and safe health professional, reflecting the extent of their role and level of proficiency.

Episode of care

The closed loop communication tool

Step	Action	Example
One	The sender verbalises/calls out an observation or required action	*I would like 10 units of Syntocinon administered intramuscularly, immediately please*
Two	The receiver of the message acknowledges and accepts receipt of the message and repeats it back to the sender: *check-back*	*You require 10 units of Syntocinon administered intramuscularly, right now*
Three	The sender confirms that the message has been heard and understood correctly and in so doing, closes the loop.	*Yes, 10 units of Syntocinon, intramuscularly right now, thanks*

Professional responsibility in emergency situations

Section 18 of the Code (NMC, 2018a) defines the professional standards regarding advising on, prescribing, supplying, dispensing and administering medicines within the limits of a registrant's training and proficiency, the law, professional statutory regulatory body (PSRB) guidance and other relevant policies, guidance and regulations. NMC (2019) refers specifically to the midwife being proficient in the safe administration of medicines in emergency situations and is detailed in the Clinical consideration.

Clinical consideration

NMC Standards of Proficiency for Midwives

6.73 demonstrate the ability to collaborate effectively with interdisciplinary teams and work in partnership with the woman to assess and provide care and support when emergency situations or clinical complications arise that ensures the safe administration of medicines; this must include:

6.73.1. safe administration of medicines in an emergency
6.73.2. manage intravenous (IV) fluids including transfusion of blood and blood products
6.73.3. manage fluid and infusion pumps and devices.

The standards for nurse and midwife prescribing programmes in the UK (NMC, 2018b) have adopted the Royal Pharmaceutical Society's (RPS) *Competency Framework for all Prescribers* (RPS, 2016) as the foundation for registrants to undertake further study and receive a recordable qualification in nurse and midwife prescribing following completion of their respective initial pre-registration programmes. Nurse and midwife prescribers are professionally accountable for prescribing decisions, actions and omissions, and cannot delegate this accountability.

Increasing the midwife's scope of practice to prescribing ultimately enhances the quality of care that a woman receives and can reduce delays in administration. However, midwives must only prescribe from the formulary linked to their recorded qualification, comply with statutory requirements related to their prescribing practice, and only ever prescribe within their own level of experience and proficiency. The prescribing of medicines should always be in line with local and national guidelines and be evidence based, with the midwife prescriber remaining up to date with prescribing knowledge and skills. It is vital that all midwife prescribers are familiar with the range of medicines they can prescribe in accordance with the legal and PRSB requirements, e.g. complementary and alternative therapies, Controlled Drugs and midwives' exemptions.

Clinical consideration

When in an emergency situation, it is usual for a second midwife or a student midwife to act as a scribe to ensure that consistent, complete, clear, accurate, secure and timely records are maintained to ensure an account of *all* care given, including the administration of medicines, is available for review by all professionals involved in the care and by the woman.

The detail of each drug should include:

- name of drug
- dose administered
- route of administration
- name of practitioner administering the drug
- time of administration
- effect of the drug (if any)

Maternal collapse

Maternal collapse is defined as an acute event involving the cardiorespiratory system and/or central nervous system, resulting in a reduced or absent conscious level (and potentially cardiac arrest and death), at any stage in pregnancy and up to 6 weeks after birth. Knight et al. (2020) recommend that any woman of reproductive age who presents in the community in a state of shock and/or collapse with no obvious cause should be transferred urgently to a hospital emergency department without delay for rapid assessment, diagnosis and treatment.

Maternal collapse is a rare but life-threatening event, with a wide-ranging aetiology. The outcome, primarily for the mother but also for the fetus, depends on prompt and effective resuscitation. Importantly, if maternal collapse which is not as the result of cardiac arrest is not treated effectively, maternal cardiac arrest can then occur. Reversible causes of maternal collapse are shown in Figure 23.1 and Table 23.1 (Chu et al., 2020).

There is a robust and effective system for maternal mortality audit in the UK in the form of the Confidential Enquiry into Maternal Deaths performed by MBRRACE-UK (Mothers and Babies: Reducing Risk through Audits and Confidential Enquiries across the UK). In the latest MBRRACE report, there were a total of 217 maternal deaths from 2 235 159 women who gave birth in the triennium 2016–2018 (Knight et al., 2020). However, the incidence of maternal collapse or severe maternal morbidity is unknown as morbidity data is not routinely collected. The incidence of cardiac arrest in pregnancy is much rarer than maternal collapse at around 1 in 36 000 maternities, with a case fatality rate of 42% (Beckett et al., 2017). In a UK study, a total of 25% of cardiac arrests in pregnancy were secondary to anaesthesia: all were associated with a 100% survival rate (Beckett et al., 2017).

Figure 23.2 shows the Royal College of Obstetricians and Gynaecologists (RCOG) algorithm (Chu et al., 2020) for treating maternal collapse commensurate with the Resuscitation Council UK (2021) guidance that indicates the procedure for cardiopulmonary resuscitation (CPR)/advanced life support (ALS) when necessary. The purpose of this guidance is to discuss the identification of women at increased risk of maternal collapse and the different causes of maternal collapse, to delineate the initial and ongoing management of maternal collapse, and review the maternal and neonatal outcomes. It covers both hospital and community settings, and includes all gestations and the postpartum period. The resuscitation team, equipment, and training requirements are also included.

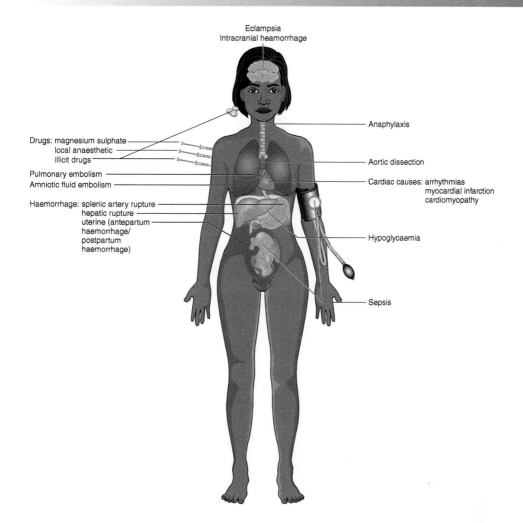

Eclampsia
Intracranial heamorrhage

Anaphylaxis

Drugs: magnesium sulphate
local anaesthetic
illicit drugs

Aortic dissection

Pulmonary embolism
Amniotic fluid embolism

Cardiac causes: arrhythmias
myocardial infarction
cardiomyopathy

Haemorrhage: splenic artery rupture
hepatic rupture
uterine (antepartum
haemorrhage/
postpartum
haemorrhage)

Hypoglycaemia

Sepsis

Figure 23.1   Causes of maternal collapse.
Source: Adapted from Chu et al. (2020)

Resuscitation in maternal collapse

Maternal collapse resuscitation should follow the Resuscitation Council UK (2021) guidelines using the standard *Airway, Breathing, Circulation, Disability, Exposure* (ABCDE) approach, with some modifications for maternal physiology, in particular relief of aortocaval compression, by manual displacement of the uterus to the left in women over 20 weeks gestation. Should cardiac arrest occur in the community, basic life support should be administered following the same guidance from the Resuscitation Council UK and *time-critical* transfer to hospital via paramedic ambulance arranged (Knight et al., 2020).

The woman should be placed in the left lateral position, obstetric review sought and the need for oxygen therapy assessed, guided by pulse oximetry to correct any hypoxia, and intravenous access should be established in order to administer any fluids or drugs. An *Alert, Verbal Stimulus, Pain Stimulus, Unresponsive* (AVPU) assessment should be undertaken as an alteration of consciousness can be a sign of critical illness. The cause of the maternal collapse should be rapidly identified and treated to prevent potential progression to maternal cardiorespiratory arrest and improve outcome. The Resuscitation Council UK (2021) divides the reversible causes of collapse into **4Ts** and **4Hs** with the addition of eclampsia and intracranial haemorrhage in pregnant women: namely *THE* (see Table 23.1).

Ongoing regular ABCDE assessment should be performed as the risk of progression to cardiac arrest remains until the cause of the collapse is treated. Focused ultrasound by a skilled operator can be used to identify reversible causes and to assess if a fetal heart rate is present. The irreversible causes of collapse and drug treatments are outlined in the following sections.

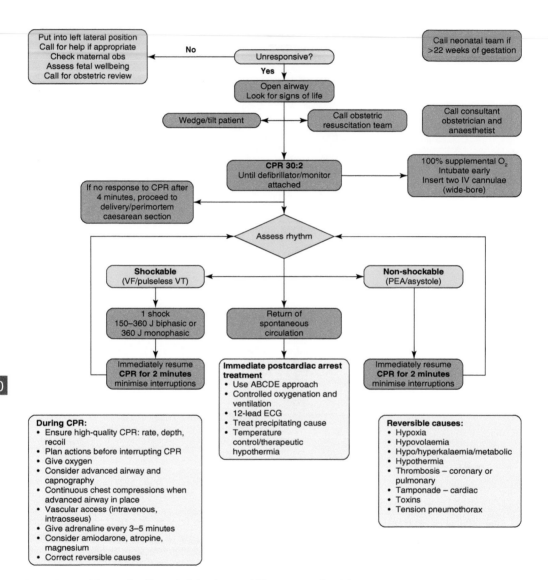

Figure 23.2 Maternal collapse/adult advanced life support algorithm.
ABCDE, airway, breathing, circulation, disability, exposure; CPR, cardiopulmonary resuscitation; ECG, electrocardiogram; PEA, pulseless electrical activity; VF, ventricular fibrillation; VT. ventricular tachycardia.
Source: Adapted from Chu et al. (2020).

Table 23.1 Causes of maternal collapse and reversible causes.

THE	Reversible cause	Cause in pregnancy
4 Ts	Thromboembolism	Amniotic fluid embolus, pulmonary embolus, air embolus, myocardial infarction
	Toxicity	Local anaesthetic, magnesium, other
	Tension pneumothorax	Following trauma/suicide attempts
	Tamponade	Following trauma/suicide attempts
4 Hs	Hypovolaemia	Bleeding (obstetric/other; may be concealed) or relative hypovolaemia of dense spinal block, septic or neurogenic block
	Hypoxia	Pregnant women can become hypoxic more quickly. Cardiac events – peripartum cardiomyopathy, myocardial infarction, aortic dissection, large vessel aneurysms
	Hypo/hyperkalaemia and hyponatraemia	Hypo- and hyperkalaemia are no more likely. Hyponatraemia may be caused by oxytocin use
	Hypothermia	No more likely
E	Eclampsia and pre-eclampsia	Includes intracranial haemorrhage

Source: Chu et al. (2020)/with permission of John Wiley & Sons.

Thrombosis and thromboembolism

Knight et al. (2020) reported that, between 2016 and 2018, there were 34 maternal deaths in the UK attributed to thrombosis and thromboembolism (the same rate as in 1985–1987), and as a consequence, this remains the leading cause of direct maternal death during or up to 6 weeks following childbirth. Increasing maternal age, obesity and the rise in operative births have had an impact on the significant static rate of thromboembolism rates despite thromboprophylaxis risk assessments and regimes being established in midwifery practice. Thromboprophylaxis involves the administration of low molecular weight heparin (LMWH) and the wearing of gradient compression stockings or TED stockings which have been discussed in Chapter 11.

A thrombus can form within a blood vessel and become detached, lodging in another blood vessel to partially or wholly occlude it, leading to a deep vein thrombosis (DVT). In pregnancy, 90% of all DVTs occur in the left leg due to the physical effect of the gravid uterus exerting pressure on the pelvic veins and the inferior vena cava, the ileofemoral veins being the most common location (Davis and Pavord, 2018).

It is advised by Knight et al. (2020) that women of reproductive age presenting to the emergency department collapsed or shocked, in whom a pulmonary embolism is suspected, should be assessed by a team of experienced clinicians, including the on-call consultant obstetrician, and have a Focused Assessment with Sonography in Trauma (FAST) scan to exclude intra-abdominal bleeding from a ruptured ectopic pregnancy, especially in the presence of anaemia. In addition, women presenting with signs and symptoms of an acute pulmonary embolism should have an electrocardiogram (ECG) and a chest x-ray (CXR). If there are also signs and symptoms of a DVT, a compression duplex ultrasound scan should be performed and if a DVT is confirmed, no further investigation is necessary and treatment for the venous thromboembolism (VTE) should continue. However, where a woman presents with a suspected pulmonary embolism without any signs and symptoms of a DVT, a ventilation/perfusion (V/Q) lung scan or a computed tomography pulmonary angiogram (CTPA) should be performed (RCOG, 2015).

In cases of massive life-threatening pulmonary embolism in pregnancy and the puerperium, the collapsed, shocked woman should be assessed and managed on an individual basis by a multidisciplinary team of experienced clinicians, including the on-call consultant obstetrician, senior physicians and radiologists. Management will consider administering intravenous unfractionated heparin

371

Table 23.2 Medicines used to treat acute pulmonary embolism.

Medicine	Administration	Distribution	Metabolism	Excretion
Unfractionated heparin (UFH)	Intravenous infusion or subcutaneous injection – dose determined by body weight	Unfractionated heparin is a long string of glycosaminoglycan molecules that can range from 3000 to 30 000 daltons. Binds with antithrombin III to enhance its ability to inhibit factor Xa and thrombin (factor IIa) (two of the body's most potent clotting factors) within minutes. The result is an increase in the activity of antithrombin, manifesting in the form of the anticoagulant effect	The liver and the reticuloendothelial system are sites of biotransformation via two mechanisms: *Saturable* – clearance by the reticuloendothelial system and endothelial cells to which heparin binds with high affinity (lower doses) *Non-saturable* – renal excretion (higher doses)	Mainly by the reticuloendothelial system. A small fraction is excreted in urine
Low molecular weight heparin, e.g. enoxaparin, dalteparin, tinzaparin	Subcutaneous injection Has an average of 15 polysaccharide units and is almost completely absorbed after subcutaneous administration. With a longer half-life, dosing is more predictable and can be less frequent than UFH, most commonly once per day. If a high body weight, higher doses will be required, depending on local administration policy	LMHW is a small fragment of a larger mucopolysaccharide, heparin. Inhibits the conversion of fibrinogen into fibrin by the activity of thrombin. Inhibits coagulation by activating antithrombin III which binds to and inhibits factor Xa only. In doing so, it prevents activation of the final common path; factor Xa inactivation means that prothrombin is not activated to thrombin, thereby not converting fibrinogen into fibrin for the formation of a clot	Partially metabolised by desulfation and depolymerisation to lower and less potent molecular weight metabolites. The affinity of plasma proteins for LMWHs is much less than for UFH so that only 10% is protein bound. This increased bioavailability ensures a more predictable anticoagulant action	Enoxaparin is mainly excreted by the kidneys. Renal clearance of active fragments represents about 10% of the administered dose and total renal excretion of active and non-active fragments, 40% of the dose

(UFH) or thrombolytic therapy or undertaking a thoracotomy and surgical embolectomy. Intravenous UFH is the preferred initial treatment in massive pulmonary embolism with cardiovascular compromise/renal impairment because of its rapid effect, extensive experience of its use in this situation and since it can be adjusted more readily if thrombolytic therapy is administered (RCOG, 2015; Scottish Intercollegiate Guidelines Network (SIGN), 2010).

One regimen for the administration of intravenous UFH is to give a loading dose of 80 units/kg, followed by a continuous intravenous infusion of 18 units/kg/h. If a woman has received thrombolysis, the loading dose of heparin should be omitted and an infusion started at 18 units/kg/h. It is mandatory to measure activated partial thromboplastin time (aPTT) level 4–6 hours after the loading dose, 6 hours after any dose change and then at least daily when in the therapeutic range. The drugs used in acute pulmonary embolism are shown in Table 23.2.

Drug toxicity/overdose

In all cases of maternal collapse occurring in any setting, drug toxicity and illicit drug overdose should be considered as a cause. The principles of observation and resuscitation already discussed in this chapter apply to such a scenario. Recreational drug use and its impact on pregnancy are covered in Chapter 22. Common sources of drug toxicity in midwifery and obstetric practice are local anaesthetic agents accidently injected intravenously and magnesium sulfate given in the presence of renal impairment (Chu et al., 2020). Toxic effects associated with local anaesthetics usually result from excessively high plasma concentrations.

Effects initially include a feeling of inebriation and light-headedness followed by sedation, circumoral paraesthesia and twitching. In cases of severe toxicity, convulsions can also occur. On intravenous injection, convulsions and cardiovascular collapse may occur very rapidly. Local anaesthetic toxicity resulting from systemic absorption of the local anaesthetic may occur sometime after the initial injection. Signs of severe toxicity include sudden loss of consciousness, with or without tonic-clonic convulsions, and cardiovascular collapse. In addition, sinus bradycardia, conduction blocks, asystole and ventricular tachyarrhythmias can all occur (Foxall et al., 2007). In terms of local anaesthetics, total spinal block or high spinal/epidural block are rarer and usually much easier to recognise as a cause of collapse.

If local anaesthetic toxicity is suspected, then the injection should be stopped immediately and lipid rescue, such as Intralipid® (a sterile fat emulsion), used in cases of maternal collapse that are secondary to local anaesthetic toxicity; the pharmacokinetics are shown in Table 23.3. This would be in the form of Intralipid 20% which should be available in all hospitals offering maternity services (Chu et al., 2020). All cases of lipid rescue should be reported to NHS Improvement and the Lipid Rescue site.

373

Table 23.3 Fat emulsion therapy.

Drug	Administration	Distribution	Metabolism	Excretion
Intralipid	20% 1.5 mL/kg over 1 minute (100 mL for a woman weighing 70 kg) followed by an intravenous infusion of Intralipid 20% 15 mL/kg/h (1000 mL/kg/h for a woman weighing 70 kg)	The mechanism by which lipids reverse local anaesthetic cardiotoxicity may be by increasing clearance from cardiac tissue. This non-specific, observed extraction of local anaesthetics from aqueous plasma or cardiac tissues is termed a 'lipid sink'	The exogenous fat particle is taken up by the low-density lipoprotein (LDL) receptors and primarily hydrolysed in the peripheral circulation which removes the triglycerides. Thus a transient triglyceride level may be elevated after Intralipid infusion	Eliminated from the circulation according to the same kinetic principles as dietary chylomicron-rich lymph

(Continued)

Table 23.3   (Continued)

Drug	Administration	Distribution	Metabolism	Excretion
	Two further 100 mL bolus injections can be repeated twice at 5-minute intervals if an adequate circulation has not been restored After another 5 minutes, the infusion rate should be increased to 30 mL/kg/h if an adequate circulation has not been restored A maximum cumulative dose of 12 mL/kg should not be exceeded (840 mL for a woman weighing 70 kg) CPR should be continued throughout this process until an adequate circulation has been restored. This may take over 1 hour	Another proposed mechanism is that lipids counteract local anaesthetic inhibition of myocardial fatty acid oxidation, thereby enabling energy production and reversing cardiac depression	The triglycerides are hydrolysed by lipoprotein lipase to fatty acids and glycerol. The free fatty acids are used by the muscle as an immediate source of energy, causing an increase in heat production, decrease in respiratory quotient and increase in oxygen consumption or reconverted into triglycerides and stored as a fat in the subcutaneous tissue for energy reserve The free fatty acids also undergo enterohepatic recycling and re-enter the systemic circulation in the form of very low-density lipoproteins (VLDL)	Both the elimination and the oxidation rates are dependent on the individual clinical condition

Major haemorrhage/hypovolaemia

374

In the UK, 20 women died from obstetric haemorrhage during or up to 6 weeks following childbirth in the triennium 2016–2018, two of which were associated with uterine inversion and six as a result of amniotic fluid embolism (Knight et al., 2020). Hypovolaemia resulting from illness or trauma can precipitate imbalances in homeostasis (the maintenance of finely balanced levels of oxygen, fluid and electrolytes) due to the loss of circulating fluid volume which can move into the tissues – the third space (Frost, 2015). By addressing hypovolaemia, homeostasis can be restored, preventing hypoperfusion and subsequent organ dysfunction.

Whenever any signs of hypovolaemia are present (tachycardia and/or agitation with hypotension), haemorrhage, which may be concealed, should always be considered (Mavrides et al., 2016). The stage in pregnancy at which major bleeding occurs will determine the action to arrest the bleeding, as in the case of a placental abruption where maternal and fetal well-being will both be of concern. The pharmacological measures to control bleeding following birth include administering an infusion of oxytocin (40 iu in 500 mL isotonic crystalloids at 125 mL/h) unless fluids are restricted, carboprost 0.25 mg by intramuscular injection at not less than 15 minutes to a maximum of eight doses and 800 micrograms sublingual misoprostol. However, as Chapter 10 has already identified the uterotonic drugs used to minimise blood loss during childbirth, i.e. oxytocin or ergometrine (contraindicated in women with hypertension), Table 23.4 relates only to those used specifically in cases of *major* haemorrhage leading to hypovolaemia.

Table 23.4 Medicines used to arrest haemorrhage.

Medicine	Administration	Distribution	Metabolism	Excretion
Carboprost tromethamine/ Hemabate®	Intramuscular injection 250 micrograms every 15 minutes for a maximum of eight doses	A synthetic prostaglandin that binds the prostaglandin E2 receptor, causing myometrial contractions, e.g. inducing labour or the expulsion of the placenta. Prostaglandins occur naturally in the body and act at several sites in the body, stimulating smooth muscle contractility. Whether or not these contractions result from a direct effect of carboprost on the myometrium has not been determined. Postpartum, the resultant myometrial contractions provide haemostasis at the site of placentation	Metabolised in the lungs and liver	Metabolites excreted in the urine
Misoprostol	*Oral:* 8-minute onset of action and action lasts approximately 2 hours *Sublingual:* 11-minute onset of action and its action lasts around 3 hours *Vaginal:* 20-minute onset of action and its action lasts approximately 4 hours	A synthetic prostaglandin E1 analogue that stimulates prostaglandin E1 receptors on parietal cells in the stomach to reduce gastric acid secretion. Mucus and bicarbonate secretion are also increased along with thickening of the mucosal bilayer so the mucosa can generate new cells.	Rapidly de-esterified in the liver to misoprostol acid, the biologically active metabolite. The de-esterified metabolite undergoes further oxidation in several body tissues	About 15% of an oral dose appears in the faeces; the balance is excreted in urine

375

(Continued)

Table 23.4 (Continued)

Medicine	Administration	Distribution	Metabolism	Excretion
Misoprostol	*Rectal*: 100-minute onset of action and its action lasts around 4 hours (for postpartum haemorrhage)	Misoprostol binds to smooth muscle cells in the uterine lining to increase the strength and frequency of contractions as well as degrade collagen and decrease cervical tone		
Tranexamic acid	Administered intravenously by injection or infusion	A synthetic derivative of lysine used as an antifibrinolytic in the treatment and prevention of major bleeding, promoting blood clotting by slowing down fibrinolysis by the binding of plasminogen to fibrin that induces fibrinolysis. The dissolution of fibrin stabilises the clot and prevents haemorrhage	Only a small fraction of tranexamic acid is metabolised	Primary means is urinary excretion. The rate of excretion is dependent on the route of administration *IV*: approximately 90% is excreted within 24 hours *Oral*: only 39% is excreted within 24 hours

Fluid volumes need to be distributed into the intracellular and extracellular spaces (the latter being further divided into the interstitial and intravascular compartments). The movement of fluid between these spaces is continual to enable cells to receive their necessary supply of electrolytes such as sodium, potassium and carbon; accompanied with oxygen, these are fundamental for cell performance (Peate and Nair, 2016). The following section presents the intravenous fluids and blood products that may be administered to replace any lost circulating volume based on the NICE (2017) guidelines and the RCOG Green-top guidelines (Mavrides et al., 2016) which are shown in Table 23.5.

Where an individual requires fluid resuscitation, NICE (2017) recommends an initial bolus of 500 mL of crystalloid solution (containing sodium in the range of 130–154 mmol/L) over less than 15 minutes. However, Frost (2015) warns this should be avoided where there is any evidence of pulmonary oedema as a result of cardiac failure. This initial fluid resuscitation should be followed by a reassessment and if further fluid resuscitation is required, then fluid boluses of 250–500 mL should be given. Further obstetric review will be required if continuous boluses of up to 2 L are required. It is important to consider potassium levels when ensuring normal electrolyte parameters are met as any alteration, either hypokalaemia or hyperkalaemia, can affect cardiac performance, causing arrhythmias, heart failure and/or cardiac arrest. Specialist intervention, such as the monitoring of central venous pressure (see Clinical consideration), kidney function tests or high-dependency care, will be required. The types of fluid replacement therapy are outlined in Table 23.5.

Crystalloids and colloids are plasma volume expanders used to increase a depleted circulating volume. Colloids carry an increased risk of anaphylaxis, are more expensive (Frost, 2015) and, as some preparations contain gelatine, would be unsuitable for vegetarian or vegan patients. However, colloid solutions are less likely to cause oedema than crystalloid solutions.

Table 23.5 Fluid replacement therapy.

Preparation	Remarks
Crystalloids, e.g. sodium chloride 0.9% (normal saline 0.9%), compound sodium lactate solutions (Ringer's lactate solution, Hartmann's solution) and glucose solutions	Crystalloid solutions are isotonic plasma volume expanders that contain electrolytes, increasing the circulatory volume without altering the chemical balance in the vascular spaces. This is due to their isotonic properties being close to those of blood circulating in the body. They are used to increase the intravascular volume when it is reduced as a result of haemorrhage, dehydration or loss of fluid during surgery. Some crystalloid preparations containing additives such as potassium or glucose are used in specific circumstances, for example in hypokalaemia and hypoglycaemia. Crystalloid solutions need to be administered in larger volumes than colloid solutions. As two-thirds of the infused volume will move into the tissues, only the remaining third will stay in the intravascular space, leaving a diminished circulating volume in need of further fluid administration. This increased volume can cause unwanted side-effects such as oedema (NICE, 2017). To reduce the risk of hyperchloraemic acidosis that may arise from excessive amounts of infused sodium chloride 0.9%, leading to renal dysfunction, resulting in a reduced glomerular filtration rate, compound sodium lactate solutions should be used
Colloids, e.g. albumin, dextran, hydroxyethyl starch (or hetastarch), Haemaccel® and Gelofusine®	Colloids are gelatinous solutions that maintain a high osmotic pressure in the blood. Particles in the colloids are too large to pass through semi-permeable membranes such as capillary membranes, so colloids stay in the intravascular spaces longer than crystalloids. When administering hetastarch, caution should be exercised as this colloid, exacerbated by the haemodilution effects of fluid administration, can negatively affect platelet count, leading to a temporary negative effect on clotting times and coagulation. In addition, hypertension and tachycardia, cardiac failure, and pulmonary and peripheral oedema are all potential side-effects of the excessive administration of albumin, dextran or hetastarch
Red cell transfusion	Red cell transfusion increases the haemoglobin and iron levels, while improving the amount of oxygen in the body. Since the central pathophysiology of haemorrhagic shock is failure of oxygen delivery, timely administration of red blood cells is the most important component of resuscitation. Blood loss greater than 25–30% usually requires transfusion of packed red blood cells in addition to crystalloids. Ensuring a ready supply of type 'O' blood that can be immediately delivered to the bedside can be life-saving in the rapidly deteriorating patient
Fresh frozen plasma (FFP)	Fresh frozen plasma is made from plasma which is separated from donor blood and frozen to minus 35 °C to preserve it and is utilised for its clotting factor content in trauma resuscitation. In the presence of massive haemorrhage or coagulopathy, 1 unit of FFP is given for every 4 or 5 units of red cells administered. Administration of FFP should be guided by serial measurement of clotting times, fibrinogen levels, prothrombin time (PT) and activated partial thromboplastin time (aPTT). FFP is not indicated just for volume expansion in trauma cases. However, a more proactive approach is beneficial in rapid bleeding to prevent the development of a coagulopathy. The timing of plasma transfusion is important. If correction is required before a haemostatic challenge such as major surgery, it should be given shortly before the procedure for maximum benefit
Cryoprecipitate	Cryoprecipitate is made from human plasma. When FFP is thawed in the cold (1–6 °C), a precipitate forms (the cryoprecipitate), after which the supernatant (cryosupernatant, cryoprecipitate-poor or cryoprecipitate-reduced plasma) is removed and the plasma is refrozen. It is rich in factor VIII, von Willebrand factor and fibrinogen. If FFP is used to supplement massive transfusion, cryoprecipitate may not be required unless the fibrinogen level falls to below 100 mg/dL

377

(Continued)

Table 23.5   (Continued)

Preparation	Remarks
Platelets (platelet concentrate)	Platelet transfusion is used to prevent or treat bleeding where there is a low platelet count or poor platelet function. In those who are bleeding, transfusion is usually carried out with a platelet count of less than 50×10^9/L with the aim of maintaining the count above 50×10^9/L. Blood group matching for ABO and RhD is typically recommended before platelets are given. Unmatched platelets, however, are often used due to the unavailability of matched platelets and are administered intravenously. However, if there is excessive bleeding, fever, infection, disseminated intravascular coagulation or splenomegaly, an increase in platelet count following transfusion may not be clearly evident
Recombinant factor VII	Recombinant clotting factors are made in a laboratory and do not originate from blood. They are made with recombinant DNA technology and are concentrated into a powder form that is then mixed with sterile water and injected. Recombinant factor VII was initially developed for the treatment of bleeding episodes in patients with haemophilia A or B, but has been known to successfully treat life-threatening postpartum haemorrhage after caesarean section

Source: Based on Mavrides et al. (2016).

Clinical consideration

Fluid replacement therapy
- The loss of circulating fluid volume can lead to imbalances in homeostasis.
- Recognising, assessing and monitoring patients' need for fluid therapy are crucial.
- The '5Rs' of intravenous fluid administration are:
  - resuscitation
  - routine maintenance
  - replacement
  - redistribution
  - reassessment (NICE, 2017).
- Crystalloids and colloids, both plasma volume expanders, are used to increase depleted circulating volumes.
- To administer intravenous fluids, health professionals must understand what crystalloids and colloids do and when to use them.

Major obstetric haemorrhage protocols must include the provision of emergency blood transfusion with immediate issue of group O, rhesus D (RhD)-negative and K-negative units, moving to group-specific blood as soon as feasible. However, until blood is available, up to 3.5 L of warmed clear fluids should be infused initially with 2 L of warmed isotonic crystalloid. Further fluid resuscitation can continue with additional isotonic crystalloid or colloid (succinylated gelatine). Hydroxyethyl starch should not be used. There are no firm criteria for initiating red cell transfusion and the decision to provide blood transfusion should be based on both clinical and haematological assessment.

If no haemostatic results are available and bleeding is continuing, then, after 4 units of red blood cells, FFP should be infused at a dose of 12–15 mL/kg until haemostatic test results are known. If no haemostatic tests are available, early FFP should be considered for conditions with a suspected coagulopathy, such as placental abruption or amniotic fluid embolism, or where detection of Post Partum Haemorrhage (PPH) has been delayed (Mavrides et al., 2016).

If prothrombin time/activated partial thromboplastin time is more than 1.5 times normal and haemorrhage is ongoing, volumes of FFP in excess of 15 mL/kg are likely to be needed to correct coagulopathy. Cryoprecipitate should be used for fibrinogen replacement to maintain a plasma fibrinogen level of greater than 2 g/L during ongoing PPH. If the platelet count falls to 75×10^9/L based on laboratory monitoring, platelets should be transfused. Consideration should also be given to using

Clinical consideration

Central venous pressure (CVP)

CVP is the pressure in the right atrium or superior vena cava and is an indicator of the volume of blood returning to the heart, reflecting the competence of the heart as a pump and the peripheral vascular resistance. Normal CVP values can vary between +5 and +10 cmH$_2$O and will change with gestation. Values within this range indicate that the vascular space is well filled and red cell transfusion would not be necessary. However, in the presence of acute peripheral circulatory failure, monitoring of CVP aids assessment of blood loss, with a negative value indicating the necessity for fluid replacement.

CVP is measured using an indwelling central venous catheter (CVC) and a pressure manometer or a transducer. Both methods are reliable when used correctly. Wards use manometers, whereas accident and emergency departments and critical care/intensive care units use transducers for measuring CVP.

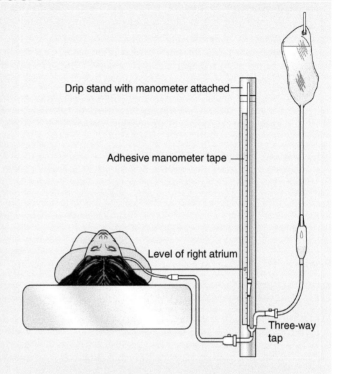

Monitoring central venous pressure with pressure manometer.

Source: Marshall & Raynor (2020)/with permission of Elsevier.

An isolated CVP recording is of little clinical value. Trends in CVP results are more useful clinically rather than an isolated reading and are interpreted in conjunction with fluid balance and peripheral perfusion.

379

intravenous tranexamic acid, an antifibrinolytic drug (1 g), to control the haemorrhage. If pharmacological measures fail, surgical interventions such as hysterectomy should be initiated sooner rather than later, especially in cases of placenta accreta or uterine rupture (Mavrides et al., 2016).

There is no proven effective therapy to manage amniotic fluid embolism (AFE) so measures should be supportive rather than specific and as a consequence, early involvement of senior experienced staff, including midwives, obstetricians, anaesthetists, haematologists and critical care experts, is essential to optimise outcome. Coagulopathy needs early, aggressive treatment, including the use of FFP. Recombinant factor VII should only be used if coagulopathy cannot be corrected by massive blood component replacement as it causes poorer outcomes in women with AFE (Chu et al., 2020).

Pre-eclampsia and eclampsia

Pre-eclampsia occurs in 3–4% of all pregnancies, with around 10% of women developing this in their first pregnancy. Action on Pre-Eclampsia (APEC, 2019) also states that black women are three times more likely to develop pre-eclampsia than white women. Although the majority of women will have a successful pregnancy outcome, some will develop multisystem complications, for example presenting as eclampsia or haemolytic elevated liver enzymes low platelets (HELLP) syndrome with no recorded changes in blood pressure and no proteinuria prior to the onset of seizures or symptoms of HELLP syndrome. In the UK, the rate of maternal deaths from hypertensive disorders of pregnancy has significantly declined and in the recent confidential enquiry into maternal deaths, a total of four women died from pre-eclampsia and eclampsia between 2016 and 2018 (Knight et al., 2020). The management and care related to hypertension in pregnancy are outlined in the NICE (2019a) guidelines.

Women who are at high risk of pre-eclampsia are advised to take a daily dose of 75–150 mg *aspirin* from 12 weeks of pregnancy until the birth of the baby. However, if the blood pressure remains above 140/90 mmHg, other pharmacological treatment should be administered with the aim of reaching a target blood pressure of 135/85 mmHg (NICE, 2019a). Furthermore, in women with severe hypertension (blood pressure 160/110 mmHg or more), pharmacological treatment should be given and blood pressure measured every 15–30 minutes.

The treatment of choice in severe pre-eclampsia is magnesium sulfate (NICE, 2019a), oral labetalol or nifedipine. However, if the blood pressure is >170/110 mmHg, bolus doses of intravenous labetalol or hydralazine should be given to lower the blood pressure and then followed by an intravenous infusion. In addition, intravenous magnesium sulfate is administered to reduce the incidence of an eclamptic seizure by around 50%. Fluids should be restricted, a low-salt diet initiated and urine output monitored and tested for proteinuria with a fluid balance chart being maintained. Magnesium toxicity may manifest with a marked reduction in urine output (<100 mL/4 h), lowered respiratory rate (<12 breaths/min) and loss of patellar reflexes. Medications used to treat pre-eclampsia/eclampsia are shown in Table 23.6.

Table 23.6 Medicines used in treating pre-eclampsia/eclampsia.

Medicine	Administration	Distribution	Metabolism	Excretion
Aspirin (acetylsalicylic acid)	*Oral*: used to treat pain, fever, inflammation and migraines, and reduce the risk of major adverse cardiovascular events	Disrupts the production of prostaglandins throughout the body by targeting cyclo-oxygenase-1 (COX-1) and COX-2, halting their action at pain receptors, preventing symptoms of pain. As an antipyretic agent, it interferes with the production of brain prostaglandin E1, an extremely powerful fever-inducing agent. The inhibition of platelet aggregation by acetylsalicylic acid occurs because of its interference with thromboxane A2 in platelets. Thromboxane A2 is an important lipid responsible for platelet aggregation, which can lead to clot formation and future risk of heart attack or stroke	The non-ionised acetylsalicylic acid passes through the stomach lining by passive diffusion and is hydrolysed in the plasma to salicylic acid in the first-hour post ingestion by esterases found in the gastrointestinal tract. Peak plasma salicylate concentrations occur between 1 and 2 hours post administration. Salicylate is mainly metabolised in the liver, although other tissues may be involved in this process. The major metabolites of acetylsalicylic acid are salicylic acid, salicyluric acid, the ether or phenolic glucuronide and the ester or acyl glucuronide. A small portion is converted to gentisic acid and other hydroxybenzoic acids	Excretion of salicylates occurs mainly through the kidney, by the processes of glomerular filtration and tubular excretion, in the form of free salicylic acid, salicyluric acid and phenolic and acyl glucuronides. Salicylate can be found in the urine soon after administration but the entire dose takes about 48 hours to be completely eliminated. The rate of salicylate excretion is often variable, ranging from 10% to 85% in the urine, and is dependent on urinary pH. Acidic urine generally aids in reabsorption of salicylate by the renal tubules, while alkaline urine increases excretion

(Continued)

Table 23.6 (Continued)

Medicine	Administration	Distribution	Metabolism	Excretion
Labetalol	Oral or intravenous	Blocks alpha and beta adrenergic receptors, resulting in decreased peripheral vascular resistance and sustained vasodilation over the long term without any significant alteration of heart rate or cardiac output	Mainly metabolised through conjugation to glucuronide metabolites such as the O-phenyl-glucuronide and the N-glucuronide present in the plasma	Metabolites are excreted in the urine and via the bile, into the faeces. Approximately 55–60% of a dose appears in the urine as conjugates or unchanged labetalol within the first 24 hours of dosing
Nifedipine	Oral	About 92–98% of circulating nifedipine is bound to plasma proteins. Blocks voltage-gated L-type calcium channels in vascular smooth muscle and myocardial cells, preventing the entry of calcium ions into cells during depolarisation, reducing peripheral arterial vascular resistance and dilating coronary arteries. These actions reduce blood pressure and increase the supply of oxygen to the heart, alleviating angina	Metabolised in the liver to highly water-soluble, inactive metabolites	Excreted in urine (60–80% of the dose) and faeces as inactive metabolites. Elimination half-life is 2–5 hours

(Continued)

Table 23.6 (Continued)

Medicine	Administration	Distribution	Metabolism	Excretion
Hydralazine	Oral. Absorbed rapidly from the gastrointestinal tract	Interferes with calcium transport in vascular smooth muscle by preventing influx of calcium into cells, preventing calcium release from intracellular compartments, directly acting on actin and myosin, or a combination of these actions. This decrease in vascular resistance leads to increased heart rate, stroke volume and cardiac output and reduction in blood pressure	Metabolised primarily by N-acetylation in the gastrointestinal mucosa and liver. It also forms hydrazones (i.e. acetone hydrazone and pyruvic acid hydrazone), which may contribute to the blood pressure-lowering effect. The rate of this N-acetylation step is genetically determined	<10% of hydralazine is recovered in the faeces; 65–90% is recovered in the urine
Magnesium sulfate (electrolyte replenisher, anticonvulsant and cathartic)	Intravenous – first-line management of eclamptic seizures. 4 g over 5–15 min, followed by an intravenous infusion of 1 g/h for 24 hours, continued for 24 hours after seizure Recurrent seizures treated with a further 2-4g administered over 5-15 min. Magnesium is the second most plentiful cat-ion of the intracellular fluids important for many systems in the body, especially the muscles and nerves	Reduces striated muscle contractions and blocks peripheral neuromuscular transmission by reducing acetylcholine release at the myoneural junction. Inhibits Ca^{2+} influx through dihydropyridine-sensitive, voltage-dependent channels, decreasing calcium availability, accounting for much of its relaxant action on vascular smooth muscle, e.g. the myocardium. Reduction in magnesium can frequently cause cardiac arrhythmias leading to cardiac arrest	Not known	Almost exclusively excreted via the kidney in the urine, at a rate proportional to the serum concentration and glomerular filtration. 90% of the dose is excreted during the first 24 hours after an intravenous infusion of $MgSO_4$

If the woman experiences worsening of symptoms, particularly headache, epigastric pain and vomiting that is accompanied by high blood pressure, it is indicative that severe pre-eclampsia is progressing to eclampsia and that a convulsion is likely to occur, necessitating emergency intervention. This will include stabilising the woman before the birth of the fetus is contemplated. Fetal outcome will be dependent on maternal resuscitation and gestational age of the pregnancy. Antihypertensive therapy will continue into the postnatal period and be adjusted according to the woman's blood pressure.

Sepsis

The World Health Organization (WHO, 2017) described maternal sepsis as *'a life-threatening condition defined as organ dysfunction resulting from infection during pregnancy, childbirth, post-abortion or postpartum period'.* Furthermore, septic shock is characterised by persistent tissue hypoperfusion despite fluid replacement therapy, leading to further complications and even death.

Sepsis has been a significant focus over the last decade with guidance produced by NICE (2019b) and the Surviving Sepsis campaign (Rhodes et al., 2017) as well as the RCOG (2012) Green-Top guidelines on bacterial sepsis in pregnancy. The recently published GLOSS study (WHO Global Maternal Sepsis Study Research Group, 2020) with data from 52 countries identified that 70.4 (95% confidence interval [CI] 67.7–73.1) hospitalised women per 1000 live births had a maternal infection, and 10.9 (95% CI 9.8–12.0) women per 1000 live births presented with infection-related severe maternal outcomes. It is estimated that at least 10.7% of maternal deaths in low- and middle-income countries and 4.7% of deaths in high-income countries are due to sepsis (Say et al., 2014).

Maternal deaths from sepsis can be due to direct causes, such as genital tract infection or wound infections, or indirect causes, such as influenza or meningitis. In the last triennial report from 2016–2018, there were 10 direct deaths in the UK from genital sepsis (Knight et al., 2020). Four of these women died from postnatal Group A streptococcus (GAS) infection, two having had a caesarean section but having had the infection prior to birth, and two women with GAS died after an unassisted vaginal birth. Six women died after midtrimester chorioamnionitis from *Escherichia coli*.

Chan (2018) emphasises that when an unwell pregnant or recently pregnant woman presents, the healthcare professional should always *Think Sepsis* at an early stage, take observations and act on them. The key actions for diagnosis and management are timely recognition and prompt administration of oxygen and intravenous broad-spectrum antibiotics (see Chapter 9 for specific drug details). NHS England (2014) affirms that involvement of experts for a senior review at an early stage is essential, along with critical care support.

To prevent further deterioration in the woman's condition, circulatory volume should be restored. By replacing fluid volume, perfusion of the vital organs will be restored and NICE (2019b) recommends an initial intravenous infusion of 500 mL of crystalloid over less than 15 minutes (see Table 23.5). Fluid replacement therapy should always be discussed with the anaesthetist and obstetrician (UK Sepsis Trust, 2018). Fluid balance is essential as fluid overload may lead to fatal pulmonary or cerebral oedema.

Cardiac arrest

When the detection of signs of life is in doubt or the signs are absent, cardiopulmonary resuscitation should be commenced following the ALS guidelines (Resuscitation Council UK, 2021), including administering high-flow oxygen, early tracheal intubation by an experienced practitioner followed by continuous chest compressions (see Figure 23.2). If feasible, a left lateral tilt of between 15° and 30° should be adopted to enable high-quality chest compressions and allow for the surgical birth of the fetus if appropriate. Electrical cardioversion is safe in all phases of pregnancy. Immediate electrical cardioversion is recommended for any woman with a tachycardia with haemodynamic instability and for pre-excited atrial fibrillation.

Ideally, early vascular access should be obtained with wide-bore intravenous cannulae inserted above the level of the diaphragm. This allows the administration of fluids to be unaffected by aortocaval compression. However, intravenous (IV)/intraosseous (IO) fluids should only be given where the cardiac arrest is caused by, or possibly caused by, hypovolaemia. The most common route of administration of drugs during CPR is through the peripheral vein as this is the most easily and safely established form of access. The circulation will be slow during cardiac resuscitation and it is therefore essential that each injection of a drug is followed by a flush of 20 mL of normal saline or 5% glucose so there is a better chance the drug will reach the heart where its action is required.

If peripheral venous access is difficult, early use of central venous access, IO access (Luck et al., 2010) or venous cut-down to aid volume replacement and drug administration should be considered. The ideal route is through a cannula placed in the central vein, in the neck or groin, from where the drugs can more easily reach the heart than from a peripheral vein. It is, however, more difficult and dangerous to place a cannula into these veins in an emergency except for experienced practitioners.

Administration of intravenous drug therapy should be expedited and include a vasopressor, such as adrenaline/epinephrine every 3–5 minutes while ALS continues and further consideration of antiarrhythmic drugs (amiodarone, atropine and magnesium sulfate – Table 23.7). Chu et al. (2020) suggest that there should be no alteration in algorithm drugs or doses used in the Resuscitation Council UK protocols when treating pregnant women, and any decision to discontinue resuscitation should be taken by the consultant obstetrician and consultant anaesthetist in collaboration with the cardiac arrest team.

Clinical consideration

Adrenaline

Adrenaline is also known as **epinephrine**.

Remember to not confuse *epinephrine* with *ephedrine* which is another sympathomimetic drug used to raise blood pressure, usually for the treatment of hypotension associated with general anaesthesia and with the use of epidural and spinal anaesthesia

1 mg of adrenaline (epinephrine) = 1 mL of *1 in 1000* adrenaline (epinephrine) or 10 mL of *1 in 10 000* adrenaline (epinephrine)

This is important to know during CPR as the concentration of adrenaline (epinephrine) is still given in this strange manner

1 in 1000 means 1 gram in a 1000 millilitres solution (1 g in 1000 mL)
The concentration of no other drug is given in this way

Perimortem caesarean section (resuscitative hysterotomy)

Assessment of fetal well-being should be undertaken after ABCDE assessment and judgement made, if the pregnancy is over 20 weeks gestation, to undertake a perimortem caesarean section (PMCS), also known as resuscitative hysterotomy (Rose et al., 2015), if there is no response to correctly performed CPR within **4 minutes** of collapse or if resuscitation is continued beyond this. This should be achieved within **5 minutes** of the collapse and undertaken to aid effective maternal resuscitation, regardless of the clinical setting. Birth of the fetus and placenta removes the cardiac impairment through mechanical and haematological adjustments. Although the outcome could be a baby with potentially severe neurological impairment (hypoxic ischaemic encephalopathy), having the neonatal emergency team awaiting the birth can improve the baby's chance of survival. However, perimortem caesarean section should be considered a resuscitative procedure to be performed primarily in the interests of maternal, *not* fetal, survival (Chu et al., 2020).

The woman should *not* be moved to an operating theatre in order to save time as a perimortem caesarean section can be performed anywhere, with only a scalpel being required. With no circulation, blood loss is minimal and no anaesthetic is required. If resuscitation is successful following the birth of the fetus, there should be prompt transfer to a high-dependency or critical care environment, to optimise continuing care, including anaesthesia and sedation to control ensuing haemorrhage and complete the operation.

Table 23.7   Medicines used in cardiac arrest.

Medicine	Administration	Distribution	Metabolism	Excretion
Oxygen	15 L/min via a reservoir/ non-rebreathing mask (variable rate if using a Venturi mask) 2–6 L/min via nasal cannulae	Ventilates the lungs, by increasing PO_2 in alveolar gas, driving more rapid diffusion of oxygen into the blood. The resultant increase in PaO_2 increases oxygen to the tissues, buying time while the underlying cause/ disease is reversed. Aim for 94–98% oxygen saturation	Although oxygen is the substrate that cells use in the greatest quantity and on which aerobic metabolism and cell integrity depend, the tissues have no storage system for oxygen. They rely on a continuous supply at a rate that precisely matches changing metabolic requirements. If this supply fails, even for a few minutes, tissue hypoxaemia may develop, resulting in anaerobic metabolism and production of lactate	From the lungs as carbon dioxide
Adrenaline/ epinephrine (sympathomimetic/ vasopressor)	1 mg IV as soon as cardiac arrest has been identified and repeated 1 mg IV every 3–5 minutes whilst ALS continues. 1 in 10 000 (100 micrograms/ mL) solution is recommended	Acts on alpha- and beta-adrenergic receptors. Stimulates the beta-adrenergic receptors in the myocardium to increase cardiac contractility and heart rate. Relaxes smooth muscle in the lungs and respiratory tract to improve inspiration and lung capacity. Stimulates liver to break down glycogen into glucose to provide energy to the brain	Rapidly inactivated mainly by the enzymes catechol-O-methyltransferase (COMT) and monoamine oxidase (MAO) to metanephrine or normetanephrine, resulting in the formation of 3-methoxy-4-hydroxy-mandelic acid (vanillylmandelic acid, VMA)	Primarily in the urine mainly as sulfate conjugates and, to a lesser extent, glucuronide conjugates. Only small amounts of the drug are excreted completely unchanged

(Continued)

385

Table 23.7 (Continued)

Medicine	Administration	Distribution	Metabolism	Excretion
Amiodarone (Class III antiarrhythmic/benzafurin)	300 mg IV (IO) given over at least 3 minutes from a prefilled syringe or diluted in 20 mL glucose 5%, after three electrical defibrillation shocks have been administered. A further dose of 150 mg IV (IO) is given following five electrical defibrillation shocks have been administered, if necessary	Relaxes smooth muscles that line vascular walls, decreases peripheral vascular resistance (afterload), and increases the cardiac index by a small amount. Blocks potassium currents that cause repolarisation of the heart muscle during the third phase of the cardiac action potential. Prolongs the QRS duration and QT interval. Decreases sinoatrial node automaticity with a decrease in atrioventricular node conduction velocity. Ectopic pacemaker automaticity is also inhibited. Increases the duration of the action potential as well as the effective refractory period for cardiac cells (myocytes). Therefore, cardiac muscle cell excitability is reduced, preventing and treating arrhythmias	Metabolised by the CYP3A4 and CYP2C8 enzymes. The CYP3A4 enzyme is found in the liver and intestines. The major metabolite of amiodarone is desethylamiodarone (DEA), which also has antiarrhythmic properties	Primarily by hepatic metabolism and biliary excretion. A small amount of DEA is excreted in the urine. There is 10–50% transfer of amiodarone and DEA in the placenta as well as a presence in breast milk
Atropine (anticholinergic or antiparasympathetic parasympatholytic/antimuscarinic agent)	1–3 mg IV. Used to correct asystole and severe bradycardia in cardiac arrest	Blocks the effect of the vagus nerve on the sinus node of the heart which normally slows heart rate or asystole. Acts on the conduction system of the heart and accelerates the transmission of electrical impulses through cardiac tissue. Antagonises the muscarine-like actions of acetylcholine and other choline esters	Is rapidly and well absorbed following administration. Disappears rapidly from the blood and is distributed throughout the various body tissues and fluids. Destroyed by enzymatic hydrolysis, particularly in the liver	13–50% is excreted unchanged in the urine
Magnesium sulfate (see Table 23.6)				

ALS, advanced life support; IO, intraosseous; IV, intravenous.
Source: Based on Chu et al. (2020).

Conclusion

This chapter has presented the specific medications and fundamental pharmacokinetics of common drugs used when an emergency arises in midwifery practice. The drugs used during cardiopulmonary resuscitation are also addressed. Midwives should be familiar with the range of these drugs within the context of their professional and legal responsibilities in administering medicines in emergency situations and utilise the specific detail in this chapter to complement contemporary national management recommendations and regimens.

Glossary

Angiogram   A type of x-ray used to examine blood vessels

Antipyretic   An agent (usually a drug) that reduces body temperature

Aortocaval compression syndrome   Compression of the abdominal aorta and inferior vena cava by the gravid uterus when a pregnant woman lies on her back

Asystole   Characterised by the complete and sustained absence of electrical activity of the heart, resulting in no contraction of the heart muscle tissue and therefore no cardiac output to the body

Cardiac tamponade   Compression of the heart due to a collection of fluid or blood in the pericardium

Cardiotoxicity   Occurs when the heart muscle has been injured

Coagulopathy   Also called a bleeding disorder, a condition where the blood's ability to coagulate is affected

Colloid   Colloids are gelatinous solutions that maintain a high osmotic pressure in the blood

Crystalloid   A crystalloid solution is an isotonic plasma volume expander that contains electrolytes

Haemodilution   Increase in the volume of plasma in relation to red blood cells; reduced concentration of red blood cells in the circulation

Hypoperfusion   An inadequate blood flow to a single organ or through the entire circulatory system

Morbidity   The state of having a specific illness or condition

Mortality rate   Refers to the number of deaths that have occurred due to a specific illness or condition

Tension pneumothorax   A life-threatening condition caused by the continuous entrance and entrapment of air into the pleural space, thereby compressing the lungs, heart, blood vessels and other structures in the chest

Tranexamic acid   A medicine that controls bleeding. It helps the blood to clot

Test yourself

Now review your learning by completing the learning activities for this chapter at ww.wiley.com/go/pharmacologyformidwives.

Find out more

The following is a list of emergencies you may encounter in midwifery practice, some being less common than others. Take some time to reflect on what you have read in this chapter and what you may have experienced in clinical practice and then write notes about each of the emergencies listed. Consider the medications that may be used to manage these emergencies and be specific about the pharmacokinetics and pharmacodynamics. Remember to include aspects of the care you provided to the woman. If you are making notes about women and families to whom you have offered care and support, you must ensure that you have adhered to the rules of confidentiality (NMC, 2018).

The emergency	Your notes
Eclampsia	
Maternal haemorrhage	
Amniotic fluid embolism	
Uterine inversion/rupture	
Pulmonary embolism	

References

Action on Pre-Eclampsia (2019) High blood pressure in pregnancy. https://action-on-pre-eclampsia.org.uk/public-area/high-blood-pressure-in-pregnancy/ (accessed February 2022).

Beckett, V.A., Knight, M., Sharpe, P. (2017) The CAPS Study: incidence, management and outcomes of cardiac arrest in pregnancy in the UK: a prospective, descriptive study. *British Journal of Obstetrics and Gynaecology*, **124**: 1374–1381.

Chan, W.S. (2018) Diagnosis of venous thromboembolism in pregnancy. *Thrombosis Research*, **163**: 221–228.

Chu, J., Johnston, T.A., Geoghegan, J. on behalf of the Royal College of Obstetricians and Gynaecologists (2020) Maternal collapse in pregnancy and the puerperium. Green-top Guideline 56. *British Journal of Obstetrics and Gynaecology*, **127**: e14–e52.

Davis, S., Pavord, S. (2018) Haematological problems in pregnancy. In: Edmunds, D.K., Lees, C., Bourne, T. (eds) *Dewhurst's Textbook of Obstetrics and Gynaecology*, 9th edn, pp.147–160. Wiley-Blackwell: Oxford.

Foxall, G., McCahon, R., Lamb, J., Hardman, J.G., Bedforth, N.M. (2007) Levobupivacaine-induced seizures and cardiovascular collapse treated with Intralipid. *Anaesthesia*, **62**: 516–518.

Frost, P. (2015) Intravenous fluid therapy in adult inpatients. *British Medical Journal*, **350**: g7620.

Haig, K.M., Sutton, S., Whittington, J. (2006) SBAR: A shared mental model for improving communication between clinicians. *Joint Commission Journal on Quality and Patient Safety*, **32**(3): 167–175.

Hargestam, M., Lindkvist, M., Brulin, C., Jacobsson, M., Hultin, M. (2013) Communication in interdisciplinary teams: exploring closed loop communication during in situ team training, *BMJ Open*, **3**: 1–8.

Knight, M., Bunch, K., Tuffnell, D. et al. (eds) on behalf of MBRRACE-UK (2020) *Saving Lives, Improving Mothers' Care – Lessons learned to inform maternity care from the UK and Ireland Confidential Enquiries into Maternal Deaths and Morbidity 2016–2018*. National Perinatal Epidemiology Unit, University of Oxford: Oxford.

Luck, R.P., Haines, C., Mull, C.C. (2010) Intraosseous access. *Journal of Emergency Medicine*, **39**: 468–475.

Marshall, J.E., Raynor, M.D. (2020) *Myles Textbook for Midwives*, 17th edn. Elsevier Churchill Livingstone: Edinburgh.

Mavrides, E., Allard, S., Chandraharan, E. et al. on behalf of the Royal College of Obstetricians and Gynaecologists (2016) Prevention and management of postpartum haemorrhage. Green-top Guideline 52. *British Journal of Obstetrics and Gynaecology*, **124**: e106–e149.

National Institute for Health and Care Excellence (2017) *Intravenous Fluid Therapy in Adults in Hospital. CG174.* NICE: London.

National Institute for Health and Care Excellence (2019a) *Hypertension in Pregnancy: Diagnosis and Management. NG133.* NICE: London.

National Institute for Health and Care Excellence (2019b) *Sepsis: Recognition, Diagnosis and Early Management. CG51.* NICE: London.

NHS England (2016) *The National Maternity Review. Better Births. Improving Outcomes in Maternity Services in England: A Five Year Forward View for Maternity Care*. NHS England: London.

NHS England (2014) *Patient Safety Alert: Resources to Support the Prompt Recognition of Sepsis and the Rapid Initiation of Treatment*. NHS England: London.

NHS Improvement (2018) Spoken communication and patient safety in the NHS. https://bmjopenquality.bmj.com/content/8/3/e000742 (accessed February 2022).

Nursing and Midwifery Council (2018a) *The Code: Standards of Practice and Behaviour for Nurses, Midwives and Nursing Associates*. NMC: London.

Nursing and Midwifery Council (2018b) *Realising Professionalism: Standards for Education and Training. Part 3: Standards for Prescribing Programmes*. NMC: London.

Nursing and Midwifery Council (2019) *Standards of Proficiency for Midwives*. NMC: London.

Ockenden D. (2022) *Findings, Conclusions and Essential Actions from the Independent Review of Maternity Services at the Shrewsbury and Telford Hospital NHS Trust*, Her Majesty's Stationary Office, London.

Peate, I., Nair, M. (2016) *Fundamentals of Anatomy and Physiology for Nursing and Healthcare Students*. Wiley-Blackwell: Chichester.

Pillay, L., Smith, L. (2019) Communicating effectively in midwifery education and practice. In: Marshall, J.E. (ed.) *Myles Professional Studies in Midwifery Education and Practice: Concepts and Challenges*, pp.37–54. Elsevier: Edinburgh.

Resuscitation Council UK (2021) Adult advanced life support guidelines. www.resus.org.uk/library/2021-resuscitation-guidelines/adult-advanced-life-support-guidelines (accessed February 2022).

Rhodes, A., Evans, L., Alhazzani, W. et al. (2017) Surviving Sepsis Campaign: international guidelines for management of sepsis and septic shock: 2016. *Intensive Care Medicine*, **43**(3): 304–377.

Rose, C.H., Faksh, A., Traynor, K.D., Cabrera, D., Arendt, K.W., Brost, B.C. (2015) Challenging the 4- to 5-minute rule: from perimortem caesarean to resuscitative hysterotomy. *American Journal of Obstetrics and Gynecology*, **213**(5): 653–656, 653.e1.

Royal College of Obstetricians and Gynaecologists (2012) *Bacterial Sepsis in Pregnancy. Green-top Guideline 64a*. RCOG: London.

Royal College of Obstetricians and Gynaecologists (2015) *Acute Management of Thrombosis and Embolism during Pregnancy and the Puerperium. Green-top Guideline 37b*. RCOG: London.

Royal Pharmaceutical Society (2016) *A Competency Framework for All Prescribers*. RPS: London.

Say, L., Chou, D., Gemmill, A. et al. (2014) Global causes of maternal death: a WHO systematic analysis. *Lancet Global Health*, **2**(6): e323–333.

Scottish Intercollegiate Guidelines Network (2010) *Prevention and Management of Venous Thromboembolism. SIGN guideline 122*. SIGN: Edinburgh.

United Kingdom Sepsis Trust (2018) *The Sepsis Manual 2017–2018*, 4th edn. UK Sepsis Trust: Birmingham.

World Health Organization (2017) *Statement on Maternal Sepsis*. WHO: Geneva.

World Health Organization Global Maternal Sepsis Study Research Group (2020) Frequency and management of maternal infection in health facilities in 52 countries (GLOSS): a 1-week inception cohort study, *Lancet Global Health*, **8**(5): e661–e671.

389

Further reading

Davey, L., Houghton, D. (2020) *The Midwife's Pocket Formulary*, 4th edn. Elsevier: Edinburgh. *An essential guide containing all the drugs midwives are likely to encounter in their sphere of practice, including emergency drugs and intravenous fluids reflecting contemporary resuscitation pathways embedded in NICE, RCOG and Resuscitation Council UK guidance. This fourth edition provides details on how to manage and administer these drugs and is written in a practical and easy-reading style.*

Medforth, J., Ball, L., Walker, A., Battersby, S., Stables, S. (eds) (2017) *Oxford Handbook of Midwifery*, 3rd edn. Oxford University Press: Oxford. *Extensively revised using the latest evidence-based guidelines and national recommendations, this third edition of the popular Oxford Handbook of Midwifery continues to provide a complete insight into the midwife's role in contemporary multidisciplinary working, including in emergency situations.*

Websites

Action on Pre-eclampsia: https://action-on-pre-eclampsia.org.uk

Mothers and Babies: Reducing Risk through Audits and Confidential Enquiries across the UK (MBRRACE-UK): www.npeu.ox.ac.uk/mbrrace-uk

NHS Improvement: https://improvement.nhs.uk/

National Institute for Health and Care Excellence: www.nice.org.uk/

Resuscitation Council UK: www.resus.org.uk/#

Royal College of Obstetricians and Gynaecologists: www.rcog.org.uk/

Royal Pharmaceutical Society: www.rpharms.com/

UK Sepsis Trust: https://sepsistrust.org/

United Kingdom Obstetric Surveillance System (UKOSS): www.npeu.ox.ac.uk/ukoss

Chapter 24

Medications used in contraception

Emma Dawson-Goodey

University of Hertfordshire, Hatfield, UK

Aim

The aim of this chapter is to provide the reader with an introduction to the various pharmacological methods of contraception available in the postnatal period and the role of the midwife.

Learning outcomes

After reading this chapter, the reader will:
- Understand the various pharmacological contraceptive methods available to women in the post-natal period
- Apply the United Kingdom Medical Eligibility Criteria for Contraceptive Use (UKMEC) guidelines
- Be able to provide women with evidence-based information
- Be able to empower women to make an informed choice regarding their sexual health.

Test your existing knowledge

- What pharmacological contraceptive methods are available to women?
- How soon can a woman start oral contraception following childbirth?
- What should a midwife consider before a woman begins a method of contraception?
- How do pharmacological contraceptive methods affect breast feeding?
- What drugs may affect the efficacy of hormonal contraceptives?

Introduction

This chapter explores the pharmacological contraceptive methods available to women. Pharmaceutical contraception includes combined hormonal contraception (CHC) which includes combined oral contraception (COC), combined transdermal patch (CTP) and combined vaginal ring (CVR).

Fundamentals of Pharmacology for Midwives, First Edition. Edited by Ian Peate and Cathy Hamilton.
© 2022 John Wiley & Sons Ltd. Published 2022 by John Wiley & Sons Ltd.
Companion website: www.wiley.com/go/pharmacologyformidwives

Other forms of pharmaceutical contraception available are the progesterone-only pill (POP), the progesterone-only injection Depo Provera® (DMPA), the progesterone implant and the intrauterine system (IUS).

Contraception may be perceived as a sensitive subject to discuss with women during the antenatal and postnatal period. However, the Faculty of Sexual & Reproductive Health (FSRH, 2020a) suggests that maternity services should provide counselling and contraception tailored to the woman's needs. Furthermore, clinicians involved in the provision of maternity care should give women the opportunity to discuss their future contraceptive requirements during the antenatal period (FSRH, 2020a). This should include those women who chose to breast feed and those who do not. Whilst midwives are not usually able to prescribe contraception, they are in a unique position to discuss the relevant methods and advise women when to start contraception and where to obtain the method of their choice.

All methods of contraception should be discussed with the woman for her to make an informed choice. The National Institute for Health and Care Excellence (2019) has published updated guidelines on long-acting reversable contraception (LARC). LARC includes those methods that are not delivered within a monthly cycle.

LARC methods include:

* copper intrauterine devices
* progesterone-only intrauterine systems
* progesterone-only injectable contraceptives
* progestogen-only subdermal implants.

Using a LARC method is more cost-effective and could also help with reducing unintended pregnancies (NICE, 2019). However, despite the effectiveness of LARC methods, women still prefer the oral contraceptive pill (NICE, 2019). It is thought that healthcare practitioners could play a key role in advising women about using LARC methods (NICE, 2019).

Consideration of the woman's medical history is essential before advising on the most appropriate methods a woman can choose from. Medical history may change following pregnancy and childbirth and therefore it may not be advisable for the woman to restart the same method of contraception that she had used prior to pregnancy. The United Kingdom Medical Eligibility Criteria for Contraceptive Use (UKMEC) (FSRH, 2019a) provide a very useful resource regarding which methods are suitable for women in relation to their medical history. The UKMEC (FSRH, 2019a) identify 'categories' and 'definitions' which in turn are applied to a medical condition and specific methods of contraception. The document provides useful evidence-based guidance criteria and gives an overview as to which method of contraception is safest to use for women with specific medical conditions or who have a history of certain medical conditions. Table 24.1 provides an overview of the various UKMEC criteria and categories.

Table 24.1 Definition of UKMEC.

Category	Definition
UKMEC 1	A condition for which there is no restriction for the use of the contraceptive method
UKMEC 2	A condition for which the advantages of using the method generally outweigh the theoretical or proven risks
UKMEC 3	A condition where the theoretical or proven risks usually outweigh the advantages of using the method. The provision of a method that requires expert clinical judgement and/or referral to a specialist contraceptive provider, since use of the method is not usually recommended unless other more appropriate methods are not available or not acceptable
UKMEC 4	A condition which represents an unacceptable health risk if the contraceptive method is used

Source: FSRH (2019a).

Clinical consideration

Access the UKMEC guidelines (FSRH, 2019a) and consider what method/methods are available in the following situations or conditions.

1. 0–6 weeks postpartum breastfeeding
2. 0-48 hours postnatal breast feeding and non-breast feeding
3. BMI over 35
4. History of high blood pressure in pregnancy

Pharmacokinetic and pharmacodynamic interactions

In addition to considering the woman's medical history, it is essential for the midwife to understand the pharmacokinetic and pharmacodynamic interactions that may impact on the efficacy of hormonal contraception.

A pharmacokinetic interaction happens when a specific drug affects the absorption, distribution, metabolism or excretion of the hormonal contraceptive and thereby may reduce the efficacy of the contraceptive (FSRH, 2019b). Drugs that affect absorption include those that induce vomiting and diarrhoea. Since the liver is the main organ for metabolising drugs, any drugs that increase metabolism, known as liver enzyme-inducing drugs, will affect contraceptive efficacy.

Levels of both circulating hormones, oestrogen and progesterone, may be reduced by 50% in those taking liver enzyme-inducing drugs (Guillebaud and MacGregor, 2017). Examples of these drugs include certain antiepileptic drugs, e.g. carbamazepine and phenytoin, the antibiotic rifampicin and certain antiretrovirals used in the treatment of HIV. However, not all antibiotics and antiretrovirals are enzyme-inducing drugs.

There are some drugs that are available over the counter which may also be enzyme inducing. The herbal remedy St John's wort, commonly used to treat depression, is also an enzyme-inducing drug. Advice should be sought from the pharmacist when buying over-the-counter medication.

In contrast, liver-enzyme inhibiting drugs may increase the level of the contraceptive hormone. These include certain antibacterials, e.g. erythromycin, and some antifungal drugs, e.g. itraconazole, specific antiretrovirals, specific immunosuppressants and some non-steroidal anti-inflammatory drugs.

Combined hormonal contraception (CHC) can also affect the metabolism of other drugs, in particular lamotrigine. The FSRH (2019b) advises that women taking lamotrigine to control their epileptic seizures should be informed that CHC can affect the circulating levels of their antiepileptic drug. This can leave the woman vulnerable to poorer control of her seizures. Furthermore, during the hormone-free interval when levels of CHC fall, lamotrigine levels may significantly increase to a toxic level (FSRH, 2019b). See Chapter 17 of this text for further discussion of antiepileptic drugs.

Pharmacodynamic interactions occur between similar drugs that compete for the same receptor sites or act on the same physiological system. The efficacy of the emergency contraceptive ulipristal acetate (UPA-EC) is reduced by progesterone-containing contraception. Similarly, the efficacy of hormonal contraception may be reduced following UPA-EC. This is because they both compete for the same progesterone receptors (FSRH, 2019b).

However, not all hormonal contraceptive methods are affected by drug interactions. Therefore, consideration of alternative methods such as the IUCD, the IUS or the injectable contraception DMPA should be offered.

See also Chapter 5 of this text for further discussion on pharmacokinetics and pharmacodynamics.

Clinical consideration

When you are in clinical placement, find out what written information regarding contraception is available to mothers:

- in the antenatal clinic or GP surgery
- on the postnatal ward
- upon discharge from the community midwife.

Combined hormonal contraception

Combined hormonal contraception (CHC) contains a combination of oestrogen and progesterone in various levels. There are three methods of delivering CHC, in the form of:

- combined oral contraception (COC)
- combined transdermal patch (CTP)
- combined vaginal ring (CVR).

Combined hormonal contraception prevents pregnancy in three ways: by inhibiting ovulation, by altering the cervical mucus, which makes it more difficult for sperm to enter the uterus, and by affecting the endometrial lining, making it unfavourable for a blastocyst to embed.

Combined hormonal contraception should be commenced during the first 5 days of the menstrual cycle and no additional contraception is required. However, if the woman begins CHC after day 5, she will need a further 7 days of additional contraception, for example condoms or abstinence from sexual intercourse. This is to allow for the level of the COC to become effective in preventing a pregnancy.

Side-effects, health risks and contraindications

Women may experience temporary side-effects when CHC is initiated. These may include, for example, nausea, breast tenderness, headache and mood swings. These effects usually resolve after the first few months.

There are specific health risks and contraindications to using CHC. CHC contains oestrogen, which alters the clotting factor levels which predispose women to an increased risk of developing blood clots, e.g. venous thromboembolism (VTE) which includes deep vein thrombosis (DVT) and pulmonary embolism (PE). Therefore, women should be advised to report if they experience symptoms such as sharp pain when breathing in, haemoptysis, pain and swelling in the calf or unusual headache or migraine. In addition, studies have shown that synthetic oestrogens increase arterial blood pressure (Guillebaud and MacGregor, 2017).

The UKMEC (FSRH, 2019a) identify certain health conditions that are associated with an increased health risk when taking CHC. these are classified into categories 3 and 4. These relate to the risk of VTE and other clotting disorders. Therefore, if a woman developed a VTE in pregnancy, she would be classified as category 4. Women who have other risk factors for cardiovascular disease and arterial disease, such as high blood pressure, smoking or a high BMI of 35 kg/m^2 or greater, should avoid using CHC as this may increase their risk further (FSRH, 2019a).

Other health risks affect women with migraine who also experience an aura. The UKMEC (FSRH, 2019a) identify this condition as category 4. Women who experience an aura with their migraine are thought to be at higher risk of experiencing an ischaemic stroke when taking CHC (Guillebaud and MacGregor, 2017).

Combined hormonal contraception contains both hormones and consequently can affect any cancer that is hormone related: women with a history of breast cancer or current breast cancer are categorised as category 3 and 4 respectively (FSRH, 2019a). Careful history taking is therefore paramount to identify those women in whom the CHC would not be appropriate. For women with additional health risks, it would be advisable to consider an alternative method of contraception.

393

Table 24.2   Pharmacokinetics of oral ethinylestradiol.

ADME	
Absorption	Absorption is via the gastrointestinal tract
Distribution	It is quickly distributed throughout the body via the bloodstream
Metabolism	This occurs primarily in the liver
Excretion	Mainly via urine, with some in faeces and in bile

Combined oral contraception

Combined oral contraception contains various amounts of ethinylestradiol (EE), which is a synthetic oestrogen, and progestogens, which are synthetic steroids similar to progesterone (Table 24.2). Modern-day pills aim to use the lowest dose of oestrogen possible to remain effective as this reduces the health risks associated with taking CHC. There are several branded COC pills available on the market. The FSRH (2020b) recommend that the first-line option for the COC pill should be one with 30 micrograms of EE and progesterone, either levonorgestrel or norethisterone; this is thought to lower the risk of cardiovascular disease. Some COCs contain desogestrel. The maximum level of EE is 35 micrograms in combination with any form of progestogen.

Combined oral contraception is effective after taking seven consecutive pills. Thereafter, the COC is taken for 21 days, followed by 7 days of no pills, known as the pill-free interval (PFI). During the PFI, the woman will experience a withdrawal bleed. The contraceptive effects of the COC continue during the PFI, provided the woman has taken 7 consecutive days of pills prior to her PFI and begins the new packet correctly after her 7th day PFI. If the more common side-effects are experienced then they may resolve with time, but it is always possible to try a different formula of the pill.

Missed pills

Combined oral contraception is user dependent and its efficacy is reduced when there is an interruption in pill taking. However, missing one pill is thought to be of no significance and it should be taken as soon as possible. The rest of the packet should be continued as per regimen. If a woman misses two or more pills in the later end of the pill packet and there are fewer than seven pills left, this can place the woman at increased risk of pregnancy. FSRH (2020b) guidance suggests that women should take the most recent pill and continue with the new packet, omitting the PFI, and also use additional contraception, e.g. condoms or abstain from sexual intercourse for 7 days.

Similarly, if the woman extends her PFI, her risk of pregnancy increases. The FSRH (2020b) guidance suggests that women who recommence the COC more than 2 days after the PFI and have had sexual intercourse should seek emergency contraception (EC) and continue taking the CHC with additional contraception, e.g. condoms or abstain from sexual intercourse for 7 days. A pregnancy test may be taken after 3 weeks to rule out a pregnancy.

If the woman requires emergency contraception, in particular UPA-EC, the FSRH (2020b) advises that CHC should not be started until 5 days following the EC and either a barrier method of contraception should be used or abstain from sexual intercourse. Once CHC has started, women should be advised to use additional contraception for the following 7 days until effective levels of CHC are reached.

Absorption of the COC can also be affected by severe diarrhoea or vomiting. Whilst the symptoms may be temporary, it is important to advise women to continue to take the COC and use an additional method of contraception for 7 days after the symptoms have resolved.

Combined transdermal patch

The CTP Evra® releases both oestrogen (ethinyloestradiol 33.9 micrograms) and progesterone (norelgestromin 203 micrograms) per day over a 7-day period. As the patch contains both oestrogen and progesterone, the same contraindications and health risks apply as with COC. In addition, it is suggested that women with a body weight of 90 kg and over should avoid the patch. Guillebaud and MacGregor (2017) suggest that this advice is based on the efficacy and safety of the drug. The efficacy of the Evra patch is reduced due to obese women having lower plasma hormone levels and a higher risk of VTE (Guillebaud and MacGregor, 2017). The patch is approximately 5 × 5 cm and is applied at the same time each week and kept in place for 7 days with a 4–7-day PFI.

Clinical consideration

The patch can be applied to areas such as the abdomen, upper arm, buttock or back. The breast area should be avoided. For the patch to remain in place, creams and oils should be avoided in the area where the patch is applied. The patch remains adherent in hot climates and on bathing.

Incorrect use of the CTP can result in reduced efficacy. If the hormone-free interval (HFI) is extended beyond 8 days, the risk of pregnancy increases. The FSRH (2020c) suggests that the woman should apply the CTP and use additional contraception, e.g. condoms or abstain from sexual intercourse for 7 days. If sexual intercourse has occurred, emergency contraception is advised and a pregnancy test should be considered.

If the CTP has been used correctly in the 7 days prior to the HFI and is removed for less than 48 hours during the first week, it should be replaced as soon as possible (FSRH, 2020c). Similarly, if the CTP has been used correctly and is removed for less than 48 hours in weeks 2 and 3 after the HFI, it should be replaced as soon as possible (FSRH, 2020c) but additional contraception must also be used.

However, if the CTP has been removed for 48 hours or more during week 1 after the HFI, in addition to the above advice. the FSRH (2020c) suggests that EC should be taken if sexual intercourse has taken place. A pregnancy test may be taken in 3 weeks to rule out a pregnancy. During weeks 2 and 3, provided that the CTP has been in place for 7 days, if it is removed for more than 48 hours it should be replaced and additional contraception used for 7 days. The CTP may be removed on the scheduled day. If it has been removed 48 hours or more in the week prior to the HFI, it should be replaced and the HFI should be avoided (FSRH, 2020c).

Combined vaginal ring

The CVR NuvaRing® releases both oestrogen (ethinylestradiol 15 micrograms) and progesterone (etonogestrel 20 micrograms) per day. As the CVR contains both oestrogen and progesterone, the same contraindications and health risks apply. It is a latex-free flexible ring 54 mm in diameter and 4 mm thick. It remains in situ for 21 days and is replaced after a 4- or 7-day break. It may be removed for up to 3 hours without the need for additional contraception. There is also the option to avoid the HFI and immediately replace it; this may be done for 3 consecutive months and is known as tricycling.

Incorrect use of the CVR can reduce its efficacy. If the HFI extends beyond 8 days, the risk of pregnancy increases. FSRH (2020c) guidance suggests that the CVR should be inserted and additional contraception used. If sexual intercourse has taken place then emergency contraception should be considered. A pregnancy test may be taken after 3 weeks.

If the CVR has been in place for 7 days prior to the HFI and is removed in the first week for less than 48 hours, then it should be inserted as soon as possible. Additional contraception should be used, e.g condoms or abstain from sexual intercourse for 7 days.

Similarly, if the CVR has been used correctly in week 1 and is removed for less than 48 hours in weeks 2 or 3, then it should be inserted as soon as possible and the woman should use additional contraception, e.g condoms or abstain from sexual intercourse for 7 days.

However, if the CVR has been removed for 48 hours or more during week 1 after the HFI and sexual intercourse has occurred then in addition to the above advice, the FSRH (2020c) suggests the use of emergency contraception. A pregnancy test may be taken in 3 weeks. During weeks 2 and 3, provided that the CVR has been in place for 7 days, if it is removed for more than 48 hours then it should be replaced and additional contraception used, e.g condoms or abstain from sexual intercourse for 7 days. The CVR may be removed on the scheduled day. If it has been removed 48 hours or more before the HFI it should be replaced and the HFI should be avoided.

Postpartum period and combined hormonal contraception

The UKMEC guidelines (FSRH, 2019a) advise that all women in the postpartum period, breastfeeding or not, should be assessed for their risk factors for VTE, prior to prescribing CHC. This includes immobility, transfusion at delivery, BMI ≥ 30 kg/m², postpartum haemorrhage, postcaesarean delivery, pre-eclampsia or smoking.

In the postpartum period, women who are 3–6 weeks postpartum and are not breast feeding and do not have any underlying risk factors for VTE are classified as category 2 (FSRH, 2019a). They may therefore commence the CHC on day 21 after birth. Contraception will be effective from this day. However, if the woman chooses to start later, she should be advised to use condoms or abstain from sexual intercourse for 7 days. Women who commence COC after 6 weeks with no risk factors for VTE will be in category 1 (FSRH, 2019a).

For women who are breast feeding and have no risk factors for VTE, the evidence suggests that they should not commence CHC until 6 weeks after birth and are category 4 (FSRH, 2019a). Breast feeding is thought to be established by 6 weeks and then the effects of oestrogen on milk production are thought to be much lower (FSRH, 2019a). Therefore, women who are breast feeding between 6 weeks and 6 months postpartum are classified as category 2, changing to category 1 after 6 months (FSRH, 2019a). If a postpartum woman who is breast feeding with no risk factors for VTE chooses to commence CHC at 6 weeks, it is important to advise her to use additional contraception, for example a barrier method or abstain from sexual intercourse, from day 21 until 7 days after she has commenced the CHC.

Episode of care

Rose is in the postnatal ward, having given birth 3 days ago. She mentions to you that she would like to restart her COC. She was diagnosed with a DVT during the antenatal period.
What advice and information would you give Rose?

Progesterone-oral pill

For those women who still prefer to take oral contraception but are unable to have the CHC due to contraindications, the POP is a reliable alternative. There are three main types of synthetic progesterone pills in use.

- Levonorgestrel
- Norethisterone
- Desogestrel

The POP works by altering the endometrial lining of the uterus, making it very thin and therefore not conducive to a blastocyst embedding. It also makes the cervical mucus much thicker which makes it more difficult for sperm to pass through into the uterus. Desogestrel can prevent ovulation. Levonorgestrel and norethisterone can also affect ovulation but the extent of this can vary between women.

The POP is designed to be taken the same time every day continuously and, unlike the oral CHC, there is no 7-day pill-free interval. If the POP is commenced during the first 5 days of the menstrual cycle, no additional contraception is required. However, if the woman begins the POP after day 5, she will need a further 2 days of additional contraception, e.g. she should be advised to use condoms or abstain from sexual intercourse. This is to allow for the level of the POP to become effective in preventing a pregnancy. Progesterone is absorbed much quicker than oestrogen and therefore the effect of progesterone on the cervical mucus is evident after just 48 hours of taking the POP.

Levonorgestrel and norethisterone POPs have a 3-hour window in which they must be taken to maintain their efficacy. Desogestrel has an extended window of 12 hours. All types of POPs are as effective as each other if taken as prescribed. The choice of which POP may therefore be reflected by the window period for remembering to take the pills as any missed pills increase the risk of pregnancy. There is no effect on returning fertility once the POP has been discontinued.

Side-effects, health risks and contraindications

Since the POP alters the endometrium after pill taking is established, the woman is likely to experience disruption to her bleeding pattern or amenorrhoea. If the POP has been taken correctly and pregnancy has been excluded then this is a normal effect of taking the POP. Other side-effects include acne, mood changes, breast pain, headache and nausea. These tend to resolve over a short period of time.

The POP does not contain oestrogen and therefore is considered to have fewer exclusion criteria. However, progesterone is contraindicated in women who have a past history of breast cancer or current breast cancer, categorised as 3 and 4 respectively (FSRH, 2019a). Further restrictions include severe liver disease category 3 and hypersensitivity to desogestrel, levonorgestrel or norethisterone (FSRH, 2019a).

Efficacy of the POP is dependent upon regular pill taking. A woman taking levonorgestrel and norethisterone POPs has a 3-hour window in which they must be taken to maintain efficacy. A woman taking a desogestrel POP has a 12-hour window; this is because of the additional benefit of suppressed ovulation. The effects of progesterone on cervical mucus decline rapidly and therefore the efficacy of this method is short-lived if pills are missed. If a woman is late taking either type of POP, she will need to take the missed pill as soon as possible and use additional contraception, e.g. condoms or abstain from sexual intercourse for 2 days. If the woman has had sexual intercourse at the time of the missed pill or within 48 hours of recommencing the POP, she should seek emergency contraception. A pregnancy test may be taken in 3 weeks.

If a woman vomits the POP within 2 hours of taking it, she should take another pill. If she does not take a further pill, she should use additional contraception.

Postpartum period and POP

A woman can commence taking the POP on any day up to day 21 of the postpartum period whether she chooses to breast feed or not, and the method would be effective immediately (FSRH, 2019c). However, if she chooses to delay starting the POP until after day 21, she should be advised to use condoms or abstain from sexual intercourse for 2 days. In addition, if she has had unprotected sexual intercourse after day 21 and before starting the POP, a pregnancy test should be done 3 weeks after the episode of sexual intercourse.

397

Progesterone injection

The typical progesterone injection used is Depo Provera (DMPA) which contains medroxyprogesterone acetate 150 mg in 1 mL; this is a progestogenic steroid (Table 24.3). It is also available as Sayana® Press which contains medroxyprogesterone acetate 160 mg in 1 mL. Both are LARC methods. The primary action of the method in preventing pregnancy is the same as CHC; it prevents ovulation. In addition, it alters the cervical mucus and alters the endometrial lining of the uterus.

Table 24.3 Pharmacokinetics of progestogen.

ADME	
Absorption	Oral progestogens are absorbed via the gastrointestinal tract. Injectable progestogens have a long duration of action due to their slow absorption from the site of injection
Distribution	It is distributed throughout the body bound to various proteins in the blood, mainly albumin
Metabolism	Oral progestogens are metabolised by the gastrointestinal tract and the liver. Injectable progestogens are only metabolised via the liver but liver enzyme-inducing drugs do not accelerate metabolism and therefore do not reduce its efficacy
Excretion	This is mainly via bile and urine

Clinical consideration

DMPA is administered as a deep intramuscular injection, preferably given in the gluteal muscle in the buttock or in the deltoid muscle of the upper arm. The site should not be massaged as this accelerates the breakdown of the drug.

Sayana Press is administered subcutaneously into the thigh or abdomen. Women are taught to self-medicate.

Liver enzyme-inducing drugs have minimal effect on the efficacy of DMPA and it is therefore the hormonal contraceptive of choice for women taking such drugs (Guillebaud and MacGregor, 2017).

DMPA can be started on day 1–5 of the menstrual cycle with no need for additional protection. It can also be started any time in the cycle if it is reasonably certain that the woman is not pregnant. Additional contraception is then required for 7 days. DMPA should be repeated 10–12 weeks after the previous dose. A repeat injection may be given up to 14 weeks after the previous dose with no additional contraception required. However, if the woman presents after 14 weeks and has not had sexual intercourse from the 14th week, DMPA may be administered and additional contraception is used for 7 days.

Side-effects, health risks and contraindications

The side-effects of DMPA include weight gain, mood changes, decreased libido and headache. The woman is likely to experience disruption to her bleeding pattern and it is difficult to predict for how long. Some women may eventually become amenorrhoeic. Women should be advised that after stopping this method, there is a potential delay in the return of fertility for up to a 1 year (NICE, 2019).

There is an exclusion criterion for this method. Since it is administered as an injection and cannot be reversed, it is imperative to rule out possible pregnancy.

Since DMPA suppresses the natural female hormone levels, particularly follicle-stimulating hormone (FSH), there is controversy over the possible negative effects of DMPA on bone health in long-term users, especially in adolescent women less than 18 years old and older women over 45 (Guillebaud and MacGregor, 2017). This differs from other progesterone methods where there is some follicular activity which aids arterial and bone health (Guillebaud and MacGregor, 2017). Therefore, a current or past history of ischaemic heart disease, stroke or multiple risk factors for cardiovascular disease (smoking, diabetes, hypertension, obesity) are a category 3 (FSRH, 2019a).

Other contraindications identified in the UKMEC (FSRH, 2019a) include:

- severe liver disease/tumours – category 3
- past breast cancer or current breast cancer – category 3 and 4 respectively
- undiagnosed abnormal vaginal bleeding – category 3.

Postpartum period and DMPA

According to the UKMEC guidelines (FSRH, 2019a), women who are breast feeding and less than 6 weeks postpartum are category 2. This changes to 1 at 6 weeks and beyond. Those women who are not breast feeding and are less than 21 days with or without risk factors for VTE are category 2. From 3 to 6 weeks postpartum, women with a risk of VTE remain in category 2; those without a risk of VTE are then classified in category 1. After 6 weeks postpartum, a woman is classified as category 1.

Progesterone implant

The progesterone implant most commonly used is Nexplanon®. It contains 68 mg of etonogestrel (ENG-IMP), a metabolite of desogesterol, in a slow-release rod, which is absorbed into the blood-stream. It is a LARC method. The primary action of the implant is stopping ovulation. The implant requires a small procedure to insert and remove, which should be undertaken by an appropriately skilled and trained professional (NICE, 2019). The implant is inserted subdermally into the inner upper section of the arm after administering local anaesthetic. Since the ENG-IMP is absorbed into the bloodstream via the subdermal route, efficacy is not reliant on daily use and is not affected by diarrhoea and vomiting. However, the efficacy of the implant is thought to be reduced by enzyme-inducing drugs (FRSH, 2021).

The implant may be inserted on day 1–5 of the menstrual cycle with no need for additional protection. It can also be inserted any time in the cycle as long as it is reasonably certain that the woman is not pregnant. Additional contraception is then required for 7 days. The efficacy of the implant lasts for 3 years. There is no delay in fertility once the implant is removed.

Side-effects, health risks and contraindications

Side-effects of the implant are primarily disruption to the uterine bleeding pattern. This may be significant in some women, and can be unpredictable and problematic. This may continue throughout use or cease; the woman may become amenorrhoeic. Additional side-effects include headache and acne. Careful aseptic technique is required to reduce the risk of infection during insertion of the implant. According to the UKMEC guidelines (FSRH, 2019a), the exclusion criteria for this method include:

- known or suspected pregnancy, severe liver disease/tumours – category 3
- past breast cancer or current breast cancer – category 3 and 4 respectively
- undiagnosed abnormal vaginal bleeding – category 3
- current and history of ischaemic heart disease – category 3 for continued use
- stroke (history of cerebrovascular accident including transient ischaemic attack) – category 3 for continued use.

Postpartum period and the implant

A woman can have the implant inserted immediately following childbirth whether she chooses to breast feed or not. It can be inserted on any day up to day 21 of the postpartum period and the method would be effective immediately. However, if the implant is inserted after day 21, she should be advised to use condoms or abstain from sexual intercourse for 7 days.

Intrauterine contraceptive (IUC)

There are two types of IUC. The intrauterine contraceptive device (IUCD) is a coil containing copper and does not contain any hormones. The intrauterine system (IUS) contains 52 mg levonorgestrel (LNG-IUS) (Mirena®) or 13.5 mg levonorgestrel (Jaydess®), a synthetic progesterone, in the coil. Both are LARC methods.

The IUS is a device inserted into the uterus via the cervix and is maintained in situ to prevent a pregnancy. There are usually two threads attached to the device which are trimmed and left visible at the external os. The threads are used to remove the IUS. Insertion and removal should be undertaken by an appropriately skilled and trained professional (NICE, 2019). The LNG-IUS primarily prevents pregnancy by interfering with the cervical mucus and uterine fluids, thereby inhibiting the flow of sperm. In addition, it causes an inflammatory effect on the endometrium, rendering it unfavourable for any potential fertilised ovum to embed. In some wome,n it is also thought to prevent ovulation. The LNG-IUS 52 mg is effective for 5 years and the LNG-IUS 13.5 mg for 3 years. Therefore, efficacy is not reliant on daily use and is not affected by diarrhoea and vomiting.

The LNG-IUS may be inserted on day 1–7 of the menstrual cycle with no need for additional protection. It can also be inserted any time in the cycle if it is reasonably certain that the woman is not pregnant. Additional contraception is then required for 7 days. Fertility returns as soon as the LNG-IUS is removed.

Side-effects, health risks and contraindications

There is some systemic absorption of progesterone with the LNG-IUS but any related side-effects are thought to resolve over a short period of time. These include headache, acne and breast tenderness. The effects of progesterone directly on the endometrium can cause a disruption to the usual bleeding pattern and in time may cause amenorrhoea.

There are associated risks with the LNG-IUS which include uterine perforation during insertion, uterine infection and expulsion of the device. To reduce the risk of infection, it is important to discuss the woman's sexual history and her risk of sexually transmitted infections, as well as a general medical history. Expulsion may occur within the first few months following insertion, particularly during menstruation as the uterus contracts. Women should be advised to feel for the threads either following menstruation or at regular intervals.

According to the UKMEC guidelines (FSRH, 2019a), the exclusion criteria for this method include:

- known or suspected pregnancy, severe liver disease/tumours – category 3
- past breast cancer or current breast cancer – category 3 and 4 respectively
- cervical and endometrial cancers – category 4 at insertion
- undiagnosed abnormal vaginal bleeding – category 4
- current and history of ischaemic heart disease – category 3 for continued use
- stroke (history of cerebrovascular accident including transient ischaemic attack) – category 3 for continued use
- specific cardiac arrhythmia, known long QT wave – category 3 at insertion
- uterine fibroids affecting the cavity of the uterus – category 3
- current pelvic inflammatory disease and specific sexually transmitted infections such as chlamydia, cervicitis and gonorrhoea – category 4 at insertion
- HIV which is dependent on the CD4 count at insertion and pelvic tuberculosis – category 4 at insertion.

Postpartum period and the IUS

According to the UKMEC guidelines (FSRH, 2019a), the IUS may be inserted up to 48 hours after childbirth. Thereafter, from 48 hours up to 4 weeks, this becomes a category 3 and should not be inserted. Women who have suffered from postpartum sepsis should not have an IUS inserted until after 4 weeks postpartum (FSRH, 2019s). However, if the device is inserted after 4 weeks, pregnancy needs to be excluded and the woman should be advised to use condoms or abstain from sexual intercourse for 7 days.

Table 24.4 provides an overview of the contraceptive methods available in the postnatal period.

Table 24.4   An overview of contraceptive methods available in the postnatal period.

Method	Postnatal period
Progesterone-only pill, progesterone-only injection, implant	Available from birth (if used after day 21, requires additional contraception for 2–7 days depending on method)
Combined hormonal contraception	Available from 21 days if not breast feeding (if used after day 21, requires additional contraception) Available from 6 weeks if breast feeding (additional contraception for 7 days)
Intrauterine system	Available from 0–48 hours or from 4 weeks postpartum (needs additional contraception for 7 days)

Source: Adapted from FSRH (2020a).

Emergency contraception

Emergency contraception (EC) is used to reduce the risk of unintended pregnancy. This may be following unprotected sexual intercourse (UPSI) or following the failure of a contraceptive method, e.g. missed pills or condom failure.

There are three methods of EC:

- the copper intrauterine device (IUCD)
- two oral emergency hormonal contraceptives (EHC).

The IUCD is the most reliable method and does not contain hormones. However, it must be fitted by a trained health professional. EC is also available over the counter from a pharmacist.

There are two EHCs: levonorgestrel (LNG) 1.5 mg and ulipristal acetate (UPA) 30 mg, each in single doses. Both methods are thought to prevent pregnancy by delaying ovulation until sperm are no longer viable. The difference between the pills correlates to the timing of the pill in relation to the luteinising hormone surge. UPA is effective within the luteinising phase, but LNG is not effective once the luteinising phase has begun (FSRH, 2020d). Ovulation is either prevented or delayed, so the woman needs to use contraception for any further sexual intercourse within the cycle. If a woman has UPSI within 5 days of her potential ovulation date, UPA is the preferred method (BNF, 2020). Both methods may interfere with and lengthen the luteal phase which can delay the menstrual phase. The menstrual bleed may also be lighter and for a shorter length of time.

There is also a time limit which affects the efficacy for each EHC method when taken after UPSI. The efficacy of levonorgestrel reduces over 72 hours following unprotected intercourse. If taken within 24 hours of UPSI, it is approximately 95% effective, within 48 hours it is 85% effective and within 72 hours it is 58% effective (FRSH, 2020d). Efficacy is also affected by the woman's weight; if a woman is more than 70 kg or has a BMI of more than 26, a double dose is recommended (FSRH, 2020d).

In contrast, UPA is effective up to 120 hours after unprotected intercourse with no decline in efficacy over this time. It is not affected by a woman's weight. If a woman vomits within 3 hours of taking EHC, a further dose is required.

Pharmacokinetic interactions can affect the efficacy of both EHCs as enzyme-inducing drugs increase the metabolism of them both (FSRH, 2020d). Antacids and any other drugs that increase gastric pH may reduce absorption of UPA and therefore decrease efficacy (FSRH, 2019a). Women with severe asthma who require oral corticosteroids should not take UPA due to its antiglucocorticoid effect (BNF, 2020).

Pharmacodynamic interactions can also affect the efficacy of UPA. As UPA is a progesterone receptor modulator, it also partially blocks the effects of progesterone (BNF, 2020). It binds to the progesterone receptors and may compete with other progesterone-containing hormonal methods. If a woman is already taking the POP, and then has missed pills and requires UPA, the efficacy of UPA may potentially be reduced (FSRH, 2020d). The efficacy of UPA itself can be reduced if hormonal contraception is started within 5 days of taking UPA (BNF, 2020). Consequently, a woman should be advised not to restart her hormonal contraception for 5 days after taking UPA and to use additional contraception, e.g. condoms or abstain, until their contraceptive method is effective. A follow-up pregnancy test is advised 3 weeks after the episode of unprotected sex.

401

Postpartum period and EHC

The FSRH (2020a) recommends that women who have had UPSI from day 21 after childbirth and do not meet the requirement of lactational amenorrhoea should receive EC. As it is not known whether UPA is excreted in breast milk, breast-feeding women are advised not to breast feed for 1 week after taking it (BNF, 2020).

Episode of care

You visit Prya in the community; she is 28 days postnatal following a normal vaginal birth. She had sexual intercourse last night and did not use any contraception. She is anxious about becoming pregnant again as she does not want another baby yet.

What advice would you give Prya?

Conclusion

Midwives are in a unique position to discuss the various methods of contraception available to women during the antenatal and postnatal period. Women may encounter health risks during their pregnancy and postnatal period which may affect their choice of method. The midwife's knowledge and understanding of contraception will help ensure that women can make informed decisions about their fertility and birth spacing.

Find out more

Consider the following conditions related to pregnancy and think about the effects they may or may not have on a woman's future contraceptive choices. Take some time and write notes about each. Remember to include aspects of care. If you are making notes about people you have offered care and support to, you must ensure that you have adhered to the rules of confidentiality.

The condition	Your notes
High blood pressure in pregnancy	
History of cholestasis (pregnancy related)	
Diabetes (history of diabetes)	
Ectopic pregnancy	
Hydatidiform mole	

Glossary

Acne   A skin condition affecting the sebaceous glands and leading to multiple whiteheads, blackheads and inflammatory skin nodules

Amenorrhoea   The absence of menstrual periods

Cervical mucus   This is the secretion found in the cervix which alters during the menstrual cycle and when women are taking contraceptive hormones

Endometrium   The layer of tissue lining the uterus which is shed each month during menstruation

Epilepsy   A neurological condition affecting the electrical activity in the brain which can result in repeated seizures.

Follicle-stimulating hormone   This is the female hormone released by the pituitary gland and is responsible for the development of ovarian follicles leading to the release of the egg

Haemoptysis   The coughing up of blood-stained sputum

Hormone-related breast cancer   This is a type of breast cancer in which the cancer is sensitive to the presence of female hormones

Ischaemic heart disease   A condition in which the coronary arteries, supplying blood to the heart muscle, become obstructed as a result of narrowing of the arteries

Ischaemic stroke   This is when a blood clot obstructs an artery to the brain, causing brain damage through lack of oxygen

Lactational amenorrhoea   This occurs following childbirth when a woman is fully breast feeding and it can result in the absence of menstrual periods and secondary infertility. In order for lactational amenorrhoea to be considered as a method of contraception, specific criteria must be met and adhered to

Libido   The sexual drive in men and women

Luteinising hormone   This is another female hormone released by the pituitary gland which is responsible for setting ovulation in motion

Migraine   A severe headache accompanied by additional sensory symptoms such as nausea, vomiting, sensitivity to light, sounds and smells

Migraine with aura   Neurological symptoms preceding the migraine lasting from 5 minutes to an hour. The symptoms include visual disturbance, flashing lights or zigzag lines. Other symptoms may include numbness or tingling, and speech and hearing may be affected

Ovulation   A specific time in the menstrual cycle when the egg is released from the ovary

Pelvic inflammatory disease   A condition caused by various infections of the uterus, fallopian tubes and ovaries which can result in pelvic pain and heavy periods and can also affect fertility

Postpartum haemorrhage   A significant blood loss suffered by the mother following childbirth. This may be immediately after birth or delayed until later

Pre-eclampsia   A disorder related to pregnancy which includes raised blood pressure and protein in the urine

Subdermal   This refers to the area underneath the deeper layers of the skin

Transdermal   This describes the absorption of medication through the skin either from patches or gel applied to the surface

Transient ischaemic attack   This occurs when there is a temporary obstruction of an artery to the brain resulting in loss of certain functions for a short period of time

Withdrawal bleed   A uterine bleed which occurs as a result of cessation of contraceptive hormones

Test yourself

Now review your learning by completing the learning activities for this chapter at www.wiley.com/go/pharmacologyformidwives.

References

British National Formulary (2020). *BNF – 78*. BMJ Group and Pharmaceutical Press: London.

Faculty of Sexual & Reproductive Healthcare (2019a) UK Medical Eligibility Criteria for Contraceptive Use (UKMEC). www.fsrh.org/documents/ukmec-2016/ (accessed February 2022).

Faculty of Sexual & Reproductive Healthcare (2019b) Drug Interactions with Hormonal Contraception. www.fsrh.org/standards-and-guidance/documents/ceu-clinical-guidance-drug-interactions-with-hormonal/ (accessed February 2022).

Faculty of Sexual & Reproductive Healthcare (2019c) Progesterone-only Pills. www.fsrh.org/standards-and-guidance/documents/cec-ceu-guidance-pop-mar-2015/ (accessed February 2022).

Faculty of Sexual & Reproductive Healthcare (2020a) Contraception After Pregnancy. www.fsrh.org/standards-and-guidance/documents/contraception-after-pregnancy-guideline-january-2017/ (accessed February 2022).

Faculty of Sexual & Reproductive Healthcare (2020b) Combined Hormonal Contraception. www.fsrh.org/standards-and-guidance/documents/combined-hormonal-contraception/ (accessed February 2022).

Faculty of Sexual & Reproductive Healthcare (2020c) Recommended Actions after Incorrect Use of Combined Hormonal Contraception. www.fsrh.org/standards-and-guidance/documents/fsrh-ceu-guidance-recommended-actions-after-incorrect-use-of/ (accessed February 2022).

Faculty of Sexual & Reproductive Healthcare (2020d) Emergency Contraception. www.fsrh.org/standards-and-guidance/documents/ceu-clinical-guidance-emergency-contraception-march-2017/ (accessed February 2022).

Faculty of Sexual & Reproductive Healthcare (2021) Clinical Guideline: Progesterone-only Implant. www.fsrh.org/standards-and-guidance/documents/cec-ceu-guidance-implants-feb-2014/ (accessed February 2022).

Guillebaud, J., MacGregor, A. (2017) *Contraception: Your Questions Answered*, 7th edn. Elsevier: Edinburgh.

National Institute for Health and Care Excellence (2019) Long-acting reversible contraception clinical guideline (CG30). www.nice.org.uk/guidance/cg30 (accessed February 2022).

Further reading

Everett, S. (2017a) *Handbook of Contraception and Sexual Health*. Taylor & Francis: London.

Glasier, A., Gebbie, A. (2008a) *Handbook of Family Planning and Reproductive Healthcare*, 5th edn. Churchill Livingstone: Edinburgh.

Neal, M.J. (2009a) *Medical Pharmacology at a Glance*, 6th edn. Wiley-Blackwell: Oxford. www.fpa.org.uk: The Family Planning Association – a useful website for women containing information and leaflets which can be downloaded.

403

Index

Note: Page numbers referring to figures in *italics* and those referring to tables in **bold**